The High Risk Foot in Diabetes Mellitus

The High Risk Foot in Diabetes Mellitus

Edited by
Robert G. Frykberg, D.P.M., F.A.C.F.S.
Attending Podiatrist
Department of Surgery
New England Deaconess Hospital
Boston, Massachusetts

Churchill Livingstone
New York, Edinburgh, London, Melbourne, Tokyo

Library of Congress Cataloging-in-Publication Data

The High risk foot in diabetes mellitus / edited by Robert G. Frykberg
p. cm.
Includes bibliographical references and index.
ISBN 0-443-08665-6
1. Foot—Diseases. 2. Diabetes—Complications and sequelae.
3. Foot—Surgery. I. Frykberg, Robert G.
[DNLM: 1. Diabetes Mellitus—complications. 2. Foot Diseases—etiology. 3. Foot Diseases—therapy. 4. Risk Factors. WK 835 H638]
RD563.H49 1991
616.4′62—dc20
DNLM/DLC
for Library of Congress 90-15028
CIP

Distributed in the United Kingdom by Churchill Livingstone, Robert Stevenson House, 1–3 Baxter's Place, Leith Walk, Edinburgh EH1 3AF, and by associated companies, branches, and representatives throughout the world.

Accurate indications, adverse reactions, and dosage schedules for drugs are provided in this book, but it is possible that they may change. The reader is urged to review the package information data of the manufacturers of the medications mentioned.

The Publishers have made every effort to trace the copyright holders for borrowed material. If they have inadvertently overlooked any, they will be pleased to make the necessary arrangements at the first opportunity.

Acquisitions Editor: *Kim Loretucci*
Copy Editor: *David Terry*
Production Designer: *Jill Little*
Production Supervisor: *Christina Hippeli*

Printed in the United States of America

First published in 1991

By learning you will teach; by teaching you will learn.

Latin proverb

Contributors

Alice N. Bessman, M.D.
Professor, Department of Medicine, University of Southern California School of Medicine, Los Angeles, California; Co-Chief, Ortho-Diabetes Service, Department of Medicine, Rancho Los Amigos Medical Center, Downey, California

James Allen Birke, M.S., P.T.
Chief, Department of Physical Therapy, Gillis W. Long Hansen's Disease Center, Carville, Louisiana; Captain, United States Public Health Service

A.J.M. Boulton, M.D., M.R.C.P.
Senior Lecturer, Department of Medicine, University of Manchester Medical School; Consultant, Department of Medicine, Manchester Royal Infirmary, Manchester, England

Jason H. Calhoun, M.D., M.Eng.
Assistant Professor, Division of Orthopedic Surgery, Department of Surgery, University of Texas Medical Branch at Galveston, Galveston, Texas

David R. Campbell, M.D.
Assistant Clinical Professor, Department of Surgery, Harvard Medical School; Attending Surgeon, Department of Vascular Surgery, New England Deaconess Hospital and Joslin Diabetes Center, Boston, Massachusetts

Ellen Cohen, D.P.M., Ph.D.
Assistant Professor, Department of Orthopedic Sciences, New York College of Podiatric Medicine; Board Eligible, American Board of Podiatric Orthopedics

Ross S. Cohen
Fourth-year student, Pennsylvania College of Podiatric Medicine, Philadelphia, Pennsylvania

William C. Coleman, D.P.M., D.A.B.P.O.
Department of Endocrinology, Ochsner Clinic, New Orleans, Louisiana; Chairman, Footwear Committee, Foot Care Council, American Diabetes Association

Lawrence B. Colen, M.D.
Associate Professor, Department of Plastic and Reconstructive Surgery, Eastern Virginia Medical School, Norfolk, Virginia

Kathleen M. Curry, P.A.-C., R.V.T.
Deputy Director, Non-invasive Vascular Laboratory, Department of Vascular Surgery, Veterans Administration Medical Center, Washington, D.C.

Mayer B. Davidson, M.D.
Professor, Department of Medicine, University of California, Los Angeles, UCLA School of Medicine; Director, Diabetes Program, Cedars-Sinai Medical Center, Los Angeles, California

Catherine F. Fix, M.S.
Senior Editor, Department of Radiology, University of California, San Diego, School of Medicine, La Jolla, California

Robert G. Frykberg, D.P.M., F.A.C.F.S.
Attending Podiatrist, Department of Surgery, New England Deaconess Hospital, Boston, Massachusetts

Gary W. Gibbons, M.D.
Associate Clinical Professor of Surgery, Harvard Medical School; Clinical Chief, Division of Vascular Surgery, Department of Surgery, New England Deaconess Hospital, Boston, Massachusetts

Flair Goldman, D.P.M.
Clinical Associate Professor, Department of Basic Medical Science, California College of Podiatric Medicine, San Francisco, California; Director, Podiatric Residency, and Chief, Division of Podiatric Surgery, Kaiser Foundation Hospital, Santa Clara, California

Des F. Gorman, M.B., Ch.B., F.A.C.O.M., Ph.D.
Senior Lecturer, Department of Anaesthesia and Intensive Care, University of Adelaide School of Medicine, Adelaide, South Australia, Australia; Director, Diving and Hyperbaric Medicine Unit, Royal New Zealand Navy, New Zealand

Lawrence B. Harkless, D.P.M.
Clinical Professor, Department of Orthopaedics, University of Texas Medical School at San Antonio; Director, Podiatry Residency Training Program, University of Texas Health Science Center, San Antonio, Texas

Kevin R. Higgins, D.P.M.
Clinical Instructor, Department of Orthopaedics, University of Texas Medical School at San Antonio; Director, Externship Program, Department of Orthopaedics, University of Texas Health Science Center, San Antonio, Texas

Allen M. Jacobs, D.P.M., F.A.C.F.S.
Director, Department of Podiatric Medicine and Surgery, Deaconess Hospital, St. Louis, Missouri

William M. Jenkin, D.P.M., D.A.B.P.S.
Professor, Department of Podiatric Surgery, California College of Podiatric Medicine; Chairman, Special Section on Diabetes, American College of Foot Surgeons, San Francisco, California

Roger Kerr, M.D.
Assistant Professor, Department of Radiology, University of Southern California School of Medicine; Chief, Division of Musculoskeletal Imaging, Department of Radiology, Los Angeles County–University of Southern California Medical Center, Los Angeles, California

Thomas J. Kirisits, D.P.M.
Assistant Director, Department of Podiatric Medicine and Surgery, Deaconess Hospital, St. Louis, Missouri

Stephen J. Kominsky, D.P.M., F.A.C.F.S., D.A.B.P.S.
Clinical Instructor, Department of Orthopedic Surgery, George Washington University School of Medicine and Health Sciences, Washington, D.C.; Adjunct Clinical Instructor, Pennsylvania College of Podiatric Medicine, Philadelphia, Pennsylvania; Director, Podiatric Medical Education, Division of Podiatry, Department of Surgery, Capitol Hill Hospital, Washington, D.C.

Ingrid Kruse-Edelman, D.P.M.
Private practice, Portland, Oregon

Leonard A. Levy, D.P.M., M.P.H.
Dean and Professor of Podiatric Medicine, College of Podiatric Medicine and Surgery, University of Osteopathic Medicine and Health Sciences, Des Moines, Iowa

H. Esterbrook Longmaid III, M.D.
Assistant Professor, Department of Radiology, Harvard Medical School; Staff Radiologist, Department of Radiology, New England Deaconess Hospital, Boston, Massachusetts

Jon T. Mader, M.D.
Professor, Division of Infectious Diseases, Department of Internal Medicine, University of Texas Medical School at Galveston, Galveston, Texas

Ewan A. Masson, M.B., M.R.C.P.
Wellcome Research Fellow, Department of Medicine, University of Manchester Medical School; Honorary Registrar, Department of Medicine, Manchester Royal Infirmary, Manchester, England

Leonard Miller, M.D., F.A.C.S., F.R.C.S.(Edin.)
Clinical Instructor in Surgery, Department of Plastic and Reconstructive Surgery, Harvard Medical School, Boston, Massachusetts

Bonnie Johng Nicklas, D.P.M., F.A.C.F.S., D.A.B.P.S.
Assistant Chairman and Assistant Professor, Department of Surgery, and Director, Residency Training Program, Ohio College of Podiatric Medicine, Cleveland, Ohio

Steven J. Palladino, D.P.M., D.A.B.P.S.
Associate Professor, Department of Podiatric Surgery, California College of Podiatric Medicine; Associate Director, Northern California Center for the Diabetic and Insensitive Foot, San Francisco, California

Frank B. Pomposelli, M.D.
Instructor, Department of Surgery, Harvard Medical School; Co-Director, Diagnostic Vascular Laboratory, Department of Vascular Surgery, New England Deaconess Hospital, Boston, Massachusetts

Hugh R. Protzel, D.P.M.
Surgical Resident, Department of Podiatric Medicine and Surgery, Deaconess Hospital, St. Louis, Missouri

Donald Resnick, M.D.
Professor, Department of Radiology, University of California, San Diego, School of Medicine, La Jolla, California; Chief, Division of Osteoradiology, Department of Radiology, Veterans Administration Medical Center, San Diego, California

Gustav Rubin, M.D., F.A.C.S.
Professor, Department of Orthopedic Sciences, New York College of Podiatric Medicine; Lecturer in Prosthetics and Orthotics, New York University Post-Graduate Medical School; Consultant, International Center for the Disabled, New York, New York

Edward C. Rzonca, D.P.M., F.A.C.F.O., D.A.B.P.O.
Professor and Chairman, Department of Orthopedic Sciences, New York College of Podiatric Medicine, New York, New York

Lee J. Sanders, D.P.M.
Clinical Professor, Department of Podiatric Medicine, College of Podiatric Medicine and Surgery, University of Osteopathic Medicine and Health Sciences, Des Moines, Iowa; Chief, Podiatry Section, Surgical Service, Department of Veterans Affairs Medical Center, Lebanon, Pennsylvania

Francisco L. Sapico, M.D., F.A.C.P.
Professor, Department of Radiology, University of California, San Diego, School of Medicine, La Jolla, California; Staff Physician, Department of Radiology, Veterans Administration Medical Center, San Diego, California

David J. Sartoris, M.D.
Associate Professor, Department of Radiology, University of California, San Diego, School of Medicine, La Jolla, California; Staff Physician, Department of Radiology, Veterans Administration Medical Center, San Diego, California

Harold D. Schoenhaus, D.P.M.
Professor, Department of Orthopedics, Pennsylvania College of Podiatric Medicine; Chief, Department of Podiatric Surgery, Graduate Hospital, Philadelphia, Pennsylvania

Ann M. Seifert, D.P.M.
Assistant Director, Department of Podiatric Medicine and Surgery, Deaconess Hospital, St. Louis, Missouri

Anton N. Sidawy, M.D., F.A.C.S.
Assistant Professor, Department of Surgery, George Washington University School of Medicine and Health Sciences; Chief, Department of Vascular Surgery, and Director, Non-invasive Vascular Laboratory, Department of Vascular Surgery, Veterans Administration Medical Center, Washington, D.C.

Isidore Steiner, D.P.M., J.D., D.A.B.P.S., F.A.C.F.S.
Past Director of Podiatric Education, Redford Community Hospital, Redford, Michigan; Member, Residency Training Committee, Botsford General Hospital, Farmington Hills, Michigan; Member, National Health Lawyers Association

Kenneth R. Stokes, M.D.
Instructor, Department of Radiology, Harvard Medical School; Director, Section of Angiography and Interventional Radiology, Department of Radiology, New England Deaconess Hospital, Boston, Massachusetts

F. William Wagner, Jr., M.D.
Clinical Professor, Department of Orthopaedic Surgery, University of Southern California School of Medicine; Chief, Foot-Ankle Clinic, Department of Orthopaedic Surgery, Los Angeles County–University of Southern California Medical Center, Los Angeles, California

Elissa Wernick, D.P.M.
Resident, Department of Podiatric Surgery, Graduate Hospital, Philadelphia, Pennsylvania

Preface

> In the thirty-ninth year of his reign Asa was afflicted with a disease in his feet. Though his disease was severe, even in his illness he did not seek help from the Lord, but only from the physicians. Then in the forty-first year of his reign Asa died and rested with his fathers.
>
> *2 Chronicles 16:12–13*

Too many limbs have needlessly been lost to the complications of diabetes mellitus. As inferred from the Biblical passage quoted above, this is an ancient disorder afflicting countless millions of people throughout history. In the United States alone approximately 6 percent of our population (12 million people) are under treatment for this disease, with an equal number estimated as having undiagnosed diabetes. Each of these people is at risk for developing a serious lesion of the foot that may threaten both limb and life.

One of the leading reasons for hospitalizing diabetic patients is for the treatment of foot ailments such as infection, ulceration, or gangrene. These lesions all too frequently result in lower extremity amputation, accounting for over 50 percent of the 120,000 nontraumatic amputations performed annually in the United States. Furthermore, the overall risk for lower extremity amputation in the diabetic population is 15 times higher than in nondiabetic individuals. With the associated costs of hospitalization and rehabilitation for these patients being in excess of $500 million per year, the impact of diabetic foot disease on our health care system is staggering. To the person with diabetes it is of vital significance.

The complications associated with diabetes mellitus are many and affect virtually all organs and systems with varying degrees of intensity. Those of greatest relevance to the pathogenesis of foot lesions, each discussed at length in the text, are neuropathy, vascular disease, and susceptibility to infection. These factors, which may act alone or in combination, predispose the diabetic foot to ulceration and infection when subjected to external traumatic forces. Commonly, it is the repetitive stress of simple walking or the wearing of tight shoes that leads to ulceration. When the lesion is neglected or remains unnoticed in the insensate foot, a cascade of events occurs that culminates in serious infection, gangrene, and eventual amputation. This catastrophic outcome so typical of the infected diabetic foot can and should be avoided.

Through an understanding of the pathophysiology involved, coupled with early, aggressive intervention, there can be at least a 50 percent reduction in the number of major lower extremity amputations necessitated by such events. Of paramount importance in this regard is the need for prevention based on thorough patient and physician education. Patients must be made aware of their disease, its potential complications, and proper preventive strategies. Physicians of all specialties and health care workers involved with such patients must attune themselves to these facts as well as to those recent advances in treatment focused on limb preservation. A multidisciplinary team approach to the care of the diabetic foot has proved itself to be the most successful way to accomplish these goals and is stressed in this book.

It is in the spirit of optimism and the belief that people with diabetes need not live with the constant fear of gangrene and obligatory limb loss that this book was conceived. Accordingly, cooperation between the patient and the treating physician(s) based on knowledge, trust, and experience is the key for effecting a reduction in the incidence of serious foot lesions and their sequelae. The value herein lies not only in the quality and content of the material presented, but also in the diversity of the contributors from across the nation and abroad. Podiatrists, physicians, surgeons, nurses, therapists, and other health care specialists have combined their expertise in one volume to provide the reader with a comprehensive resource to state of the art management of these patients. It is our sincere hope that this text will be enlightening in its content and foster a heightened interest in the enigmatic high risk foot in diabetes mellitus.

Robert G. Frykberg, D.P.M., F.A.C.F.S.

Acknowledgments

I am deeply indebted to my colleagues at the New England Deaconess Hospital and to all the contributors, from England to Australia, who selflessly agreed to participate in this very worthwhile project. Their enthusiasm was encouraging from the very beginning. Many of these men and women had never met nor heard of me when I approached them in solicitation of their contributions. Nevertheless, the importance of this work was readily apparent to them and each person was eager to make the effort to see it through to completion. The quality of their efforts illuminates the pages that follow and will stimulate us to strive harder in our attempts to preserve the feet and legs of our diabetic patients.

My sincere thanks go to Kim Loretucci, Acquisitions Editor and taskmaster, who was convinced of the need for such a text. Her enthusiasm and quest for excellence are written into each line. David Terry, Carol Bader, Leslie Burgess, and others at Churchill Livingstone also have my gratitude for their untiring efforts in assisting in the publication of this project.

It is with profound regret that I note that my mother, Marguerite, did not live to see my vision come to fruition in these pages. She and my father, Walter, have always been my strength and my impetus to strive to be the very best that I can be. The solid foundation that they provided for me in concert with the innate desire to seek higher goals has now been transformed into a tangible work that can potentially benefit thousands of people.

And finally, my deepest thanks and love go to my wife, Heather, and children, Ian, Ashley, and Reid, who allowed me to devote interminable hours to this project at their own expense. Their constant love, devotion, and belief in me and the value of this work was not only essential, but inspirational.

Contents

1

An Overview of Diabetes Mellitus

Mayer B. Davidson, M.D.

Most of the readers of this volume are primarily concerned with foot problems in diabetic patients. These problems, usually the result of diabetic peripheral neuropathy and/or peripheral vascular disease, are just one of a host of difficulties to which these patients are prone. The purpose of this introductory chapter is to give the reader an overview of the syndrome of diabetes mellitus: its definition, cost, pathophysiology of signs and symptoms of hyperglycemia and ketosis, classification, diagnosis, pathogenesis, genetics, clinical manifestations of small vessel and neuropathic complications, and treatment of the hyperglycemia.

DEFINITION

Diabetes mellitus is a syndrome with metabolic, vascular, and neuropathic components that are interrelated. The metabolic syndrome is characterized by alterations in carbohydrate, fat, and protein metabolism secondary to absent or markedly diminished insulin secretion and/or to ineffective insulin action. Hyperglycemia is the sine qua non of the metabolic syndrome and is the parameter most closely followed to make the diagnosis and to judge therapy. The vascular syndrome consists of abnormalities in both large vessels (macroangiopathy) and small vessels (microangiopathy). The macroangiopathic changes cause cerebral vascular accidents (strokes), myocardial infarctions (heart attacks), and peripheral vascular disease. Although these large vessel sequelae all occur in people without diabetes, they appear earlier and are more severe in diabetic patients. The clinical expressions of the microangiopathic changes are diabetic retinopathy (eye disease) and nephropathy (kidney disease). Finally, a variety of abnormalities in the peripheral nervous system are also part of the diabetic syndrome. Most of these neuropathic changes are due to metabolic alterations, although a few of them may be secondary to vascular causes.

COST

Diabetes mellitus has a tremendous impact, not only on the health of individuals, but also on the health care system in the United States. According to the National Commission of Diabetes, this syndrome now affects 6 percent of the overall population of this country (approximately 12 million people), and it is estimated that a similar number of patients remain undiagnosed. The prevalence of diabetes rises with age with a major increase starting after the age of 40 years, reaching 15 to 20 percent after the age of 65. Diabetes and its associated vascular complications are the third leading cause of death in this country. Diabetes is the leading cause of blindness in individuals between 20 and 74 years of age in industrialized countries. One in three patients on dialysis are there because of diabetic nephropathy. Over half of all lower extremity amputations take place in diabetic patients. On a relative basis, people with diabetes are 25 times more likely to develop blindness, 17 times more likely to develop kidney disease, 20 times more likely to develop gangrene, 30 to 40 times more likely to undergo a major amputation, and twice as likely to develop coronary artery disease or suffer a stroke than are individuals without diabetes. The total economic impact of diabetes in the United States was estimated by the Center of Economic Studies in Medicine to be $20.4 billion in 1987. It certainly is not less now.

PATHOPHYSIOLOGY OF THE SIGNS AND SYMPTOMS

To understand the signs and symptoms of diabetes mellitus, it is helpful to relate them to the abnormal metabolism associated with this syndrome. For this purpose, it is necessary to summarize normal metabolism against which the alterations in diabetes can be compared. Although many tissues in the body can utilize glucose, only a few have an absolute requirement for it, the most important of which are the central nervous system and the red blood cells. In the postabsorptive state, for instance after an overnight fast, glucose concentrations are regulated within a narrow range (70 to 100 mg/dl). This is accomplished by very precise mechanisms whereby the liver releases almost the exact amount of glucose that the brain, red blood cells, and a few other tissues require. The glucose is produced by the liver through two separate pathways, glycogenolysis and gluconeogenesis. *Glycogenolysis* is the breakdown of glycogen, the storage form of glucose. After an overnight fast, approximately 75 percent of the glucose supplied by the liver is derived from this pathway. *Gluconeogenesis* is the synthesis of new glucose from noncarbohydrate precursors delivered to the liver. The rate-determining step for gluconeogenesis seems to be the amount of these substrates presented to the liver. Although only 25 percent of hepatic glucose production derives from gluconeogenesis after an overnight fast, the contribution from glycogen decreases considerably as the period of fasting lengthens and gluconeogenesis becomes the predominant pathway. The moment-to-moment control of glucose production by the liver is regulated by insulin, which decreases it; by glucagon, which increases it; and by autoregulation, a process by which the glucose concentration mediates glucose production by the liver independent of any external hormonal stimuli. As one would expect, insulin concentrations tend to fall while glucagon levels rise as the fasting period increases.

This situation changes rapidly following a meal. The increasing concentration of glucose in the circulation stimulates the β cells of the islets of Langerhans, located in the pancreas, to release insulin while glucagon production by the α cells of the islets is suppressed. The newly secreted insulin traverses the liver first where approximately 50 percent is degraded on each passage. The remainder escapes into the general circulation, where its half-life is approximately 5 minutes. Insulin binds to specific receptors located on the cell surfaces of liver, muscle, and fat tissue, where it may exert an effect for several hours following its binding.

The metabolic result of these hormonal changes is that glucose production by the liver is markedly suppressed and the carbohydrate content of the meal (which had been broken down by cells located in the wall of the intestine to simple sugars—mostly glucose) is stored in the three tissues. Approximately 25 percent ends up in the liver and the remainder in the peripheral tissues, mostly muscle. In people without diabetes, glucose levels usually rise between 20 to 50 mg/dl after a meal. Two hours after eating, glucose concentrations have mostly returned to baseline in younger people. As one ages, there is an increasing resistance to insulin action so that postprandial glucose concentrations rise approximately 5 mg/dl with each decade. Fasting glucose concentrations change little during aging—1 to 2 mg/dl per decade. Insulin secretion remains intact so that postprandial insulin concentrations are often increased due to the higher glucose levels.

As carbohydrate metabolism starts to worsen, regardless of age, the postprandial glucose concentrations fail to return to the preprandial level until 3 to 5 hours after eating. There are no signs or symptoms at this point as long as glucose concentrations do not exceed the renal threshold. Along with all other small molecules in the blood, glucose is filtered at the renal glomerulus and reabsorbed almost completely back into the circulation so that virtually no glucose is normally excreted in the urine. However, the ability of the proximal tubule to reabsorb glucose is limited. If the amount of glucose presented to the cells of the proximal tubule exceeds the capacity for reabsorption, glucose will be lost into the urine. This is termed *glucosuria* or, less accurately, *glycosuria*. With normal glomerular filtration rates (i.e., normal kidney function), the glucose concentration in the plasma above which glucosuria will usually appear is approximately 180 mg/dl. This value is called the renal threshold for glucose. It is usually less in children, young adults, and pregnant women and often higher in older people. Renal disease can also cause an elevated renal threshold for glucose.

If the postprandial rise in glucose levels exceeds the renal threshold, glucosuria will occur and the test for glucose will be positive in urine formed following meals. However, these tests will be negative in urine formed just prior to meals when glucose concentrations will have fallen below the renal threshold. Thus, patients are only intermittently glucosuric and usually do not have any symptoms.

As the carbohydrate abnormality worsens, glucose concentrations take even longer to fall to preprandial levels and often remain above the renal threshold during longer parts of the day. Although patients have persistent glucosuria during this period, they are most often not aware of any symptoms except possibly, and usually in retrospect, some fatigue.

The next stage of deteriorating carbohydrate metabolism is the loss of normal regulation of hepatic glucose production. This causes fasting hyperglycemia, which, as it increases, leads to glucose levels exceeding the renal threshold during the day and evening. This persistent glucosuria will usually cause an osmotic diuresis (increased urine volume) because the excess glucose in the fluid traversing the kidney prevents the reabsorption of fluids by the kidney back into the circulation. Thus, the patient will notice increased urination , or *polyuria*. The resultant renal loss of fluid leads to dehydration, which causes increased thirst, or *polydipsia*. If the glucose concentrations continue to exceed the renal threshold overnight, the patient will urinate during this period *(nocturia)* as well. As insulin becomes increasingly unavailable and/or ineffective, the body is unable to utilize sufficient calories. This leads to weight loss even though patients have increased hunger, or *polyphagia*. These patients may also complain of *blurring of vision*. This is due to alterations in the shape of the ocular lens due to the osmotic changes induced by hyperglycemia. Finally, patients may show an increased susceptibility to certain infections. Especially prominent are *fungus infections*, usually moniliasis *(Candida)*, which appear as vaginitis, nail infections, or, occasionally, a mouth infection (oral thrush) as well as infections due to *Staphyloccus aureus*, which are marked by recurrent furuncles or carbuncles.

The next stage in the deterioration of carbohydrate metabolism is the appearance of ketosis. The presence of ketone bodies in the urine reflects the fact that the effect of insulin on body tissues is either completely absent or almost so. Ketone bodies are synthesized in the liver from the breakdown products of free fatty acids. The most important factor determining hepatic ketone body production is the amount of free fatty acids presented to the liver. Free fatty acids are released into the circulation from adipose tissue following lipolysis, which is the breakdown of triglycerides, the storage form of fat. Insulin has an important effect on retarding lipolysis, a pathway very sensitive to insulin. It takes 10 to 50 times higher concentrations of insulin to affect carbohydrate metabolism than to inhibit lipolysis. Therefore, only when almost no effective insulin is available does uncontrolled lipolysis occur, flooding the liver with free fatty acids and leading to an overproduction of ketone bodies. Ketone bodies can be utilized only to a limited extent by the peripheral tissues. The excess is excreted by the kidneys. This is the biochemical explanation as to why the presence of ketone bodies in the urine signifies an almost complete lack of effective insulin.

As more and more ketone bodies are produced by the liver, their disposal by peripheral tissue utilization and renal excretion becomes inadequate and they start to accumulate in the blood. The only change in the signs and symptoms at this point is that polyphagia is no longer present because ketone bodies cause anorexia and occasionally nausea. Ketone bodies are acidic and therefore must be buffered. As the body bases become depleted, the patient builds up an excess of acid and thus becomes acidotic. Since the acidosis is caused by an accumulation of ketone bodies, the patient now has ketoacidosis. When ketoacidosis is present, it almost always is due to diabetes mellitus. If the patient is not treated quickly and appropriately, death will ensue. The hallmarks of *diabetic ketoacidosis*[1] are electrolyte depletion, dehydration, and acidosis; their pathogenesis is depicted in Figure 1-1.

Thus, deterioration from normal metabolism through postprandial hyperglycemia, fasting hyperglycemia, ketosis, and finally to complete decompensation, ketoacidosis, has been described. It should be pointed out that most patients with diabetes do not progress to ketosis or ketoacidosis and that the rate at which their carbohydrate metabolism deteriorates is variable. For instance, some patients may never progress beyond postprandial hyperglycemia, while others may decompensate to fasting hyperglycemia over a period of years. On the other hand, most ketosis-prone diabetic patients probably go from normal metabolism to ketoacidosis in a matter of weeks to a few months. Almost all of these patients will have the signs and symptoms of uncontrolled diabetes at the time of diagnosis.

In sharp contrast, in approximately 75 percent of patients the diagnosis of ketosis-resistant diabetes is made while undergoing routine screening during a physical exam or in conjunction with another medical problem. In only a minority of ketosis-resistant patients (the other 25 percent) do symptoms appear. In a few (often the elderly), the polyuria and polydipsia are ignored and symptomatic hyperglycemia is tolerated for many weeks. In this situation, hyperglycemia is so profound and prolonged that the patient can become extremely dehydrated with glucose levels exceeding 1,000 mg/dl; the patient thereby suffers decreased mentation, which can progress to coma. The pathophysiology for this condition, termed *hyperosmolar, nonketotic syndrome*, is also shown in Figure 1-1. If enough insulin is present to regulate lipolysis, the chain of events shown on the right side of

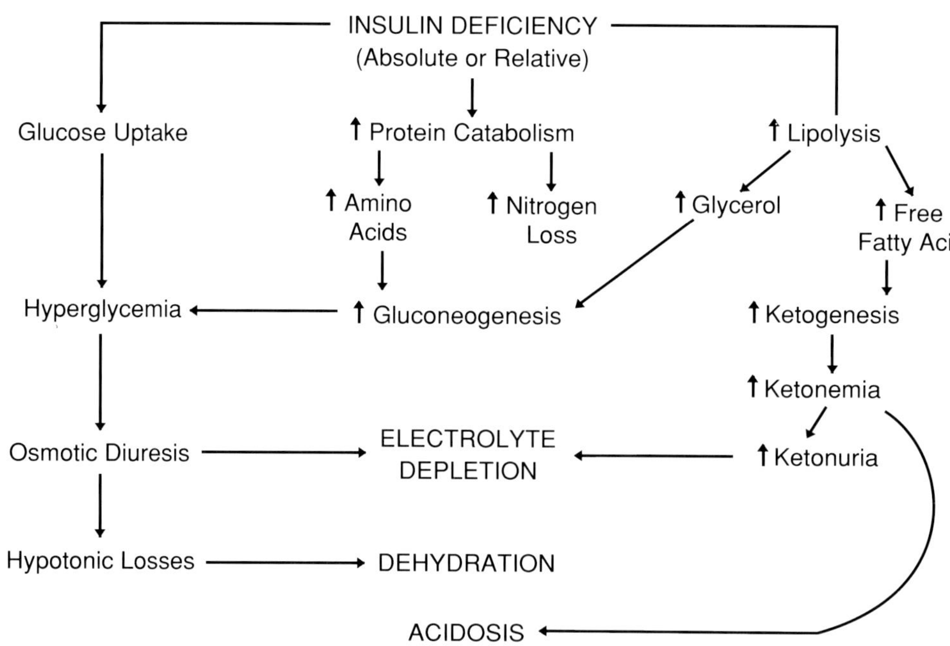

Fig. 1-1. Pathophysiology for diabetic ketoacidosis. See text for discussion. (From Davidson,[1] with permission.)

the figure (i.e., increased lipolysis leading to ketogenesis and ketonuria with subsequent development of acidosis) does not occur. Insulin lack would affect carbohydrate and protein metabolism and would lead only to electrolyte depletion and dehydration. In the absence of the gastrointestinal symptoms caused by ketosis and ketoacidosis, patients may not seek medical attention. Then this sequence of events (hyperglycemia leading to dehydration and electrolyte depletion) occurs over a much longer period of time and leads to severe dehydration, which eventually impairs renal plasma flow. Less glucose is presented to the kidney and renal losses of glucose do not keep pace with hepatic overproduction. Glucose concentrations may become extremely high, occasionally exceeding 2,000 mg/dl.[1]

CLASSIFICATION

Diabetes mellitus can be divided into five general types (Table 1-1).[2,3] One kind is called *type 1 diabetes*, or insulin-dependent diabetes mellitus (IDDM). These patients are defined by the presence of ketosis. For reasons just discussed, this signifies the almost complete lack of effective insulin, and without insulin therapy, these patients will usually progress to diabetic ketoacidosis and die. Although most of these patients are children and young adults (i.e., less than 30 years of age), the older terminology, juvenile-onset diabetes, was not entirely accurate since some lean adult and elderly patients can also have ketosis-prone diabetes. Of the 6 percent of the total population, or approximately 12 million Americans, who have diabetes, only 10 percent, or approximately 1 million, have type 1 diabetes mellitus.

Table 1-1. Classification of Disorders of Carbohydrate Metabolism

A. Diabetes mellitus
   1. Insulin-dependent (IDDM), type 1
   2. Non-insulin-dependent (NIDDM), type 2
   3. Other types
   4. Gestational
   5. Malnutrition-related
B. Impaired glucose tolerance
C. Increased statistical risk for diabetes mellitus
   1. Previous abnormality of glucose tolerance
   2. Potential abnormality of glucose tolerance

The second kind of diabetes is called *type 2 diabetes*, or non-insulin-dependent diabetes mellitus (NIDDM). The important metabolic characteristic of this type of diabetes is the absence of ketosis. Older terms included adult-onset, maturity-onset, or ketosis-resistant diabetes. The fact that these patients do not have ketone bodies in their urine signifies that they have at least some effective insulin. Eighty to ninety percent of type 2 diabetic patients are obese. The term non-insulin-dependent diabetes mellitus may be confusing since approximately 25 percent of these patients receive insulin. The difference is that they do not need insulin to sustain life as the type 1 diabetic patients do. Obesity and older age are two independent risk factors for this kind of diabetes. It is estimated that the chances of developing type 2 diabetes double for every 20 percent increase over ideal body weight and for each decade after the fourth, regardless of weight. The prevalence of diabetes mellitus in persons aged 65 to 74 years is approximately 20 percent. It is likely that a higher percentage of people in the ninth and tenth decades have diabetes mellitus.

The third kind of diabetes is now termed *other types*. Formerly called secondary diabetes, this type includes the following:

1. Diseases of the pancreas that destroy the β cells (e.g., hemochromatosis, pancreatitis, cystic fibrosis)
2. Hormonal syndromes (e.g., acromegaly, Cushing's syndrome, pheochromocytoma) that interfere with insulin secretion and/or inhibit insulin action
3. Drugs that may interfere with insulin secretion (e.g., phenytoin [Dilantin]) or may inhibit insulin action (e.g., glucocorticoids, estrogens)
4. Rare conditions involving abnormalities of the insulin receptor
5. A variety of rare genetic syndromes in which diabetes mellitus inexplicably occurs more frequently than in normal persons
6. Several recently described families in which point mutations in the insulin gene caused amino acid substitution at sites in the insulin

structure necessary for hormonal binding to its receptor leading to an ineffective insulin molecule and diabetes mellitus

Gestational diabetes is really impaired glucose tolerance (see below) that occurs in pregnancy. Thus, diabetic patients who subsequently become pregnant are not included in this class. In normal pregnancy, insulin-antagonistic hormones are produced by the placenta. In 2 to 5 percent of pregnant women, the increased demands on the pancreatic β cell to produce more insulin cannot be met and abnormal carbohydrate metabolism ensues. Gestational diabetes is associated with increased perinatal risks to the offspring and an increased risk to the mother for progression to diabetes mellitus within the next 10 to 15 years. When the pregnancy ends, these patients require reclassification into (1) previous abnormality of glucose tolerance; (2) impaired glucose tolerance; or (3) diabetes mellitus, depending on the results of their postpartum evaluation.

The World Health Organization (WHO) has added another category of diabetes that is noted in underdeveloped countries, *malnutrition-related diabetes mellitus*. The afflicted individuals are usually young, between 10 and 40 years, at onset. They are symptomatic with marked polyuria, polydipsia, and weight loss. Insulin is usually required to control their hyperglycemia, although they remain ketosis-resistant even when insulin is withdrawn. Some of these patients experience antecedent abdominal pain radiating to the back, suggesting pancreatitis. Indeed, at autopsy some of them show pancreatic calcifications on radiograph and exocrine and endocrine destruction and fibrosis as well as calcium stones in the exocrine ducts. However, chronic pancreatitis does not account for their diabetes since insulin requirements are high (patients with diabetes secondary to pancreatic inflammation are usually sensitive to insulin) and many of these patients have no clinical or autopsy evidence of pancreatitis. The role of malnutrition in causing this kind of diabetes is unknown.

The results of oral glucose tolerance tests that are higher than normal but fail to meet the criteria for diabetes mellitus are classified as *impaired glucose tolerance* (IGT). Ten to thirty percent of the population over 65 years of age have IGT (in addition to the 15 to 20 percent with diabetes mellitus). Former terminology included chemical, latent, subclinical, borderline, and asymptomatic diabetes. When the subjects are retested with an oral glucose challenge, even after many years, approximately 30 percent will have reverted to normal, 50 percent will continue to show IGT, and the remaining 20 percent will be diabetic. Progression to overt diabetes in this latter population occurs at a low rate, 1 to 5 percent per year. Recent evidence suggests that patients with IGT are unlikely to develop the neuropathic and microangiopathic complications (retinopathy and nephropathy) of diabetes. However, these patients are especially prone to macroangiopathic complications: coronary artery, peripheral vascular, and cerebrovascular disease.

The classification of *previous abnormality of glucose tolerance* is restricted to persons whose glucose tolerance test at one time fulfilled the criteria for IGT or diabetes mellitus, either spontaneously or in response to an identifiable stress, but who are currently normal. This group was formerly described as having latent diabetes or prediabetes. Gestational diabetic patients are an obvious source for this class, as are formerly obese patients who have lost weight. Subjects undergoing acute stress due to trauma or illness may experience transient hyperglycemia and would fit into this category as well. With the exception of gestational diabetic patients, there has been little systematic study of the propensity of these subjects to subsequently develop diabetes mellitus. It is likely that the risk is increased, and these individuals should be monitored closely when they are in stressful situations.

The classification of *potential abnormality of glucose tolerance* is reserved for individuals who have never exhibited abnormal glucose tolerance but who have a substantially increased risk for the development of diabetes mellitus. The former term for this class was prediabetes or potential diabetes. Subjects who are at increased risk for type 1 diabetes include (in decreasing order of risk) persons with islet cell antibodies (see below); the monozygotic twin of a type 1 diabetic patient; the sibling of a type 1 diabetic patient, especially one with an identical human leukocyte antigen (HLA) genotype (see below); and the offspring of a type 1 diabetic patient.

Individuals who are at increased risk for type 2 diabetes include (in decreasing order of risk) the monozygotic twin of a type 2 diabetic patient; a first degree relative (sibling, parent, or offspring) of a type 2 diabetic patient; the mother of a baby weighing more than 9 pounds at birth; obese subjects; and members of racial or ethnic groups with a very high prevalence of type 2 diabetes (such as certain Indian tribes). The actual degree of risk for any of these circumstances is not well established at the present time, except for the monozygotic twins who are virtually certain to develop type 2 diabetes.

DIAGNOSIS

According to the WHO,[3] any one of three criteria is sufficient to diagnose diabetes mellitus: (1) random plasma glucose concentrations more than or equal to 200 mg/dl (whether associated with symptoms of uncontrolled diabetes or not); (2) fasting plasma glucose concentrations more than or equal to 140 mg/dl; or (3) plasma glucose concentrations more than or equal to 200 mg/dl 2 hours after oral glucose (Table 1-2). (For whole blood glucose levels, the numbers would be decreased 10 to 15 percent [i.e., to 180 and 120 mg/dl].) The National Diabetes Data Group[2] has promulgated similar, but more complex, criteria, which can result in a "nondiagnostic" category. For this reason, I prefer the WHO approach to diagnosis.

It is important to confirm these abnormal values so that an erroneous diagnosis due to lab error is not made. Persons with abnormalities of glucose tolerance that lie between normal (fasting <115 mg/dl and 2 h after glucose <140 mg/dl) and diabetes are designated as having impaired glucose tolerance (Table 1-1). Because even minor abnormalities of glucose tolerance in pregnant women can be associated with large fetuses, leading to increased risk at delivery as well as in the neonatal period, the criteria accepted in this country for gestational diabetes (glucose intolerance of pregnancy) are more sensitive (Table 1-3) than those for impaired glucose tolerance in nonpregnant adults (Table 1-2). Treatment with insulin of pregnant women with these relatively mild abnormalities of carbohydrate metabolism has been associated with fewer complications at delivery.

Table 1-2. World Health Organization Criteria for Diabetes Mellitus and Impaired Glucose Tolerance (IGT)

	Venous Plasma Glucose Concentration (mg/dl)		
	Fasting		*2 Hours*[a]
Diabetes mellitus	≥140	or	≥200
IGT	<140	and	140–199

[a] After ingesting 75 g of glucose.

PATHOGENESIS

Type 1 Diabetes

The evolution of type 1 diabetes[4–6] in a given individual can be divided into stages. These are depicted in Figure 1-2 where the hypothetical pancreatic β-cell mass is plotted against time. Genetic, immunologic, and probably environmental (e.g., possibly viral) influences are involved, which eventually lead to total exhaustion of the β cell. The major genetic risk factor for the development of type 1 diabetes is the HLA genes located on the short arm of the sixth chromosome. Their identification requires testing white blood cells which accounts for their name. These genes determine which surface antigens are produced by nucleated cells. The surface antigens are involved in a host of

Table 1-3. Criteria[a] for the Diagnosis of Gestational Diabetes

Venous Plasma (Whole Blood) Glucose Concentrations (mg/dl)
Fasting 105 (90)
1 h 190 (170)
2 h 165 (145)
3 h 145 (125)

[a] Two or more of the listed values after a 100-g glucose challenge must be met or exceeded to make the diagnosis.

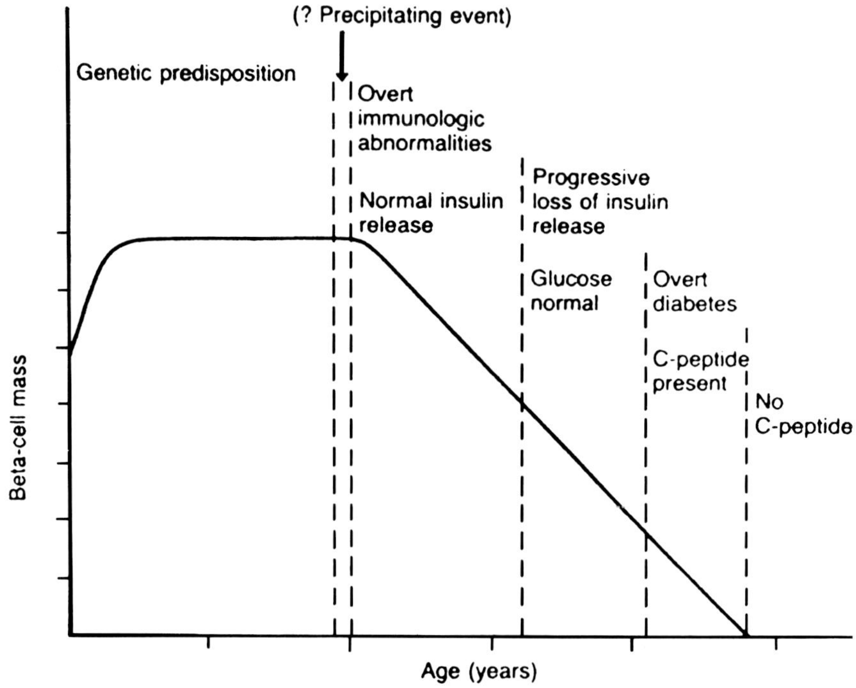

Fig. 1-2. Stages in the development of type 1 diabetes mellitus. The stages are portrayed from left to right. β-Cell mass (hypothetical) is plotted against time. (From Eisenbarth,[17] with permission.)

cell-to-cell interactions, one of which includes the rejection process (i.e., the reaction when tissue from one host is transplanted into another). Since many different surface antigens are possible in a population, a large number of separate genes are responsible for them. Two HLA types, DR3 and DR4, are common in white patients with type 1 diabetes. This means that certain genes, the ones whose expression produces these HLA types, are also common in these patients and provide a marker for the genetic background that increases susceptibility to type 1 diabetes.

Each parent furnishes a gene that codes for different DR antigens. If an offspring should be so unfortunate to have a genotype of DR3/DR4, receiving a DR3 from one parent and a DR4 from the other, the lifetime risk for developing type 1 diabetes in that individual is 1 : 45. If the genotype is DR3/DR3 or DR4/DR4, the lifetime risk is reduced to 1 : 125 to 150. If the haplotype (set of closely related genes) of an individual contains just one HLA type that confirms susceptibility for type 1 diabetes (i.e., DR3 or DR4), the lifetime risk is 1 : 500. If neither DR3 nor DR4 is present, there is only a 1 : 5,000 chance of getting type 1 diabetes. However, it is unlikely that the HLA antigens themselves confer the susceptibility. Rather, they either act as inert "markers" for the existence of disease susceptibility or immune response genes (see discussion following) that are in linkage disequilibrium with the HLA system, or more specific subtypes of the DR alleles (one of a possible group of genes located at the same site on a chromosome) are responsible. (Linkage disequilibrium is the tendency in a population for some alleles at closely linked loci to occur together in the same haplotype [i.e., on the same chromosome] more often than expected by chance.)

The HLA system in humans is the analog of the major histocompatibility system that occurs in all animals. This chromosomal region consists of loci that not only control the synthesis of transplantation (surface) antigens, but also have fundamental roles in the immune process. Indeed, good evidence suggests that an immune process is active at the onset of type 1 diabetes. Lymphocytic infiltrates are seen in the islets of Langerhans of patients on whom an autopsy is performed soon after the diagnosis. Antibodies against islet cells are present in the sera of over 80 percent of type 1 patients if they are tested near the onset of their disease; a gradual reduction in antibody titers occurs over the ensuing year in most patients. Furthermore, it has been recently found that these patients also have autoantibodies against the insulin molecule at the time of diagnosis. (Although it is common for patients treated with insulin to develop antibodies against the hormone, these individuals have not been exposed to exogenous insulin and their antibodies have been made against their own insulin). In addition, both the islet cell antibodies and the insulin autoantibodies have been shown to precede the clinical appearance of type 1 diabetes, sometimes for a period of years.

During this period preceding the development of diabetes, oral glucose tolerance is normal and the insulin response to oral glucose is either normal or only subtle changes can be detected. However, the insulin response to intravenous glucose may show a progressive decline. After a bolus of glucose is injected, there is a rapid (within 1 to 3 minutes) rise in insulin. This acute phase of insulin release has been measured serially in patients with normal oral glucose tolerance who harbor the islet cell and insulin autoantibodies. When the acute phase of insulin release falls below 5 percent of the response in a normal population in these individuals (even though they still maintain relatively normal glucose and insulin responses to oral glucose), type 1 diabetes can appear soon afterward (within weeks to months). Even with overt diabetes, these patients initially retain some insulin secretion (as assessed by C-peptide, a polypeptide packaged with insulin in β-cell granules and secreted along with insulin). Within a year, however, the β cell is completely exhausted and incapable of secreting any C-peptide or insulin.

There is controversy concerning possible environmental "stresses" that may trigger the events leading to type 1 diabetes. Although viral infections may play a role in some cases, the evidence for a viral influence on the onset of type 1 diabetes is indirect and weaker than the case for genetic and immunologic factors. First, there are a number of isolated case reports of different viral syndromes preceding the onset of ketosis-prone diabetes by several weeks. Second, direct epidemiologic data relate the prevalence of new cases of type 1 diabetes in the winter months to seasonal changes of viral illnesses. Third, a similar direct relation exists between antibody titers to Coxsackie B virus (after viral infections, titers rise acutely and then fall) and the onset of new cases of type 1 diabetes. Fourth, certain strains of mice develop diabetes after infection with several different viruses. It seems certain, however, that whatever initiates the chronic autoimmune process, be it viral agent, toxin, or random immunologic event, it occurs because of genetic susceptibility. At the present time, the HLA types DR3 and DR4 are the best identifying characteristics of these individuals in the population at large.

Type 2 Diabetes and IGT

The pathogenesis of type 2 diabetes[7,8] involves both relative insulin deficiency and resistance to insulin action. The insulin response to intravenous and oral glucose is impaired, although insulin concentrations after meals are normal or only slightly decreased. Since postprandial glucose levels are elevated, one might expect higher insulin concentrations, hence, a relative insulin deficiency. On the other hand, the combination of normal insulin concentrations and hyperglycemia implies the presence of insulin resistance. Indeed, sophisticated methods of evaluating insulin action have directly shown that insulin works ineffectively in the target tissues (muscle and liver) in patients with type 2 diabetes mellitus. Studies of insulin action in a large number of normal (nondiabetic) subjects have revealed a wide range of sensitivity to insulin. Some normal people have as much insulin resistance as those with type 2 diabetes. The former, however, are able to secrete more insulin than the latter.

The following temporal relationship between insulin secretion and sensitivity to insulin is now accepted by most investigators. Insulin resistance occurs in those patients who may develop type 2 diabetes mellitus. In those in whom the pancreatic β-cell reserve is sufficient, normal glucose levels are preserved at the expense of hyperinsulinemia (high insulin levels in the blood). In those in whom the β-cell reserve is inadequate to maintain normal glucose levels, IGT appears. Hyperinsulinemia initially continues. However, as the β cells start to fail, glucose concentrations increase to values consistent with diabetes and insulin concentrations fall to "normal" or below. Presumably, those individuals who progress from hyperinsulinemia and normal glucose tolerance to hyperinsulinemia and IGT to overt diabetes have a genetic susceptibility for a decreased β-cell reserve. Those with an adequate reserve for insulin secretion will maintain normal or impaired glucose tolerance at the expense of continued hyperinsulinemia. This scenario is supported by considering two groups of people who are at an increased risk for type 2 diabetes (i.e., the obese and the elderly). Not only has insulin resistance and hyperinsulinemia been documented in both, but IGT is also more common. If enhanced insulin secretion were unable to continue to overcome their insulin resistance, diabetes would ensue, thus accounting for the fact that 80 percent of type 2 patients are obese and the prevalence of diabetes in people over 65 years of age may be as high as 20 percent.

Why β-cell reserve is not maintained in those individuals developing type 2 diabetes is completely unknown. The mechanism of the insulin resistance is almost as enigmatic. The critical first step of insulin action is binding to receptors located on the cell surface. This triggers a signal (or signals) within the cell, which enables insulin to carry out a myriad of effects. However, insulin binding is normal in type 2 diabetic patients. Therefore, the site of the insulin resistance must be at a postbinding step. At the moment, that is all that can be said with certainty.

GENETICS

The inheritance[9] of diabetes mellitus is probably the most controversial of all the many uncertainties surrounding this enigmatic syndrome. Indeed, it has been termed the "geneticist's nightmare." Familial aggregation (the tendency for diabetes to run in families) was first recorded in 1628. Modern studies have shown that overall the prevalence of diabetes is approximately fourfold higher in the parents and ninefold higher in the siblings of diabetic as compared to nondiabetic patients. However, the inheritance of type 1 and type 2 diabetes is clearly different.

Monozygotic twins are genetically identical, whereas the genetic constitution of dizygotic twins is like that of any two siblings. A number of twinships have been identified in which one member has diabetes. If the other twin also has the disease, they are concordant for diabetes; if diabetes is not present, they are discordant for the trait. Monozygotic twins have a much higher concordance for diabetes than dizygotic twins. However, concordance is very different in identical twinships with type 1 and type 2 diabetes. In type 1 twinships, concordance is only 30 to 50 percent. Many of the nondiabetic twins have remained normal for 20 or 30 years suggesting that most of these twins will never develop diabetes.

It seems probable that in type 1 diabetes, there is a genetic predisposition related to the HLA locus as discussed previously. However, in order for diabetes to occur, an outside cause is required. In recent years, family studies have provided some information concerning the probabilities of developing type 1 diabetes. Offspring of a type 1 diabetic patient have a 5 percent chance of developing the disease, while the siblings of such patients have a 5 to 10 percent chance. These statistics can be refined in the siblings if the HLA haplotypes are known. Those siblings who do not share either of the HLA haplotypes of the type 1 diabetic patient have only a 1 percent chance; if one HLA haplotype is common to both of them, there is a 5 to 7 percent chance; and if both HLA haplotypes are similar, there is a 20 percent chance of developing type 1 diabetes at some time in the future.

In regard to type 2 diabetes, concordance in identical twinships approaches 100 percent with the second twin developing diabetes shortly after the first one. As these twins usually live apart for many years before the onset of type 2 diabetes, genetic, rather than environmental, factors must play the predominant role. Except for the unusual patient who inherits type 2 diabetes as an autosomal dominant trait (see below), the empiric risk for a first degree relative (i.e., sibling, parent, offspring) of a ketosis-resistant diabetic patient to develop diabetes is 10 to 15 percent. There is a 20 to 30 percent risk for first degree relatives to develop IGT. Avoidance of obesity will prevent the abnormal carbohydrate metabolism in many of these individuals at risk.

Thus, although the evidence is overwhelming that diabetes mellitus is "inherited," the heterogeneous nature of this disorder prevents a clearer understanding of its mode of transmission. Progress will only be made when homogeneous subsets of this syndrome can be identified and studied. This type of study is possible with young type 2 diabetic patients in whom ketosis-resistant diabetes could be traced back through three generations. This finding indicates an autosomal dominant inheritance in this small group of type 2 patients. The original appellation for these patients was maturity-onset diabetes of youth (MODY), now termed non-insulin-dependent diabetes of youth (NIDDMY). In addition to heterogeneity complicating the genetic analysis of the remaining type 2 patients, certain environmental stresses (e.g., obesity, age, pregnancy, infection) seem to be important in the phenotypic expression of the genetic trait. This environmental influence could prevent the identification of all patients who may carry the gene(s). Until these problems can be resolved, diabetes mellitus will remain the "geneticist's nightmare."

COMPLICATIONS OF DIABETES MELLITUS

The complications of diabetes are best considered in three separate groups: (1) macrovascular (large vessel or atherosclerotic) disease, the clinical manifestations of which are angina and myocardial infarctions (heart attacks), cerebral vascular accidents (strokes), and peripheral vascular disease; (2) microvascular (small vessel) disease, the clinical manifestations of which are diabetic retinopathy (eye disease) and diabetic nephropathy, also called diabetic glomerulosclerosis (kidney disease); and (3) neuropathy (involvement of both the peripheral and autonomic nervous systems), the clinical manifestations of which can lead to a variety of problems.

There are six independent risk factors for *macrovascular* disease in the general population (Table 1-4), of which diabetes is only one. Whatever the degree of risk an individual has, smoking will approximately double it. Smoking is obviously a reversible risk factor.

Although appropriate treatment of hypertension will eliminate it as a risk factor, it is estimated that at least 25 percent of patients do not take their medications. Like diabetes, hypertension is a "silent killer" without symptoms. Many patients will not bother with treatment. However, if the patient complies with proper treatment, hypertension is also a reversible risk factor.

The evidence regarding elevated cholesterol levels as a risk factor for macrovascular disease is very strong. To be more specific, it is the increased low density lipoproteins that carry cholesterol (LDL cholesterol) that shows the strongest association with macrovascular disease. Low levels of high density lipoproteins that carry cholesterol (HDL cholesterol) also seem to be associated with macrovascular disease. This may be an important factor in regard to the possible association of elevated triglyceride concentrations with macrovascular disease. Some studies show a positive correlation between hypertriglyceridemia and large vessel disease; others do not. In recent years, it has become apparent that low HDL cholesterol levels usually occur in conjunction with high triglyceride levels. Therefore, the primary risk factor may lie with the former rather than the latter. Hyperlipidemia is usually a reversible risk factor since there are both dietary and drug treatments for elevated cholesterol and triglyceride concentrations. Furthermore, since both obesity and uncontrolled dia-

Table 1-4. Risk Factors for Macrovascular Disease

1. Smoking
2. Hypertension
3. Hyperlipidemia (elevated cholesterol and/or triglyceride levels)
4. Obesity
5. Family history (genetic)
6. Diabetes mellitus

betes can cause hypertriglyceridemia, successful therapy for increased glucose levels and body weight will help decrease hypertriglyceridemia.

Although hypertension and hypertriglyceridemia are associated with obesity, increased body fat has been shown to be an independent risk factor as well. For completely unknown reasons, those who carry their excess weight around their waists (android or "apple" obesity) seem to be at much more risk than those whose excess weight is concentrated around their hips (gynecoid or "pear" obesity). Although successful long term treatment is not easy after an initial weight loss (recidivism rates can range up to 90 percent), obesity is also a reversible risk factor.

Each of us inherits a genetic susceptibility for developing atherosclerosis. Since macrovascular disease is usually expressed earlier in males, the past medical history of one's father, grandfather, brothers, and uncles furnishes a clue to the seriousness of the risk factor. Obviously, it is not a reversible one.

Diabetes mellitus is the final independent risk factor for macrovascular disease. It approximately doubles the chances of developing coronary artery, cerebrovascular, or peripheral vascular disease. Patients with diabetes who also smoke are particularly prone to develop peripheral vascular disease. Thus, diabetes increases the risk for peripheral vascular disease in smokers approximately five times as opposed to doubling the risk for coronary artery and cerebrovascular disease. Although epidemiologic studies have established a positive correlation between hyperglycemia and macrovascular disease, there is little current evidence to suggest that lowering glucose levels in patients with diabetes will lessen their chances of developing large vessel disease. This may be due to the fact that there are five other risk factors involved and it is difficult to isolate a separate effect of better diabetic control. Therefore, at the present time, diabetes must be considered an irreversible risk factor for macrovascular disease. In sharp contrast, there is very good evidence (summarized under "Treatment") for a beneficial effect of strict diabetic control (near euglycemia) on the eye, kidney, and neuropathic complications of diabetes.

Diabetic eye disease[10] (commonly called *diabetic retinopathy*, although other structures are sometimes involved) is a potentially very serious complication. As stated above, it is the leading cause of blindness in people between the ages of 20 and 74 years of age. Diabetes can affect the outer (lens), middle (vitreous), and inner (retina) parts of the eye. The temporary change in the shape of the lens due to hyperglycemia with resultant blurring of vision has already been described. The lens is also more prone to cataract formation in diabetic patients. A rare occurrence is a "snowflake" or "Christmas tree" type of cataract (sometimes called the *diabetic cataract*) in which a pattern resembling these kinds of structures can be seen in the middle of the lens. Since this type of cataract was usually associated with episodes of severe diabetic ketoacidosis, it is rarely seen today.

Although more typical "senile" cataracts may not be more common in the diabetic population, they are approximately 5 times more likely to develop at a younger age than in the normal population. Diabetic control (as reflected in glucose levels) does not seem to play a role.

The first observable diabetic changes on the retina are a subtle dilation of the major retinal veins. Normally the retinal veins are 1.5 times the size of the retinal arteries (a 2 : 3 artery to vein ratio). In these early changes, the arteries remain normal, but the veins become distended and may become 2 to 3 times the size of the arteries. This phase is termed *preretinopathy* and is generally present for less than 2 years before the retinal changes progress to the classic background stage.

The next phase is called *background, simple,* or *nonproliferative diabetic retinopathy*. It is characterized by microaneurysms, hemorrhages, and hard exudates (Fig. 1-3). Microaneurysms, usually the first sign of background retinopathy, appear as tiny, round, red dots which, as the name implies, are small aneurysmal outpouchings or sacculations of the retinal capillaries. If hemorrhage from these weakened areas of the capillary occurs in the superficial retinal layers, they appear flame-shaped. Those occurring in the deeper retinal layers have the appearance of "dots and blots." Although the smaller ones may be difficult to distinguish from microaneurysms, most are large enough to be differentiated. In addition, the capillaries become permeable to plasma, which leaks out and precipitates in the retinal layers. This leads to the forma-

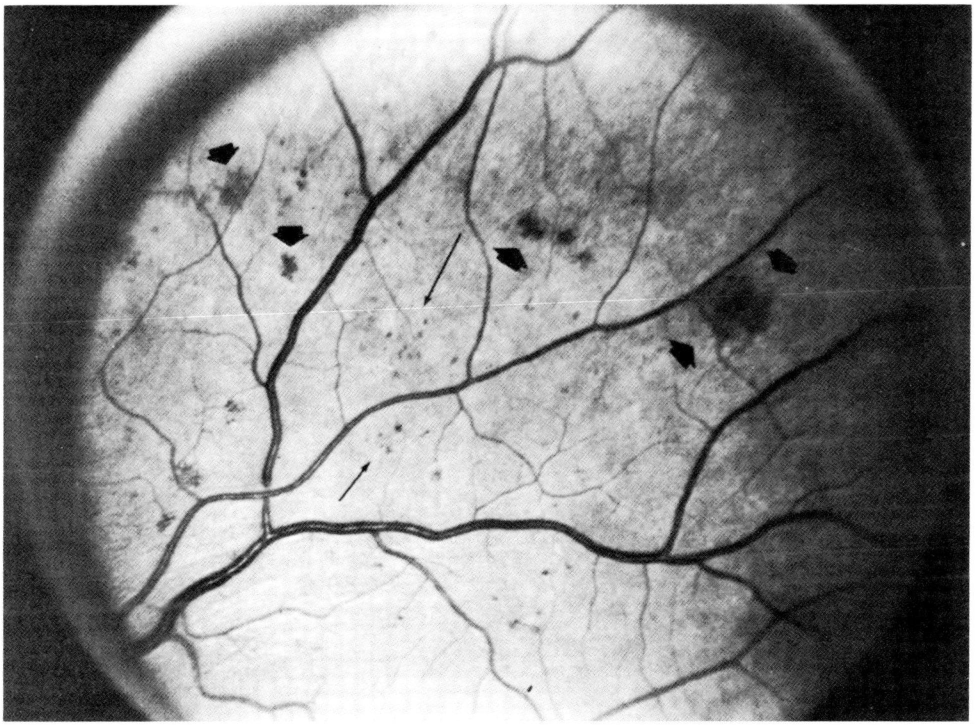

Fig. 1-3. Nonproliferative (background, simple) diabetic retinopathy characterized by microaneurysms (long dark arrows) and "blot" hemorrhages (short thick arrows). See text for discussion. (From Klein,[18] with permission.)

tion of hard exudates, which are seen as sharply defined, glistening, yellowish deposits. Such leakage involves only plasma, not red blood cells. These changes (microaneurysms, hemorrhages, and exudates) wax and wane. They do not impair vision unless the plasma leakage occurs near the macular areas. There, the pattern is often of a ring of hard exudates surrounding the macula. Since this is the central vision area, exudates here with the associated swelling (termed *macular edema*) can diminish vision. Macular edema is much more common in older patients. Background retinopathy is not usually seen until approximately 10 years after the diagnosis of diabetes. With our current methods of controlling glucose levels, it will eventually appear in up to 80 percent of diabetic patients.

The next stage is called *preproliferative diabetic retinopathy*. The veins now have an irregular caliber, often looking like a string of sausages. A particularly important sign is the appearance of cotton wool spots or soft exudates. They represent evidence of capillary closure with resultant hypoxia (lack of oxygen) to parts of the retina. Soft exudates are pale, yellow patches with poorly defined margins that do not contrast well with the normal retina (i.e., they may be difficult to see with the ophthalmoscope). The other finding of particular significance is intraretinal microvascular abnormalities (IRMAs). IRMAs are tufts of new capillaries that are still located beneath the inner limiting membrane (i.e., they have not yet broken out to lie on the surface of the retina). Although it may be difficult (except by special tests) to distinguish between IRMAs and neovascularization (i.e., new vessels that either lie on the surface of the retina or are growing out into the vitreous [the middle part of the eye]), the differentiation is not clinically important since either one should trigger an immediate referral to a qualified ophthalmologist.

These preproliferative changes are the immediate forerunner to proliferative diabetic retinopathy, which occurs in 5 to 10 percent of patients with diabetic retinopathy. New vessel growth occurring on the surface of the retina or growing from there into the vitreous is its distinguishing feature. These new vessels (Fig. 1-4) are structurally weak and liable to hemorrhage, thereby obscuring vision. This often leads to formation of fibrous (scar) tissue as the blood is resorbed. This scar tissue puts traction on the retina and can cause a retinal detachment (i.e., pulling the retina off the back of the eye). If the process is allowed to continue untreated, the neovascularization can eventually involve the front part of the eye. A fluid normally

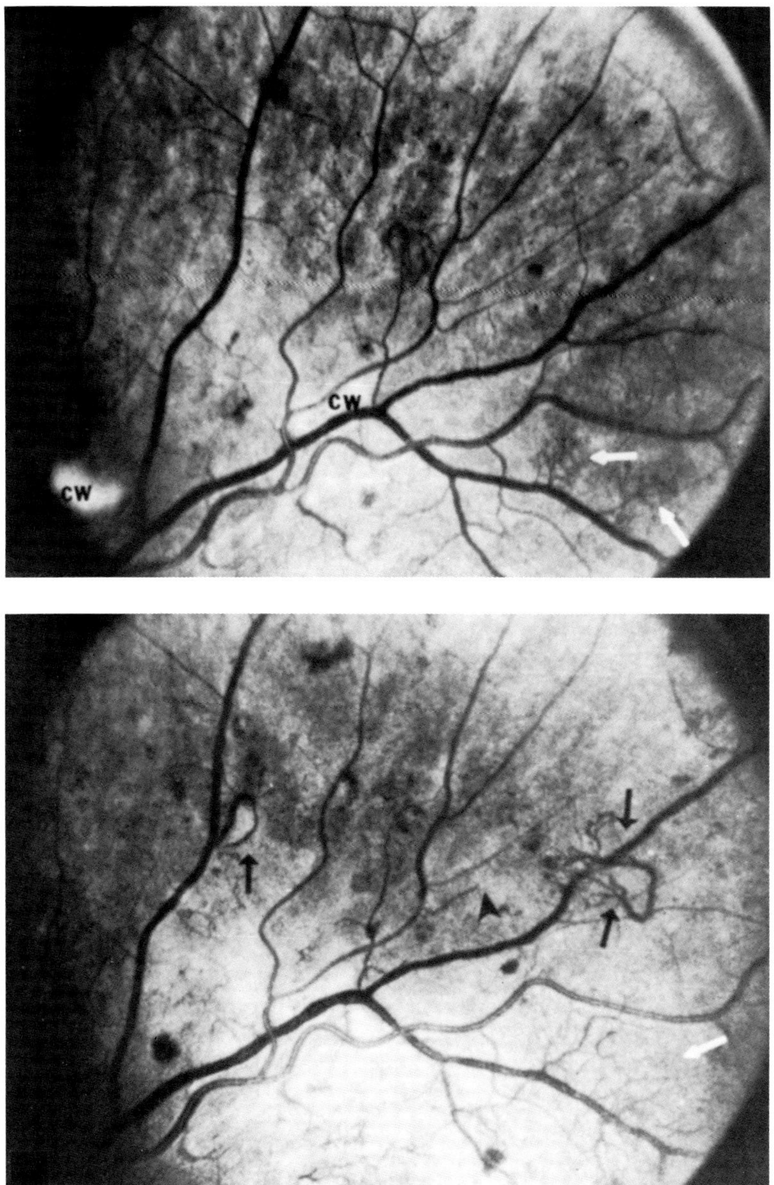

A

B

Fig. 1-4. (**A & B**) Proliferative diabetic retinopathy characterized by IRMAs (white arrows), cotton wool spots (CW), neovascularization (black arrows), and abrupt termination of the arterioles (black arrowhead). See text for discussion. (From Klein,[10] with permission.)

circulates around the eye keeping it lubricated. The neovascular process reaching the front of the eye can interfere with the channels used for circulation of this fluid. If that should happen, the pressure within the eye increases dramatically and usually leads to a very painful blindness.

Fortunately, the latter is a rare outcome since appropriate treatment usually arrests this process. Diabetic patients should be examined routinely by an ophthalmologist. Recent studies have shown convincingly that laser photocoagulation treatment for preproliferative and proliferative diabetic retinopathy as well as macular edema has been associated with markedly less vision loss. Recent surgical techniques now enable eye surgeons to restore retinal detachments and remove blood and blood products from the vitreous. No dietary or drug treatments have yet been shown to be helpful for diabetic retinopathy.

The clinical course of *diabetic nephropathy*[11,12] for type 1 patients is depicted in Figure 1-5. Although less information is available on type 2 patients, it is assumed that the sequence of events is similar since the prevalence of overt diabetic nephropathy is the same in the two types of diabetes for a given duration of disease. Approximately 40 percent of patients develop clinical renal disease. Therefore, there must be either a protective factor in the other 60 percent who remain free of renal disease or a sensitizing one in those who do develop it, either of which could be genetically related.

Diabetic nephropathy may be divided in five stages. Stage 1 occurs at the onset of the disease (and is not shown in Fig. 1-5). It is characterized by a 30 to 40 percent increase in the glomerular filtration rate (GFR) above normal. The GFR is a measure of how well the kidney filters the blood, which is the first step in ridding the body of toxic wastes. It is used as a test to judge how well the kidney is functioning. The increased GFR often returns to normal within a few weeks to a few months with treatment that lowers glucose levels.

Stage 2 is characterized by normal excretion of albumin by the kidney (<20 μg/min or 30 mg/24 h) regardless of the duration of diabetes. Exercise increases albumin excretion in general, but in some stage 2 patients, the levels attained are higher than normal. This is termed *microalbuminuria* (induced

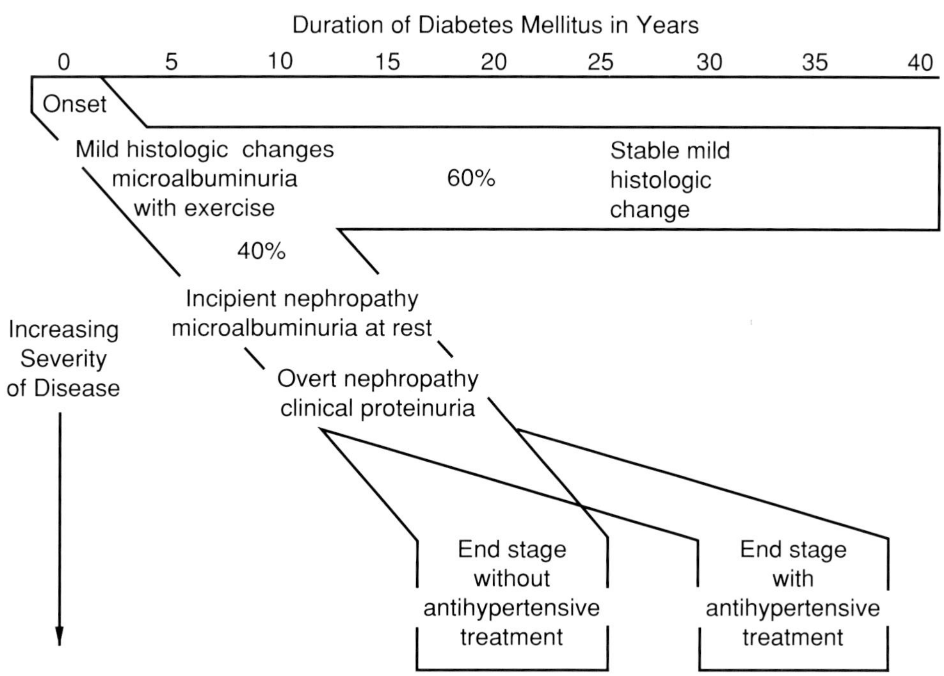

Fig. 1-5. Clinical course of diabetic nephropathy. See text for discussion. (From Omachi,[11] with permission.)

in this case by exercise). In addition, those patients that remain in poor metabolic control may retain their elevated GFR. Recent studies have suggested that the latter may be a poor prognostic factor for eventual progression to clinical renal disease.

Stage 3, or incipient diabetic nephropathy, is characterized by microalbuminuria at rest. This is defined as elevated excretion rates of albumin between 20 and 200 μg/min (30 to 300 mg/24 h). In general, patients with lower amounts of microalbuminuria (20 to 70 μg/min) have either an elevated or normal GFR which is higher than those with more microalbuminuria (70 to 200 μg/min). This suggests that GFR (kidney function) begins to decline during the incipient stage of diabetic nephropathy. At this stage, blood pressures are often higher (although in the normal range) compared to nondiabetic subjects and may increase to abnormally high levels during exercise. In general, blood pressures will increase 3 to 4 mmHg per year. Without treatment, approximately 80 percent of patients with microalbuminuria will progress within 7 to 14 years to clinical proteinuria or overt diabetic nephropathy (see below); only 5 percent without microalbuminuria will do so. Although control of glucose levels and blood pressure will reduce or eliminate microalbuminuria, it is too early to tell if these measures will forestall the progression of incipient diabetic nephropathy.

Stage 4, or overt diabetic nephropathy, is characterized by clinical proteinuria, (i.e., a level of urinary proteins that is detectable [Albustix-positive]) by tests performed in clinical laboratories. These methods are much less sensitive than the specially developed ones used to measure microalbuminuria. Thus, overt diabetic nephropathy is defined by urinary protein excretion exceeding 0.5 g/24 h. Since albumin is not the only protein excreted at this stage, clinical proteinuria corresponds to albumin excretion rates exceeding 200 μg/min or 300 mg (0.3 g)/24 h. Early in the clinical course of overt diabetic nephropathy, the GFR may be in the normal range but usually falls slowly but steadily. During this stage of diabetic nephropathy, blood pressure increases approximately 7 mmHg per year so that hypertension eventually occurs in almost all patients. Control of blood pressure will slow the rate of decline of the GFR. At this point, lowering glucose levels will not. Almost all of these patients will have diabetic retinopathy and many of them will have the proliferative type.

Stage 5, or end stage renal disease, is similar to kidney failure from any other cause. Signs and symptoms include progressive weakness, lethargy, fluid retention (possibly leading to congestive heart failure), anorexia, nausea, possibly vomiting, diarrhea, hiccups, pruritis, difficult to control hypertension, anemia, and electrolyte disturbances. There is a clinical impression, however, that patients with end stage renal disease due to diabetes are more symptomatic at higher levels of GFR than patients with nondiabetic causes of kidney failure (i.e., the GFR does not have to be as low for diabetic patients to start experiencing difficulties). Therefore, dialysis is usually started earlier in patients with diabetes. Diabetic patients on dialysis have a worse prognosis than nondiabetic patients. For this reason, kidney transplantation is considered the preferred method of treatment, especially if a close relative will donate a kidney. In spite of successful treatment for end stage renal disease, many of these patients succumb to their associated macrovascular disease.

Diabetic neuropathy[13] has a wide-ranging (Table 1-5) and serious impact on the health of people with diabetes. Although the exact mechanism(s) is (are) not known, it is generally believed that long-term hyperglycemia is the cause (except as noted).

Peripheral neuropathy is the earliest, most widely recognized, and probably most common form of diabetic neuropathy. It is a generalized, sensory-motor polyneuropathy of gradual onset, which is usually progressive. The legs are almost

Table 1-5. Classification of Diabetic Neuropathy

1. Peripheral neuropathy
2. Autonomic neuropathy
   a. Cardiovascular
   b. Gastrointestinal
   c. Genitourinary
   d. Sudomotor
   e. Hypoglycemia unawareness
3. Acute onset neuropathies
   a. Mononeuropathy
   b. Mononeuropathy multiplex
   c. Radiculopathy
   d. Plexopathy
4. Neuropathic diabetic cachexia

always affected earlier than the hands. Patients initially experience sensory manifestations (e.g., tingling [paresthesias], burning sensation, and hypesthesia [uncomfortable feeling when the skin is touched]). These symptoms can be quite uncomfortable. On examination, there is an early loss of tendon reflexes and a decreased vibration sense and sense of touch. As the peripheral neuropathy progresses, the feet become numb and the patient is unable to appreciate trauma (i.e., to feel any pain in the feet). Additionally, involvement of motor fibers can cause muscle weakness and atrophy. This leads to deformities of the feet, causing areas that receive increased pressure (manifested by callous formation). A further serious cause of foot deformities and areas receiving increased pressure is Charcot's arthropathy. Repeated unrecognized trauma to the foot may destroy the joint structures with subsequent flattening of the foot arch. Since the patient has decreased sensation in the foot, these areas can ulcerate. Once the integrity of the skin has been broached, the chances for a serious infection are increased, especially if the patient has high glucose levels. Any impairment of circulation to the foot because of peripheral vascular disease compounds the problem. The combination of loss of sensation leading to ulceration of the skin (whether foot deformities are involved or not) and diminished circulation is the root cause of the large number of lower extremity amputations in diabetic patients.

Although various tests may reveal abnormalities in the functioning of the autonomic nervous system (both sympathetic and parasympathetic) early in the course of diabetes, clinical signs and symptoms appear much later and almost always after peripheral neuropathy is established. Parasympathetic activity decreases the heart rate. Sympathetic activity increases the heart rate and its force of contraction (leading to a rise in cardiac output) and redirects blood flow from the viscera (internal organs) to skeletal muscle by increasing peripheral resistance. The parasympathetic arm of the autonomic nervous system is often affected earlier and more profoundly than the sympathetic one. Therefore, a resting tachycardia is usually the initial clinical cardiovascular effect of autonomic neuropathy. Exercise intolerance may occur when the sympathetic nervous system is affected since the necessary increase in cardiac output and skeletal blood flow is blunted. When one moves from a lying to a sitting to a standing position, the sympathetic nervous system is responsible for the maintenance of the blood pressure via stimuli from the baroreceptors. Therefore, autonomic neuropathy may cause postural (orthostatic) hypotension, which has been defined in two ways: either a 30-mmHg decrease in systolic blood pressure or a 10-mmHg decrease in diastolic blood pressure 2 minutes after standing. Clinically, patients complain of sudden dizziness, lightheadedness, weakness, nausea, occasionally vomiting and even passing out (syncope) after standing up.

Autonomic neuropathy can involve all parts of the gastrointestinal tract: esophagus, stomach, gallbladder, small intestine, and large intestine. Esophageal and gallbladder dysfunction do not usually cause any symptoms.

In patients with gastric involvement (gastroparesis diabeticorum), the stomach is large, dilated, and hypotonic. (Smooth muscle contractions of the gastrointestinal tract are mediated by the parasympathetic nervous system.) Symptoms include anorexia, nausea, vomiting, postprandial fullness (bloated feeling), early satiety, and gastric reflux. Essentially, the ingested food remains in the stomach and is delayed in entering the small intestine; the vomitus may include undigested food eaten hours earlier. This problem is a particularly difficult one for insulin-requiring patients who need a predictable response to meals to cover the action of the injected insulin. Autonomic neuropathy of the intestine leads to constipation (most common) or diarrhea or alternating constipation and diarrhea. Diabetic diarrhea is often nocturnal and can be associated with fecal incontinence (due to neurogenic impairment of rectal sensation).

Bladder dysfunction and, in males, retrograde ejaculation and impotence are the result of autonomic neuropathy involving the genitourinary tract. As in the intestinal tract, the parasympathetic nervous system mediates the sensation of bladder fullness and contraction. The necessary involuntary relaxation of the bladder sphincters during urination is under control of the sympathetic nervous system. The initial symptom is decreased frequency of urination as the bladder becomes larger and larger before contraction occurs. This progresses to overflow incontinence associated with urgency and dribbling, incomplete emptying of the bladder, and finally, inability to void. The retained urine is a prime source for infection, which, if it travels in a retrograde fashion up the ureter, can lead to serious kidney infections.

Unfortunately impotence (erectile dysfunction) is a common problem in male diabetic patients, eventually occurring in up to 50 percent. The usual situation is a slowly progressive inability initially to maintain and eventually to achieve a satisfactory erection. This usually occurs (at least initially) in association with normal libido (sexual drive) and ejaculation. However, as satisfactory intercourse becomes more difficult, the accompaning anxiety and depression may secondarily impair libido. Other causes of impotence must be ruled out, especially a primary psychogenic cause, and importantly in the diabetic patient, vascular insufficiency. Certain antihypertensive medications may be a contributing factor, especially since hypertension will eventually occur in approximately 50 percent of people with diabetes.

Normal functioning of the parasympathetic nervous system is necessary for an erection by dilating the penile blood vessels. The sympathetic nervous system is responsible for muscle contractions resulting in ejaculation. If the internal bladder sphincter (which is innervated by the sympathetic nervous system) does not close appropriately during orgasm, the ejaculate (sperm and accompanying fluid) enters the bladder, a situation termed retrograde ejaculation. The sensory component of orgasm (as opposed to the ejaculatory aspect) is mediated by nervous pathways that are not part of the autonomic nervous system. Thus, the pleasurable sensation of orgasm remains intact. Involvement of the parasympathetic nervous system occurs more readily than impairment of the sympathetic component. Therefore, the inability to achieve a satisfactory erection to complete successfully the act of sexual intercourse is much more common than retrograde ejaculation. The latter is uncommon by itself. When it does occur, it is almost always in conjunction with erectile dysfunction.

Patients with autonomic dysfunction may also have sudomotor dysfunction (sweating disorder). Usually there are areas of anhidrosis (lack of sweating) and hyperhidrosis (excessive sweating) over the body, with the former more common in the lower extremities and the latter usually occurring over the trunk and face. The probable explanation is that a lack of perspiration over one area leads to a compensatory increase over other areas to accomplish overall heat regulation. Regrowth of damaged autonomic nerve fibers has also been suggested. Excessive sweating often occurs at mealtime, at night, or under stress. Although sudomotor dysfunction is usually not bothersome, an uncommon, but troublesome symptom is profuse facial perspiration when the patient starts to eat (gustatory sweating).

The final manifestation of autonomic dysfunction may be hypoglycemia unawareness. Hypoglycemia unawareness occurs only in type 1 diabetic patients for the following reason. The normal hormonal counterregulatory responses to hypoglycemia are a secretion of glucagon from the α cells in the pancreatic islets of Langerhans, epinephrine (adrenaline) from the adrenal medulla, cortisol from the adrenal cortex, and growth hormone from the pituitary gland. The first two are secreted rapidly and have immediate, but short-lived, effects to restore glucose levels toward normal. Not only is there an approximately 30-minute delay before the latter two are secreted, but their effects are also delayed and prolonged. As long as the glucagon response is intact, glucose concentrations will be restored. If glucagon is not secreted, epinephrine will raise glucose levels. If both of these normal responses are absent, hypoglycemic levels will be maintained (or continue to drop) since the effects of growth hormone and cortisol are too delayed to reverse the situation.

For unknown reasons, the glucagon response to hypoglycemia starts to wane shortly after the onset of type 1 (but not type 2) diabetes and is mostly gone 5 years later. Epinephrine remains as the patient's only effective counterregulatory response to combat hypoglycemia. The secretion of epinephrine also causes the adrenergic signs and symptoms (weakness, sweating, tachycardia, palpitations, hunger, tremor, nervousness, tingling of mouth and fingers) of hypoglycemia. These alert the patient to the need to treat the hypoglycemia by eating. Since epinephrine secretion by the adrenal medulla is mediated by autonomic innervations, autonomic neuropathy blunts and eventually abolishes this counterregulatory response. Not only does this leave patients without any warning of hypoglycemia so that they may eat to counteract it, but also epinephrine is not present to raise the glucose concentration. Therefore, the neuroglucopenic signs and symptoms (i.e., those due to the depressed activity of the central nervous system) often occur without warning in these patients. These include visual disturbances, bizarre behavior, mental dullness, confusion, amnesia, seizures, and coma. This is a frightening, and occasionally, life-threatening situation. Since the harder one tries to achieve near euglycemia, the more likely one is to encounter hypoglycemia, strict diabetic control (see "Treatment") should be compromised in these patients to avoid hypoglycemia unawareness.

Certain neuropathies seem to devolop rapidly. In addition to their rather acute onset, they are usually associated with pain and a self-limited course of 1 to 3 months' duration (occasionally longer) with spontaneous resolution. They may occur in patients without peripheral or autonomic neuropathy. Indeed, the most common one, a cranial nerve palsy (usually the 3rd, but sometimes the 4th, 6th, or rarely the 7th) may herald the onset of diabetes. Also classified under acute onset neuropathies are lesions of several nerves ("mononeuropathy multiplex") and focal lesions of the brachial or lumbosacral plexis ("plexopathy") or of the nerve roots ("radiculopathy"). In addition to the pain in the distribution of the affected nerve structures, motor weakness in the muscles innervated by involved nerve(s) also commonly occurs. The descriptive term *amyotrophy* is sometimes used to describe a syndrome of asymmetric pain and weakness usually involving the pelvic girdle and thigh muscles. It is usually seen in older individuals and could be the result of lesions classified as a mononeuropathy, mononeuropathy multiplex, or plexopathy. The acute onset neuropathies are likely caused by acute thrombosis or ischemia of the vessels nourishing the particular nervous system structures involved rather than by chronic hyperglycemia.

A very unusual syndrome occurring mostly in older males with relatively mild type 2 diabetes consists of anorexia, painful neuropathy, depression, and profound weight loss (neuropathic diabetic cachexia). The weight loss is so dramatic that an occult malignancy is usually suspected. Spontaneous recovery occurs gradually within 12 to 18 months.

TREATMENT

Before describing the general principles of treatment, a brief discussion of the goals and monitoring of treatment is in order. Briefly stated, the goal of therapy is to bring glucose concentrations to as near normal as possible without a serious disruption of patients' life-styles. The reason to attempt to achieve near normal blood glucose concentrations (euglycemia) is the very persuasive evidence linking strict diabetic control with beneficial effects on the diabetic complications of retinopathy, nephropathy, and neuropathy. Prospective studies, some involving thousands of patients, have demonstrated that the better the control (good, tight, or strict diabetic control are terms denoting lower glucose concentrations), the less chance there is of developing these complications. Moreover, the early changes occurring in these complications (e.g., increased widths of the capillary basement membranes, leaking of plasma from retinal vessels, microalbuminuria, painful peripheral neuropathy) are all reversible when strict diabetic control is instituted. Unfortunately, later changes (e.g., structural retinal alterations observable by the ophthalmoscope, larger amounts of albuminuria, and loss of sensation due to damaged peripheral nerves) are not reversible. This, of course, emphasizes the importance of maintaining strict diabetic control when patients are not having symptoms related to their diabetes.

Although the goal of treatment is easily stated, achieving it may not be so easy since various disruptions of patients' usual life-styles invariably occur. Near euglycemia can only be approached in insulin-requiring patients if they use home glucose monitoring at least several times a day. This is a procedure in which the patient obtains a drop of blood by pricking the finger and places it on a specially treated strip where a chemical reaction takes place which allows the glucose concentration in the blood to be measured. Armed with this information obtained in patients' daily environments, they (under the guidance of their physician) can adjust their insulin doses to try to achieve euglycemia. As they approach this goal, episodes of hypoglycemia may occur, which can be troublesome. A marked disruption of life-style occurs in obese patients, all of whom must lose weight for proper management of their diabetes. This change in their usual eating pattern is often very difficult for them. Exercise is often helpful, but altering the sedentary habits of many patients (especially obese ones) is not easily achieved.

Monitoring long-term diabetes control can be easily accomplished by measuring glycosylated (also called glucosylated or glycated) hemoglobin levels. Other tests, which are not as accurate, but which allegedly measure the same thing, are the hemoglobin A_{1C} and the hemoglobin A_1 tests. Glucose reacts with proteins throughout the body in a manner that does not depend on enzymes. The glycated product formed is simply a function of the glucose concentration and the length of time the protein had been exposed to glucose. Hemoglobin is the protein in the red blood cell that transports oxygen. The life of a normal human red blood cell is 120 days. At any given time, red cells of varying ages will be present in the circulation. Thus, the level of glycosylated hemoglobin reflects the amount of glucose to which the red cells were exposed for the previous 2 to 3 months. Other glycosylated products can also be measured, the most common of which is glycosylated serum albumin. Since the half-life of albumin is approximately 17 days, these values reflect diabetic control over the previous 2 to 4 weeks.

The treatment of diabetes mellitus involves diet,[14] exercise (especially for the obese patient), oral hypoglycemic agents,[15] and insulin.[16] Although there is some controversy concerning diets for diabetic patients, three principles have been established beyond any doubt. First, obese patients need hypocaloric diets since weight loss is their most effective treatment. Second, in patients taking insulin, carbohydrate intake needs to be reasonably consistent in regard to both the timing and amount. The absorption and effect of insulin will depend on the dose, time, and type of insulin injected. Therefore, food must be ingested at the appropriate times, not only to counteract the hypoglycemic effects of insulin during the period in which insulin is working, but also to avoid hyperglycemia before insulin becomes effective or after its effect has waned. Third, a low saturated fat intake is important. Dietary saturated fat will raise serum cholesterol levels, which are a major risk factor for macrovascular disease (Table 1-4). Since atherosclerosis is so prevalent in people with diabetes, a low fat diet is particularly important. Unresolved controversies concern the amount and type of fiber, the form of dietary carbohydrate (complex versus simple), the propensity of individual carbohydrate-containing foods to increase postprandial glucose levels (glycemic index), and a permissible amount of dietary sucrose, all of which are beyond the scope of this chapter.

Several principles concerning exercise are important. Although the psychological benefits of exercise are helpful, weight loss through exercise alone is extremely difficult. Decreased food intake must accompany it. Intense exercise (i.e., a minimum of 30 minutes at least three times a week at levels that will raise the heart rate to 70 to 85 percent of maximum [defined as 220 minus age]), is necessary to increase insulin sensitivity and improve glucose utilization. Unfortunately, this effect is lost quickly (by 1 week) after exercise is stopped. Similarly, the maximal cardiovascular benefits of exercise require this level of intense exercise.

In this country, the only oral hypoglycemic medications available at the current time are the sulfonylurea agents (Table 1-6). There are few important differences among them. The first four in Table 1-6 are termed first generation agents, while the last two, introduced into this country in 1984 after many years of use in Europe and Canada, are called second generation agents. Although the second generation agents are more potent than the first generation agents (i.e., lower doses are effective), this is clinically irrelevant since their effectiveness at maximal doses is similar to chlorpropamide and tolazamide. The primary mechanism of action of these agents is to increase insulin secretion by the pancreatic β cell, but they also improve

Table 1-6. Selected Properties of Sulfonylurea Agents

Generic Name	*Trade Name*	*Tablet Size(s) (mg)*	*Usual Daily Dose Range (mg)*	*Maximal Dose (mg)*	*Duration of Action (h)*
Tolbutamide	Orinase	250, 500	500–2,000 (divided)	3,000	6–12
Chlorpropamide	Diabinese	100, 250	100–500 (single)	750	60
Acetohexamide	Dymelor	250, 500	250–1,500 (single or divided)	1,500	12–24
Tolazamide	Tolinase	100, 250, 500	100–750 (single or divided)	1,000	12–24
Glyburide	Micronase, Diabeta	1.25, 2.5, 5.0	2.5–10 (single or divided)	20	12–24
Glipizide	Glucotrol	5.0, 10.0	5–25 (single or divided)	40	10–24

the action of the secreted insulin in the insulin-sensitive tissues (liver, muscle, and fat). Therefore, these agents are only useful in patients with type 2 diabetes and are completely ineffective in type 1 diabetes.

Since the majority (approximately 75 percent) of type 2 diabetic patients have little or no symptoms when the diagnosis is made, these patients should be treated with diet first. If diet is not effective, a small dose of a sulfonylurea agent is introduced and gradually increased every week or two until a satisfactory response is obtained or until a maximal dose is reached. Type 2 patients who have the symptoms of uncontrolled diabetes (polyuria, polydypsia, weight loss) at diagnosis are often placed on higher (even maximal doses) of a sulfonylurea agent from the outset. All patients (whether symptomatic or not) who fail to respond satisfactorily to maximal doses of sulfonylurea agents should be treated with insulin.

All type 1 diabetic patients (and, as just mentioned, those with type 2 diabetes who have failed on maximal doses of sulfonylurea agents) are treated with insulin. The most important difference among insulin's various preparations concerns their time-activity relations (i.e., onset, peak, and duration of action [Table 1-7]). They also differ in regard to their species (beef, pork, human) and purity, but these matter relatively little clinically. To gain effective insulin coverage throughout the 24-hour period, short-acting insulin is usually mixed in the same syringe with intermediate-acting, or occasionally, long-acting insulin. Few patients can be satisfactorily controlled with only one injection per day. Most require at least two, with some patients taking three or even four daily injections. In general, patients taking three or more injections of insulin per day are using regular insulin before each meal (the intermediate-acting or long-acting insulin covers the overnight period) and are able to have a more flexible life-style in regard to eating and exercise patterns.

Table 1-7. Approximate Time-Activity Relation of Various Insulins

Kind of Insulin	*Preparation*	*Onset of Action (h)*	*Maximal Action (h)*	*Total Duration of Action (h)*
Short-acting	Regular[a]	0.5–1	2–4[b]	4–6
	Semilente	1–2	3–6	8–12
Intermediate-acting	NPH[c]	3–4	10–16	20–24
	Lente	3–4	10–16	20–24
Long-acting	PZI[d]	6–8	14–20	>32
	Ultralente	6–8	14–20	>32

[a] Also called crystalline zinc insulin (CZI).
[b] In some patients, the action of regular insulin may peak later than indicated here (between 4 and 8 h) and last considerably longer.
[c] Neutral protamine Hagedorn.
[d] Protamine zinc insulin.

CONCLUSION

Diabetes is a complex syndrome with marked implications for many of those who have it. The readers of this volume will mainly be interested in the impact of diabetes and some of its complications on the foot, an often neglected part of the body. This impact on the foot can be profound, leading to major morbidity and, not infrequently, mortality. Although the remaining chapters in this volume will focus on the diabetic foot (or more accurately, the feet of patients with diabetes), this introduction should give this audience some perspective concerning the overall problems that patients with diabetes face.

REFERENCES

1. Davidson MB: Diabetic ketoacidosis and hyperosmolar nonketotic coma. p. 175. In: Diabetes Mellitus: Diagnosis and Treatment. 3rd Ed. Churchill Livingstone, New York, 1991
2. National Diabetes Data Group: Classification and diagnosis of diabetes mellitus and other categories of glucose intolerance. Diabetes 28:1039, 1979
3. Diabetes Mellitus: report of a WHO study group. WHO Tech Rep Ser 727:1, 1985
4. Eisenbarth GS: Type I diabetes mellitus: a chronic autoimmune disease. N Engl J Med 314:1360, 1986
5. Eisenbarth GS: Type I diabetes: clinical implications of autoimmunity. Hosp Pract Sept 15: 167, 1987
6. Gorsuch AN: The immunogenetics of diabetes. Diabet Med 4:510, 1987
7. Davidson MB: Review: pathogenesis of type 2 diabetes mellitus: an interpretation of current data. Am J Med Sci 292:35, 1986
8. Olefsky JM: Cellular mechanisms of insulin resistance in non-insulin-dependent (type II) diabetes. Am J Med, suppl. 5A, 85:86, 1988
9. Rotter JI, Rimoin DL: The genetics of diabetes. Hosp Pract 79, May 15, 1987
10. Klein R: Retinopathy and other ocular complications in diabetes. p. 101. In Olefsky JM, Sherwin RS, (eds): Diabetes Mellitus: Management and Complications. Churchill Livingstone, New York, 1985
11. Omachi R: The pathogenesis and prevention of diabetic nephropathy. West J Med 145:222, 1986
12. Mogensen CE, Schmitz O: The diabetic kidney: from hyperfiltration and microalbuminuria to end-stage renal failure. Med Clin North Am 72:1465, 1988
13. Greene AD, Pfeifer MA: Diabetic neuropathy. p. 223. In Olefsky JM, Sherwin RS (eds): Contemporary Issues of Endocrinology and Metabolism. Vol 1. Diabetes Mellitus. Management and Complications. Churchill Livingstone, New York, 1985
14. Davidson MB: Dietary therapy. p. 35. In: Diabetes Mellitus: Diagnosis and Treatment. 3rd Ed. Churchill Livingstone, New York, 1991
15. Davidson MB: Oral hypoglycemic sulfonylurea agents. p. 147. In: Diabetes Mellitus: Diagnosis and Treatment. 3rd Ed. Churchill Livingstone, New York, 1991
16. Davidson MB: Insulin therapy. p. 95. In: Diabetes Mellitus: Diagnosis and Treatment. 3rd Ed. Churchill Livingstone, New York, 1991
17. Eisenbarth GS: Type 1 diabetes: a chronic autoimmune disease. Triangle 23: 111, 1984
18. Klein R: Management of eye disease in the insulin-dependent diabetic patient. In MacDonald M: Managing Diabetes Mellitus in Children and Adolescents. WB Saunders, Philadelphia, 1983

2

Epidemiology and Prevention of Diabetic Foot Disease

Leonard A. Levy, D.P.M., M.P.H.

With the exception of trauma, lower extremity amputations in the United States are most frequently due to complications of diabetes mellitus. One of the ultimate goals of the physician should then be the prevention of such occurrences. While amputation is one of the most serious complications of diabetes, goals far earlier in the natural history of this disease should have high priority. Indeed the most desirable goal is to maintain the pedal extremity in a healthy state so that it is not vulnerable to the sometimes devastating complications too often seen in the diabetic.

SPECIFIC EPIDEMIOLOGY AND ECONOMIC IMPACT

It is estimated that persons with diabetes undergo over half of the approximately 125,000 lower extremity amputations in the United States annually. The risk for lower extremity amputation is fifteen times greater in those with diabetes than in other individuals. However, the National Diabetes Advisory Board of the National Institutes of Health, which reported these figures, also concluded that despite a number of patient care programs that suggest reductions in amputations would be possible with intensive prevention-oriented foot care, available preventive and therapeutic strategies are not used fully in public or private health care delivery settings.

The same board also remarks that while much improvement has been made in reducing perioperative mortality associated with lower extremity amputation, much less progress has been made in preventing amputations. Furthermore, it also indicated that the extent of the problem may be understated because of the absence of a surveillance system to monitor care practices and all hospital discharge data. With a goal set by the advisory board to reduce the incidence of lower extremity amputation in persons with diabetes 30 percent by the year 1995 and by 40 percent by the year 2000, in effect a major challenge has been extended to practitioners concerned with the care of the diabetic foot.[1]

The National Diabetes Data Group points out that arteriosclerosis obliterans (ASO) affecting the feet and legs is present in 8 percent of adult diabetic patients at diagnosis and in 45 percent after 20 years. The incidence of ASO in diabetic men and women is four to seven times greater than their nondiabetic counterparts. In addition, about 15 percent of diabetic patients have experienced ulcers of the feet or ankles. The incidence of gangrene is 4.5 cases per 1,000 diabetic patients per year, and survival of diabetic patients with gangrene is only about 45 percent of expected. Diabetic patients account for 40 to 45 percent of all nontraumatic amputations. This amounts to about 60 per 10,000 diabetics annually. Survival for 3 years after an amputation is only about 50 percent of expected.[2]

Data from the 1974 National Health Interview Survey indicated that while 6.6 percent of the general population over age 65 saw a podiatrist, 11.4 percent of those in the same age category who were diabetics visited a podiatric physician.[3]

While there are few data on the costs of specific complications of diabetes, in 1980 the number of lower extremity amputations was estimated at 40,381. There was an average length of stay of approximately 30.5 days or about 1.2 million days in hospital for these procedures. At an average cost of $245 per day in 1983, the total hospitalization cost for lower extremity amputation was about $302 million excluding rehabilitation, premature mortality, or disability costs.[2]

THE NATURAL HISTORY OF DISEASE AND DIABETES

The natural history of any disease is the total course of that condition (Fig. 2-1). It begins when the individual is well and in equilibrium with the environment and disease-producing agents. As long as this equilibrium is maintained, no disease occurs. We refer to this as the period of prepathogenesis. If this equilibrium is disturbed in favor of the agent, the disease process begins, and the patient is said to be in the period of pathogenesis. The early phase of the period of pathogenesis may have no discernible signs and symptoms even when the most sophisticated examinations are employed. Therefore, at that time it is beyond anyone's capability to diagnose clinically. The goal of the health provider ought then to be to promote health and prevent any disease process. Should this not be successful, then the second goal should be to apply measures as early as possible during the period of pathogenesis to arrest further development of the disease.

In most patients and most diseases prevention or early detection is possible. Obviously there still are certain diseases in which our level of knowledge is not yet sophisticated enough to arrest the natural history from running its full course. Some patients may not present to a health care provider until late in the natural history of a disease. In other situations patients may fail to follow prescribed preventive or therapeutic measures and become victims of the late manifestations of a disease and many of its complications. Finally, health care providers too often fail to give appropriate emphasis to prevention or treatment of the earlier, often minor problems associated with a disease so that the serious complications of such conditions are more likely to occur.

In order to place health promotion and disease prevention regarding the foot of the diabetic patient in appropriate perspective it is important to outline the natural history of the complications that may occur in the lower extremity. The concept of thinking of a single cause of a disease or disorder often clouds the approach of clinicians with their patients. For example, too often, as soon as a specific agent is identified, such as a particular bacterium found in an infected ulcer, antibiotic therapy is introduced with too little emphasis on other factors contributing to the cause of the condition. Failure of the ulcer to heal is often blamed on the ineffectiveness of the antibiotic. Additional causes of the problem lie in the environment, habits, customs, vascular and neurologic status, inherent constitution, and nutrition of those affected. Clinicians should, therefore, consider the causes of all diseases and disorders as being multifactoral including agent, host, and environmental factors.[4]

In the patient with diabetes mellitus, foot problems that can occur provide examples of the phenomenon of multifactoral causation. Being able to identify and understand the agent, host, and environmental factors leading to these conditions improves our ability to appreciate the pathogenesis of such problems as well as increases our capability of determining and employing the most effective methods of intervention. Ideally these interventions should occur as early as possible in the natural history of the various foot problems that may affect diabetic patients. It is hoped that they should take place before a foot problem is present while the diabetic patient's feet are considered to be normal. The objective of the physician and the person with diabetes at that point in time should be the maintenance of healthy feet. Such an objective is not specific to any foot disorder but is entirely health oriented. It is a classic example of primary prevention

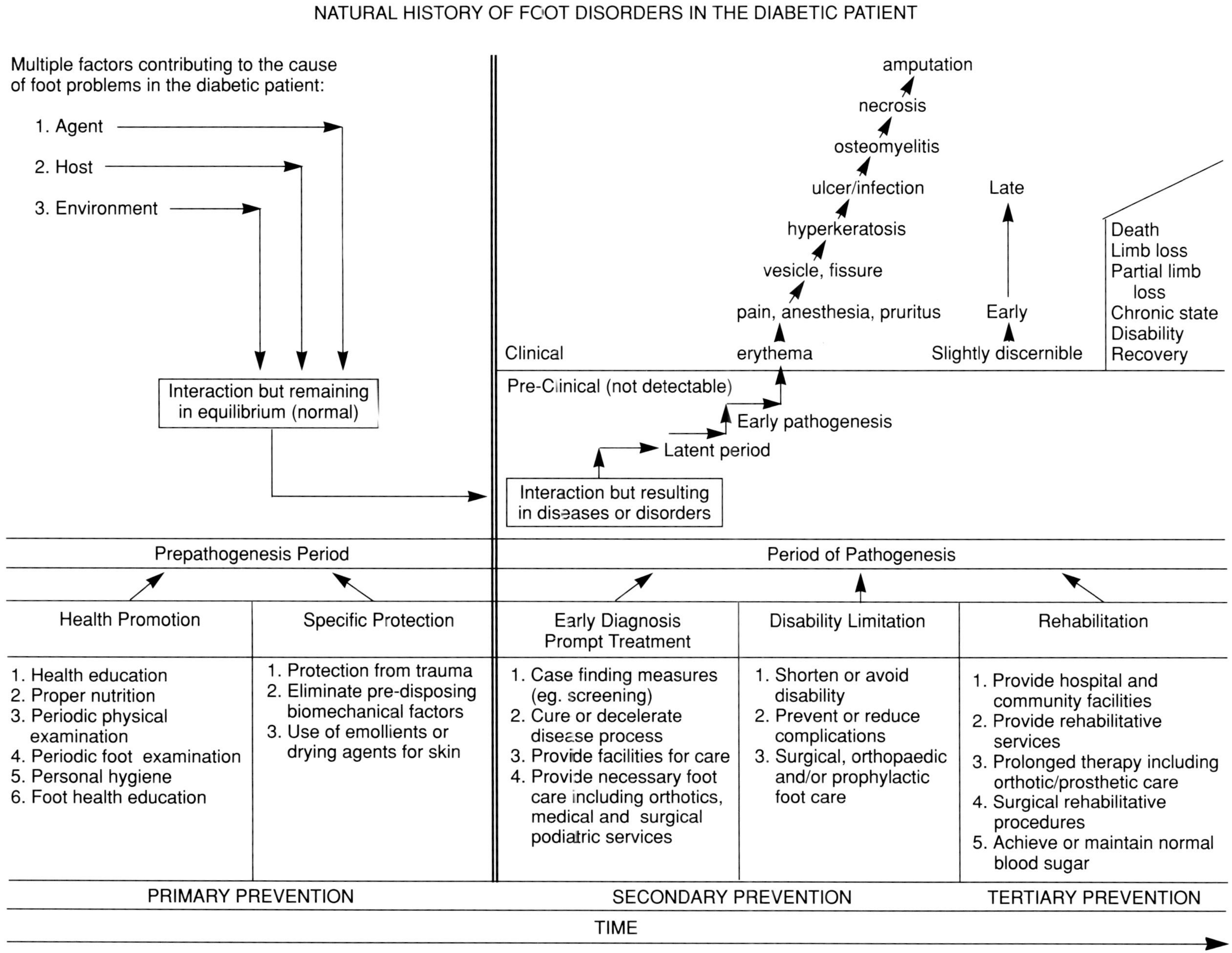

Fig. 2-1. Natural history of foot disorders in the diabetic patient.

and includes such activities as those outlined below.

Podiatric Primary Prevention in Diabetes

1. Health education
   A. General health education
   B. Education about diabetes and its complications
   C. Foot health education
2. Proper nutrition for general health and diabetic control
3. Periodic physical examination (as provided by family practice physician, internist, pediatrician)
4. Periodic foot examination (as provided by podiatric physician)
5. Protection from trauma at home and the workplace
6. Attention to personal hygiene
7. Elimination of biomechanical factors that may predispose to foot disorders

Primary prevention, however, while the ideal goal to which clinicians should strive, is only one aspect of prevention in the diabetic patient with regard to foot health. In the event that a diabetic patient does develop a podiatric medical problem because of such factors as patient neglect or recalcitrance, previously undiagnosed diabetes, inability to control blood glucose levels, vascular disease, neuropathy, systemic infection or trauma, the goal of the health care provider should then be early diagnosis and prompt treatment as well as disability limitations. This is referred to as secondary prevention, which can be outlined in the following manner.

Podiatric Secondary Prevention In Diabetes

1. Case-finding measures—individual and mass (e.g., foot examination of groups of known diabetic patients, foot examinations of groups of elderly persons who are known to be diabetic and those not yet identified as being diabetic.
2. Cure or prevention of disease process; palliative or nonsurgical measures; surgical measures.
3. Prevention or reduction of extent of complications.
4. Shortening or avoidance of disability.
5. Providing of facilities and personnel for care.

In addition to primary and secondary prevention there is still another level of intervention referred to as tertiary prevention. Tertiary prevention takes place further along the natural history of a disease process. This usually is after significant anatomic and physiologic changes have occurred. In the diabetic patient it could be after an amputation of all or part of an extremity. The goal of tertiary prevention here would be to prevent complete disability by providing programs for patients to make maximum use of their remaining capacities and to prevent further destruction or amputations if possible. Examples of activities that can be included under the designation of tertiary pevention include the following.

Podiatric Tertiary Prevention In Diabetes

1. Hospital and community facilities with podiatric medical, general medical, and rehabilitative services providing patient education and training for maximum use of remaining capacities.
2. Prolonged therapy and periodic evaluation on a regular basis to prevent additional tissue damage and/or further amputation, and/or further disability
   A. Orthotic and/or prosthetic devices
   B. Surgical rehabilitative procedures
3. General and/or speciality medical care to achieve or maintain as normal blood sugar levels as possible

For factors associated with the natural history of foot disorders in the diabetic patient, see Table 2-1.

Table 2-1. Multiple Factors Associated with the Natural History of Foot Disorders in the Diabetic Patient

Host Factors
- Age, sex, ethnicity
- Occupation
- Deformities
  - Congenital
    - Varus or valgus deformities—digital, forefoot, tarsal
    - Shape and length of toes/metatarsals
    - Overlapping digits
  - Acquired
    - Arthritides—rheumatoid, osteoarthritis, gout, other
    - Exostosis
    - Hallux valgus
    - Hammer toes or mallet toes, other digital deformities
- Circulatory abnormalities—occlusive, vasospastic, microangiopathy, vasculitis
- Neuropathy
- Post cerebrovascular accident
- Muscular imbalances
- Hereditary conditions
- Obesity
- Mental and psychological state
- Personal habits and customs—hygiene, attitudes toward health, alcohol abuse, smoking
- Dermatologic conditions
  - Hyperhidrosis or anhidrosis
  - Eczematoid disorders
  - Predisposition for or presence of tineal disease
  - Nail disorders—incurvated, hypertrophic, onychomycotic, psoriatic, post-traumatic, etc.
  - Other skin conditions
- Coexisting, apparently non-diabetic-related disease—blood disorders, infections, neuropsychiatric problems, neoplasms, etc.

Agent Factors
- Loose- or tight-fitting shoes and inappropriate shoe design—pointed shoes
- Improperly fitting hose
- Shoe or sock dyes or other chemicals—glues, detergents
- Soaps, perfumes
- Primary irritants—chemicals in workplace or at home
- Sun—sunburn
- Foreign bodies
- Topical medications—salicyclic acid plasters and solutions
- Factitial—knives or other instruments for self-treatment, use of hot-water bottle and other heating devices, scratching due to intense pruritus

Environmental Factors
- Socioeconomic
  - Customs—shoe styles
  - Low income—cost of health care, cost of food, costs of shoes, socks
  - Availability of podiatric and other health facilities
  - Level of education
  - Nutritional habits
  - Awareness of importance of foot care and other health services
  - Type of occupation
  - Recreational activities
- Cultural barriers
- Physical
  - Climate and seasons—extremes in temperature and humidity
  - Floor covering
  - Type of terrain
- Diagnostic and treatment facility adequacy

FOCUS OF HEALTH EDUCATION

By identifying and understanding the implications of the numerous agent, host, and environmental factors that can potentially affect the natural history of foot problems in the diabetic, clinicians are in the position to be able to interrupt that process or slow it down considerably. By using this multifactorial approach, the possibility of helping the diabetic patient avoid many foot problems is often very great. Most frequently the interventions available to the physician and patient are remarkably simple and inexpensive. Perhaps because of that very fact the patient often feels that these activities are not useful, which is reinforced by the doctor failing to emphasize their importance. For example, asymptomatic maceration or fissuring due to tinea or hyperhidrosis found between one or two toes is often overlooked by the patient and regrettably even the podiatric physician. Other examples include minimal irritations or blisters from a poorly fitting shoe, stepping on a small foreign body, and other seemingly trivial injuries. While this may not be of any major significance in most people, in the diabetic, particularly when there is some peripheral vascular embarrassment, these minor insults to the integrity of the skin become portals of entry for disease-producing agents leading to serious infection. Such a scenario emphasizes the importance of preventing the seemingly minor defects in the skin of the foot and the need to identify and seriously treat such conditions before they contribute to the natural history of a disease process that can lead to amputations and even death.

Much of these efforts can be employed by patients themselves, provided they are educated about the importance of foot health care. If the physician fails to give major emphasis to this phase of patient management, a message of unimportance is transmitted to the patient and the likelihood of the diabetic patient failing to put a high priority on preventive foot care is great. This educational process should not consist of simply passing out colorful brochures about diabetic foot care, although that certainly is potentially helpful and should be encouraged. In addition to printed material, additional reinforcement should be provided by the physician and other members of the staff who see the patient in the clinical environment. This could be a major duty of a properly trained office assistant. In a busy practice patients could be given a separate appointment to visit with the assistant for this purpose alone. For the purpose of health education, a single encounter with a patient should not be considered adequate. Follow-up activities might include mailings about the importance of preventive foot care in the diabetic patient, and occasional discussions by the podiatrist, physician, nurse, or assistant that emphasize this aspect of foot health.

The efforts of the individual practitioner in diabetic foot health education can be greatly assisted if communitywide programs also are instituted. Public education campaigns from private and public groups such as the national and local chapters of the American Diabetes Association, American Podiatric Medical Association, U.S. Public Health Service, local health departments, nursing organizations, and other groups can add credibility and reinforcement to diabetic foot health education. To the highest degree possible, health care providers who see diabetic patients and their respective professional organizations should become involved with these various groups or communicate with them to increase the priority of foot health education and the likelihood of campaigns that emphasize or include diabetic foot health. Such activities should be supplemented by articles in frequently read magazines and with radio and television public service announcements. Such a multipronged organized effort has a greater likelihood of succeeding than an isolated, infrequent focus on this problem. Figure 2-2 diagrams the delivery of foot care information to the diabetic patient.

EFFORTS TO CHANGE BEHAVIOR

While the control of blood sugar levels with diet, oral medications, and insulin are vital factors in delaying some of the complications due to disorders of the vessels and nerves in the foot, many so-called controlled diabetic patients still are plagued with these serious difficulties. It is axiomatic, then, that all diabetic patients, no matter what the level of their blood sugar, require that attention be given to their foot health. Fortunuately, there is much that can be done to prevent most of the sequellae of the pathologic changes occurring in or affecting the

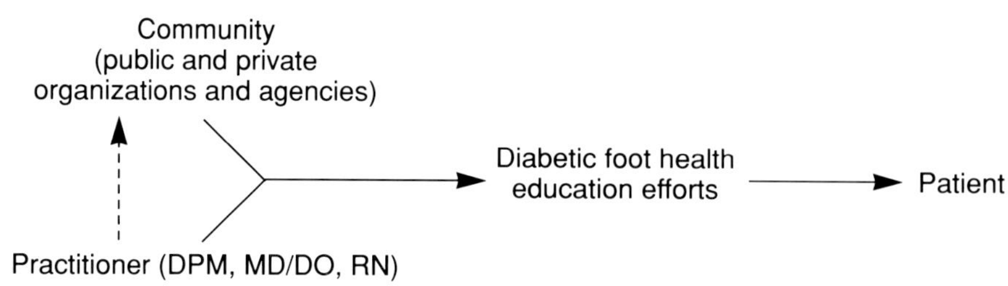

Fig. 2-2. The role of communitywide programs in diabetic foot health education.

foot. Furthermore, most of these efforts require very little time and are often at minimal or no expense. The key is to transmit to the patient an awareness of the importance of such attention. However, no single mention about the importance of foot health care to the diabetic patient, even if accompanied with several pieces of advice about how to prevent foot problems, will guarantee that a communication will be successful and that the patient's behavior will change. Like most other efforts to change human behavior, a sustained effort and carefully planned program are necessary. To assume that a single patient encounter is all that is necessary is unreasonable and inappropriate; single encounters will have little effect on reducing potentially serious foot complications.

The value of screening foot examinations on an annual basis can pay high yields in an adult diabetic population, even among those who are asymptomatic. Not only does this provide a means to identify foot problems early in the patients natural history, but it also brings more attention to the importance of the feet to the patients and their families. Because diabetic patients not infrequently also have problems with their eyes, they may have difficulty reading labels on over-the-counter foot remedies. This may be dangerous for them and make regular foot inspections difficult. A family member or close friend who is well informed can in such instances be most helpful in preventing serious foot complications in the diabetic patient. In any event, relatively simple preventive measures can be extremely important for the growing population of diabetic persons who are vulnerable to foot problems.

A listing of objectives of a diabetic foot health education program that can be used as guide for diabetic patients, perhaps in a simple brochure, is provided below. However, it should be re-emphasized that this is only an adjunct to the education of patients and should be supplemented by additional activities such as individual and/or group conferences, demonstrations, films, or other instructional methods.

In developing a program in foot health designed for the individual diabetic patient or for groups, it would be helpful to establish its expectations to the greatest degree of specificity possible. This can be done by stating in behavioral terms the objectives of such activities. It is also a useful technique in evaluating the success of the program.

Objectives of a Diabetic Foot Health Education Program

The diabetic patient, after a properly planned health education program, should be able to do the following:

1. Describe the role of blood circulation problems as it relates to the feet
2. Describe the role of nerve problems (neuropathy) as it relates to foot complications
3. Describe the types of the problems that may be seen in the feet such as
   A. Infection
   B. Numbness
   C. Nail problems
   D. Skin ulcers
   E. Gangrene
4. Describe what can be done to prevent foot problems such as
   A. Avoid extreme cold or heat
   B. Avoid smoking
   C. Avoid pressure on blood vessels (e.g., garters, leg-crossing)
   D. Avoid breaks in skin
   E. Avoid corn plasters or medications
   F. Avoid "bathroom surgery" (i.e., self-cutting of corns or calluses)
   G. Avoid cutting nails too short or digging into corners
   H. Avoid tight or loose shoes
   I. Wash feet daily with mild soap and dry between toes with cotton
   J. Inspect feet daily (i.e., self inspection or inspection by family member or friend)
   K. Follow advice of general physicians regarding diabetic control and control of other health problems
   L. Follow advice of podiatric physician
   M. Have periodic foot examinations (frequency to be determined by podiatric physician)
   N. Contact podiatric physician in the event of any change in feeling or appearance of feet

THE YOUNG DIABETIC PATIENT AND FOOT HEALTH

While serious vascular disease of the lower extremities is not typically seen in the diabetic child, foot health education efforts should begin early in this group of patients. Establishing good habits *before* bad ones are adopted will help to avoid many of the complications seen during the adult years. Smoking is an excellent example of a habit that may be prevented through comprehensive long-term educational campaigns. The diabetic person who is more vulnerable to peripheral occlusive vascular disease but who is a nonsmoker is far less likely to be the victim of an amputation. If educational efforts are focused on young people, including those who are diabetic, the potential for reducing the incidence of lower extremity amputations can be considerable. Diabetic foot health education should not be considered within the exclusive domain of adults, but an activity that should encompass all age groups. While it may be more difficult to convince children and younger diabetic patients about the importance of foot health care because of their perceived invulnerability, even a small percentage of success can be rewarding. If diabetic patients can be educated prior to the ages when they may be at higher risk for the development of foot complications and prior to the time that they develop poor habits, many lower extremity amputations would be prevented. Indeed, developing sound general health and foot health habits among young nondiabetic individuals who in later years may develop diabetes mellitus also could result in reducing the frequency of complications of this disease including those affecting the foot.

TEACHING AND LEARNING RESOURCES

In developing comprehensive foot health education programs for individual diabetic patients or groups, a number of resources are available. I have identified some of which represent the broad area of diabetes education rather than that focused on foot health. This is to underline the fact that diabetes mellitus is a disease requiring the involvement of many different health professionals. Failure to be sensitive to this would result in a less than effective foot health education program. Because of the often long-term relationship that the podiatrist and physician develop with patients, they are in the position to reinforce with the diabetic individual not only the importance of good foot health but also health promotion and disease prevention in general. Indeed, this should be among the obligations of the foot health practitioner since individuals who neglect their health in general are more likely to adversely affect their diabetic state, thus becoming at higher risk for developing complications, including those affecting the foot.

Some of the various resources available to physicians and other professionals interested in the foot health of the diabetic is provided in the appendix.

REFERENCES

1. National Diabetes Advisory Board: The National Long-Range Plan to Combat Diabetes. p. 24. U.S. Department of Health and Human Services, Public Health Services, National Institutes of Health, NIH Publication No. 88-1587, September 1987
2. National Diabetes Data Group: Diabetes in America, Diabetes Data Compiled 1984. pp. 1–3, xxx11–11. U.S. Department of Health and Human Services, Public Health Service, National Institutes of Health, National Institute of Arthritis, Diabetes, and Digestive and Kidney Diseases, NIH Publication No. 80-1468, 1984
3. Drury TF: National Health Interview Survey. National Center for Health Statistics, 1974
4. Levy, LA: Epidemiology of Podiatric Medical Diseases and Disorders. p. 91. In Helfand A.E. (ed): Public Health and Podiatric Medicine. Williams & Wilkins, Baltimore, 1987

APPENDIX

Resources for Diabetes Education

ORGANIZATIONS

American Diabetes Association
1660 Duke Street
P.O. Box 25757
Alexandria, VA 22313

Juvenile Diabetes Foundation
23 East 26th Street
New York, NY 10010

American Association of Diabetes Educators
North Woobury Road, Box 56
Pitman, NJ 08071

American Podiatric Medical Association
9312 Old Georgetown Road
Bethesda, MD 20814-1621

U.S. Department of Health and Human Services
Public Health Service
National Institutes of Arthritis, Diabetes, and Digestive Diseases
Bethesda, MD 20892

National Diabetes Information Clearing House
Box ND1C
Bethesda, MD 20892

International Diabetes Center
5000 West 39th Street
Minneapolis, MN 55416

U.S. Department of Health and Human Services
Public Health Service
National Institutes of Health
National Institute on Aging—Information Office, Bldg. 31
Bethesda, MD 20205

SPECIFIC INFORMATION AND MATERIALS

Foot Care and Diabetes: Selected Annotations
This publication, prepared by the National Diabetes Clearinghouse, provides the sources of numerous materials suitable for patients as well as providers interested in educating patients about diabetic foot care. It is one of the most comprehensive bibliographies, and most items listed were produced since 1983. It includes journal articles, audiovisual materials, pamphlets, and brochures, many of which are either free or at low cost. This publication is obtainable from

National Institute of Diabetes and Digestive and Kidney Disease
National Institues of Health
Bethesda, MD 20892
Re: NIH Publication No. 89-1870, May 1989

Audiovisual Resources for Diabetes Education, 7th Ed.
This is a guide for nonprinted materials for patients and health professionals. It includes descriptions of materials from commercial and nonprofit sources as well as how they may be obtained and is available from

Learning Resource Center
University of Michigan Diabetes Research and Training Center
1135 East Catherine Street
Ann Arbor, MI 48109

3

Diabetic Vascular Disease

David R. Campbell, M.D.

Diabetic vascular disease is the major cause of morbidity and mortality in the diabetic patient. It is responsible for the increased incidence of death from myocardial infarction and stroke disease as well as the major cause of limb loss in the diabetic patient.

For many diabetic patients, the greatest fear is losing their legs. Many have known relatives with diabetes who develop gangrene of their toes and underwent progressive amputations of their extremity until after an above knee amputation they finally died of a myocardial infarction. In the last decade there has been an improvement in understanding and treating the infectious and neuropathic complications of diabetes, and consequently more of the major limb loss is now secondary to peripheral vascular disease. In 1963 Hoar and Torres reported that 90 percent of consecutive below knee amputations had significant peripheral vascular disease.[1] In 1984 Fearon et al. reported a further series of consecutive below knee amputations, and at this time 90 percent of the patients had significant peripheral vascular disease.[2] Both of these reports were from the New England Deaconess Hospital and Joslin Clinic. Since then management of the diabetic foot has improved significantly at the community level, and even fewer patients now lose their legs because of infection and neuropathy alone.

The magnitude of the problem is well demonstrated by a report from the National Diabetes Advisory Board, in which diabetic vascular disease was noted to account for 17,000 to 20,000 amputations of the lower extremity per year in the United States, representing 50 to 70 percent of all nontraumatic amputations. It is estimated that peripheral vascular disease is 20 times more common in the diabetic patient.[3]

Diabetic vascular disease is also the major cause of death in the diabetic patient. Data from the Joslin Clinic[4] reveal that diabetic vascular disease is responsible for 70 percent of the deaths in non-insulin-dependent diabetes mellitus (NIDDM) and a smaller but rising proportion in insulin-dependent diabetes mellitus (IDDM). For men there was no increase in mortality until after age 50, but for women there was a noticeable increase in mortality before age 45 that was unrelated to childbirth or pregnancy. After age 50, survival for both sexes declined rapidly so that the median survival was reached at age 65 for women and 66 for men. This is 12 years earlier than in the general population for women and 5 years earlier for men. Thus, while survival for both sexes is similar, these statistics represent a greater impact of diabetes on women than men. Figure 3-1 demonstrates the survival of diabetic patients in the Joslin study diagnosed before the age of 30. While few deaths occurred by age 25, survival among diabetic patients was already appreciably below that of the general population by age 30 and then went on to decrease rapidly after age 35 so that survival at age 50 was only 52 percent for women and 46 percent for men. The major causes of death were coronary artery disease and renal failure.

The Whitehall study in England showed 3.9 deaths from coronary artery disease per 100 men per 100 years compared to 6.1 deaths for insulin-dependent diabetic patients and 8.3 deaths for non-insulin-dependent diabetic patients.[5] A Ruma-

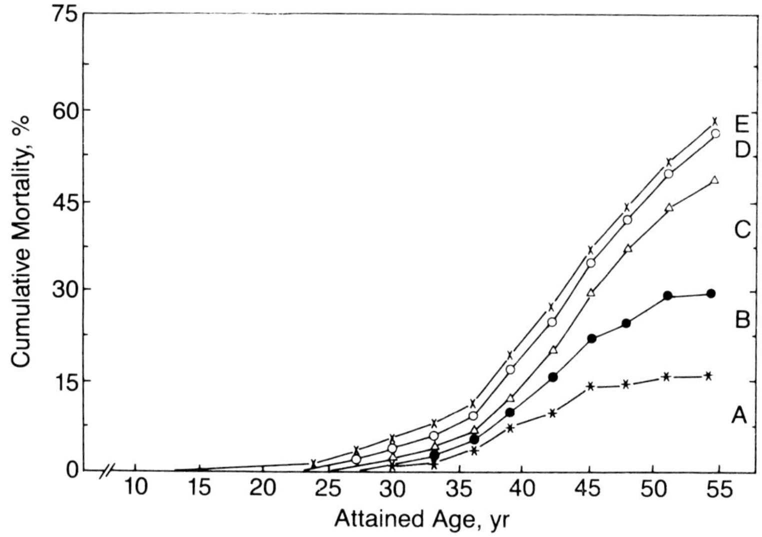

Fig. 3-1. Mortality of diabetic patients with juvenile-onset diabetes. A, renal failure; B, coronary heart disease preceded by nephropathy; C, coronary heart disease; D, other causes; E, diabetic ketoacidosis. (From Campbell et al.,[9] with permission.)

nian study has shown that by 10 years of duration half of all diabetic patients have evidence of diabetic vascular disease and that this has risen to 100 percent by 26 years.[6]

The most widely quoted study in the United States is the Framingham study, in which an entire population has been followed for 30 years.[7] This study confirms the increased cardiovascular risk for diabetic patients. It shows that the protective effect of female gender in developing cardiovascular disease is lost in the diabetic patient so that diabetic men and women have an equal risk. The study also shows that besides having a higher incidence of cardiovascular disease, diabetic patients tend to survive less well with a 40 percent mortality from congestive cardiac failure compared with 25 percent among nondiabetic patients. A number of reported patient series following peripheral vascular surgery and carotid artery surgery have shown that at the 5-year follow-up, 50 percent of the diabetic patients have died compared to 25 percent of the nondiabetic patients.[8,9]

PERIPHERAL VASCULAR DISEASE

The high incidence of gangrene and recurrent foot ulceration in the diabetic patient was noted soon after the introduction of insulin in the 1920s. When Dr. Elliot Joslin set up his clinic for diabetic patients at the New England Deaconess Hospital, he asked a prominent surgeon, Dr. Leland McKittrick, to help with the management of diabetic foot problems. Dr. McKittrick set up the "foot room" with its own nursing team, and initially they were concerned with basic foot care and patient education. Since then the team has expanded to include vascular surgeons, podiatric and orthopaedic surgeons, and plastic surgeons as well as the diabetologist. It should be kept in mind that the diabetic foot lesion is usually a multifactorial lesion, and throughout this discussion of diabetic vascular disease the impact of neuropathy and infection has to be considered.

SMALL VESSEL DISEASE

Because of some misleading work published in the late 1950s, there has been much confusion about the nature of diabetic vascular disease. A study involving pathologic examination of amputated limbs was published by Goldenberg et al. in 1959.[10] This appeared to show an increase in occlusive disease in the small vessels of the diabetic patient. This finding was well received as it appeared to explain the observed fact of gangrene in the presence of good distal pulses. Two subsequent prospective studies reported by Strandness et al. in 1964[11] and Conrad in 1967[12] failed to demonstrate any increase in arteriolar occlusive disease in the diabetic patient. It was also noted that there was no endothelial proliferation at the capillary level. The only change that has been well documented is the basement membrane thickening associated with diabetic microangiopathy. The degree of basement membrane thickening varies considerably. In one study in which needle biopsies of the quadriceps muscle were studied by electron microscopy, the average thickness of nondiabetic basement membranes was 1,080 Å compared to 1,373 Å for prediabetic and 2,403 Å for diabetic patients.[13] There is also evidence to suggest that there may be functional abnormalities of these capillaries. The loss of albumin to the extracellular fluid appears to be increased, and other abnormalities have been reported, although the significance is not clear.[14] The argument against the existence of small vessel disease has been recently reviewed by LoGerfo and Coffman and is now gaining universal acceptance.[15]

How then does one explain the existence of gangrene in the presence of good distal pulses? It should be remembered that gangrene is the final event in a number of disease processes. Thus, infection may lead to thrombosis of the digital vessels and consequently to gangrene. This is particularly likely to happen in a closed-space infection. Another common cause of gangrene in the presence of good circulation is pressure necrosis. Severely neuropathic patients may wear a shoe that is too small or leave a sock in the toe of the shoe, and because they have no feeling, the first indication of a problem may be gangrene of the toes. Diabetic vascular disease is therefore not thought to involve small vessel disease but may be considered under the categories of microangiopathy and macroangiopathy.

MICROANGIOPATHY

All of the recent studies of the pathogenesis of diabetic vascular disease have demonstrated the presence of basement membrane thickening in diabetic patients. The degree of thickening is variable but is most prominent in type 1 or insulin-dependent diabetic patients and is associated with the major microangiopathic complications of diabetes, namely retinopathy, nephropathy, and neuropathy. The changes resulting in basement membrane thickening are felt to be directly related to hyperglycemia rather than to a separate metabolic abnormality.[16] Such thickened basement membranes have been shown to leak albumin[14] and are thought possibly to interfere with the transfer of nutrients and the migration of leukocytes and thus to impair wound healing. Although the focus of this chapter is on the consequences of macrovascular disease, it must be remembered that all diabetic patients have some degree of microangiopathy, and this may severely affect the presentation and clinical effects of macrovascular disease. For this reason it is relevant to consider some of the microangiopathic complications in more detail.

Retinopathy

Retinopathy is the most common microangiopathic complication of diabetes, being found in 100 percent of type 1 and 65 percent of type 2 diabetic patients after they have had diabetes for over 15 years. Proliferative retinopathy leading to blindness is found in 5 percent of type 1 and only rarely in type 2 diabetic patients.[4] For those patients with a history of retinal bleeds, long-term anticoagulation therapy for peripheral vascular problems is generally contraindicated, although most ophthalmologists will permit aspirin therapy.

Nephropathy

Nephropathy is the most feared complication of diabetes, as it carries a poor prognosis. Again, its prevalence is related to the duration of the diabetes, and it is much more common in type 1 diabetic patients. About 25 percent of type 1 diabetic patients will go on to develop a proliferative nephropathy resulting in azotemia with the prevalence slowly increasing with the duration of the diabetes. Of interest is that while the incidence of nephropathy increases with the duration of the diabetes, the rapid acceleration of macrovascular disease associated with it does not start until the patient has reached about 30 years of age. Insulin-dependent diabetic patients without nephropathy have a 4-fold risk of developing macrovascular disease, whereas those with nephropathy have a 12-fold risk. The reason for this increased risk is not clear. Presumably diabetic nephropathy accelerates a naturally occurring process rather than initiating it.[4] Nephropathy is much less common in type 2 patients but still occurs in 8 percent of patients with long-standing diabetes. Milder degrees of renal impairment are, however, quite common and need to be carefully considered when giving a dye load as in angiography.

Neuropathy

Neuropathy is the microangiopathic complication that most impacts on the diagnosis and management of macrovascular disease in the diabetic patient. In its most common form it is a distal symmetric polyneuropathy affecting the extremities. This neuropathy is felt to be due to a metabolic abnormality resulting in segmental demyelination and axon loss.[16] As with other microangiopathic complications, its severity tends to be related to the duration of the diabetes, and it is therefore much more prevalent in type 1 diabetic patients. It affects macrovascular disease in a number of ways. First, loss of sensation and the normal flare response results in increased trauma and may mask the symptoms of claudication and ischemic rest pain. Parkhouse and LeQuesne drew attention to the importance of the absence of the Lewis flare in the development of neuropathic foot lesions. This is an axon reflex dependent on the integrity of nociceptive C fibers, which secrete vasodilator peptides such as substance P to initiate neurogenic inflammation. The absence of this reflex was more common in diabetic patients with foot lesions than in diabetic patients with neuropathy but with no foot lesions.[17]

The motor neuropathy causes intrinsic muscle wasting, which results in clawing of the foot, further predisposing the foot to trauma. Thirty percent of patients with neuropathy have an autonomic neuropathy as well. This causes shunting of blood to the skin away from the nutrient vessels due to an abnormally high degree of arteriovenous shunting within the foot. Studies confirm the consequent increase in venous oxygen in these patients and distended veins on the dorsum of the foot when recumbent.[18] Recent studies suggest that these changes in blood flow, which mimic a surgical sympathectomy, may not actually be related to the degree of autonomic nerve dysfunction in the diabetic patient.[19] Paralysis of the sudomotor system results in a dry foot, and this may further predispose to trauma.

Medial Calcific Sclerosis

One of the prominent features of the arteries in the diabetic patient is the presence of medial arterial calcification. This was originally felt to be part of the picture of atherosclerosis in the diabetic patient, but it is becoming increasingly clear that it is a microangiopathic complication most closely associated with neuropathy.[20] A study by Edmonds et al. suggests that denervation of the smooth muscle of the tunica media may be important in the etiology. As the name implies, calcification occurs in and around the smooth muscle cells of the media. Initially, calcium is deposited in fine granules, which eventually fuse to form a large, homogeneous, structureless, basophilic mass.[21] These deposits tend to form incomplete rings around the vessel, resulting in the characteristic "goose trachea" nodularity on palpation. As this progresses, the artery may become one long, rigid tube of calcium giving the classic "pipestem" appearance on radiograph (Fig. 3-2).

Uncomplicated medial calcification does not compromise the lumen of the artery, and there is no significant intimal injury. The calcification is continuous and irregular, whereas in atherosclerosis it is regular and discontinuous. In older patients there is often superimposed atherosclerosis, and the presence of medial calcification may make the noninvasive diagnosis of ischemia more difficult. The rigid vessels also pose a problem for the vascular surgeon trying to occlude the vessels, as regular clamps are either ineffective or crush the vessel.

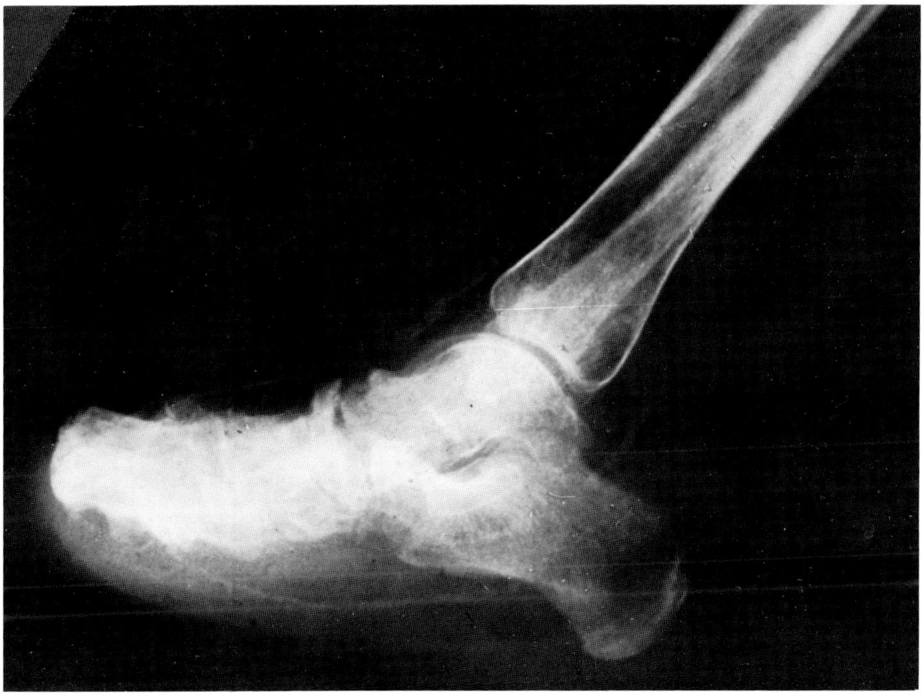

Fig. 3-2. Progression of calcium deposits along the artery giving the classic "pipestem" appearance on radiograph.

MACROANGIOPATHY

The macroangiopathy of diabetic patients is no different from the atherosclerotic process seen in nondiabetic patients. It differs only in the location of the lesions and the frequency with which it occurs. As noted in type 1 diabetic patients, neuropathic and metabolic complications are much more prominent initially and are then followed by rapid acceleration of the atherosclerotic process, resulting in gangrene, stroke, and death from myocardial infarction. In type 2 diabetic patients, microangiopathic and metabolic complications are much less frequent, but macroangiopathic complications are correspondingly more frequent and appear to be unrelated to the duration of the diabetes or how well the blood sugar is controlled. The protective effect of female gender is lost, and in peripheral vascular disease, coronary artery disease, and stroke disease, diabetic patients seem to fare poorly compared to nondiabetic patients.

ROLE OF RISK FACTORS IN THE DIABETIC PATIENT

The usual risk factors for macrovascular disease include hypertension, lipid abnormalities, and smoking. In diabetes other factors may also be involved, including obesity, impaired glucose tolerance, hyperglycemia, hyperinsulinemia, microalbuminuria, elevated fibrinogen levels, and altered platelet function. There is a mass of research data on these factors, and a nice summary is contained in the consensus statement from the American Diabetes Association conference on the role of cardiovascular risk factors in the prevention and treatment of macrovascular disease in diabetes held in May 1989.[22] The presence of diabetes without other major risk factors results in a substantially increased risk of developing macrovascular disease in both males and females (Fig. 3-3). In most epidemiologic studies the prevalence of hypertension, lipid abnormalities, and cigarette smoking is the

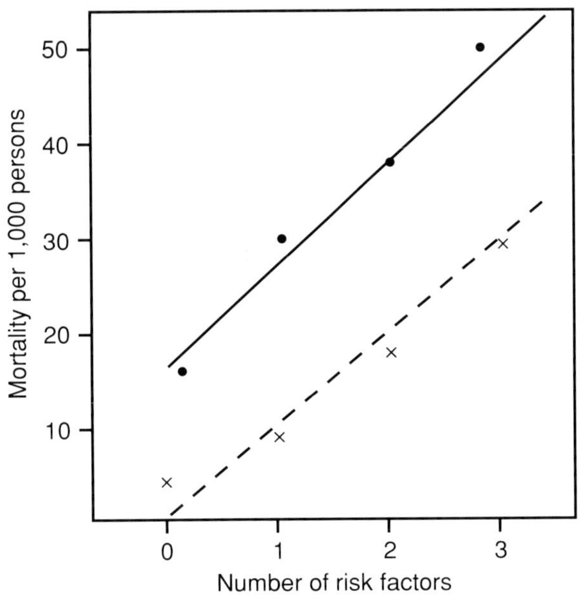

Fig. 3-3. Effects of three major risk factors (hypercholesterolemia, smoking, and diabetic hypertension) on age-standardized cardiovascular mortality in 5,245 diabetic subjects (solid line) and 350,977 nondiabetic subjects. (From Consensus Statement,[22] with permission.)

same in diabetic as in nondiabetic patients. The Framingham study[23] and Multiple Risk Factor Intervention Trial[24] suggest that in non-insulin-dependent diabetic patients, at least, these factors have the same adverse impact on the development of macrovascular disease as they do in the nondiabetic patient. Cross-population studies show that not all diabetic patients are subject to the same risk. Thus Pima Indian and Japanese diabetic people have a lower risk of vascular disease than white diabetic patients, suggesting that genetic or environmental factors may play a role.[22] The risk of macrovascular disease is directly proportional to low density lipoprotein (LDL) cholesterol and inversely proportional to high density lipoprotein (HDL) cholesterol. Hypertriglyceridemia is extremely common in NIDDM, but its significance as an independent risk factor is not clear.

Another factor that has been shown to be important in nondiabetic patients is obesity. This is especially important in NIDDM patients as 60 to 85 percent are obese and this group has a high morbidity from macrovascular disease. Hypertension, hyperinsulinemia, diabetes, increased very low density lipoprotein (VLDL), and low HDL are highly associated with abdominal obesity, measured as an increased waist to hip ratio. In contrast femoral and gluteal obesity appears to have less impact on these risks. There is also a suggestion that exercise may be beneficial in preventing macrovascular disease as well as in assisting weight loss.[22]

Impaired glucose tolerance has been found to be a risk factor in a number of epidemiologic studies, and as these patients are hyperinsulinemic, it raises the question of hyperinsulinemia as a factor in the development of macrovascular disease. There is no evidence as yet that exogenous insulin can have an adverse effect, although many are wondering whether obese type 2 diabetic patients should be treated with high dose insulin rather then strict weight control.[22] IDDM is also associated with an increased risk of macrovascular disease unrelated to lipid abnormalities, which is dramatically increased to 12 times normal when nephropathy is present.[4] The reasons for this are unclear.

Much work has been done evaluating whether treating these risk factors in nondiabetic patients prevents macrovascular disease, but there are not many data available relating to diabetic patients as a separate group. Treating abnormal lipids has been shown to reduce the number of subsequent myocardial events but has yet to result in improvement in mortality. Control of hypertension has been well shown to reduce cardiovascular mortality. The Oslo heart study found that a reduction in cigarette smoking lowered the incidence of myocardial infarction and sudden death. Anecdotally it has certainly been the impression of most vascular surgeons that the patients who continue to smoke do much worse than those who are successful at stopping.[22]

Aggressive treatment of hyperglycemia has not been shown to reduce the incidence of macrovascular complications as it has for microangiopathic complications (University Group Diabetes Program). Indeed, there is evidence that the pathogenic mechanisms leading to macrovascular disease among NIDDM patients begin long before the onset of diabetes during the prediabetic period.[22] Although hyperglycemia is not important in the genesis of macrovascular disease, it may be responsible for the increased incidence of thrombolic complications reported in diabetes. It has been well demonstrated that a significant increase in platelet aggregation exists in hyperglycemic patients. This disappears when the blood glucose is kept within normal limits. High blood sugar levels have also been shown to result in increased thromboxane production by the platelets and decreased prostacyclin production by the vessel wall. This is an area of great research interest as it is felt by many that these platelet and vessel wall abnormalities may be the primary reason for the increase in macrovascular disease seen in the diabetic patient.[25] Since the hypersensitivity of platelets from diabetic patients is abolished by adequate control of the concentration of glucose in plasma, good control of the patient's blood sugar may be important in reducing the incidence of thrombotic complications. Low dose aspirin therapy has been shown to reduce the frequency and severity of myocardial events in men over 50, and although unproved, it may make sense to treat all type 2 diabetic patients over 50.

PATHOLOGY

The pathology of atherosclerotic plaque is believed to be the same in the diabetic as in the nondiabetic patient (Fig. 3-4). The traditional theory entails injury to the endothelium as the primary lesion. The next event is the aggregation of platelets around the lesion with the release of platelet-derived factors. These in turn would stimulate

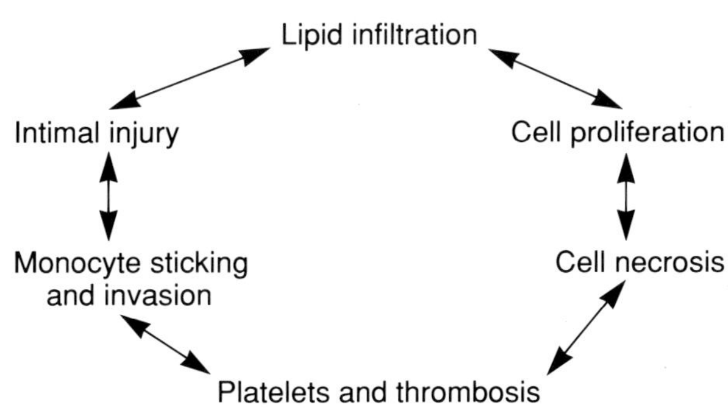

Fig. 3-4. Probable pathologic processes in progression of atherosclerotic plaque. (From Vinicor,[46] with permission.)

smooth muscle proliferation and the deposition of cholesterol.[26] Recently Ross has proposed a modification of this theory, suggesting that monocyte adherence to the endothelium is the initial lesion and that platelet adherence comes later, depending on the host response.[27] Once the plaque is formed, the damaged endothelium remains a potential site for thrombosis and here the hyperglycemic diabetic patient may be at a greater risk than the nondiabetic patient. Recent studies of the progression of lesions in the carotid[28] suggest that intraplaque hemorrhage may play a role in sudden expansion of the lesion with ulceration of the intima and distal embolization of the contents of the plaque. This may explain why anticoagulants have not been consistently effective.

Despite the fact that the pathologic process is the same as in nondiabetic patients, the effects of the process are clearly different. The likelihood of gangrene in vascular disease has been reported to be 38 to 71 times more likely in diabetic than in nondiabetic patients.[29] In the fifth decade of life the incidence of gangrene has been reported to be 156 times greater in diabetic patients with vascular disease than in nondiabetic patients with vascular disease.[30] Why are diabetic patients much more likely to sustain tissue loss than nondiabetic patients? Conrad[31] had looked at this question in some detail.

It has often been suggested that the severity of the disease is greater in the diabetic patient. This is certainly true in the type 1 or IDDM patients, particularly in those patients with nephropathy. These patients with severe microangiopathy are often blind and have already had a renal transplant when they develop rapidly progressive macrovascular disease. This results in their demise from myocardial infarction or stroke, but often not before major amputations have been required. However, IDDM patients represent less then 10 percent of all diabetic patients, and the 55 percent who die before age 55 cannot account for the massive increase in tissue loss seen. For the vast majority of diabetic patients who are non-insulin-dependent, it has been shown that macrovascular disease often precedes the diagnosis of diabetes and is unrelated to control of hyperglycemia. Studies of major amputations[32] and peripheral vascular and carotid artery surgery[9] fail to show a significantly reduced age for these patients. This does not support the thesis that more severe disease is responsible for the excess tissue loss in the majority of diabetic patients.

While the pathology of the atherosclerotic plaque is identical to that in the nondiabetic patient, the distribution is certainly quite different. Inflow disease, or obstruction of the aortoiliac segment, is much less common in the diabetic patient, while outflow disease, or obstruction of the femoropopliteal-tibial segment, is much more frequent.[11] Involvement of the tibial segment is particularly characteristic of the diabetic patient, and as many as a third of the patients with symptomatic ischemia have palpable popliteal pulses.[33] There does, however, seem to be relative sparing of the foot vessels, and as noted earlier, small vessel disease is not felt to exist. There is certainly a clinical impression that more distal disease is likely to be associated with tissue loss, and this different distribution of atherosclerosis may be partly responsible. The reasons for the differences in the distribution of atherosclerosis are, however, entirely unknown.

One reason commonly given for the worse prognosis in diabetic patients was that they were unable to develop an effective collateral circulation. However, there is little evidence to support this position. In fact, studies measuring runoff pressures at the time of vascular reconstruction show no difference between the diabetic and the nondiabetic patient.[34] Furthermore, reports on the results of vascular surgery in the diabetic patient from the New England Deaconess Hospital and other institutions have shown that the diabetic patients do just as well as far as graft patency is concerned. If the runoff was less because of poor collaterals, then the results should be worse.

There is much attention currently being focused on the role of basement membrane thickening in leading to necrosis. It is not hard to imagine that basement membrane thickening could lead to problems with the passage of nutrients and white blood cells, which in turn could require a higher perfusion pressure to maintain tissue viability. However, this remains to be proved. It should also be remembered that frequently the patient does not have a pure ischemic lesion but also may have severe neuropathy and infection, and as noted earlier, both of these factors are capable of causing tissue loss on their own. The combination of neuropathy and ischemia may result in tissue breakdown at higher perfusion pressures than ischemia alone.

CLINICAL PRESENTATION OF PERIPHERAL VASCULAR ISCHEMIA

The classic symptoms of peripheral vascular disease, namely intermittent claudication and ischemic rest pain, are often the presenting features of ischemia in the diabetic patient. However, the symptoms may be modified by the presence of neuropathy. Thus, patients with severe sensory neuropathy may simply complain that their legs get tired when they walk a certain distance. Occasionally, patients will deny any discomfort in their calves on walking but then tell you that they avoid walking at all costs. As inflow disease is relatively uncommon in diabetic patients, calf claudication rather than thigh or buttock claudication is usually the presenting symptom.

As the degree of obstruction progresses, patients may find that without the help of gravity they cannot get enough blood to their feet and so develop ischemic rest pain, usually in the toes. The usual complaint is the patients awaken after a couple hours of sleep with severe pain in the feet that is only relieved by getting up and hanging the feet down. This is a serious problem, as it is usually quickly followed by tissue loss. However, with severe sensory neuropathy there often is no rest pain, and tissue loss may be the presenting feature.

Patients with neuropathy may also have neuritic pain, which may be extremely difficult to distinguish from ischemic pain. Neuropathic patients may complain that their feet feel cold or that they feel like they are walking on bricks. They often complain of "shooting," "burning," or "knifelike" pains that characteristically involve the front of the leg and do not seem to be related to exercise or dependency. They complain of cramps and foot pain at night that are not relieved by any particular position. Whereas ischemic pain tends to be consistent in that it occurs whenever the patient walks a certain distance or has the feet elevated a certain amount of time, neuropathic pain is usually quite variable. The patient may be pain-free for days or weeks at a time.

Physical examination may also be confusing because of the coexistence of neuropathy. Both ischemia and neuropathy may be associated with muscle wasting and hair loss. Purely ischemic lesions tend to occur at the most distal part of the extremity, while neuropathic lesions occur on weight-bearing areas or areas that are traumatized. However, in patients with both neuropathy and ischemia the lesion may occur on a weight-bearing area as a result of trauma and then fail to heal because of ischemia. Of particular significance is the fact that 30 percent of patients with neuropathy also have an autonomic neuropathy. This has the same effect as a surgical sympathectomy with shunting of the blood from the nutrient vessels to the skin so that the skin feels warm to the touch. Thus it is possible to have an asymptomatic patient with warm feet who is critically ischemic. Under these circumstances a small podiatric procedure may result in gangrene.

Often on physical examination the patient is noted to have a good popliteal pulse but no pedal pulses, and the question is raised as to whether the patient has significant ischemia. A useful test is to elevate the legs for 30 seconds. If there is significant ischemia, the elevation will produce acute ischemia and at the same time empty the legs of blood. The ischemia results in capillary vasodilation, which, however, cannot be seen as the legs are empty of blood. Next the feet are allowed to hang down, and the veins on the dorsum of the foot are watched to determine how long it takes the veins to fill. A venous filling time of over 15 seconds is considered significant. The feet are then watched further to see if they become red as the vasodilated capillaries fill with blood. The longer it takes the dependent rubor to develop, the worse the ischemia, although any rubor at all is significant.

Office Doppler examination is a useful adjunct to the usual physical examination. Measuring the ankle-brachial ratio is less helpful than in the nondiabetic patient because medial calcific stenosis may result in artifactually elevated pressures. However, it is still worth doing as low readings are accurate, and it provides a baseline so that the results of therapeutic intervention may be followed. The normal Doppler pulse is triphasic, but below a major obstruction it becomes monophasic, and this can be readily detected audibly. If a patient seen in the office is obese with ankle edema, it may not be possible to palpate distal pulses. However, if all the foot pulses are triphasic by Doppler, then one can rest assured that the patient does not have significant ischemia. If the pulses are monophasic, then formal noninvasive evaluation is indicated.

TREATMENT OF DIABETIC VASCULAR DISEASE

It is interesting to first review the history of the management of diabetic vascular disease, as it permits us to put our current position in perspective. When Dr. McKittrick first set up the foot room at the New England Deaconess Hospital in the 1930s, there was no vascular surgery or antibiotics. Treatment consisted of local debridement and then minor or major closed amputation, depending on the circulation. Dr. McKittrick realized that patients with palpable popliteal pulses and ischemic lesions on their toes would often heal following a transmetatarsal amputation (TMA), and in the late 1940s he published the first reported series.[35] In the 1950s the specialty of vascular surgery was born, and in particular the femoral popliteal bypass was introduced by Jean Kunlin[36] and its use rapidly spread. Between 1960 and 1983 a tremendous experience in the use of the femoral popliteal bypass was developed at Deaconess Hospital, and published series showed that isolated femoral popliteal disease could be successfully bypassed as long as autogenous vein was used.[8] When saphenous vein was not available, then arm vein was found to work as well (Fig. 3-5).[37] Patients with isolated tibial disease were not considered candidates for reconstruction, and they were evaluated clinically to determine if they would heal from a TMA or a below knee amputation. If rubor extended to the proposed incision site for a TMA, they were not considered candidates and a below knee amputation was performed. The advent of the noninvasive vascular lab did not help predict which patients would heal from a major amputation, but a good forefoot tracing on the pulse volume recording did suggest that the patient would heal from a TMA.[38] Bypass to the tibial vessels was rarely performed and then only with moderate success.[39]

In the early 1980s, Leather et al. considered that

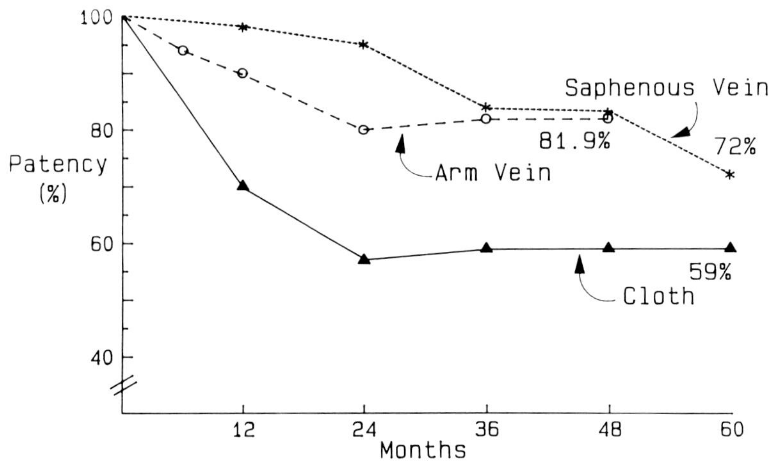

Fig. 3-5. Comparison of conduits for femoral popliteal bypass grafts.

the lack of success with the tibial bypass was due to a size mismatch between the reversed saphenous vein and the tibial vessel. Often the surgeon would be sewing a 3-mm vein to a 15-mm femoral artery and a 7-to 10-mm vein to a 2-mm artery. They therefore introduced a modified Mills valvulotome to enable the valves to be cut and the vein to be kept in situ with a better size match. This produced impressive results, and there was some experimental work to suggest that minimal vein handling was also important.[40] Many patients, however, were still considered unreconstructible, as current radiologic techniques prevented adequate visualization of the distal vessels. Failure to visualize the distal posterior tibial (PT) and dorsalis pedis (DP) arteries led to many bypasses being done to the peroneal artery, which frequently worked nicely. However, on occasion a major amputation had to be performed despite a functioning graft.

The introduction of arterial digital subtraction arteriography in the early 1980s was a tremendous help in visualizing arteries that could not previously be seen, and in the last few years surgeons have been going progressively lower down the leg so that bypass to the foot has become routine. Those patients with palpable popliteal pulses and ischemia now receive an arterial digital subtraction arteriogram (DSA) and if an open DP or distal PT artery is visualized, then a bypass is performed from the popliteal to the distal vessel (Fig. 3-6). Because the foot vessels are often spared, it is now extremely rare that a TMA has to be performed for a purely ischemic lesion. It does, however, remain a useful procedure to close a foot after revascularization when there has been extensive tissue loss. It has also become clear that size match is the important feature rather than not dissecting out the vein. Therefore, we will use the in situ vein, reversed saphenous vein or nonreversed saphenous vein, depending on the size match and what is technically the easiest. The introduction of intraluminal vessel occluders has made it possible to occlude the flow in the small calcified tibial vessels without damaging them by attempting to clamp them. Our experience with 97 bypasses to the DP artery has recently been published, and although the follow-up is short, the grafts do appear to be durable (Fig. 3-7).[33] Long term success in the diabetic patient is more difficult to evaluate, as 50 percent of the patients die within 5 years from coronary artery disease.

With all of this improved technology it is reasonable to ask what this has meant in terms of limb salvage. We compared the fate of all patients presenting with ischemia secondary to outflow disease from July 1984 to June 1985 with the 12-month period before the introduction of the in situ technique in May of 1983. The most significant data was the reduction of the primary amputation rate from just under 30 percent to just under 10 percent without an increase in the secondary amputation rate. Since then the primary amputation

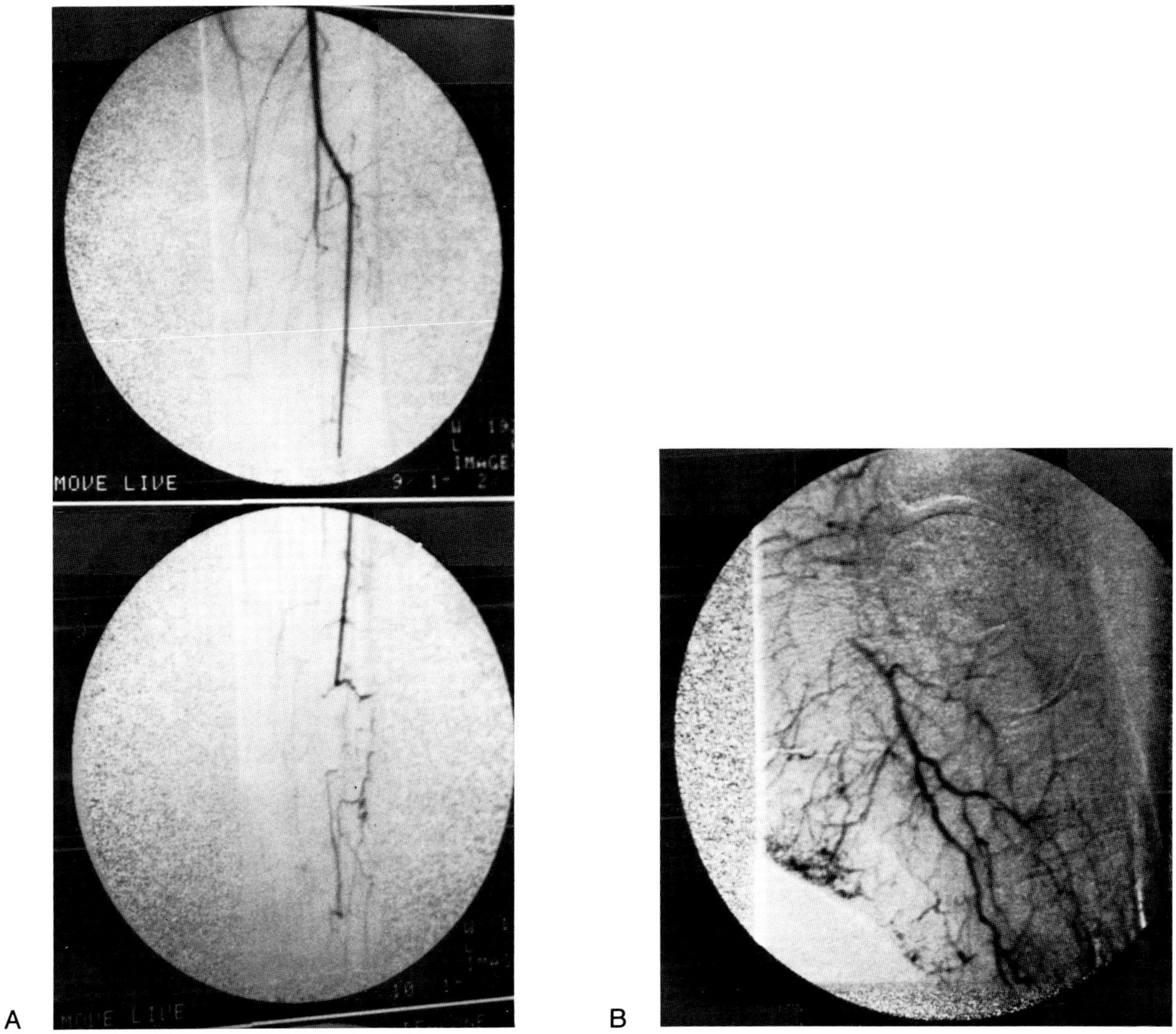

Fig. 3-6. (**A & B**) Digital subtraction arteriogram showing severe tibial disease with reconstitution of the plantar artery.

rate has continued to decline and is currently around 6 percent. During the same period there have been tremendous improvements in anesthesia, monitoring, and postoperative care. With these advances and routine use of the Swan-Ganz catheter our operative mortality has dropped from 8.9 to 0.7 percent. Thus, we feel that an elderly diabetic patient in her 90s who lives at home and who presents with ischemic lesion is better served by reconstruction and a return to home in a week or two, than by a major amputation that would sentence her to a nursing home for the rest of her life.

With so many advances in the last decade it is tempting to predict where we will go from here. Angioscopy has proved a useful tool at our institution, particularly for detecting uncut valves when using the in situ technique. We have recently started to cut the valves under direct vision to see if this reduces the trauma to the vein. We are, however, starting a prospective randomized trial to see whether the expense of the procedure can be justified by improved results. With the development of a broad range of new technology there is also a tremendous interest in endovascular procedures.

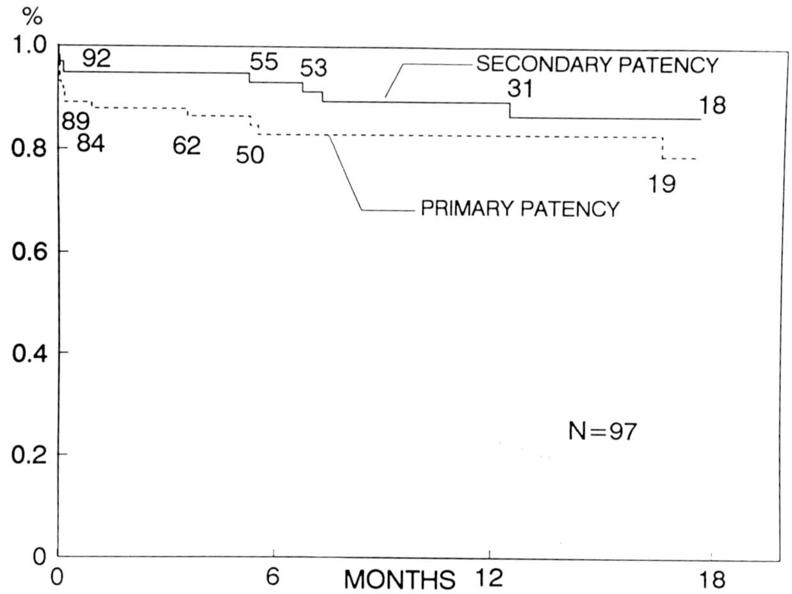

Fig. 3-7. Patency after DP bypass.

Transluminal angioplasty has proved to be useful for localized lesions in large arteries, but this is less commonly indicated in diabetic patients with diffuse distal disease. All major series report worse results as the disease becomes more distal and worse in the diabetic patient at all levels.[41] The increased thrombogenicity noted in the diabetic patient may be a factor here. Recently developed technologies include the use of lasers and atherectomy devices to remove localized occlusions. It remains to be seen what their role will be. Twenty years ago surgical endarterectomy was extremely popular for treating local lesions but was gradually abandoned as it was found that particularly for outflow disease this was not as effective as bypass grafting. It appeared that there was a definite relationship between the amount of intima that could be removed and the blood flow in the area that defined whether thrombosis would occur. It is my perspective that the same limitations will apply to the new endovascular techniques, and that unless something can be done to reduce the tendency of damaged intima to produce thrombosis, then the value of the new techniques will be limited.

Treatment of the Purely Vascular Lesion

The indications for surgery in the diabetic patient remain the same as in the nondiabetic patient. Ischemic rest pain and nonhealing lesions are absolute indications, and disabling claudication is a relative indication. As diabetes is so likely to produce gangrene, diabetic patients are more likely to be operated on for limb salvage than are nondiabetic patients. For patients presenting with stable claudication, conservative measures include cessation of smoking, exercise, and pentoxyfylline.

The role of pentoxyfylline remains unclear. Pentoxifylline is a substituted methylxanthine similar to caffeine and theophylline, but unlike these it has been shown to alter the hemorrheologic properties of blood. When first introduced it was felt that its major therapeutic effect was brought about by increasing red cell flexibility and reducing whole blood viscosity. It also has an aspirinlike effect in that it decreases platelet aggregation and reduces plasma fibrinogen levels.[42] Recently, studies have suggested that its therapeutic effect is not related to blood viscosity, and this may explain why second generation rheologic drugs such as ketanserin have not been found to be effective.[43] Pentoxifylline has, however, been demonstrated to improve the distance some of the patients can walk in a number of controlled trials.[44] I routinely offer it to my patients with stable claudication, and about 25 percent continue to take it long term. I also try it in those few unreconstructible patients who are not yet ready for a major amputation. In view of the increased platelet activity reported in diabetic patients, it makes sense to put the patient on low dose aspirin, although there is no evidence to prove that this is effective in preventing worsening of their symptoms.

Treatment of the Complex Lesion

Frequently patients do not present with pure ischemia, but a combination of infection, ischemia, and neuropathy. These patients can be extremely challenging, requiring the attention of the whole team of physicians. As a general rule, acute infection needs to be controlled first with incision and drainage and broad spectrum antibiotics as indicated. The patient should be at bed rest to take neuropathy out of the equation. Once the acute infection and cellulitis has resolved, then arteriography and revascularization should be performed expeditiously. Extensive debridement, except where necessary to control acute infection, should be avoided prior to revascularization if at all possible, as it may result in extension of the tissue loss. Once infection has been controlled and the foot revascularized, then attention can be directed to creating a walking foot. This may require minor amputation, skin grafting, or even local or distant pedicle flaps. Even if there is not much tissue loss, there may be sufficient deformity secondary to motor neuropathy to require osteotomy or tenotomy to improve the mechanical status of the foot. Chronic infection of the foot such as is seen in osteomyelitis secondary to neuropathic ulceration should be surgically debrided after revascularization. It can be quite difficult sometimes to know whether a patient needs wide incision and drainage first and then revascularization or the reverse. As a general rule, revascularization is not recommended in the face of active cellulitis or free pus. Sometimes the patient does poorly despite adequate treatment of infection and yet has palpable distal pulses. In this case arteriography may be indicated because there have been cases reported where in the face of tibial disease there was sufficient collateral circulation to produce distal pulses but not enough to heal the lesion.[45] In this series prompt healing occurred once revascularization was performed.

SUMMARY

The management of diabetic vascular disease is an exciting field that has made tremendous advances over the last decade. The future promises to be even more interesting with further gains being made in the fight to reduce limb loss. As this brief review has demonstrated, there are many questions yet to be answered. While proper management of diabetic vascular disease now requires a large team of specialists, it is very important that the vascular surgeon leading the team has a clear understanding of the problems to be faced.

REFERENCES

1. Hoar CS, Torres J: Evaluation of below-the-knee amputations in the treatment of diabetic gangrene. N Engl J Med 266:440, 1962
2. Fearon J, Campbell DR, Hoar CS et al: Improved results with diabetic below-knee amputations. Arch Surg 120:777, 1985
3. National Diabetes Advisory Board: The prevention and treatment of five complications of diabetes: a guide for primary care practitioners. HHS publ. no. 83-8392. Centers for Disease Control, Atlanta, GA, 1983
4. Krolewski AS, Warran JH: Epidemiology of diabetes mellitus. p. 12. In Marble A, Krall LP, Bradley RF et al (eds): Joslin Diabetes Mellitus. 12th Ed. Lea & Febiger, Philadelphia, 1985
5. Fuller J, McCartney P, Jarrett R et al: Hyperglycemia and coronary heart disease: the Whitehall studies. J Chronic Dis 32:721, 1979

6. Mincu L: Diabetic Macro and Microangiopathy. DeGruyter, Berlin, 1975
7. Lerner D, Kannel W: Patterns of coronary heart disease morbidity and mortality in the sexes: a twenty-six year followup of the Framingham population. Am Heart J 111: 383, 1986
8. Wheelock FC, Filtzer HS: Femoral grafts in diabetics. Arch Surg 99:776, 1979
9. Campbell DR, Hoar CS, Wheelock FC: Carotid artery surgery in diabetic patients. Arch Surg 119:1405, 1984
10. Goldenberg SG, Alen M, Joshi RA, Blumental HT: Nonatheromatous peripheral vascular disease of the lower extremity in diabetes mellitus. Diabetes 8:201, 1959
11. Strandness DE, Priest RE, Gibbons GW: Combined clinical and pathological study of diabetic and non-diabetic peripheral arterial disease. Diabetes 13:366, 1964
12. Conrad MC: Large and small artery occlusion in diabetics and non-diabetics with severe vascular disease. Circulation 36:83, 1967
13. Siperstein MD, Unger RH, Medison LL: Studies of muscle capillary basement membrane in normal subjects, diabetic and pre-diabetic patients. J Clin Invest 47:1973, 1968
14. Parving HH, Rasmussen SM: Transcapillary escape rate of albumen and plasma volume in short and long term juvenile diabetics. Scand J Clin Lab Invest 32:81, 1973
15. LoGerfo FW, Coffman JD: Vascular and microvascular disease of the foot in diabetes, implications for foot care. N Engl J Med 311:1615, 1984
16. Delbridge L, Cterctekoy G, Fowler C et al: The aetiology of diabetic neuropathic ulceration of the foot. Br J Surg 72:1, 1985
17. Parkhouse N, LeQuesne PM: Impaired neurogenic vascular response in patients with diabetes and neuropathic foot lesions. N Engl J Med 318:1306, 1988
18. Boulton AJM, Scarpello JHB, Ward JD: Venous oxygenation in the diabetic neuropathic foot: evidence of arteriovenous shunting. Diabetologia 22:6, 1982
19. Corbin DOC, Young RJ, Morrison DC et al: Blood flow in the foot, polyneuropathy and foot ulceration in diabetes mellitus. Diabetologia 30:468, 1987
20. Edmonds ME, Morrison N, Laws JW, Watkins PJ: Medial arterial calcification and diabetic neuropathy. Br J Surg 284:928, 1982
21. Khettry U: Pathology of the diabetic foot. p. 27. In Kozak GP et al (eds): Management of the Diabetic Foot. WB Saunders, Philadelphia, 1984
22. Consensus statement. American Diabetes Association. Role of cardiovascular risk factors in prevention and treatment of macrovascular disease in diabetes. Diabetes Care 12:573, September 1989
23. Kannel WB, McGee DC: Update of some epidemiological features of intermittent claudication: the Framingham study. J Am Geritr Soc 33:13, 1985
24. Watkins LD, Neaton JD, Kuller LH: Racial differences in high density lipoprotein, cholesterol and coronary heart disease incidence in the usual care group of the multiple risk factor intervention trial. Am J Cardiol 57:538, 1986
25. Mustard JF, Pachan MA: Platelets and diabetes mellitus. N Engl J Med 311:665, 1984
26. Colwell J, Lopes, Virella M et al: New concepts about the pathogenesis of atherosclerosis in diabetes mellitus. p. 51. In Levin ME, O'Neil LW (eds): The Diabetic Foot. CV Mosby, St. Louis, 1988
27. Ross R: The pathogenesis of atherosclerosis—an update. N Engl J Med 314:488, 1986
28. Imparato AM, Riles TS, Mintzer R et al: The importance of hemorrhage in the relationship between gross morphologic characteristics and cerebral symptoms in 376 carotid artery plaques. Ann Surg 197:195, 1983
29. Bell ET: Incidence of gangrene of the extremities in non-diabetic and in diabetic persons. Arch Pathol Lab Med 49:469, 1950
30. Bell ET: Diabetes Mellitus. Charles C Thomas, Springfield, IL, 1960
31. Conrad MC: Contributions of large and small vessel disease to severe ischemia of the lower extremities in diabetics and non-diabetics. Vascular Diagnosis and Treatment 17:26, Oct/Nov, 1981
32. Lisa JR, Magidan M, Hart JF: Peripheral arteriosclerosis in the diabetic and the non-diabetic. JAMA 118:1353, 1942
33. Pomposelli FB, Jepsen SJ, Gibbons GW et al: Efficacy of the dorsalis pedis bypass for limb salvage in diabetic patients. J Vasc Surg 11:745, 1990
34. Berner HB, Kaiser EC, Willmar VC: Blood flow in the diabetic leg. Circulation 43:391, 1971
35. McKittrick LE, McKittrick JB, Risley TS: Transmetatarsal amputation for infection or gangrene in patients with diabetes mellitus. Ann Surg 130:826, 1949
36. Kunlin J: Le traitment de l'arterite obliterante par la greffe veineuse longue. Arch Mal Coeur 42:371, 1949
37. Campbell DR, Hoar CS, Gibbons GW: The use of arm veins in femoral popliteal bypass grafts. Ann Surg 190:740, 1979
38. Gibbons GW, Wheelock FC, Siembieda C et al: Non-invasive prediction of amputation level in diabetic patients. Arch Surg 113:1253, 1979
39. Mannick JA, Jackson BT, Coffman JD, Hume DM:

Success of vein bypass grafts in patients with isolated popliteal artery segments. Surgery 61:17, 1967
40. Leather RP, Shah DM, Karmody AM: Infrapopliteal arterial bypass for limb salvage: increased patency and utilization of the saphenous vein used insitu. Surgery 90:1000, 1981
41. Morin JF, Johnston KW, Wasserman L, Andrews D: Factors that determine the long term results of percutaneous transluminal dilatation for peripheral arterial occlusive disease. J Vasc Surg 4:68, 1988
42. Strano A, Davi G, Avellone G et al: Double-blind crossover study of the clinical efficiency and hemorrheological effects of pentoxifylline in patients with occlusive arterial disease of the lower limbs. Angiology 35:439, 1984
43. Bounameaux H, Holditch T, Hellemans H et al: Placebo-controlled double-blind, two centre trial of ketanserin in intermittent claudication. Lancet 2(8467):1268, 1985
44. Porter JM, Cutler BC, Lee BY et al: Pentoxifylline efficiency in the treatment of intermittent claudication. Multicenter controlled double-blind trial with objective assessment of chronic occlusive arterial disease patients. Am Heart J 104:66, 1982
45. Andros G, Harris RW, Dulawa LG, et al: The need for arteriography in diabetic patients with gangrene and palpable foot pulses. Arch Surg 119:1260, 1989
46. Vinicor F: Atherosclerosis and diabetes mellitus. Diabetes Spectrum 1(5):321, 1989

4

Diabetic Neuropathy

A.J.M. Boulton, M.D., M.R.C.P.

Diabetes mellitus has been recognized for thousands of years, but the long-term complications of this chronic condition have a much shorter history. Although some authorities consider that an Old Testament biblical passage was referring to diabetic gangrene,[1] the important and frequent connection between diabetic nerve disease and foot ulceration and gangrene has only been recognized in the last 40 years. One exception to this is found in a paper by Auche in 1890,[2] who described classic neuropathic foot ulceration and concluded that this was due to some alteration in the peripheral nerve function. However, subsequent extensive reviews on diabetic neuropathy made little mention of foot problems,[3,4] and it was not until 1957 when Oakley and colleagues[5] listed neuropathy as a major etiologic factor in foot ulceration that the link between these two problems was firmly established. It is now believed that the neuropathic diabetic foot is at high risk of ulceration, and that education of such "high risk" individuals might play a major role in reducing the morbidity of diabetic foot disease.[6]

The clinical features of diabetic neuropathy were first described about 200 years ago, and the diverse manifestations of this condition have been summarized in several recent reviews.[7–9] Early descriptions were mainly confined to the most common type of diabetic nerve disease, that is, the distal symmetric polyneuropathy. However, as almost any area of the somatic or autonomic nervous system may be involved in diabetic patients, it is necessary to classify the diabetic neuropathies into several subgroups.

The classification, prevalence, natural history, etiopathogenesis, assessment, and management of the diabetic neuropathies will be discussed in this chapter. Finally, the relationship between peripheral neuropathy and foot problems will be outlined.

CLASSIFICATION OF THE DIABETIC NEUROPATHIES

An ideal classification would be based upon clinical and pathologic features of the neuropathies, but until our understanding of the etiopathogenesis is complete, such a classification is not possible. Some investigators have proposed a classification based upon presumed etiology[10] or topography.[11] If electrophysiologic abnormalities alone were considered to be sufficient evidence to diagnose neuropathy, then a very high prevalence would be found: Skillman and colleagues reported that 70 percent of their patients had such abnormalities.[12] Conversely, if pathologic criteria were applied, a very different classification would result. It is therefore the belief of that author that, at the present time, a simple clinical classification should be used as outlined in Table 4-1.

Diabetic Mononeuropathies

Isolated and Multiple

Although isolated, multiple mononeuropathies are relatively uncommon, it is important to recognize

Table 4-1. Clinical Classification of Diabetic Neuropathies

Mononeuropathies	*Polyneuropathies*
Isolated	Sensory
	Acute
	Chronic sensorimotor
Multiple	Autonomic
Cranial	Proximal motor

mononeuropathy in diabetic patients with other neuropathic syndromes as the mononeuropathy may be treatable or reversible. In a study of diabetic neuropathy, Mulder et al. found that 11 percent of patients had clinical evidence of a mononeuropathy with the median and peroneal nerves most commonly affected.[13] Involvement of the peroneal nerve gives rise to foot drop that may require management with a dropped foot splint. Such a mononeuropathy may be the presenting feature of type 2 diabetes,[14] and it should be remembered that mononeuropathies may frequently occur in the absence of other diabetic complications. Mononeuritis multiplex describes the involvement of more than one peripheral nerve in the same patient: this would appear to be a common occurrence according to Mulder et al.,[13] who found 29 nerves to be affected among the 16 patients with mononeuropathies in their series.

Cranial

Involvement of most of the cranial nerves in diabetic mononeuropathy has been described, but extraocular mononeuropathies, especially those involving the third cranial nerve, are the most common.[15] As with other mononeuropathies, the prognosis for recovery is generally good.

Diabetic Polyneuropathies

Autonomic

Dysfunction of the autonomic nervous system is common in diabetes and may affect any tissues receiving autonomic innervation.[8,9,16] It is fortunate that symptoms of such dysfunction are relatively infrequent, as, when present, they may be severely disabling. Objective evidence of autonomic neuropathy is frequently found in patients with sensorimotor neuropathy, whether or not it is symptomatic. The main clinical manifestations of autonomic neuropathy are listed in Table 4-2, with a more detailed discussion of autonomic dysfunction in the lower limb in the following section.

Anhidrosis of the lower limbs due to involvement of the postganglionic sympathetic fibers to the sweat glands is common in diabetic patients with the distal sensorimotor neuropathy.[17,18] Although the patients rarely have any specific complaints, clinical assessment will reveal dry skin that cracks or splits easily and is liable to form callous tissue under weight-bearing areas. Some patients may also exhibit a compensatory increase in sweating in the upper body: in its extreme form this is known as gustatory sweating, and patients with this condition sweat profusely in the head and neck region after eating certain foodstuffs.

A further consequence of peripheral sympathetic neuropathy ("autosympathectomy") in the absence of peripheral vascular disease is an increase in blood flow to the lower limb with shunting of blood through pre-existing arteriovenous shunts, leading to an increase in skin temperature. It was for this very reason that the surgical operation of sympathectomy was performed, and consequently, there is virtually no indication today for this procedure in diabetic patients. There is strong evidence that arteriovenous shunting is a common occurrence in the diabetic neuropathic leg[19–21] and is contributory to the etiology of neuropathic foot ulceration.

Table 4-2. Some Clinical Manifestations of Diabetic Autonomic Neuropathies

Cardiovascular	Gastrointestinal
Resting, fixed tachyardia	Gastroparesis diabeticorum
Postural hypotension	Motility disturbances (diarrhea or constipation)
Painless myocardial ischemia	Anorectal dysfunction (fecal incontinence)
Peripheral	Pupillary disturbances
Reduced sweating in lower limbs	Miosis
Neuropathic edema	Disturbances of dilation
Genitourinary	
Impotence or ejaculatory disturbance	
Cystopathy (bladder dysfunction)	

A further consequence of autonomic dysfunction in the lower limb is the well-documented though relatively rare neuropathic edema.[4,22] This is probably also related to sympathetic dysfunction as profound vasodilation and arteriovenous shunting lead to venous pooling and ultimately peripheral edema.

Proximal Motor Neuropathy

The term *proximal motor neuropathy* is used to describe both symmetric and asymmetric forms of the motor neuropathy that has previously been referred to as "amyotrophy."[23,24] The condition is most commonly seen in middle-aged or elderly type 2 diabetic patients who describe a relatively acute (days or weeks) onset of deep, aching pain in one or both thighs, which is associated with wasting and weakness of the affected muscles. In some patients the diabetes is biochemically mild or undetected when the neuropathy presents, although evidence of a distal sensorimotor neuropathy is usually found in addition to the proximal muscle wasting. A further frequent associated feature is weight loss, which may be so marked that it simulates neuropathic cachexia.[25] Clearly this diagnosis is therefore one of exclusion of more serious causes such as underlying malignancy. If the motor neuropathy is indeed secondary to the diabetes, then the prognosis for recovery is good.[26]

Diabetic Sensory Neuropathies

The most common peripheral nerve disorder in diabetes is a symmetric polyneuropathy of insidious onset involving predominantly the lower limbs. However, there are two distinct forms of these sensory neuropathies — the chronic form, with gradual onset of symptoms and abnormalities of both sensory and motor function on examination, and the acute form, with severe symptoms of rapid onset but few abnormal signs on examination. The main differences between these two forms are summarized in Table 4-3.

Chronic Sensorimotor

In the series reported by Mulder and colleagues,[13] over two-thirds of neuropathic patients had this form of neuropathy. Patients usually complain of a gradual onset of paresthetic and painful symptoms, which may be positive (burning discomfort, pins and needles, stabbing pain, hyperesthesias) or negative (numbness, "feet feel dead"). In addition, nonspecific experiences such as tingling, itching, or vague alterations in temperature perception may be described. All these symptoms are prone to nocturnal exacerbation. However, some patients may present with signs of this neuropathy but with no history of any symptoms.[27] A particularly dangerous situation is to be found in the patient with the "painful-painless leg,"[28] that is, who experiences painful symptoms but who, on examination, has lost the ability to perceive painful stimuli: such patients are at great risk of neuropathic foot ulceration.

Examination of the patient with this type of neuropathy usually reveals a sensory deficit in a stocking-and-glove distribution with predominant dys-

Table 4-3. Contrasts Between Acute Sensory and Chronic Sensorimotor Neuropathies

	Acute Sensory	*Chronic Sensorimotor*
Duration of diabetes	May be short	Variable
Precipitating factor	Often present (e.g., recent ketoacidosis)	Unusual
Mode of onset	Relatively rapid (days, weeks)	Insidious
Neuropathic symptoms	Severe, often accompanied by weight loss	Variable intensity
Signs	May be absent, or mild	Variable sensory loss; small muscle wasting
Other diabetic complications	Unusual	Often present
Quantitative sensory testing	Mild abnormalities; occasionally all tests may be normal	Abnormalities of thermal and vibration testing
Natural history	Complete recovery usual within a year	Symptoms may persist; insensitive foot may develop

function with small muscle wasting and absent ankle reflexes. In addition to the neurologic findings, patients with sensorimotor neuropathy are more likely to have evidence of other microvascular complications (retinopathy, nephropathy) than nonneuropathic patients.[29]

Acute Sensory Neuropathy

Acute sensory neuropathy is less common. It is often precipitated by an event such as ketoacidosis, sudden change in diabetic control, or even treatment of newly diagnosed diabetes. The symptoms are severe and of acute onset, which is in contrast to the signs, which are usually few, occasionally none. Positive symptoms are usually prominent, with marked sleep disturbance.

EPIDEMIOLOGY OF DIABETIC POLYNEUROPATHIES

Prevalence

The true prevalence of this common complication will remain unknown until agreement is reached on the classification of this condition. Thus, the quoted prevalence of neuropathy has varied widely in the literature[7]: those studies that have accepted minor symptoms and signs as evidence of neuropathy have quoted a high prevalence, while those that have included duration of symptoms and abnormalities of multiple quantitative tests have reported a much lower prevalence. Moreover, there are very few such reports that are based on true population studies. As symptoms and signs indistinguishable from those of diabetic neuropathy are not uncommon in the older, nondiabetic population,[30] the need for strict diagnostic criteria for any prevalence study is apparent. In a cross-sectional study of an insulin-treated population attending a British hospital clinic, the prevalence of symptomatic sensorimotor neuropathy was shown to be 11 percent, when vascular disease was excluded and the diagnosis was confirmed by objective measurements.[29] It is well recognized that diabetic complications are related to duration of disease, and in a more recent study of long-standing type 1 diabetic patients, the prevalence of symptomatic sensorimotor neuropathy was found to be 58 percent.[31]

The prevalence of autonomic dysfunction is even more difficult to assess as symptoms are vague and nonspecific; however, abnormalities of cardiovascular autonomic function tests may be present at diagnosis[32] and are frequently found in long-standing type 1 diabetes.[31]

Natural History of the Polyneuropathies

There is a paucity of observations in the literature on the natural history and prognosis of the sensory neuropathies. Knowledge of such data is essential if effective trials of potential interventions, such as the aldose reductase inhibitors,[33] are to be successful. It is now generally agreed that the prognosis for the acute sensory neuropathies is good (Table 4-3), with complete recovery occurring in most cases within a year.[34,35] In contrast, the more common sensorimotor neuropathy of insidious onset has a less favorable prognosis, with many patients suffering from persistent or intermittent symptoms for several years.[36,37] It is important to remember that a gradual improvement of painful symptoms in a diabetic patient with established neuropathy does not necessarily indicate structural improvement. There may be further loss of function during this time, leaving the patient with a numb, insensitive foot that is at great risk of painless injury.[6]

The natural history of autonomic neuropathy is less clear, although in patients with multiple abnormalities of autonomic function tests the prognosis is poor,[38] with cardiorespiratory arrests having been described in patients with severe autonomic neuropathy during a general anesthetic.[39]

ETIOLOGY AND PATHOGENESIS OF DIABETIC NEUROPATHY

The etiology of the diabetic neuropathies has been an area of active research this century, with two main schools of thought, one favoring a metabolic hypothesis and the other proposing a vascular etiology. However, it is becoming increasingly apparent that no single mechanism is likely to be able to explain all the special characteristics of human diabetic neuropathy. It is my view that both metabolic and vascular mechanisms are contributory to the pathogenesis of neuropathy, and evidence for both theories will be presented.

Metabolic Theories

Various features of diabetic neuropathy make a metabolic background likely: the morphologic picture is nonspecific with axonopathic degenerative changes affecting all fiber types, and segmental demyelination and remyelination. Neuropathy occurs in both major types of diabetes, with a prevalence that increases with duration of diabetes.[40] A relationship between nerve function (measured by electrophysiologic tests) and glycemic control has been demonstrated in many studies,[7,41] and moreover, the incidence of neuropathy appears to be higher in patients with poor glycemic control.[40,41] Despite the fact that some patients never develop neuropathy regardless of their metabolic control, to date, no measurable genetic predictors of neuropathy have been identified.[41]

It therefore seems likely that a variety of metabolic insults to peripheral nerve occur as a consequence of chronic hyperglycemia, and one of the prime candidate mechanisms involves the activation of the polyol pathway (Fig. 4-1) and the subsequent accumulation of sorbitol and associated depletion of myoinositol in peripheral nerve.[42] It is now over 30 years since the first demonstration of sorbitol accumulation in the lens of diabetic rats with cataracts, an observation that led to the investigation of polyol metabolism and its rate-limiting enzyme aldose reductase (Fig. 4-1) as a possible etiologic mechanism for diabetic complications. Aldose reductase has now been demonstrated in all

$$\text{D-Glucose} + \text{NADPH} + \text{H}^{+} \xrightarrow[\text{Reductase}]{\text{Aldose}} \text{Sorbitol} + \text{NADP}$$

$$\text{Sorbitol} + \text{NAD} \xrightarrow[\text{Dehydrogenase}]{\text{Sorbitol}} \text{D-Fructose} + \text{NADH} + \text{H}$$

Fig. 4-1. The Sorbitol (polyol) pathway. Aldose reductase inhibitors prevent the conversion of glucose to sorbitol.

the important target tissues for diabetic complications and was first demonstrated in the nerve over 20 years ago.[43] In animal models of diabetes, polyol pathway overactivity has been linked with depletion of endoneurial myoinositol[44] and is associated with reduced sodium-potassium ATPase activity, which may be prevented by the administration of an aldose reductase inhibitor (ARI). The central role of myoinositol depletion associated with increased polyol pathway activity is further supported by the observation that treatment with either myoinositol supplementation or an ARI may restore nerve conduction velocities in diabetic animals.[45]

CLINICAL TRIALS OF ALDOSE REDUCTASE INHIBITORS IN DIABETIC NEUROPATHY

At the time of writing, the clinical experience with ARIs has failed to meet the high expectations provided by the earlier experimental studies.[33] The main reason for this is probably that whereas in nearly all the trials in animal models, the ARI was introduced at or soon after the induction of diabetes, in clinical trials, the ARIs were administered much later in the history of diabetes and after the complication in question was well established. In this situation in neuropathy, for example, it is unlikely that major structural repair will follow ARI administration, although a recent trial has suggested that some nerve fiber regeneration might occur in neuropathic patients treated with the ARI Sorbinil.[46] However, the majority of trials of ARIs in diabetic neuropathy have been too short in duration and conducted too late in the disease process.[47] As many such trials show some minor objective improvement, there appears to be an urgent need for an early intervention or even a prevention study of ARIs in diabetes.

Vascular Theories

In addition to the metabolic abnormalities described above, there is also much evidence from both experimental and human diabetic neuropathies to implicate microvascular abnormalities in its etiology.[48] It is postulated that either rheologic abnormalities or microvascular disease leads to increased endoneurial vascular resistance and to reduced nerve blood flow and oxygen delivery, and that the remitting endoneurial hypoxia is of major importance in the pathogenesis of neuropathy.[48,49] Reduced nerve blood flow and endoneurial hypoxia have been demonstrated in experimental diabetes,[50] a state that has been confirmed in established human diabetic neuropathy.[51] Experiments with nondiabetic rats reared in hypoxic conditions have produced nerve abnormalities similar to those seen in experimental diabetes,[52] and several of the cardinal features of human diabetic neuropathy have been shown in nondiabetic patients with chronic hypoxia secondary to pulmonary disease.[53] More recently, clinical, electrophysiologic, and morphologic changes similar to those seen in diabetic neuropathy have been demonstrated in nondiabetic patients with chronic hypoxia secondary to obstructive airways disease.[54] Thus it appears that chronic hypoxia of whatever etiology may be associated with peripheral neuropathy in both experimental animals and humans.

In summary, there is evidence from this brief review to implicate both metabolic and vascular mechanisms in the etiopathogenesis of diabetic neuropathy. It is likely that these interact in the pathogenesis, and a suggested scheme to summarize all these points is provided in Figure 4-2.

CLINICAL ASSESSMENT AND MEASUREMENT OF DIABETIC NEUROPATHY

A detailed discussion of the assessment and quantification of diabetic polyneuropathy is included to enable the reader to be familiar with the large number of investigations that are available. It must be emphasized, however, that most patients who are at risk of neuropathic foot ulceration can

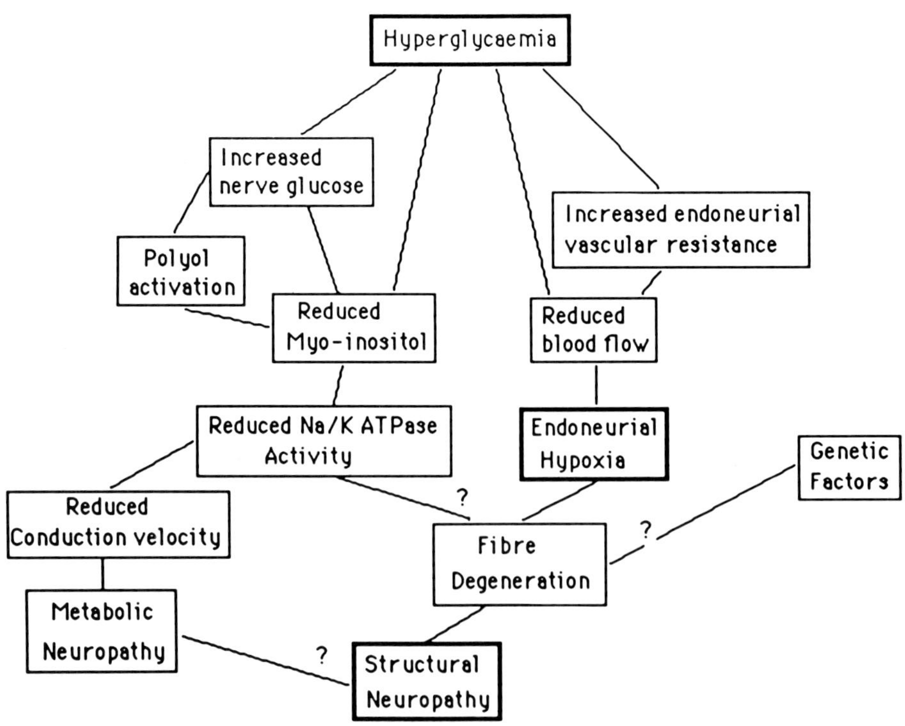

Fig. 4-2. Probable etiologic mechanisms for diabetic neuropathy.

be identified by a simple clinical examination that is outlined in the last section of the chapter.

The full assessment of diabetic neuropathy can present the practicing physician with a number of problems, including the following:

1. Neuropathic symptoms can be transient or prolonged, and many nondiabetic individuals report occasional symptoms typical of neuropathy.
2. The clinical examination may be abnormal in many asymptomatic patients.
3. Conventional nerve conduction studies are often abnormal in diabetic patients with no clinical evidence of neuropathy.

A consensus panel of neurologists and diabetologists who met to discuss the assessment of diabetic neuropathy recommended focusing on at least one measure from the following categories in order to fully classify diabetic neuropathy[55]:

Neuropathic symptom assessment
Clinical examination
Electrodiagnostic studies
Quantitative sensory testing
Autonomic function tests

Symptoms

It must be remembered that it is usually the symptoms that bring the patient to the doctor, although it is recognized that symptomatic assessment of neuropathy is highly subjective. The symptoms must be directly evaluated and cannot be inferred from any measurement. For clinical trials, a neuropathy symptom score can be derived from the neurologic history,[56] or another detailed questionnaire such as the McGill may be applied.[57]

Clinical Examination

The routine clinical examination is useful in clinical diagnoses, but because it lacks precision and is somewhat subjective, it is of limited use in clinical trials. However, a careful examination is essential and should include an assessment of small and large fiber sensory function (e.g., pain sensation and vibration perception using a 128 tuning fork), together with an examination of motor function and reflexes. A thorough clinical assessment will also help to exclude other potential causes of symptoms such as lumbar root disease or significant peripheral vascular disease. Neurologic deficits may be scored in order to quantify neuromuscular dysfunction,[58] remembering that the sensory deficit may be very patchy.

Electrodiagnostic Studies

Electrophysiologic measures of nerve function have been used for many years to assess neurologic deficits in diabetic patients. However, although an abnormal result of a nerve conduction study may help to diagnose a neuropathy, it will not confirm that diabetes is the underlying cause. Despite this caveat, nerve conduction studies can provide much information on nerve function if proper attention is paid to technique.[55] As with symptoms and signs, the results of multiple electrophysiologic tests of nerve function may be combined to give a score of neurophysiologic dysfunction,[27] a variable that can be followed in longitudinal studies of the natural history of diabetic neuropathy.

Quantitative Sensory Testing

Instruments that test for vibration perception, temperature appreciation, and current perception threshold will be summarized. As all these tests generally evaluate sensations evoked by stimulation of cutaneous receptors, they depend on a subjective response. However, these are relatively sensitive tests that may be abnormal early in neuropathy, and their use was strongly recommended by the recent consensus meeting.[55]

Vibration Perception

The biothesiometer (Biomedical Instrument Co. Inc., Newbury, OH) is the most widely used instrument to test for vibration perception, and reduction in the ability to perceive vibration has been strongly associated with a risk for neuropathic foot ulceration.[59] Other instruments that assess vibration perception, a large fiber sensory modality, include the Vibrameter (Somedic, Stockholm, Sweden) and the computer-assisted sensory exam.[60]

Thermal Testing

Several instruments are available to test thermal sensation, a small fiber sensory modality that is usually impaired early in diabetic neuropathy. However, these may not be as useful in the identification of the high risk foot.[6]

Neurometer

The neurometer is a new device employing a constant current sine wave generator that may test different nerve fiber populations at varying frequencies of stimulation. Preliminary studies with this device suggest that it may be useful in the identification of subjects at high risk of neuropathic ulceration.[61]

Autonomic Function Testing

Noninvasive testing of autonomic nerve function is widely applied and most commonly assesses the cardiovascular reflexes (e.g., beat-to-beat variations, Valsalva maneuver); ideally, at least one test of sympathetic and parasympathetic systems should be used.[9,55] Detection of peripheral autonomic dysfunction involving the lower limb may help in the identification of the high risk foot.[62] Reduced or absent peripheral sweating, as measured by galvanic skin response, may help to identify those patients with an autosympathectomy.

MANAGEMENT OF CHRONIC SYMPTOMATIC DIABETIC PERIPHERAL POLYNEUROPATHY

An approach to the patient complaining of neuropathic symptoms in the lower limbs is summarized in this section and also in Tables 4-4 and 4-5. Particular attention should be paid in the history to the nature and mode of onset of symptoms. A careful enquiry should be made into any symptoms of peripheral vascular disease as it may sometimes be difficult to differentiate between vascular and neuropathic pain, and not infrequently they may coexist.[63] Most patients do not present problems with diagnosis as a patchy neurologic deficit is usually present with small muscle wasting in the foot together with reduced sensation in a stocking distribution and absent ankle reflexes. After other causes have been excluded (Table 4-4), the level of metabolic control should be assessed, with an aim to achieve optimal control in neuropathic patients. This does not necessarily mean insulin is required in all patients: there is no evidence to suggest that a patient with good glycemic control on oral hypoglycemic drugs would have less severe symptoms if transferred to insulin therapy. Although it is generally agreed that good control may alleviate symptoms in some patients, transient symptomatic deterioration may be experienced during this time.[7]

Table 4-4. Assessment of the Patient with Presumed Diabetic Neuropathy

1. Are the symptoms and signs consistent with the diagnosis?
   If not, exclude:
   - Unusual presentation of vascular disease
   - Lumbar root or cauda equina lesion
2. Exclude other causes of neuropathy
   Common alternative causes:
   - Malignant disease
   - Toxins (e.g., alcohol)
   - Metabolic (e.g., B_{12} deficiency)
   - Infections (e.g., AIDS)
   - Iatrogenic (e.g., vincristine, hydantoins)
3. Assess level of diabetic control
   - Blood glucose profiles
   - Glycosylated hemoglobin
4. Aim for optimal, stable metabolic control

Table 4-5. Drug Therapy of Symptomatic Neuropathy

Simple analgesics:
- Aspirin
- Acetaminophen
- Nonsteroidal anti-inflamatory drugs

Tricyclic drugs:
- Imipramine
- Amitriptyline
- Mianserin

Other medications:
- Phenytoin
- Carbamazepine
- Mexilitene
- Clonazepam

The majority of patients with symptomatic neuropathy will also require medications for symptomatic relief: those more commonly used are listed in Table 4-5. Although simple analgesics may help in some cases, the tricyclic drugs should be regarded as first line therapy for those who fail to obtain relief with analgesics.[7] The mode of action of the tricyclic drugs is peripheral rather than central, as suggested by the relatively rapid onset of action, and two controlled trials have confirmed their efficacy in diabetic neuropathy.[64,65] Other drugs that may be helpful include phenytoin, carbamazepine, clonazepam, and more recently proposed, mexilitene.[66]

Despite their popularity, there is no strong evidence that vitamin preparations are of benefit, whereas addictive drugs such as narcotic analgesics should be avoided for the management of diabetic neuropathy.

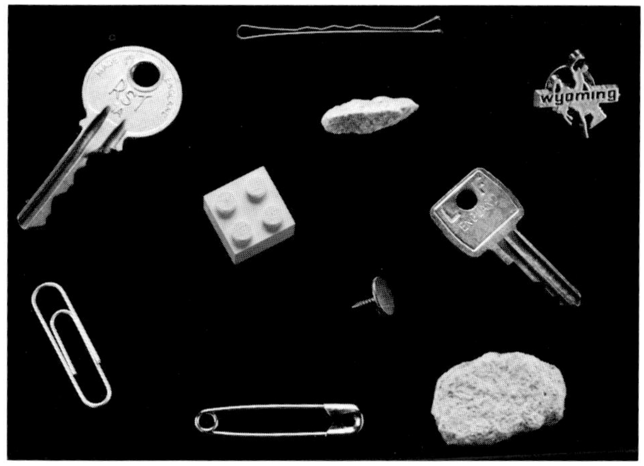

Fig. 4-3. Objects found in shoes of patients with diabetic neuropathy, the presence of which the patients were unaware.

IDENTIFICATION OF THE PATIENT AT RISK OF NEUROPATHIC FOOT ULCERATION

The aim of screening diabetic patients for foot problems is to identify those who are at greater risk of ulceration. Such patients can then receive specific education and more frequent follow-up in the hope of preventing the development of such ulcers. It is essential to recognize those with reduced sensation because education and regular reinforcement are so important in these patients, who need never develop ulcers. It is difficult for those of us with normal sensation to envisage what it is like to have insensitive feet, for pain is a protective sensation. It has therefore been suggested that such patients "reject" the insensitive part and that denial of the dangers of insensitivity is common.[67] The most significant contribution that health care professionals can make toward the reduction in the incidence of diabetic foot ulceration is to inspect our patients' feet when they attend the clinic— if we fail to do this once or twice a year, can we honestly expect our patients to do this on a daily basis?[6,67]

Although there is no direct proof that neuropathy can lead to foot ulcers, there is strong evidence from cross-sectional studies.[6] Any evidence of reduced sensation to pinprick or vibration on clinical examination or finding muscle wasting in the feet, dry skin, or thick callus would place the patient in the high risk category. Use of the Semmes-Weinstein monofilaments to quantify sensation may help in the identification of the high risk foot.[68] As stated above, use of other simple devices to quantify sensory loss, such as the biothesiometer for vibration testing,[59] may also help in the screening process. The degree of insensitivity that some patients may experience is demonstrated by the objects shown in Figure 4-3: all these were found in patients' shoes, although the patients themselves had been unaware of their presence.

In conclusion, two key facts should be remembered when trying to identify the at risk foot: first, the warm, insensitive foot is as much at risk of ulceration as the cold, ischemic foot, and second, any patient who walks without a limp but with a foot ulcer must have neuropathy even if the clinical examination is relatively normal.

ACKNOWLEDGMENT

The author is supported by the Wellcome Trust.

REFERENCES

1. II Chronicles XVI:12
2. Auche MB: Des alterations des nerfs peripheques chez les diabetiques. Arch Med Exper 2:635, 1890
3. Jordan WR: Neuritic manifestations in diabetes mellitus. Arch Int Med 57:307, 1936
4. Rundles RW: Diabetic neuropathy: general review with report of 125 cases. Medicine 24:111, 1945
5. Oakley W, Catterall RCF, Martin MM: Aetiology and management of lesions of the feet in diabetes. Br Med J 2:953, 1956
6. Boulton AJM: The diabetic foot. Med Clin North Am 72:1513, 1988
7. Boulton AJM, Ward JD: Diabetic neuropathies and pain. Clin Endocrinol Metab 15:917, 1986
8. Harati Y: Diabetic peripheral neuropathies. Ann Intern Med 107:546, 1987
9. Bays HE, Pfeifer MA: Peripheral diabetic neuropathy. Med Clin North Am 72:1439, 1988
10. Clements RS, Bell DSH: Diagnostic, pathogenetic and therapeutic aspects of diabetic neuropathy. Special topics. Endocrinol Metab 3:1, 1982
11. Brown MJ, Asbury AK: Diabetic neuropathy. Ann Neurol 15:2, 1984
12. Skillman TG, Johnson EW, Hamwi GJ, Driskill JH: Motor nerve conduction velocity in diabetes mellitus. Diabetes 10:46, 1961
13. Mulder DW, Lambert EH, Bastron JA, Sprague RG: The neuropathies associated with diabetes mellitus: a clinical and electromyographic study of 103 unselected patients. Neurology 11:275, 1961
14. Shahani B, Spalding JM: Diabetes mellitus presenting with bilateral foot drop. Lancet 2:930, 1969
15. Fraser DM, Campbell IW, Ewing DJ, Clarke BF. Mononeuropathy in diabetes mellitus. Diabetes 28:96, 1979
16. Ewing DJ, Clarke BF: Diabetic autonomic neuropathy: present insights and future prospects. Diabetes Care 9:648, 1986
17. Ozeran RS, Wagner GR, Reimer TR, Hill RA. Neuropathy of the sympathetic nervous system associated with diabetes mellitus. Surgery 68:953, 1970
18. Boulton AJM, Hardisty CA, Betts RP et al: Dynamic foot pressure and other studies as diagnostic and management aids in diabetic neuropathy. Diabetes Care 6:26, 1983
19. Partsch H: Neuropathies vom ulzero-mutilienden typ: klinik, klassifikation durchblutungsmerssungen. Vasa, suppl. 6:1, 1977
20. Boulton AJM, Scarpello JHB, Ward JD: Venous oxygenation in the diabetic neuropathic foot: evidence of arterio-venous shunting? Diabetologia 22:6, 1982
21. Edmonds ME, Roberts VC, Watkins PJ: Blood flow in the diabetic neuropathic foot. Diabetologia 22:9, 1982
22. Edmonds ME, Archer AG, Watkins PJ: Ephedrine: a new treatment for diabetic neuropathic oedema. Lancet 1:548, 1983
23. Bastron JA, Thomas JE: Diabetic polyradiculoneuropathy: clinical and electromyographic findings in 105 patients. Mayo Clin Proc 56:725, 1981
24. Asbury AK: Focal and multifocal neuropathies of diabetes. p. 48. In Dyck PJ et al (eds): Diabetic Neuropathy. WB Saunders, Philadelphia, 1987
25. Ellenberg M: Diabetic neuropathic cachexia. Diabetes 23:418, 1974
26. Casey EG, Harrison MJG: Diabetic amyotrophy: a follow-up study. Br Med J 1:656, 1972
27. Young RJ, Zhou YQ, Rodriguez E et al: Variable relationship between peripheral somatic and autonomic neuropathy in patients with different syndromes of diabetic polyneuropathy. Diabetes 35:192, 1986
28. Ward JD: The diabetic leg. Diabetologia 22:141, 1982
29. Boulton AJM, Knight G, Drury J, Ward JD: The prevalence of symptomatic diabetic neuropathy in an insulin-treated population. Diabetes Care 8:125, 1985
30. Mayne N: Neuropathy in the diabetic and non-diabetic population. Lancet 2:1313, 1965
31. Ziegler D, Cicmir I, Wiefels K, Berger H, Gries FA: Peripheral and autonomic nerve function in long-term insulin dependent diabetes. Diabetes Res 4:9, 1987
32. Ziegler D, Cicmir I, Mayer P, Wiefels K, Gries FA: Peripheral and autonomic nerve function in newly-diagnosed insulin-dependent diabetes. Transplant Proc 18:1593, 1986
33. Masson EA, Boulton AJM: Aldose reductase inhibitors in the treatment of diabetic neuropathy: a review of the rationale and clinical evidence. Drugs 39:190, 1990
34. Archer AG, Watkins PJ, Thomas PK et al: The natural history of acute painful neuropathy in diabetes. J Neurol Neurosurg Psychiatry 46:491, 1983
35. Young RJ, Ewing DJ, Clarke BF: Chronic and remitting painful diabetic neuropathy. Diabetes Care 11:34, 1988
36. Bischoff A: The natural course of diabetic neuropathy: a follow-up. Horm Metab Res, 9 suppl. 1, 9:98, 1980
37. Boulton AJM, Armstrong WD, Scarpello JHB, Ward JD: The natural history of painful diabetic neuropathy, a four year study. Postgrad Med J 59:556, 1983

38. Ewing DJ, Campbell IW, Clarke BF: The natural history of diabetic autonomic neuropathy. Q J Med 49:95, 1980
39. Page MB, Watkins PJ: Cardiorespiratory arrest and diabetic neuropathy. Lancet 1:7, 1978
40. Pirart J: Diabetes mellitus and its degenerative complications: a prospective study of 4400 patients between 1947 and 1973. Diabetes Care 1:168, 252, 1978
41. Boulton AJM, Worth RC, Drury J et al: Genetic and metabolic studies in diabetic neuropathy. Diabetologia 26:15, 1984
42. Greene DA, Latimer SA, Sima AAF: Sorbitol, phosphoinositides and sodium-potassium ATPase in the pathogenesis of diabetic complications. N Engl J Med 316:599, 1987
43. Gabbay KH, Merola LO, Field RA: Sorbitol pathway: presence in nerve and cord with substrate accumulation in diabetes. Science 151:209, 1966
44. Greene DA, Latimer SA: Action of sorbinil in diabetic peripheral nerve: relationship of polyol (sorbitol) pathway inhibition to a myo-inositol-mediated defect in sodium-potassium ATPase activity. Diabetes 33:712, 1984
45. Mayer JH, Tomlinson DR: Prevention of defects of axonal transport and nerve conduction velocity by oral administration of myo-inositol or an aldose reductase inhibitor in streptozotocin diabetic rats. Diabetologia 25:433, 1983
46. Sima AAF, Bril V, Nathaniel V et al: Regeneration and repair of myelinated fibres in sural nerve biopsy specimens from patients with diabetic neuropathy treated with Sorbinil. N Engl J Med 319:548, 1988
47. Zimerman BR: Current status of aldose reductase inhibitors (editorial). Diabetes Care 10:123, 1987
48. Low PA: Recent advances in the pathogenesis of diabetic neuropathy. Muscle Nerve 10:121, 1987
49. Dyck PJ: Hypoxic neuropathy: does hypoxia play a role in diabetic neuropathy? 39:111, 1989
50. Tuck RR, Schmelzer JD, Low PA: Endoneurial blood flow and oxygen tension in the sciatic nerves of rats with experimental diabetic neuropathy. Brain 107:935, 1984
51. Newrick PG, Wilson AJ, Jakubowski JJ et al: Sural nerve oxygen tension in diabetes. Br Med J 293:1093, 1986
52. Low PA, Schmelzer JD, Ward KK, Yao JK: Experimental chronic hypoxic neuropathy: relevance to diabetic neuropathy. Am J Physiol 250:E94, 1986
53. Masson EA, Church SE, Woodcock AA et al: Is resistance to ischaemic conduction failure induced by hypoxia? Diabetologia 31:762, 1988
54. Masson EA, Malik RA, Sharma AK et al: Aetiology of diabetic neuropathy—lessons from human hypoxia. In Ward JD (ed): Proceedings of the 13th International Diabetes Federation Satellite symposium on diabetic neuropathy. John Wiley & Sons, Chichester, 1990 (in press)
55. Consensus statement: report and recommendations of the San Antonio conference on diabetic neuropathy. Diabetes 37:1000, 1988
56. Dyck PJ, Sherman WR, Hallcher LM et al: Human diabetic endoneurial sorbitol, fructose and myo-inositol related to sural nerve morphometry. Ann Neurol 8:590, 1980
57. Masson EA, Gem J, Hunt L, Boulton AJM: A novel approach to the diagnosis and assessment of symptomatic diabetic neuropathy. Pain 38:25, 1989
58. Dyck PJ: Detection, characterization and staging of polyneuropathy assessed in diabetics. Muscle Nerve 11:21, 1988
59. Boulton AJM, Kubrusly D, Bowker JH et al: Impaired vibratory perception and diabetic foot ulceration. Diabetic Med 3:335, 1986
60. Dyck PJ, Karnes JL, Daube J et al: Clinical and neuropathologic criteria for the diagnosis and staging of diabetic polyneuropathy. Brain 108:861, 1985
61. Masson EA, Fernando DJS, Veves A, Boulton AJM: Current perception thresholds: a new, quick and reproducible method for the assessment of peripheral neuropathy in diabetes mellitus. Diabetologia 32:724, 1989
62. Ahmed ME, Delbridge L, Le Quesne LP: The role of autonomic neuropathy in diabetic foot ulceration. J Neurol Neurosurg Psychiatry 49:1002, 1986
63. Ward JD, Boulton AJM: Peripheral vascular abnormalities in diabetic neuropathy. p. 89. In Dyck PJ et al (eds): Diabetic Neuropathy. WB Saunders, Philadelphia, 1987
64. Kvinesdal BB, Molin J, Froland A, Gram LF: Imipramine treatment of painful diabetic neuropathy. JAMA 215:1727, 1984
65. Young RJ, Clarke BF: Pain relief in diabetic neuropathy: the effectiveness of imipramine and related drugs. Diabetic Med 2:262, 1985
66. Dejgard A, Petersen P, Kastrup J: Mexilitene for treatment of chronic painful diabetic neuropathy. Lancet 1:9, 1988
67. Brand PW: The diabetic foot. p. 829. In Ellenberg M, Rifkin H (eds): Diabetes Mellitus: Theory and Practice. Medical Examination Publishing, New York, 1983
68. Birke JA, Sims DS: Plantar sensory thresholds in the ulcerative foot. Lepr Rev 57:262, 1986

5

Evaluation of the Diabetic Foot and Leg

Lawrence B. Harkless, D.P.M.
Kevin R. Higgins, D.P.M.

Recognizing important risk factors and making a comprehensive assessment of the diabetic foot and leg requires a thorough and consistent diagnostic approach. Without such a method, the practitioner is more likely to overlook information critical to the limb viability and the treatment outcome. A useful evaluation of the diabetic foot and leg will involve identification of the contributory problems and assignment of relative risk. Only then can an effective treatment plan be designed and implemented. This chapter focuses on the clinical aspects of this evaluation.

PATIENT HISTORY

The first step, as always, is the development of a good patient history. Factors to be considered are diabetes control, wound healing, previous amputations and the events leading up to them, relevant symptoms, and patient orientation to the disease process as it relates to the lower extremities.

A background understanding of the patient and collation of prognostic indicators must take the patient's diabetes control into account. Current evidence suggests that the extent of peripheral neurovascular deficits are linked to glycemic control.[1–4] Some studies show that impaired wound healing in the presence of hyperglycemia can be improved with better glycemic control.[5–7] Rubenstein, Pierce, and Bloomgarden present two cases where restoration of tighter glycemic control through continuous subcutaneous insulin infusion dramatically affected the healing response.[8]

Most patients with diabetes are those with type 2, and it should be remembered that several years of uncontrolled disease often precedes the diagnosis.[9] A practitioner who is mindful of this fact will be less likely to perform a cursory examination, thereby missing significant findings in a patient with recently diagnosed diabetes. The misconception that the time of diagnosis coincides with the onset and duration of the disease can otherwise lower the physician's index of suspicion and increase the patient's overall risk.

Social habits of smoking and drinking must be discussed and quantified using the necessary tact. Each of these dramatically accelerates the respective vascular and neurologic disease processes.[10] Therefore, every attempt to encourage the patient to be open, nondefensive, and complete should be made. It is generally not acceptable to simply ask a patient if he or she smokes or drinks. Quite commonly a patient will state, "No, I don't smoke," while only further questioning will reveal a previous 40 pack-year history.

Perhaps the most practical information will be gleaned from a discussion of the patient's wound history. Attention to locations, recurrences, infections, hospitalizations, wound care, surgeries, accommodative measures, and the patient's responses to these treatments will prove crucial to establishing an accurate prognosis. The clinician should try to assess the efficacy of previous treatments and understand why each led to success or failure. A history of healing an ulcer or a distal amputation site in the vicinity of a new wound can be as important in quantifying viability and healing potential as a battery of diagnostic tests. This history cannot, however, cause the investigator to ignore the results of these tests, as new or progressive arterial lesions may have changed the clinical picture. On the other hand, a poor healing response in the past should not automatically be attributed to patient-related factors without first scrutinizing the past treatment plans, as well as the patient's understanding of and compliance with these plans. Questions that the physician might entertain could be as follows:

1. If an amputation was performed in the past, was a bypass necessary to achieve a successful level?
2. Were other modalities, such as hyperbaric oxygen therapy, required (or considered) to promote healing?
3. After surgery, did the patient alter social, work, or ambulation activities to preserve the amputation level and minimize complications?
4. Did the patient use a walker?
5. Did the patient obtain the appropriate shoes?
6. What sort of prosthesis was provided?
7. How frequent were the follow-up visits?
8. What level of diabetes teaching was involved in the patient's overall care?
9. Was the patient compliant? The answer to this last question is best found in the pattern of response to previous questions. The patient will usually have a perception of compliance and have a genuine desire to be a "good" patient but may have underestimated the importance of some of the treatment measures.

Particularly in cases with poor previous outcomes other factors such as death or illness in the family may have played important roles in the patient's ability to follow the treatment plan. Once these questions are asked the physician can begin to sort the volume of information that contributes to an accurate assessment of the patient's risk factors and the prognosis for healing and long-term limb salvage.

Special attention must be directed to the relevant symptoms of the patient's disease. Clues relating to ischemia, such as claudication cramps, should be identified if present. Care must be taken to distinguish the pains characteristic of ischemia from cramps caused by electrolytic imbalance or biomechanical fatigue. Generally, pain from claudication will dissipate in 3 to 5 minutes with the limb rested in a dependent position. Other cramps and pain of neuropathic origin will not fade as predictably. When suffering the pains of symptomatic neuropathy, the patient will usually relate radiating, shooting, or burning pains in one or both legs or the soles of the feet. The pains are usually most symptomatic at night and during periods of rest. The symptoms tend to subside during the day and with activity. They may, however, be constant and without pattern. If these symptoms are present, the patient often relates other supportive symptoms such as loss of lower extremity muscle strength or numbness in the feet. These diagnoses will usually be supported by physical findings correlating to the system involved.

Finally, a discussion of the patient's understanding of his or her diabetes and its impact on the lower extremities should take place. The patient's perception and how it is altered or improved by the physician will have tremendous effect on the treatment outcome.[11] Delbridge and associates found a significant difference when comparing education and understanding in patients with ulcerative foot disease to those without it. Patients without ulcers showed higher knowledge about diabetes and foot care.[12]

The physician should find out the following:

1. Does the patient or a well-sighted significant other examine the patient's feet daily? In our experience it is not rare for a patient to be brought into the clinic, in the care of the family,

several days after a puncture wound to a neuropathic foot. We commonly hear family members state that they were concerned by the appearance of blood on "grandpa's" (or grandma's) sock. Like many foot problems in diabetes, the timely viewing of the feet by someone other than the patient will tend to bring the patient more quickly to proper care.
2. Does the patient walk barefoot? Is the patient aware of risks such as insulin needle puncture that commonly take place in the "safety" of the home?
3. Does the patient inspect shoes before putting them on? Does the patient shake them to remove foreign objects?
4. Is the patient aware of some of the possible foot complications of diabetes?
5. Does the patient know what to look for when checking the feet?
6. When the patient identifies a possible problem, is the physician called immediately? Commonly, a patient with diabetes can recognize the presence of a problem, but usually the medical team is not alerted until the condition has become quite serious. The patient's perception of problem severity almost always lags well behind the actual clinical severity. The classic example of this is the pinch callus of the hallux that evolves into an ulceration. We often find that the patient will generally identify this as a serious condition and begin to experience significant pain only when the ulceration has reached the flexor tendon sheath or osteomyelitis has lead to engorgement of the toe.

Questions like these should help the practitioner to assess the patient's level of concern, education, and orientation regarding the disease process. If possible, the practitioner should also attempt to discern the level of understanding the patient's family has regarding diabetes and its potential effect on the extremities. Particularly for patients who may be unable to take complete care of themselves, the orientation of the family members can have substantial impact on the patient's outcome.

CLINICAL EXAMINATION

All patients with diabetes visiting the physician's office for either an initial or follow-up visit require a careful examination. The examination should be performed systematically so that important aspects are not overlooked. First, take a good look at the patient and his or her extremities (Fig. 5-1). Any obvious problem can then receive closer scrutiny with examination. In this overview make note of the patterns of color and texture changes in the feet and legs. Is there a brown pigmentation consistent with venous stasis hyperpigmentation about the ankles or dorsums of the feet? Are the soles and toes ruborous, pale, or normal in appearance? Are any toenails darkened, suggesting subungual hematoma? Look carefully for any asymmetries in the overall foot appearance. Is one foot swollen while the other is not? Does one have an arch while the other does not? Is one erythematous or cellulitic while the other is not? Are ulcerations present (Figs. 5-2 to 5-4)? Once this background assessment is accomplished a systematic examination can be performed.

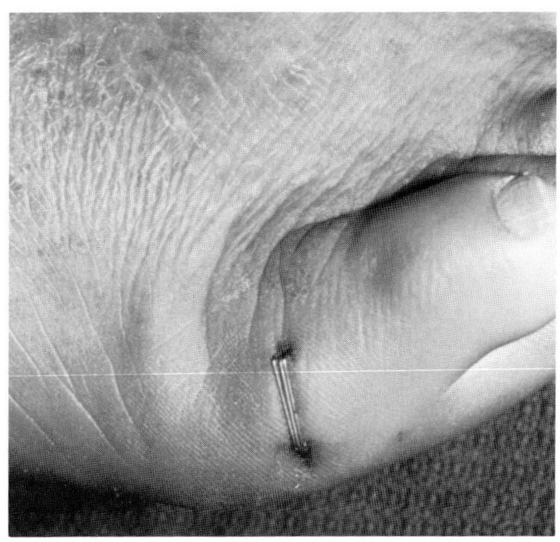

Fig. 5-1. Incidental finding of staples in the foot of this neuropathic patient highlights the importance of taking a good look at both feet.

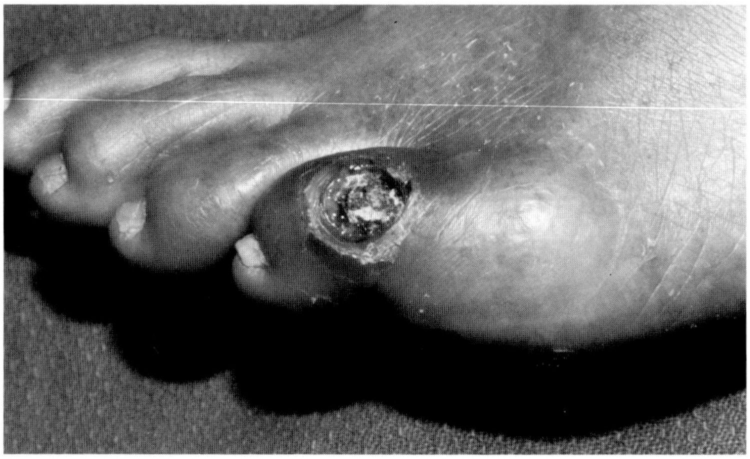

Fig. 5-2. Necrotic ulceration over prominent proximal interphalangeal joint of the fifth toe with purulence seeping from distal rim.

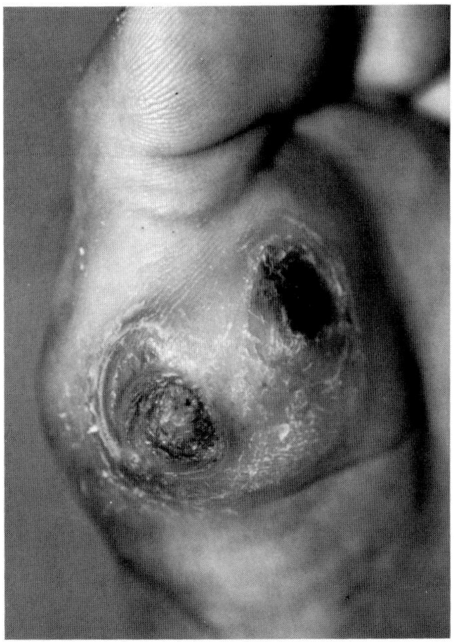

Fig. 5-3. Ulcerations beneath the first metatarsal head.

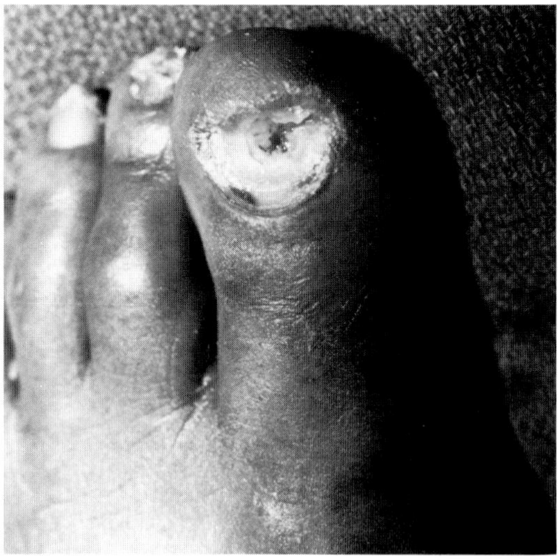

Fig. 5-4. Nail-bed ulceration.

VASCULAR EXAMINATION

Beginning with the vascular examination, an attempt should be made to answer questions about the patient's extremity health that may have arisen from the foregoing visual examination. Is the ruborous appearance of the toes and soles a result of congestion from diminished arterial flow or from impaired venous return? Look at and feel the texture of the skin in the feet and legs. The functional efficiency of the blood supply is usually manifested in the quality of this end organ (Figs. 5-5 and 5-6). Make note of the temperature gradient, any skin atrophy, color changes, abnormal wrinkling, diminished pedal hair, or nail changes that might be attributable to arterial insufficiency. Atrophy in the subcutaneous tissue layer often gives the overlying skin a "baked-potato skin" feel due to the diminution of underlying support.

After making note of the level of functional impairment that is clinically evident in the skin and subcutaneous tissues, palpate the pedal and extremity pulses, including the popliteal pulses on a routine basis. The pulses should be palpated using the "pulps" of the fingers and not the sharp nail ends of the fingers. Best results are obtained using several fingertips from both hands placed gently over the course of the vessel in an interlocking fashion. If there is evidence of impairment at any of these levels, the femoral, iliac, and abdominal aorta should also be palpated. The subpapillary venous plexus filling time, venous filling time, and temperature gradient should be assessed. Assessment of the subpapillary venous plexus filling time is really an attempt to quickly assess capillary bed filling from the arteriolar blood supply. The feet should be slightly elevated to remove the venous reflux component. Fingertip pressure is then used to "blanche" the toe pulps. The time to return of normal color is then counted in seconds. Three seconds or less may be considered the normal range while greater time periods are considered "delayed."

Calculation of venous filling time is accomplished by first marking or identifying a prominent

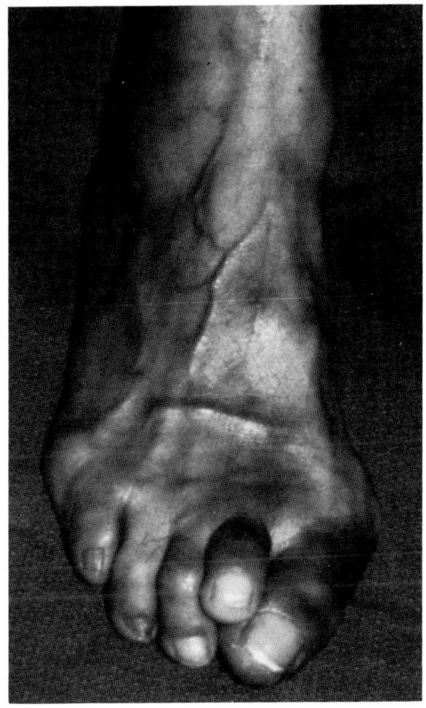

Fig. 5-6. Prominent dorsal veins that may correspond to arteriovenous shunting.

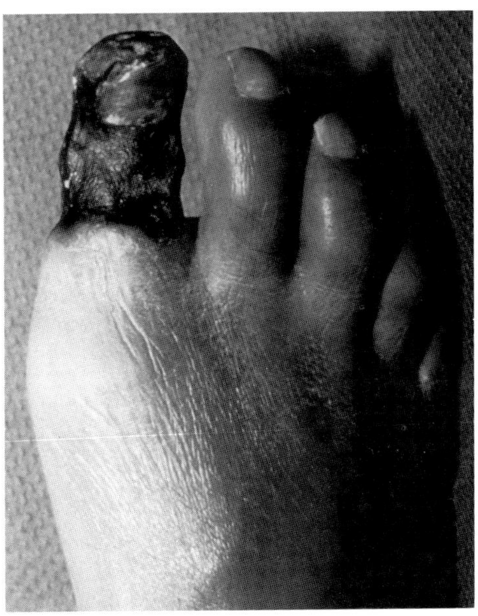

Fig. 5-5. Necrotic hallux that evolved following "trivial" trauma to an unprotected foot.

pedal vein such as the great saphenous or one of the marginal branches while the leg is dependent. The extremity is then elevated above the heart for exsanguination. When returned directly to the dependent position and observed, veins with competent valvular structure will fill in 10 to 20 seconds while those that fill rapidly may be consistent with valvular incompetency.

The temperature gradient is checked by using the backs of the hands and gently moving them from the pretibial region of the leg distally over the dorsum of the feet to the toes while keeping in contact with the patient's skin. Of course, a temperature probe is a more objective measure, but the hands are sensitive tools and may be more practical in sorting out "gross" pathology. A temperature difference of 10°F can be normal (warm-cool) but more than this could be consistent with ischemia. An asymmetric gradient may indicate either unilateral ischemia on the colder side or unilateral inflammatory response (such as Charcot joint or infection) on the warmer side. If an ulcer is present, the appearance of the ulcer base should be checked. Ischemic wounds are characterized by an appearance of irregular borders, necrotic base, tenderness with examination, and a location that may correlate better with an event of trivial trauma than with a neuropathic location. For all extremity wounds in diabetes the location is particularly important and usually correlates well with the underlying cause. Abnormal findings in these areas or the presence of an ulceration are indications for further workup and vascular consultation.

The most readily available and productive information can be gleaned from a thorough Doppler examination, which includes digital photoplethysmography (PPG), with calculation of the digital systolic blood pressure (SBP), Doppler analysis of the pulses with calculation of the ankle-brachial indices, segmental pressures, and venous examination (Figs. 5-7 to 5-11).[13] Historically, the ankle-brachial indices have served a dominant role in predicting amputation healing in diabetes.[14,15] Gibbon's group, however, urged closer attention to clinical judgment in preference to the use of segmental systolic measurements.[16] More current

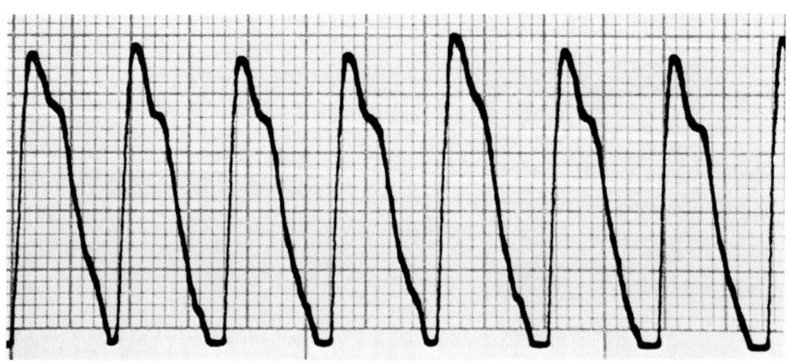

Fig. 5-7. Photoplethysmograph showing good perfusion.

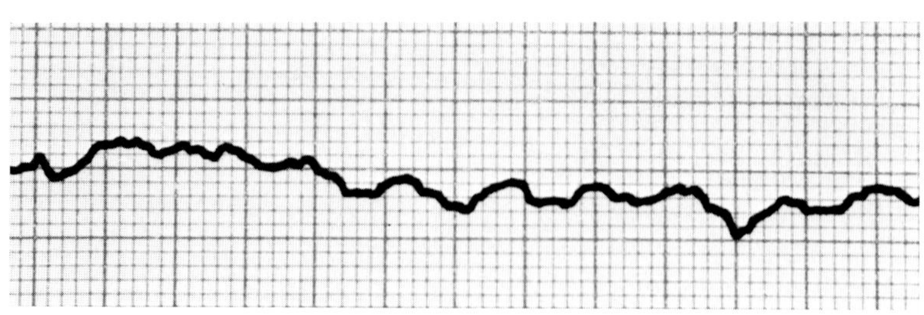

Fig. 5-8. Photoplethysmograph showing poor perfusion.

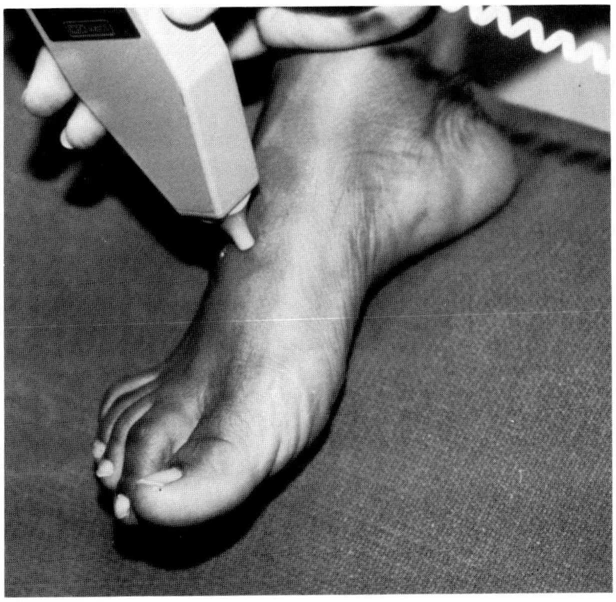

Fig. 5-9. Doppler unit.

methods using the digital SBP and transcutaneous oxygen appear to be gaining more favor. Bone and Pomajzl reported their results comparing the predictive value of digital systolic pressure to the ankle systolic pressure in 27 patients who underwent 30 forefoot amputations.[17] The digital pressure was measured with PPG placed distal to an occluding digital cuff. Ankle pressures were obtained with the Doppler and ankle cuff. The Doppler values for the ankle level of perfusion were not found to be significantly different when comparing wounds that healed primarily to those that did not. The value of toe pressures among those that healed, 86 ± 39 mmHg, were significantly greater than those that did not heal, 25 ± 18 mmHg. It was also a consistent finding that failure to heal occurred in all eight limbs with toe pressures less than 45 mmHg.

Barnes and co-workers found that the presence of digital pulsation with PPG correlated better with healing than did ankle systolic pressures and that

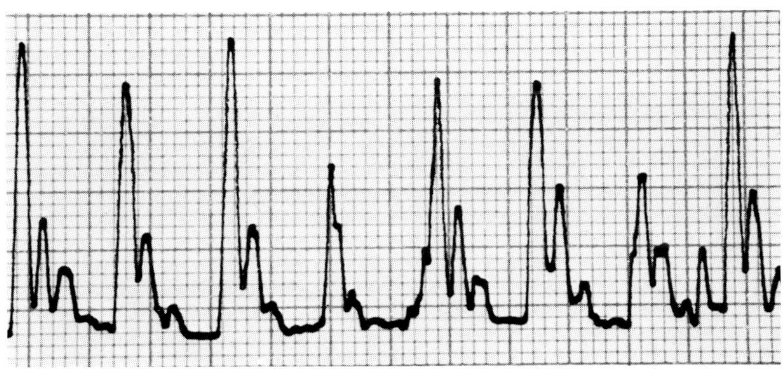

Fig. 5-10. Dorsalis pedis Doppler pulse waveform demonstrating patency and elasticity.

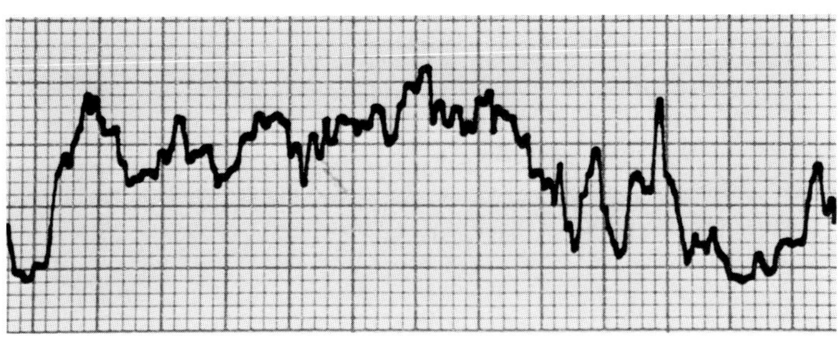

Fig. 5-11. Doppler waveform demonstrating poor flow.

limb segmental pressures could be misleading in predicting healing.[18] Holstein's work also identified and reaffirmed the higher level of distal healing predictability of digital SBPs compared to ankle Doppler pressures.[19] In his group, healing was most likely with toe pressures above 30 mmHg. Apelqvist and co-workers examined the roles of systolic ankle and toe blood pressure levels in predicting healing outcomes for ulcers rather than amputations.[20] They found that no patient in their group healed with an ankle pressure less than 40 mmHg. Primary healing occurred in 85 percent of those with a toe pressure level above 45 mmHg. They found a combination of these methods to be useful in predicting primary healing of diabetic foot ulcers.

Transcutaneous oxygen measurements, when taken in a controlled setting, can prove a useful overall predictor of healing (Figs. 5-12 to 5-14). Transcutaneous oxygen tension measurements may provide better predictability and correlation of prognostic factors than the other noninvasive methods of evaluating diabetic limbs at risk.[21,22] The sensors are placed on the involved foot and at the subclavicular or precordial chest region. Hauser and associates found values of 62 to 68 mmHg for the supine normal foot (or 90 to 92 percent of chest value), 36 to 44 with claudication, 14 to 22 with rest pain, and 12 to 18 with Frank gangrene.[21] The values of pedal and chest measurements can be related with the regional perfusion index (RPI), which is calculated as the ratio of foot transcutaneous oxygen pressure ($tcPO_2$)/chest $tcPO_2 \times 100$ in the supine, standing, and leg-elevated positions. This method provides more accurate comparison. Limbs with compromised perfusion will show more dramatic changes with measurements taken in the elevated, supine, and dependent positions. Bongard and Krahenbuhl found that patients whose $tcPO_2$ changed less than 10 mmHg when inhaling 100 percent oxygen were at the highest risk for impending amputation.[22] In their group, the digital SBP also proved to be a useful indicator where no patient with a digital SBP above 30 mmHg required amputation.

Oishi and associates found transcutaneous oxy-

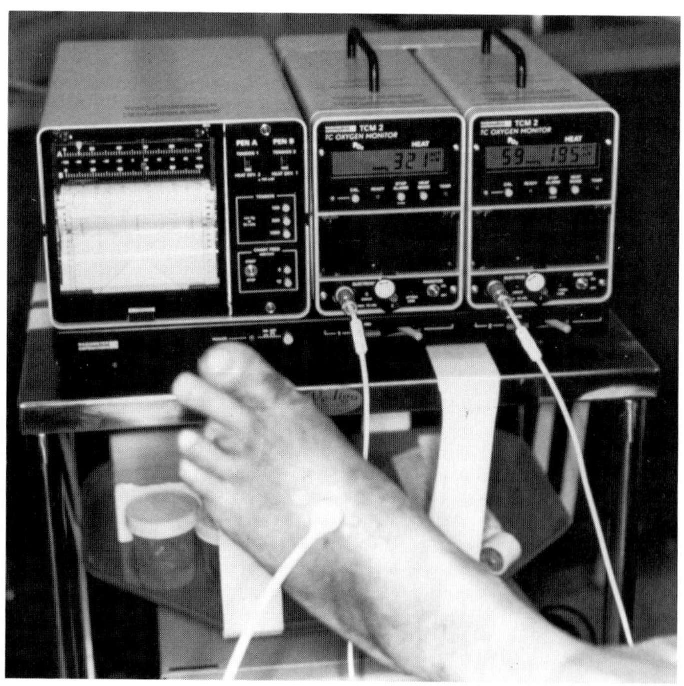

Fig. 5-12. Transcutaneous oxygen monitor.

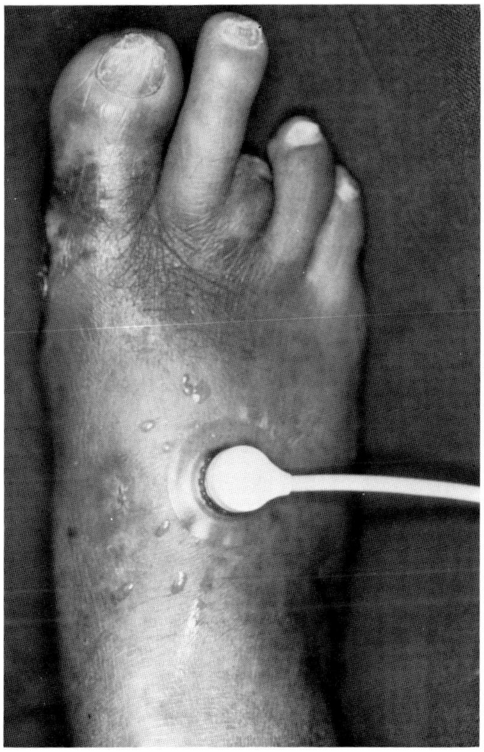

Fig. 5-13. Placement of pedal transcutaneous oxygen probe.

gen measurements more accurate in predicting amputation healing than either Doppler methods or skin temperature evaluation in their group of 80 patients who underwent 90 amputations. When the initial $tcPO_2$ value rose 10 mmHg or more with inhalation of oxygen, it predicted healing of the amputation stump with a sensitivity of 98 percent.[23]

In the course of the workup and treatment, further vascular evaluation provided by a vascular surgeon, such as arteriography, will play a role in evaluating the patient's candidacy for arterial bypass grafting should this consideration arise. Owing to the more recent availability of microvascular grafting, these radiographic findings may not absolutely eliminate the patient's candidacy for arterial bypass grafting as an attempt at limb salvage.

NEUROLOGIC EXAMINATION

Of equal importance to the vascular assessment is the neurologic examination. The role of neuropathy in mediating diabetes-related foot pathology cannot be overstated. It has been our experience that neuropathy is the dominant underlying feature of the high risk diabetic foot lesions that pre-

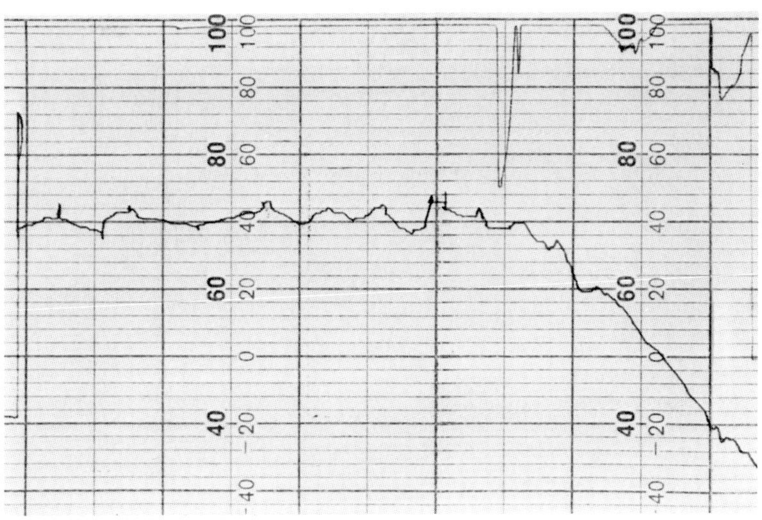

Fig. 5-14. Transcutaneous oxygen graphic recording. Left portion of the graph represents stable reading while right portion with slope is equilibrating.

dominate in the forefoot pressure areas either related to weight-bearing stress or external pressure (e.g., from shoes at the toe box or from the bed in the case of decubiti about the heels). These relationships are well documented.[24-26] In their excellent review, Bays and Pfeifer describe the prevalence of diabetic neuropathy to be as high as 62 percent if defined by subjective complaints, 55 percent if based on signs, and 100 percent if based on motor conduction velocities.[27] They note that prevalence of progressive involvement may be a cumulative 8 percent a year from the time of diagnosis. At diagnosis, measurable autonomic involvement may be 17 to 60 percent.

Too often we think of this as an all or none entity: "Are your feet numb? No? Then you must be okay." However, most patients have a level of neuropathy difficult to elicit with close examination and commonly normal results of peripheral nerve studies. The San Antonio conference on diabetic neuropathy recognized that normal results in electrodiagnostic testing do not rule out neuropathy.[28] The conference suggested that consistent identification and classification of diabetic neuropathy is more likely with a combination of measures, including clinical symptoms, clinical examination, electrodiagnostic studies, quantitative sensory testing (vibration, thermoreception, and nociception), and autonomic function testing (heart rate and blood pressure responses to stimuli). The need for broad testing to accurately quantify diabetes-related neuropathy likely relates to variables including but not limited to age, duration of diabetes, glycemic control, and type of nerve fiber involvement. These factors tend to make consistent research and clinical diagnosis difficult. Performing a battery of nerve tests on each patient may not prove to be time-efficient either. Some authors are attempting to use tests such as the current perception threshold (CPT) to map diabetes sensory deficits ordinarily quantified with a combination of subjective assessment and physical tests. Rendell and associates' work using this constant sine wave-alternating current suggests that this is a useful technique and may approach the accuracy of a combination of measures.[29]

We must always remember that many diabetes-related problems evolve in an incremental (low pressure over long periods of time), insidious fashion. The types of stresses involved would generally not bother normal sensate persons either, at least over short periods of time. Pressure-related ulcers require only a greater tolerance of a bothersome pressure to persist for a few weeks or months to evolve. It is especially important therefore to be meticulous in the neurologic examination and to identify subtle deficits where they exist.

Above and beyond elaborate neurologic tests, the practitioner should not fail to identify obvious signs of neurologic deficit when evident on inspec-

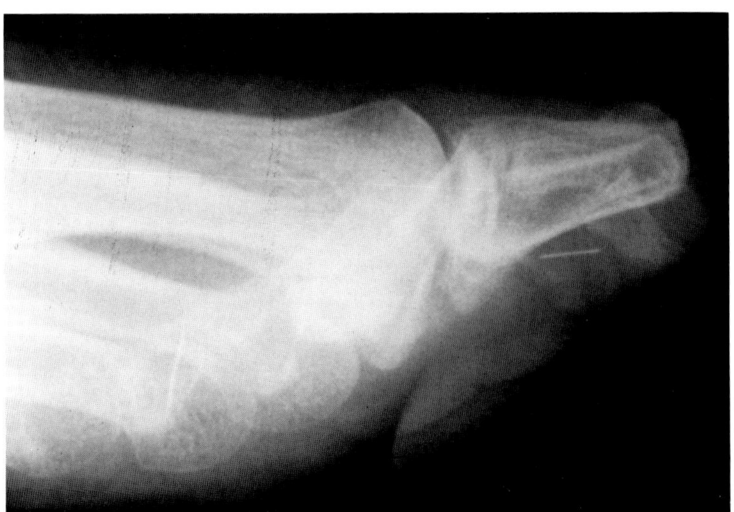

Fig. 5-15. Lateral radiograph with incidental finding of insulin needles.

tion (Fig. 5-15). If the patient has any findings, including an intrinsic minus foot,[30] multiple subungual hematomas without a direct traumatic cause, hemorrhage within calluses or corns, plantar forefoot ulcerations, decubitus heel ulcerations, ulceration over a bony prominence, or a foot deformity suggestive of neuroarthropathy, then the patient is likely to be neuropathic, regardless of the test results. The physician should not be above suspecting that an anhydrous foot with or without fissures may be caused by sweat gland atrophy as a result of autonomic neuropathy (Figs. 5-16 to 5-22). Clearly, if a patient is so neuropathic as to tolerate shoe pressure on fungal nails long enough to manifest subungual hematoma or to evolve a painless ulceration, then that patient is neuropathic enough to tolerate these conditions until the limb is severely threatened. The examiner should always ask him or herself, "What would my foot feel like if it looked this way? Could I possibly tolerate this condition this long?" Hemorrhage within calluses or corns will generally be found with either the neuropathic patient or a very stoic person. People with pressure-callused areas who have normal sensation will always effect some activity or footwear change long before bleeding occurs at the dermal level. A person who does not make these adjustments is at definite risk.

On the other hand, the presence of pain about a lesion should not cause the practitioner to overlook the underlying neuropathic cause. It should always be remembered that once an ulceration has occurred, the ensuing progression, which is often accompanied by infection, will likely involve an inflammatory response that will surpass the patient's elevated pain (or protective sensory) threshold. Ulceration of a purely ischemic cause will tend to be more painful earlier in the course. It may be helpful for the physician to note that if a known neuropathic patient presents in pain, immediate considerations should include a new ischemic event, progression of Charcot's arthropathy, infection, or a combination of these possibilities.

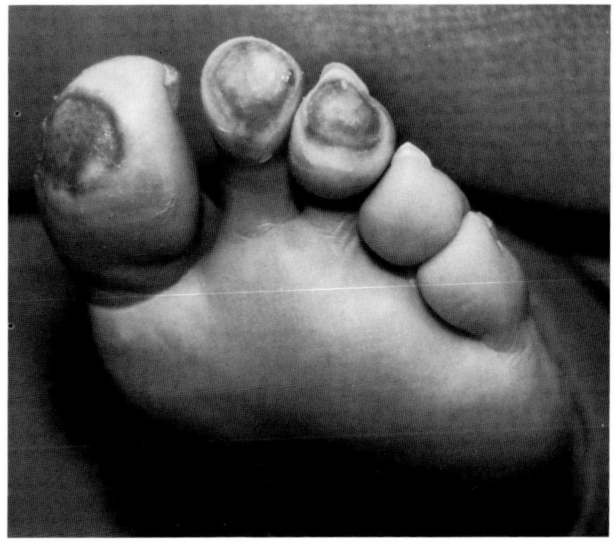

Fig. 5-17. Ulcerations secondary to burns sustained when this neuropathic patient attempted to warm the foot in close proximity to the radiator.

In their staging of diabetic polyneuropathy,

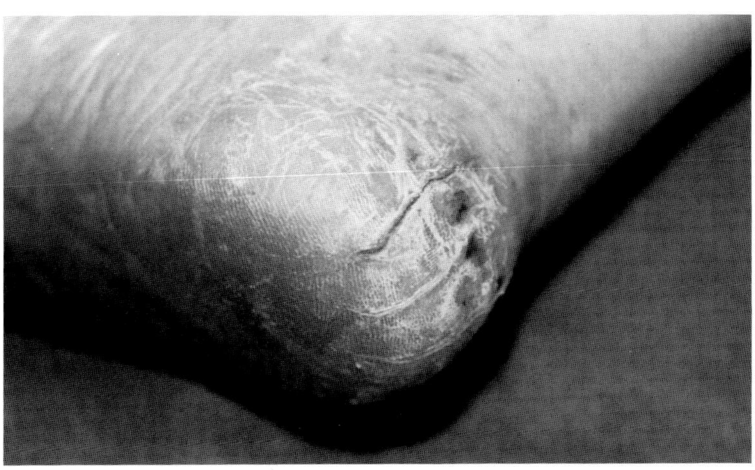

Fig. 5-16. Dry, fissured skin of the posterior heel consistent with anhidrosis of autonomic neuropathy.

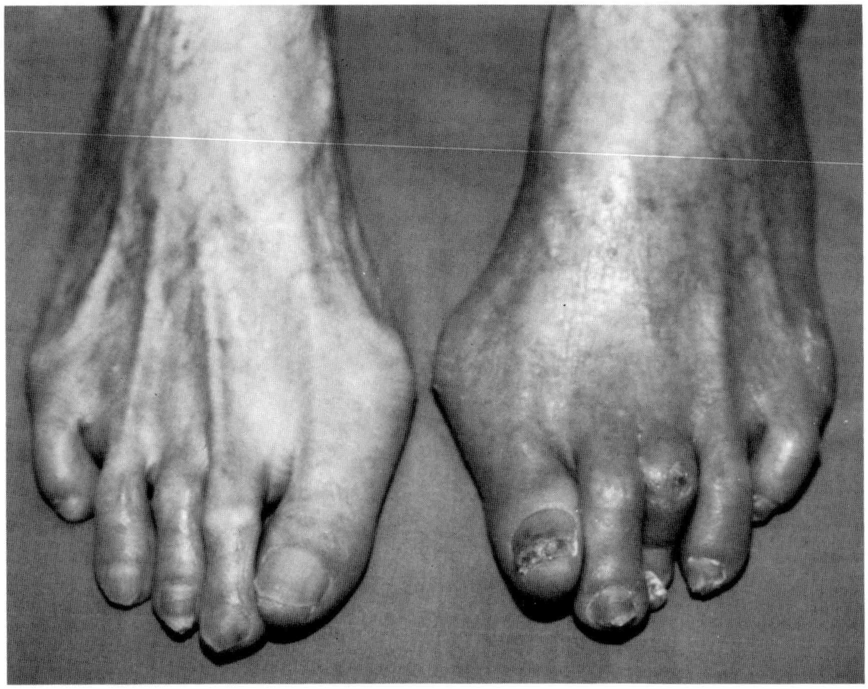

Fig. 5-18. Classic intrinsic minus foot appearance of neuropathy with digital contractures, intrinsic muscle wasting, and prominent appearance of long extensor tendons.

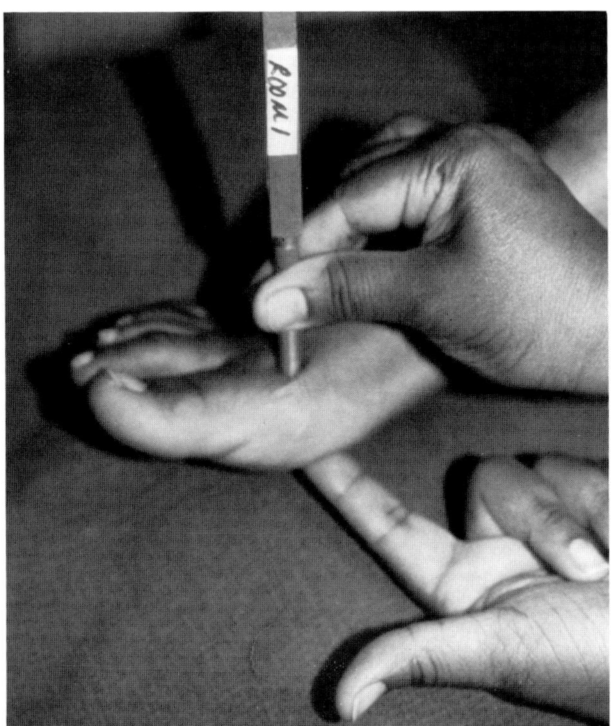

Fig. 5-19. Use of the tuning fork.

Dyck and co-workers found vibratory sense to be more sensitive than touch-pressure or thermal cooling.[31] Abnormalities of nerve conduction were sensitive and reliable with velocity most frequently abnormal, followed by F-wave latency and amplitude. (F-wave nerve conduction involves stimulation of distal efferent motor fibers resulting in antidromic impulses. These enter the spinal cord and return by the normal efferent pathway. The difference between stimulation and return of the impulse is known as the F-wave latency.[32])

When using electrodiagnosis to evaluate diabetic neuropathy, nerve conduction velocity studies will best identify large fiber sensory and motor pathology (skeletal motor, vibratory, skeletal muscle sensory, and proprioceptive) while electromyography will help assess large fiber motor function involvement.[32]

Quantitative sensory testing is the testing of large fiber function with methods such as vibratory perception or small fiber function with thermal and tactile perception thresholds. Steiness advocated the use of a biothesiometer, an electrical vibrating machine set within the range of maximum sensitiv-

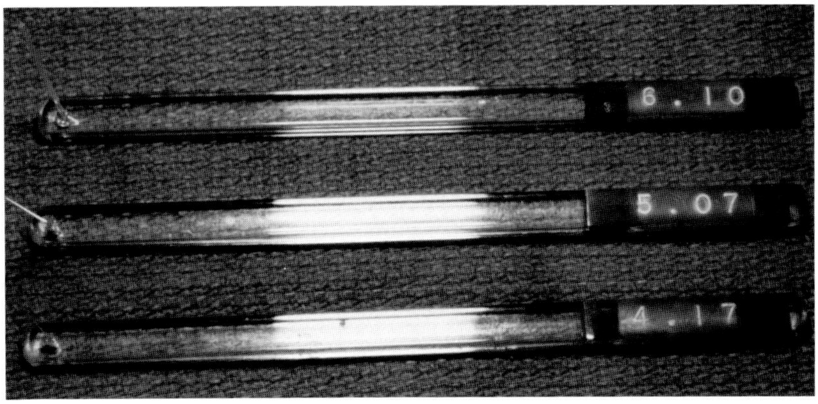

Fig. 5-20. Semmes-Weinstein monofilaments.

ity (100 to 600 cycles per second), for better reproducibility in vibratory examination.[33] His recommendations are well taken; however, we find that in a busy clinical setting and certainly in preference to no assessment at all, the tuning fork can provide meaningful information especially with repetitive experience by the same examiner. Used this way, impairment is considered when the patient perceives the vibratory end point 10 seconds or more before the examiner's perceived end point. The examination is most useful at the functional level (metatarsophalangeal joints) and should measure both the first and fifth bilaterally. While quantifying this test remains one of the continued difficulties in consistently diagnosing and staging diabetic neuropathy, vibratory threshold abnormalities are likely more sensitive than cooling detection thresholds (although whether this is due to a higher prevalence to large diameter efference fiber disease or not remains unclear).[34]

Sophisticated methods for evaluation of touch-pressure and thermal cutaneous sensation have been recommended[35] but may not be practical. On the other hand, Semmes-Weinstein monofilaments are easy to use, highly predictable,[36] and provide meaningful clinical assessment of ulcerative risk.[37] Birke and Sims identified the lowest threshold sur-

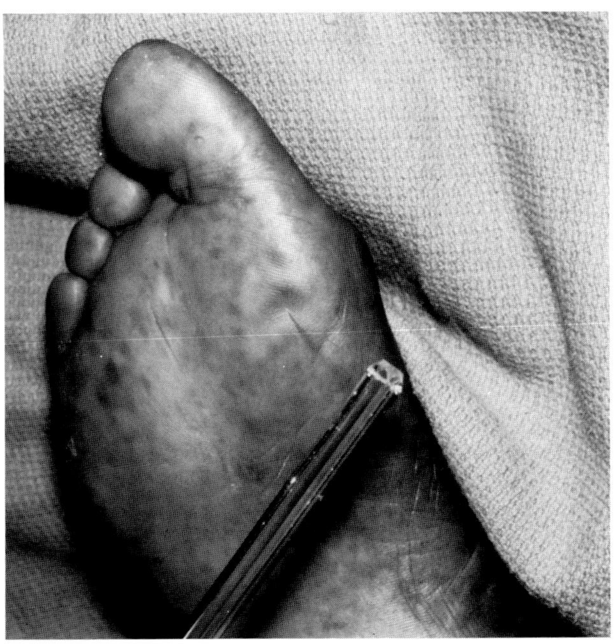

Fig. 5-21. Use of the Semmes-Weinstein monofilaments.

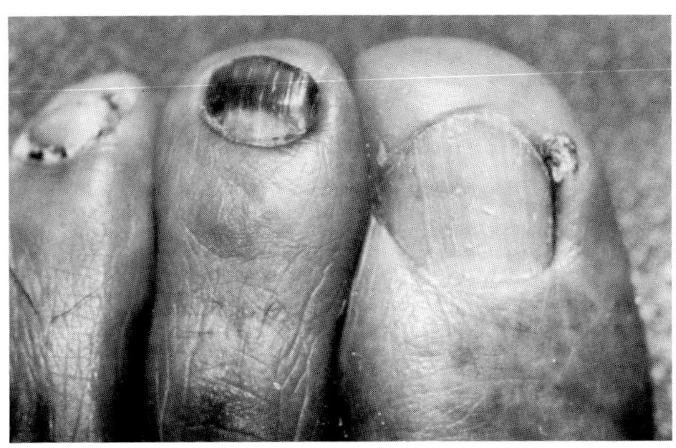

Fig. 5-22. Subungual hematoma of the second toe.

rounding an ulcer site with the 6.10 filament.[37] They suggested that patients who can perceive the 5.07 filament have enough protective sensation to be unlikely to sustain major foot injuries. The filaments, which are made of nylon of increasing diameter (1.65 to 6.65) set at right angles into acrylic rods, are applied to a force that just buckles the nylon filament. Patients are asked to respond as to whether they perceive the touch and must demonstrate fair accuracy in their perception.

When performing the objective neurologic examination, the most predictive identification or risk will likely result when two or more measures are combined.

MUSCULOSKELETAL EXAMINATION

While performing the musculoskeletal examination, as with other examinations, as much information as possible should be obtained by an overview of the foot and the attitude of the lower limb. In static examination look for relationships that tie into previous findings, such as sub-first metatarsal head ulceration, an anterior equinus foot type, or medial hallux ulceration with hallux abductus interphalangeus deformity. Overt unilateral Lisfranc or other pedal deformity of the rearfoot should be examined with an eye toward the probability of neuroarthropathy. Unilateral pedal temperature increase, especially in the absence of ulceration and even without associated symptoms, is best presumed neuroarthropathy until proven otherwise. Thermography may help to identify soft-tissue inflammation early at plantar pressure areas of high risk, may help identify evolving arthropathy, or allow improved follow-up on the resolution of these conditions.[38] An assessment of the clinical severity of this entity can be made by coupling the patient's perceived history of the deformity and the patient's treatment of it with the local findings. All pedal deformities, including hammer toe contractures and areas of bony prominence, should be noted. Then an assessment of the patient's muscle power using a standardized grading system can be made with both static and gait examinations. A gross evaluation can be made by first asking the patient to walk on the heels and then on the toes for respective evaluation of the dorsiflexors and plantar flexors at the ankle. Each foot should then be examined separately, muscle group by muscle group. It is best to allow the patient to use the group actively before resisting the muscle force. This allows the examiner to see how that muscle group works in relation to gravity without further stress.

Duckworth and co-workers found that sophisticated measures of dynamic force such as obtained with the pedobarograph are useful and may even identify high risk areas missed by clinical judgment.[39] The practicality and usefulness of these approaches may, however, be best limited to patients who have demonstrated risk, such as vibratory deficit. Use of the Harris mat appears to be a valid method of pressure assessment, particularly at the higher pressures associated with increased risk.[40] Although it may lack some of the precision of the pedobarograph, it has more practical availability to wider use in the clinical setting.

In addition to established patterns of diabetic foot deformity (such as intrinsic muscular wasting and progressive forefoot contracture associated with higher risk),[30] other phenomena, such as the limited joint mobility believed related to progressive soft-tissue glycosylation, may also be considered.[41] This entity is described as a painless stiffening beginning in the smaller joints, possibly preceded by a waxy, scleroderma-like skin hypertrophy. Musculoskeletal processes such as fibromatosis should also be looked for, as they may have a higher incidence in the diabetic population.

The musculoskeletal portion of the examination is not complete without firm palpation examination of the sole of the foot. Although it may only reveal a plantar fascial inflammation, in the presence of ulceration and possible infection it is a very useful indicator of deep plantar space involvement.

DERMATOLOGIC EXAMINATION

The dermatologic examination will mirror the findings from other systems and in this way serves as a reminder that the isolated findings from any of the systems should be related to the others and to the patient as a whole. Only after looking between the toes, observing all nail beds, and examining all surfaces of the feet and legs with good lighting can a more detailed dermatologic examination begin. Too often a physician examining an obvious toe ulceration (such as in a hospitalized patient in the supine position) will neglect the developing decubitus heel ulceration. Ulcer assessment should include documentation of location, depth, diameters, odor, drainage, quality of tissue in the wound, quality of peripheral tissues, and local inflammatory response. The wound examination is not complete until careful probing for sinus tracts has been made. Commonly, beefy red-appearing ulcerations will hide a deep sinus tract leading to an abscess.

Thickened, mycotic, hypertrophic nails, paronychia, tinea pedis, web-space maceration, xerosis and scaling, fissuring, corns, calluses, ulcers, shin spots (diabetic dermopathy), xanthochromia, and necrobiosis lipoidica diabeticorum (NLD) are the more common skin lesions of diabetes. Shin spots are very common, of debated origin, and benign in their course whereas NLD may be considered a rare phenomenon.[42] Neither is limited to the diabetic population. The lesions of NLD predispose to the lower extremities, tend to be bilateral, and evolve to ulceration about one-third of the time. They are characterized as well-circumscribed red papules that extend radially with waxy, atrophic, telangiectatic centers. The round or oval macular hyperpigmented lesions of diabetic dermopathy are usually found in the anterior tibial region and have been produced by experimental trauma.[43]

Fungal infections of the toenails are the most common skin condition affecting the diabetic patient. In the nondiabetic patient, fungus is most commonly seen with hyperhidrosis or nail trauma. A subungual hematoma that goes undrained, untreated, or without avulsion will often serve as an excellent medium for fungus and often results in a mycotic, hypertrophic nail. The etiology of fungal nails in diabetes is unclear; however, diabetic neuropathy may predispose to subungual hemorrhage increasing the chance of fungal infections. Diabetic vascular disease works in conjunction with diabetic neuropathy and immunopathy by decreasing the patient's intrinsic ability to combat infection. The fungus usually invades the nail bed and lifts the nail plate dorsally causing onycholysis. The hallux is the most common nail affected. It will generally start in one corner, and over a period of years it will spread to involve the entire toenail as well as the lesser toes. As the nail thickens the pressure from the shoe gear will increase and in the trophic foot may lead to subungual hematoma and even ulceration.

Paronychia is another common infection of the nail. This is usually associated with a nail that has a convexed nail bed with tendency to incurvate in the corners. Repetitive pressure in the insensitive foot can cause repetitive microtrauma in the nail groove, therefore causing the nail to act as a foreign body, creating a foreign body inflammatory response with secondary inflammation and localized infection. With aggressive diagnosis and treatment, the prevention of sequella such as possible osteomyelitis and amputation is more likely. If the circulation is adequate, a partial matrixectomy of the involved ingrown border or a total matrixectomy of the hallux nail are excellent procedures. These should prevent the recurrence of this particular problem, especially in the patient who is noncompliant or unable to come in for routine diabetic foot care every 2 months.

The lower extremity examination is not complete without an evaluation of the patient's footwear. The practitioner should note if the footwear accommodates existing deformities, provides protection from plantar puncture, and compensates for loss of propulsion if needed. Existing inlays should be fabricated so as to occupy any space left from previous digital amputation. Holstein and coworkers found accommodative insoles such as Plastazote to be helpful in the healing of 37 of 38 neuropathic ulcers.[44] Plastazote and Spenco have been suggested to be superior to other materials used for this purpose.[45] We find that materials that contour the sole of the foot, such as heat-molded Plastazote, are most effective. Even protective hosiery may prove to be of benefit in reducing risk, especially when used in conjunction with conventional methods.[46]

Attention to shoe wear patterns will give important clues to the patient's biomechanical function and may suggest areas of high pressure and risk. The shoes should be examined for lining wear, areas that may prove irritating and warrant replacement (Fig. 5-23). Any foreign bodies potentially present in the shoes should be identified and removed.

Evaluation of the diabetic foot and leg is more than the summary of the component examinations suggested herein. In a practical sense this evalua-

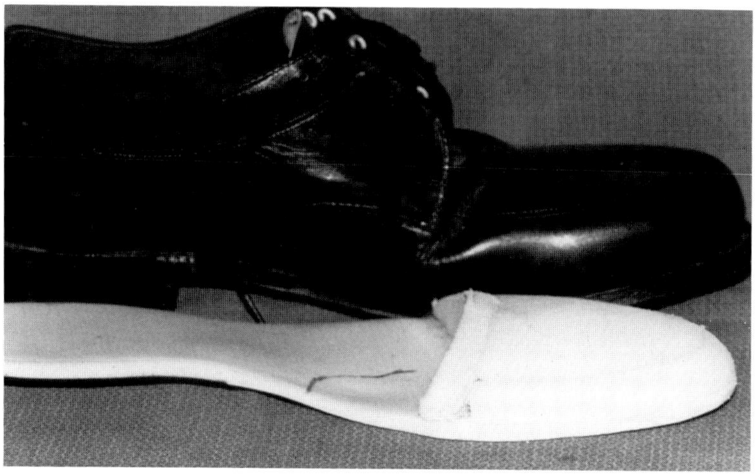

Fig. 5-23. Leather shoe with Plastazote inlay and toe filler.

tion is really an assessment of the patient's risk for extremity complications. The patient with no overt clinical pathology but lacking the necessary visual acuity to give him or herself a daily foot examination represents a patient at risk. The same is true for patients in poor diabetic control, those who live alone, those who do not have an understanding of at least some of the disease processes, or those who do not perceive themselves to be at risk. Assignment of the extremity risk therefore is a complex clinical summary of the patient's condition including factors beyond the extremities.

REFERENCES

1. Winegrad AI, Simmons DA, Martin DB: Has one diabetic complication been explained? N Engl J Med 303:152, 1983
2. Harati Y: Diabetic peripheral neuropathies. Ann Intern Med 107:546, 1987
3. Young RJ, Macintryre CCA, Martyn CN et al: Progression of subclinical polyneuropathy in young patients with type I (insulin-dependent) diabetes: associations with glycemic control and microangiopathy (microvascular complications). Diabetologia 29:156, 1986
4. Pirart J: Diabetes mellitus and its degenerative complications: a prospective study of 4,400 patients observed between 1947 and 1978. Diabetes Care 1:168, 1978
5. Goodson WH III, Hunt TK: Wound healing and the diabetic patient. Surg Gynecol Obstet 149:600, 1979
6. Gottrup F, Andreassen TT: Healing of incisional wounds in stomach and duodenum: the influence of experimental diabetes. J Surg Res 31:61, 1981
7. Taitelman U, Reece EA, Bessman AN: Insulin in the management of the diabetic surgical patient, continuous infusion vs. subcutaneous administration. JAMA 237:658, 1977
8. Rubenstein A, Pierce CE, Bloomgarden Z: Rapid healing of diabetic foot ulcers with continuous subcutaneous insulin perfusion. Am J Med 75:161, 1983
9. Bild DE, Selby JV, Sinnock P et al: Lower-extremity amputation in people with diabetes: epidemiology and prevention. Diabetes Care 12:27, 1989
10. Lithner F: Is tobacco of importance for the development and progression of diabetic vascular complications? Acta Med Scand [Suppl] 687:33, 1984
11. Assal JP, Muhlhauser I, Pernat A et al: Patient education as the basis for diabetes care in clinical practice. Diabetologia 28:602, 1985
12. Delbridge L, Appleberg M, Reeve TS: Factors associated with development of foot lesions in the diabetic. Surgery 93:78, 1983
13. Hershey FB, Barnes RW, Sumner DS: Noninvasive Diagnosis of Vascular Disease. pp. 16, 24. Appleton Davies, Pasadena, CA, 1984
14. Wagner FW: Transcutaneous Doppler ultrasound in the prediction of healing and the selection of surgical level for lesions of the toes and forefoot. Clin Orthop 142:110, 1979

15. Verta MJ, Gross WS, VenBellin B et al: Amputation for gangrene. Surgery 80:729, 1976
16. Gibbons GW, Wheelock FC, Siembieda C et al: Noninvasive prediction of amputation level in diabetic patients. Arch Surg 114:1253, 1979
17. Bone GE, Pomajzl MJ: Toe blood pressure by photophlethysmography: an index of healing in forefoot amputation. Surgery 5:569, 1981
18. Barnes RW, Thornhill B, Nix L et al: Prediction of amputation wound healing: roles of Doppler ultrasound and digit photoplethysmography. Arch Surg 116:80, 1981
19. Holstein P: The distal blood pressure predicts healing of amputations on the feet. Acta Orthop Scand 55:227, 1984
20. Apelqvist J, Castenfors J, Larsson J et al: Prognostic value of systolic ankle and toe blood pressure levels in outcome of diabetic foot ulcer. Diabetes Care 12:373, 1989
21. Hauser CJ, Klein SR, Mehringer CM et al: Assessment of perfusion in the diabetic foot by regional transcutaneous oxymetry. Diabetes 33:527, 1984
22. Bongard O, Krahenbuhl B: Predicting amputation in severe ischemia: the value of transcutaneous PO_2 measurement. J Bone Joint Surg 70B:465, 1988
23. Oishi CS, Fronek A, Golbranson FL: The role of non-invasive vascular studies in determining levels of amputation. J Bone Joint Surg 70A:1520, 1988
24. Lang-Stevenson AI, Sharrard WJ et al: Neuropathic ulcers of the foot. J Bone Joint Surg 67(B):438, 1985
25. Hall DC, Brand PW: The etiology of the neuropathic ulcer. J Am Podiatry Assoc 69:173, 1979
26. Ctercteko GC, Dhanendran M, Hutton WC, LeQuesne LP: Vertical forces acting on the feet of diabetic patients with neuropathic ulceration. Br J Surg 68:608, 1981
27. Bays HE, Pfeifer MA: Peripheral diabetic neuropathy. Med Clin North Am 72(6):1439, 1988
28. American Diabetes Association and American Academy of Neurology consensus statement. Report and recommendations of the San Antonio conference on diabetic neuropathy. Diabetes Care 11:592, 1988
29. Rendell MS, Dovgan DJ, Bergman TF et al: Mapping diabetic sensory neuropathy by current perception threshold testing. Diabetes Care 12:636, 1989
30. Lippman HI, Perrotto A, Farrar R: The neuropathic foot of the diabetic. Bull NY Acad Med 52:1159, 1976
31. Dyck PJ, Karnes JL, Daube J et al: Clinical and neuropathological criteria for the diagnosis and staging of diabetic polyneuropathy. Brain 108:861, 1985
32. Daube JR: Electrophysiologic testing in diabetic neuropathy. p. 162. In Dyck PJ, Thomas PK, Asbury AK et al (eds): Diabetic Neuropathy. WB Saunders, Philadelphia, 1987
33. Steiness IB: Vibratory perception in normal subjects: a biothesiometric study. Acta Med Scand 158:315, 1957
34. Dyck PJ, Bushek W, Spring EM et al: Vibratory and cooling detection thresholds compared with other tests in diagnosing and staging diabetic neuropathy. Diabetes Care 10:432, 1987
35. Dyck PJ, Zimmerman IR, O'Brien PC et al: Introduction of automated systems to evaluate touch-pressure, vibration, and thermal cutaneous sensation in man. Ann Neurol 4:502, 1978
36. Bell-Krotoski J, Tomancik E: The repeatability of testing with Semmes-Weinstein monofilaments. J Hand Surg 12A:155, 1987
37. Birke JA, Sims DS: Plantar sensory threshold in the ulcerative foot. Lepr Rev 57:261, 1986
38. Bergtholdt HT, Brand PW: Temperature assessment and plantar inflammation. Lepr Rev 47:211, 1976
39. Duckworth T, Boulton AJM, Betts RP et al: Plantar pressure measurements and the prevention of ulceration in the diabetic foot. J Bone Joint Surg 67:79, 1985
40. Silvino N, Evanski PM, Waugh TR: The Harris and Beath footprinting mat: diagnostic validity and clinical use. Clin Ortho Rel Res 151:265–269, 1980
41. Brink SJ: Limited joint mobility as a risk factor for diabetes complications. Clinical Diabetes 5:122, 1987
42. Sibbald RG, Schachter RK: The skin and diabetes mellitus. Int J Dermatol 23:567, 1984
43. Huntley AC: The cutaneous manifestations of diabetes mellitus. J Am Acad Dermatol 7:427, 1982
44. Holstein P, Larsen K, Sager P: Decompression with the aid of insoles in the treatment of diabetic neuropathic ulcers. Acta Orthop Scand 47:463, 1976
45. Leber C, Evanksi PM: A comparison of shoe insole materials in plantar pressure relief. Prosthet Orthot Int 10:135, 1986
46. Veves A, Masson EA, Fernando DJS, Boulton AJM: Use of experimental padded hosiery to reduce abnormal foot pressures in diabetic neuropathy. Diabetes Care 12:653, 1989

6

Imaging of the Diabetic Foot

Roger Kerr, M.D.
David J. Sartoris, M.D.
Catherine F. Fix, M.S.
Donald Resnick, M.D.

PLAIN FILM RADIOGRAPHY

Diabetes mellitus predisposes the patient to certain complications involving the feet. Vascular problems (ischemia, increased peripheral blood flow, or arteriovenous shunting) and neuropathy may occur unpredictably and can be irreversible.[1] Once these problems develop, the foot becomes vulnerable to injury. Moreover, the tendency for these predisposing conditions to coexist increases the likelihood that foot lesions will occur. Impairments in sensation (from neurologic defects) may allow minor wounds or infections to go unrecognized and progress to severe proportions; in addition, the impaired blood supply may result in delayed healing. Thus, although infections presumably are complications rather than primary causes of the "diabetic foot," they may initiate a fulminating destructive process that would otherwise have remained latent.[2]

In general, abnormalities of the foot consist of painless soft tissue swelling with or without bone deformity in the tarsometatarsal group of bones. Often the forefoot is involved bilaterally. The superimposition of neuropathy, infection, or both often complicates the interpretation of films.

Radiographs of the foot in patients with diabetes commonly reveal a combination of bone alterations, including gross destruction, fragmentation, periosteal new bone formation, and pointed bone deformity—changes that are believed to represent different phases of the same pathologic process.[3,4]

Infections

Infections of the foot are quite common in persons with diabetes mellitus, and early recognition is extremely important to avoid amputation of the foot or leg. Over 80 percent of leg amputations carried out annually in the United States are performed on diabetic patients,[5] most often because of infection. Even seemingly minor infections in diabetes can result in the loss of a foot.[6] Given the seriousness of this circumstance, it is crucial to identify infectious processes as early as possible.

Several factors—anatomic, vascular, and neuropathic—combine to make foot infections a prominent feature of diabetes mellitus. Soft tissue ulceration over certain pressure points (particularly the metatarsal heads and calcaneus), associated with circulatory and neurologic defects, leads to conditions favorable to bacterial contamination and growth. The resulting infections may spread within the soft tissue compartments and cause osteitis, osteomyelitis, and septic arthritis. Normal anatomic pathways of spread of infection are important in understanding the radiographic manifestations of foot infections.

Pathways of Infection

The three plantar muscle compartments — medial, intermediate, and lateral — are separated from each other by the medial and lateral intermuscular septa, which extend from the plantar fascia to the overlying bones (Fig. 6-1A). The three compartments differ in amount of potential space, which has a bearing on how infections will disseminate in the soft tissues.

In general, processes that begin in a given compartment tend to spread proximally within that compartment along the path of least resistance.[5] The two intermuscular septa are the major potential barriers to intercompartmental dissemination, but at specific sites these septa are traversed by muscles and tendons, constituting regions where spread of infection is more likely to occur.

In the intermediate compartment, which has the greatest amount of potential space, fluids (and by extension other material, such as infectious processes) were found experimentally to extravasate or spread from this compartment along four pathways (Fig. 6-1B): (1) along the tendon sheath of the flexor hallucis longus muscle into the deep posterior compartment of the leg; (2) into the medial compartment through the medial intermuscular septum at the midportion of the first metatarsal; (3) into the lateral compartment via spread along the fascial plane of the plantar arterial arch and plantar metatarsal artery; and (4) into the plantar fat through the aponeurosis at the proximal end of the second metatarsal bone.[6]

The medial compartment has the second greatest amount of potential space. Infectious processes originating in this compartment would tend to spread through the midportion of the medial intermuscular septum (not along the flexor hallucis longus tendon or the insertion of the adductor hallucis muscle, as had been previously thought). Spread would then occur along the fascial planes of the adductor hallucis and flexor muscles in the intermediate compartment.

The lateral compartment has the least amount of potential space. This compartment also has weak fascial boundaries, and as a result infections could spread to the dorsal compartment or into the plantar fat of the foot.

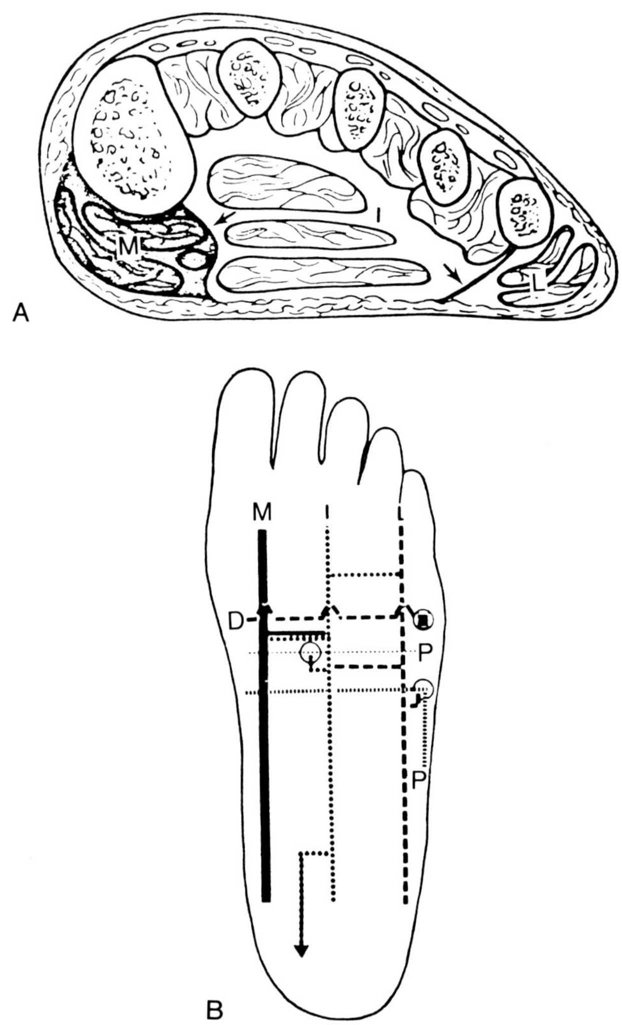

Fig. 6-1. (**A**) Cross section of the foot, showing the medial (M), intermediate (I), and lateral (L) compartments, separated by the medial and lateral intermuscular septa (arrows). The medial compartment contains the muscles to the great toe; the lateral compartment contains those to the fifth toe; and the intermediate compartment contains the remaining muscles. (**B**) Potential routes for spread of infection in the foot. The arrow pointing toward the heel connotes spread to the lower leg; dotted and dashed lines indicate pathways of dissemination. D, dorsum of foot; P, plantar fat. (From Feingold,[6] with permission.)

These pathways of spread have implications for the radiographic evaluation of soft tissue infections in the plantar aspect of the foot. Initial contamination at pressure points can spread to adjacent bones and joints; in addition, osteomyelitis and septic arthritis can occur at sites remote from the initial site of soft tissue contamination. Neglected foot infections may eventually require that the leg be amputated at a level above or below the knee as a result of spread from the intermediate compartment to the lower leg.

Plain Film Findings In Infection

The early findings in infection are defects in soft tissue contour and loss of tissue planes. Edema or swelling is common. The initial soft tissue changes occur particularly frequently beneath the first and fifth metatarsophalangeal joints and calcaneus at pressure points. Soft tissue involvement may be severe, owing to a combination of decreased host resistance to infection, vascular alterations, and neuropathy.

Soft tissue infections frequently spread to adjacent bones or joints, in which case the features of osteomyelitis or septic arthritis become evident on plain films. Bone changes associated with osteomyelitis may not be seen on plain films until 7 to 15 days after the onset of infection.[7]

The radiographic features of bone involvement in diabetic patients are complicated by coexisting problems, including neuropathy and vascular alterations (Fig. 6-2). Significant soft tissue swelling and mottled osteolysis are common. Other findings include osteosclerosis, fragmentation, periostitis, and radiolucent areas within the soft tissues. These radiolucent areas may result either from introduction of air during dissection or debridement or from production of gas by microorganisms. In some patients, pathologic fractures and subluxations—which also are characteristics of diabetic neuroarthropathy—are prominent. Because neuroarthropathy and infection frequently coexist in the midfoot and forefoot of diabetic patients, differentiation between infections and neurologic processes may be difficult. In such cases, the most helpful radiographic clue to the presence of osteomyelitis is poorly defined bone contours.

Certain features of osteomyelitis and septic arthritis, such as periosteal new bone formation and osteopenia, may not be seen in the diabetic foot if blood supply is inadequate (i.e., in the presence of ischemia). However, several authors[8-10] have reported an increased peripheral blood flow to the foot in diabetes, and extensive lesions usually are

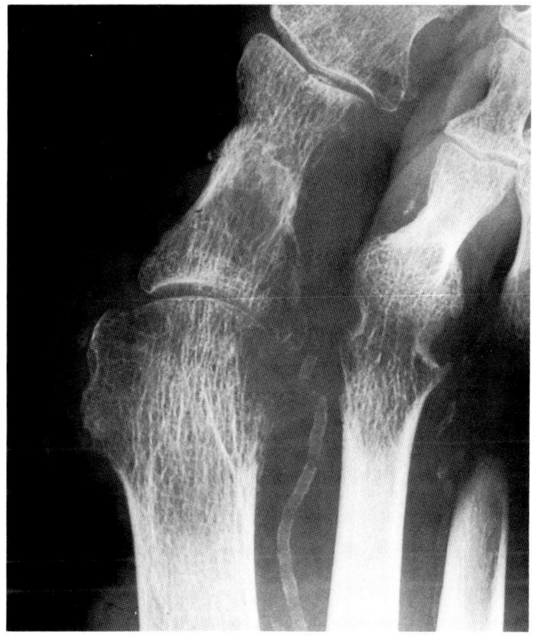

Fig. 6-2. Spread of soft tissue infection in the foot in diabetes mellitus. Soft tissue infection is present about the first metatarsophalangeal joint with ulcerations and with erosion of bone. Observe vascular calcifications at the second and third metatarsophalangeal joints. (From Resnick,[61] with permission.)

seen in feet with good circulation.[2] When osteoporosis does occur, it may progress to cortical erosion, medullary destruction, loss of the subchondral bone plate, and joint space narrowing. Often the patient has spontaneous fractures, subluxations, or dislocations.

A possibly unique feature of diabetes is that infection may lead either to rapid and marked dissolution of bone or to remarkable restoration of bone architecture, even in bones that appear almost completely destroyed. Radiographs taken during the course of infections therefore should be interpreted with caution, keeping in mind that "irreversible" bone destruction is difficult to define.

Production of gas by infecting microorganisms is common in the diabetic foot. Although gangrene from infection with *Clostridium* is responsible for some cases (and gangrene is more common in diabetic persons than in the general population), nonclostridial organisms, particularly *Escherichia coli*, also cause gas formation in infected tissues. Other organisms known for gas production are *Aerobacter aerogenes, Klebsiella pneumoniae,* nonhemolytic streptococci, *Bacteroides,* and anaerobic streptococci.

Neuroarthropathy

Diabetes has now overtaken both syphilis and syringomyelia as the leading cause of neuroarthropathy. The incidence rates are difficult to determine, in part because the joint lesions tend to be asymptomatic.

Patients may reveal painless soft tissue swelling, skin ulceration, and joint deformity, which can involve either a single joint or multiple articulations. At times, the clinical and radiographic manifestations at one site may resolve spontaneously, to be followed by the appearance and progression of alterations at a previously unaffected site.

Many theories have been advanced to explain the neuroarthropathy that commonly accompanies diabetes, which most likely involves both mechanical and physiologic factors: neurologic impairment leads to loss of the protective sensations of pain and proprioception, which in turn results in relaxation of the supporting structures of the joints. Chronic instability of the joint ensues, and repeated micro- and macrotrauma (such as occur with normal daily stresses) produce injury, malalignment, and abnormal joint loading. Vascular alterations and superimposed infection frequently complicate the situation. Increased blood flow may promote both lysis and sclerosis in a neuropathic joint. Continued weight bearing then leads to progressive degeneration and disorganization of the joint.

Typically, the tarsometatarsal, intertarsal, and metatarsophalangeal joints are involved; less frequently, changes may be seen at the ankle and interphalangeal joints. Patients tend to be middle-aged and to have had long-standing diabetes, but persons of younger or older age groups also can be affected. The radiographic and pathologic pictures may reveal alterations characteristic of both neuroarthropathy and infection. Early features may simulate the changes of osteoarthritis. Depending on the location of the neuroarthropathy, osteolysis and resorption may predominate over fragmentation and bone proliferation. Spontaneous fractures and dislocations sometimes occur.

The intertarsal and tarsometatarsal joints may show prominent bone fragmentation, sclerosis, and dislocation or subluxation. One or more tarsal bones may disintegrate completely over a rapid period of time—in a matter of days or weeks—possibly because of microfractures that have evolved quickly into gross fragmentation. Characteristically, the metartarsal bones are displaced dorsolaterally in relation to the cuneiforms and cuboid bone, with a talar disruption, leading to a radiographic picture resembling an acute Lisfranc's fracture-dislocaton at the tarsometatarsal joints (Fig. 6-3).

The metatarsophalangeal joints frequently reveal partial or complete resorption of the metatarsal heads and proximal phalanges (Fig. 6-4). Tapering ("pencil-pointing") of the phalangeal and metatarsal shafts is common. This appearance is thought to signify repair of a tubular bone after destruction.[3] The metatarsal heads may be flattened and show fragmentation, simulating a Freiberg's infraction. Broadening of the bases of the proximal phalanges occasionally occurs, leading to a characteristic radiographic picture variously termed a "mortar and pestle," "pencil and cup," or "balancing pagoda." These changes represent different phases of the same pathologic process, and they are seen in other conditions associated with sensory neuropathy. Continued involvement of the forefoot results in progressive resorption of the phalanges, dorsiflexion, and shortening of the toes. Ulceration of the soft tissues over bony prominences is frequent and may cause infection that may progress to osteomyelitis or septic arthritis. Superimposed suppurative processes, such as gangrene, can accentuate and accelerate the joint destruction in neuroarthropathy. However, as already noted, recovery from the infection sometimes is followed by remarkable reconstitution of bone architecture.

Vascular Calcification

Calcification of the arteries (also known as medial arterial calcification or Mönckeberg's arteriosclerosis) is a common finding in patients with diabetes mellitus; the feet are the most frequent site of involvement and usually are the earliest to be affected.[11] Involvement of the interdigital arteries of the feet can be a helpful diagnostic clue in clinically unsuspected diabetes, as these vessels are rarely

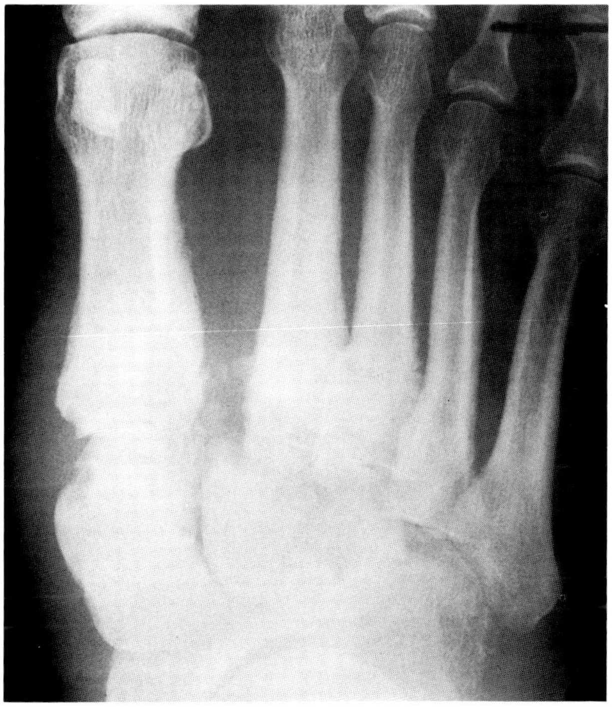

Fig. 6-3. Tarsometatarsal joint in diabetes mellitus. Note the lateral displacement of the bases of the metatarsals with respect to the tarsals. This finding, combined with soft tissue swelling and fragmentation of bone, resembles a Lisfranc's fracture-dislocation. (From Resnick,[61] with permission.)

calcified in nondiabetic persons. Usually the calcific deposits accumulate in the tunica media rather than the tunica intima of the vessels, and radiographically they appear as regular, diffuse, fine-grained collections typically affecting the entire circumference of the vessel, appearing circumferential on cross-sectional radiographs and like railroad tracks on longitudinal views (Fig. 6-2).[11] Calcified vessels may reveal fractures with callus formation.

Some physicians view such a condition as clinically insignificant, but Everhart and colleagues[11] found that medial arterial calcification was associated with a marked increase in the risk of amputation.

Although the arterial calcifications rarely impinge on the lumen and therefore do not produce occlusion, they may cause increased rigidity of the wall, resulting in an inability to adjust to circulatory demands. This may explain the more frequent arterial calcifications in diabetic patients with gangrene than in those without gangrene.

Pathogenetically, the calcific deposits may be related to neuroarthropathy, as similar alterations are observed in patients with familial amyloidosis and neuropathy.

Forefoot Osteolysis

Patients with diabetes mellitus may develop a distinct form of osteolysis involving the distal metatarsal bones and proximal phalanges. The lesions occur primarily in the bones, and usually the joint surfaces are spared initially. This condition is characterized by generalized or patchy osteoporosis, which closely resembles the changes of osteomyelitis. Juxta-articular cortical defects may not be easy to identify on radiographs, and more than one

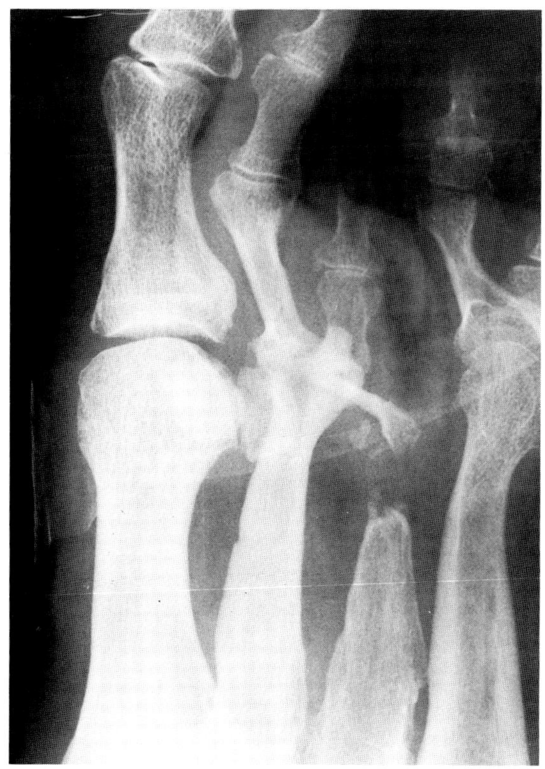

Fig. 6-4. Metatarsophalangeal and interphalangeal joints in diabetes mellitus. Neuroarthropathy and infection in the forefoot of a diabetic patient can combine to produce bizarre abnormalities consisting of osteolysis of distal metatarsals and proximal phalanges, with tapering of bone contours. (From Resnick,[61] with permission.)

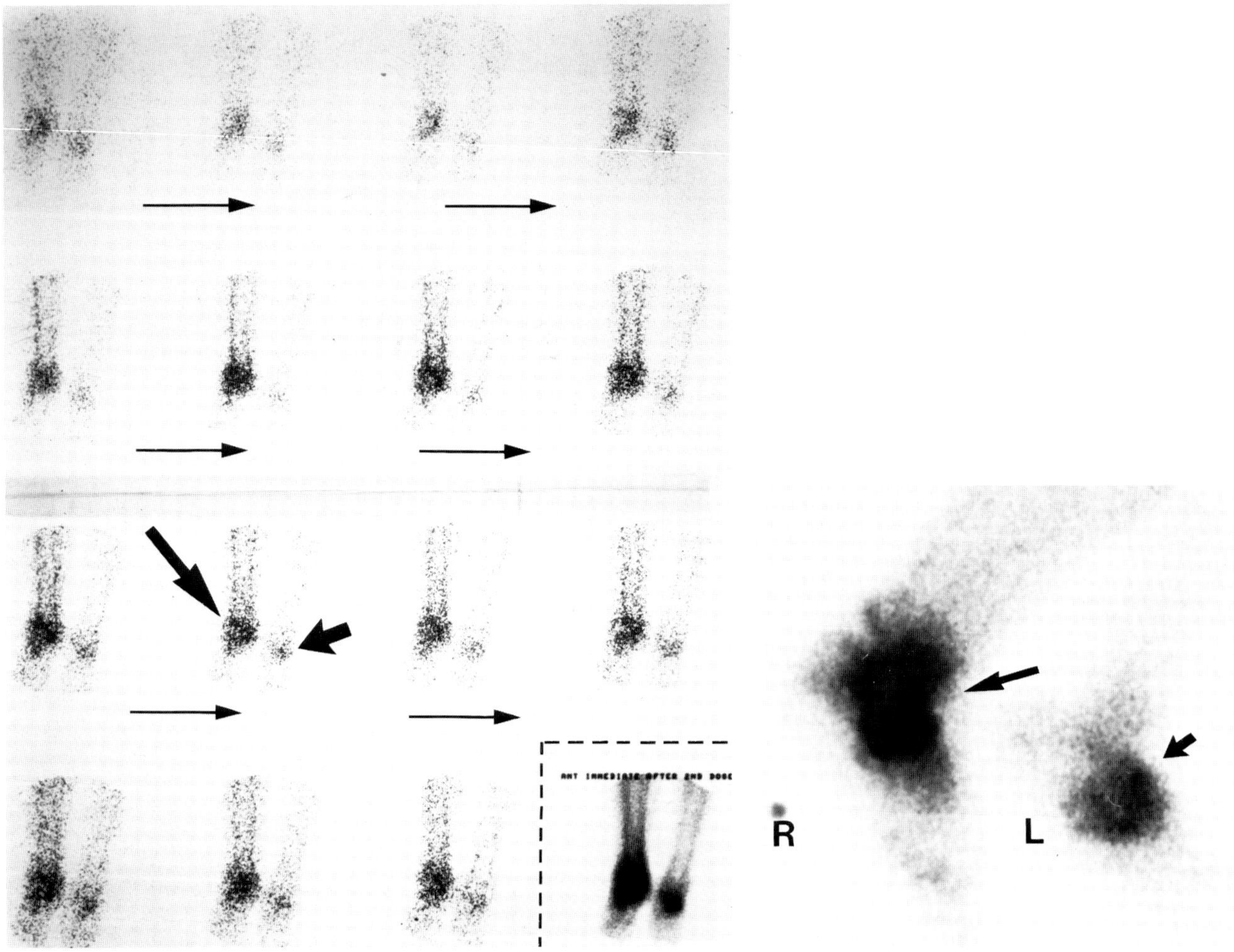

A B

Fig. 6-5. Comparison of bone scan and gallium scan. (**A**) Serial flow phase images in the anteroposterior projection reveal mild increased activity in the left hindfoot (short arrow) and moderate increased activity in the right ankle/hindfoot (long arrow). The blood pool image (box, lower right) demonstrates a similar pattern of uptake. (**B**) Lateral blood pool image. *(Figure continues.)*

projection or even magnification techniques may be required to demonstrate the lesions.

Sometimes the osteolysis is progressive, but the process may terminate spontaneously at any stage, with partial or complete restoration of bone.[9] The cause of the condition is not clear; some patients with forefoot osteolysis reveal no evidence of either neurologic deficit, ischemia, or infection. Nevertheless, a similar radiographic appearance may be seen in diabetic neuroarthropathy, and it is possible that sympathetic nerve dysfunction is involved in the pathogenesis.

SCINTIGRAPHY

Radiographic evaluation of the diabetic foot is often made difficult by the presence of neuroarthropathy, cellulitis, or soft tissue ulceration. The patient with cellulitis or neuroarthropathy may present with a warm, swollen foot suggestive of osteomyelitis. Accurate detection or exclusion of osteomyelitis has important treatment implications, and a variety of imaging procedures have been utilized to this end.

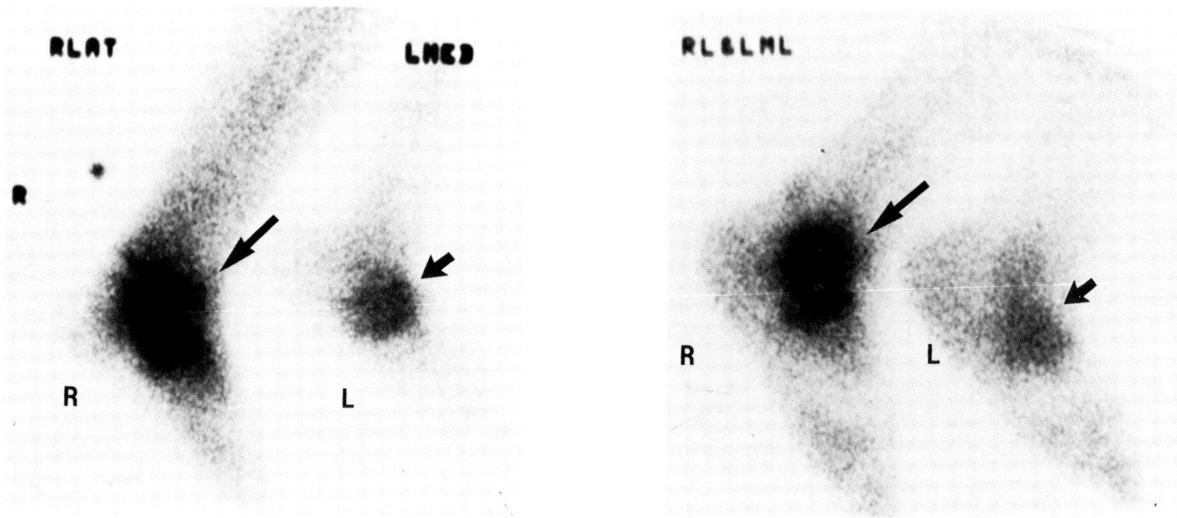

C D

Fig. 6-5. *(Continued).* (**C**) lateral delayed image reveal mild activity in the left hindfoot/midfoot region (short arrow) and moderate activity in the right hindfoot/ankle (long arrow). (**D**) A 48-hour gallium scan demonstrates increased activity in the right tibia and talus of equal intensity to that on the bone scan in a concordant, although slightly more focal, distribution (long arrow). This was confirmed to represent osteomyelitis. The activity on the left (short arrow) was less intense than on the bone scan and was secondary to neuropathic disease. Radiographs only revealed neuropathic changes in both feet. R, right; L, left. (Courtesy of Charles A. Stewart, M.D., Los Angeles, CA.)

Imaging in cases of a suspected diabetic foot infecton begins with conventional radiography and magnification views, but additional imaging techniques often are necessary. In the neuropathic foot, early radiographic changes of osteolysis, osteopenia, and periosteal reaction can simulate acute osteomyelitis. More advanced destructive neuropathic changes of fragmentation, collapse, pathologic fracture, and sclerosis can resemble chronic osteomyelitis and mask a focus of osteomyelitis. Conversely, radiographs are typically negative during the first 10 to 14 days of acute osteomyelitis. Therefore, unless plain films demonstrate unequivocal active osteomyelitis, further imaging is required and is usually accomplished with scintigraphic techniques. It must be noted that although radiographs may be nondiagnostic of infection, they provide valuable information with regard to the presence of diabetic osteoarthropathy or degenerative joint disease. Knowledge of such changes is required for accurate interpretation of scintigraphic or other subsequent studies.

^{99m}Tc-MDP Bone Scan

In patients without clinical or radiographic evidence of peripheral neuropathy or other significant underlying bone or joint disease, a technetium 99m methylene diphosphonate (^{99m}Tc-MDP) bone scan is useful for diagnosing osteomyelitis. A bone scan may be positive 2 to 3 days after the onset of osteomyelitis. Often, the goal of imaging is to distinguish osteomyelitis from septic arthritis or cellulitis. This is accomplished with a three-phase bone scan consisting of (1) a radionuclide angiogram or flow phase; (2) a blood-pool image; and (3) delayed static images. The first two phases are useful for the detection of abnormal perfusion to bone, whereas the third phase reflects abnormal bone turnover. After the intravenous injection of 20 mCi of ^{99m}Tc-MDP, a series of 12 to 20 flow phase images is obtained every 3 seconds. At 3 to 10 minutes after injection, a blood-pool image is acquired. Delayed static images are obtained 3 to 4 hours after injection (Fig. 6-5).

The chief advantage of the three-phase technique over delayed static imaging in the diagnosis of osteomyelitis is a reduction in the number of false positive studies.[12] Osteomyelitis is readily distinguished from disorders that reveal concentration of radionuclide but have no significant hyperemia, such as fractures, degenerative disease, and avascular necrosis. A retrospective study of diabetic patients with foot problems requiring surgery reported a sensitivity of 83 percent and specificity of 75 percent for the diagnosis of osteomyelitis with the three-phase technique.[13] The accuracy of this technique in evaluating early or low-grade diabetic foot infections has not, however, been determined.

On a three-phase bone scan, cellulitis, osteomyelitis, and septic arthritis demonstrate increased activity on the radionuclide angiogram and blood-pool images. On delayed images, acute osteomyelitis reveals focal enhanced activity, whereas cellulitis and septic arthritis exhibit normal or low-grade uptake. Chronic osteomyelitis typically reveals a diffuse, nonfocal pattern of increased activity on delayed images. Ischemia of the toes is characterized by the absence of radionuclide uptake.[14]

Alazraki et al. advocate the use of a four-phase bone scan wherein a 24-hour static image is added to the three-phase study.[15] Osteomyelitis is diagnosed when the lesion-to-background ratio of activity increases on the 24-hour image in comparison to the 2-hour image. Using this technique, accuracy was slightly improved (85 percent versus 80 percent) and there were fewer false positive studies (specificity of 87 percent versus 73 percent). Degenerative disease was a cause of false positive three- and four-phase studies. Israel et al. obtained similar results using a quantitative four-phase technique.[16]

As stated earlier, increased activity, reflecting hyperemia, in the radionuclide angiogram and blood-pool images enhances the diagnostic specificity for osteomyelitis. Inflammatory or infectious soft tissue processes, such as cellulitis and ulceration, however, are also associated with a vascular response on these early images. Alazraki et al. were unable to distinguish between osteomyelitis and cellulitis on the basis of the pattern of hypervascular response and instead relied on delayed static images for diagnosis.

In contrast, Seldin et al. were able to distinguish between osteomyelitis and cellulitis or ulceration in diabetic feet according to the pattern of hyperemia on the flow phase of the study.[17] They defined arterial hyperemia as the appearance of activity before or at the same time as in the surrounding tissues and venous hyperemia as activity developing after that seen in the surrounding tissues. Focal arterial hyperemia combined with focally increased activity on blood-pool and delayed images was interpreted as acute osteomyelitis. A pattern of venous hyperemia corresponded to soft tissue pathology without osteomyelitis and was seen even in the presence of peripheral vascular disease. Using this approach, the sensitivity and specificity for osteomyelitis were 94 percent and 79 percent, respectively. Seldin et al.'s data confirmed a previous report that more than 2 weeks of antibiotic therapy is necessary before hyperemia to infected bone is significantly diminished.[18] Noninfected neuropathic joints demonstrated intense activity on all phases and were distinguished from osteomyelitis by the diffuse, nonfocal pattern of abnormality. The authors recognized, however, that it would be difficult, if not impossible, to confidently diagnose osteomyelitis superimposed on a neuropathic joint using this technique.

Bone scintigraphy may be used for the early diagnosis of diabetic neuroarthropathy. Scintigraphy often reveals more extensive abnormalities than radiography and, interestingly, may show abnormal activity when radiographs are normal.[4,19] In a recent study of 27 diabetic patients with clinical evidence of neuropathy, radiographs and bone scans were both abnormal in 37 percent of patients.[4] In 19 percent of patients, abnormalities were only seen on the bone scan. Abnormal activity was seen on both blood-pool and delayed images. Neuropathic disease may produce diffuse or focal concentrations of radionuclide on all phases of a three-phase study.[4,19] These results indicate a potential role for scintigraphy in identifying patients at risk to develop progressive foot deformity who would benefit from early treatment. Conversely, the abnormal radionuclide uptake seen with neuropathy may also occur with bone or soft tissue infection and must be correlated with the clinical findings. These results indicate that accurate diagnosis of the presence and extent of infection in a

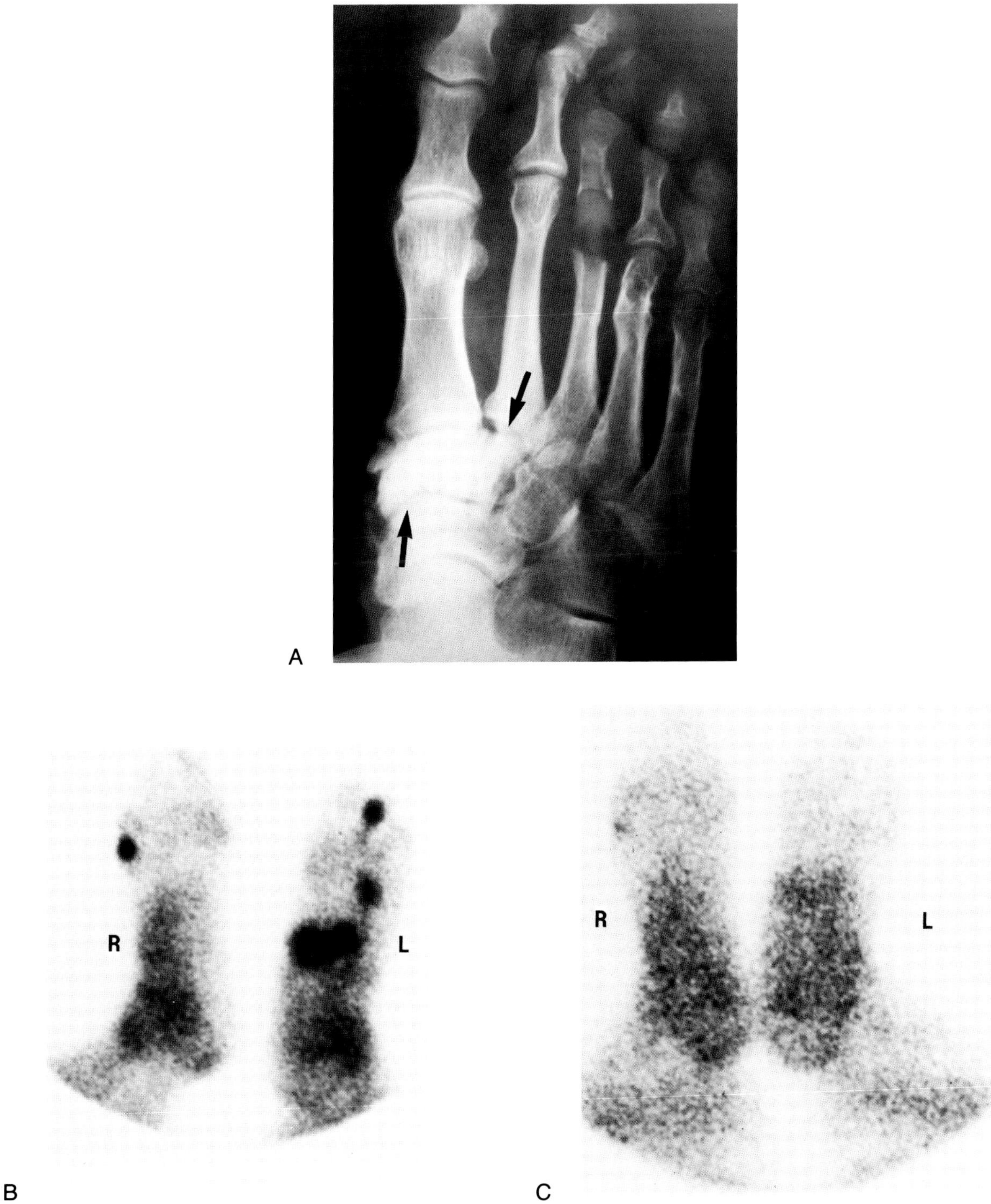

Fig. 6-6. Use of gallium scan in diabetic neuropathy. (**A**) A dorsoplantar radiograph reveals sclerosis and fragmentation of the medial and intermediate cuneiform with degenerative changes in adjacent joints consistent with neuroarthropathy (arrows). Degenerative, post-traumatic, and postsurgical changes are noted in the forefoot. (**B**) A bone scan reveals focal increased activity in the left midfoot and forefoot corresponding to the radiographic abnormalities noted above. R, right; L, left. (**C**) A 48-hour gallium scan demonstrates no focal abnormal activity, confirming the absence of infection. R, right; L, left. (Courtesy of Charles A. Stewart, M.D., Los Angeles, CA.)

patient with early or established peripheral neuropathy cannot be accomplished by a bone scan alone. In a broader context, any form of pre-existing osseous disease will almost invariably be positive on a bone scan and supplementary scintigraphic techniques are needed to exclude infection.

^{67}Ga Scan

The combination of gallium 67 (^{67}Ga) and bone scintigraphy has been shown to improve accuracy in the diagnosis of uncomplicated osteomyelitis.[14,20] Gallium imaging has been most valuable, however, in improving the specificity of diagnosis in subacute and chronic bone infections and when infection is superimposed on bone, joint, or soft tissue pathology (Fig. 6-6).[21,22] As stated earlier, the major limitation of ^{99m}Tc-MDP is that it is nonspecific; it accumulates wherever there is increased perfusion to bone or increased bone turnover. Although it has a mild affinity for bone, gallium accumulates primarily at sites of inflammation. The mechanism of gallium localization is multifactorial and includes binding to leukocytes in circulation and at the septic focus, binding to a plasma protein (lactoferrin) excreted by leukocytes at the infected site, and accumulation due to increased vascular permeability and direct bacterial uptake.[23-25]

For accurate diagnosis, the gallium scan must be compared to the bone scan. Osteomyelitis is diagnosed (1) when the pattern of gallium uptake in bone is discordant to that of ^{99m}Tc-MDP (i.e., in a different distribution); or (2) when there is a concordant pattern of gallium and ^{99m}Tc-MDP uptake in which the intensity of gallium uptake equals or exceeds that of Tc-MDP (Figs. 6-5 and 6-7). Cellulitis is characterized by the uptake of gallium in a pattern that does not correspond in configuration to any bony structures (Fig. 6-7). Due to limited resolution it may be difficult to distinguish osteomyelitis from cellulitis in the small digits of the foot.[14]

Gallium scanning is useful in the clinical follow-up of acute and chronic osteomyelitis.[26,27] With a favorable response to antibiotic treatment, gallium concentration decreases and eventually reverts to normal. Persistent low-grade uptake may be seen with an incomplete response and is not an indication for prolonged antibiotic therapy. Failure of therapy is indicated by persistently elevated gallium uptake on serial scans. Serial bone scans are less useful, revealing persistent abnormal activity secondary to remodeling long after the septic focus has been eradicated.

Unfortunately, there are significant limitations to the use of gallium in the diagnosis of muculoskeletal infection. Gallium may be taken up at sites of bone repair, by inflamed synovium, and by tumors, and mild to intense uptake may be observed in association with noninfected neuroarthropathy (Fig. 6-5D).[4,28] Furthermore, a gallium scan may be normal in the presence of osteomyelitis, and gallium uptake in osteomyelitis is suppressed by prior antibiotic therapy.[14] The overall accuracy of combined bone and gallium scanning for diagnosing osteomyelitis in traumatized bone is less than that in nontraumatized bone. Diminished accuracy is also seen in evaluating infected joint prostheses.[29,30] An additional drawback of gallium imaging is that the study is usually not complete until a 48-hour postinjection scan has been obtained. The overall accuracy of combined bone and gallium scanning for diagnosing osteomyelitis is approximately 70 to 80 percent.[31,32]

^{111}In-Labeled Leukocyte Scan

Indium 111 (^{111}In)-labeled leukocytes have also been used for the evaluation of osteomyelitis complicating diabetic osteoarthropathy. The theoretical advantage of this technique over gallium scintigraphy is that ^{111}In-labeled leukocytes do not accumulate at sites of increased bone turnover and would not be expected to accumulate in neuropathic bone. This property of ^{111}In-labeled leukocytes is brought into question, however, by a recent report of a 30 percent rate of false positive uptake of ^{111}In-labeled leukocytes at sites of rapidly progressing osteoarthropathy.[23] This uptake[33] is probably due to an acute inflammatory reaction that is less intense or absent in chronic neuroarthropathy.

Prior studies have shown an absence of such uptake in noninfected neuropathic bone.[34-36] Two studies of the use of ^{111}In-labeled leukocyte scans

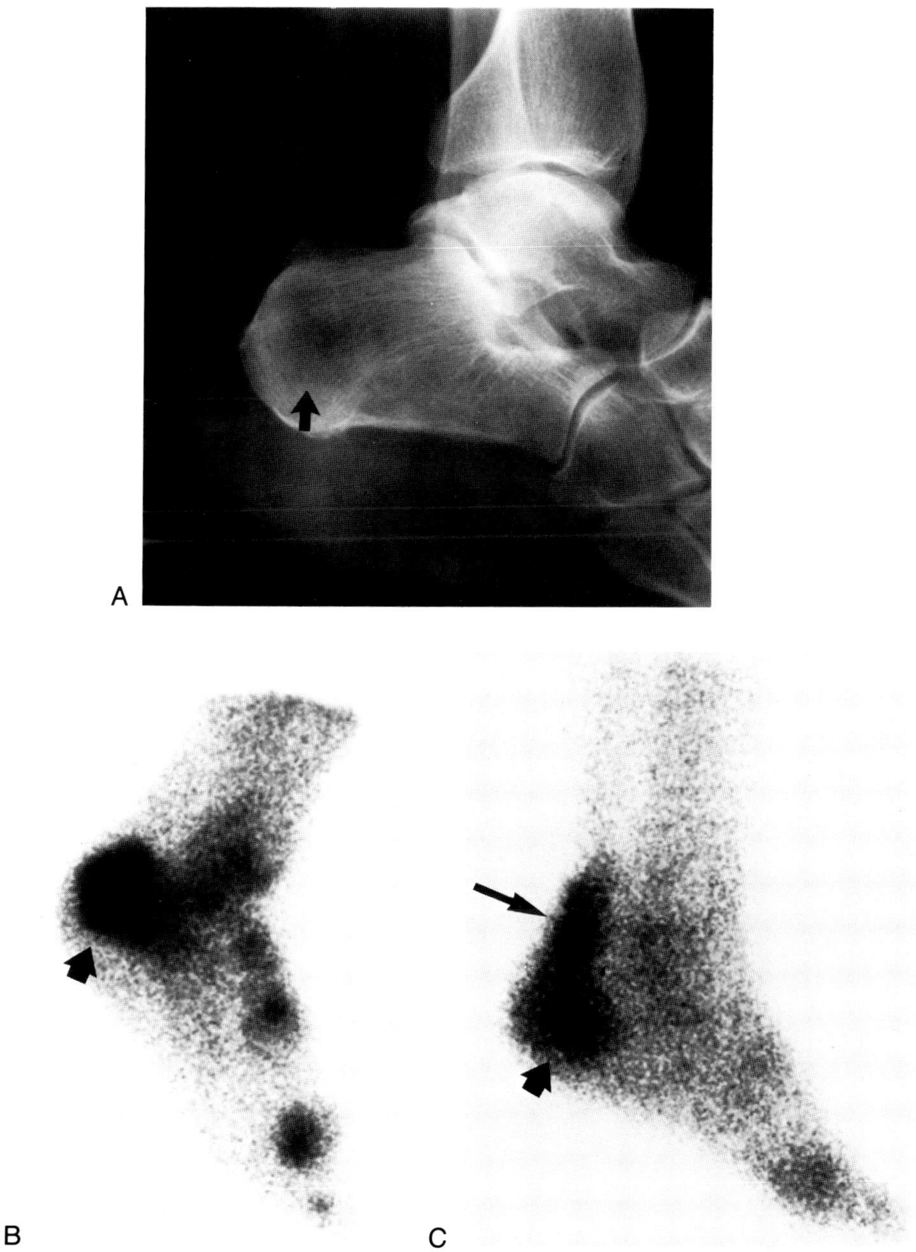

Fig. 6-7. Use of gallium scan in osteomyelitis and cellulitis. (**A**) A lateral radiograph reveals focal osteolysis of the calcaneus (arrow). (**B**) A bone scan reveals focal intense activity within the calcaneus consistent with osteomyelitis (arrow). Other foci of mild increased activity were due to degenerative disease. (**C**) A 48-hour gallium scan demonstrates focal increased activity within the calcaneus (short arrow) and in the posterosuperior soft tissues about the Achilles tendon (long arrow). These changes were due to calcaneal osteomyelitis and adjacent cellulitis. (Courtesy of Charles A. Stewart, M.D., Los Angeles, CA.)

in diagnosing osteomyelitis in neuropathic foot disease reported a sensitivity of 75 and 100 percent and a specificity of 89 and 83 percent, respectively.[34,35] False positive results were not due to neuroarthropathy, but instead were a result of the poor spatial resolution of this technique wherein a soft tissue infection was mistakenly attributed to bone. The greatest value of leukocyte scanning was its high negative predictive value; the absence of leukocyte activity in osteopathic bone excludes active infection.[34]

Because of its limited spatial resolution, correlation of an ^{111}In-labeled leukocyte scan with a bone scan is recommended to determine if abnormal activity arises from bone or adjacent soft tissues.[35] Detection of osteomyelitis, however, can be difficult when there is an adjacent soft tissue infection.[34]

An early report on a small number of patients indicated that gallium imaging was superior to ^{111}In-labeled leukocyte imaging in the diagnosis of chronic infection.[37] The sensitivity of the ^{111}In-labeled leukocyte scan fell from 100 percent for infections less than 2 weeks in duration to 73 percent for those present for more than 2 weeks. This finding was refuted by a study of 290 patients in which the sensitivity of leukocyte scanning was 90 and 86 percent, respectively, for infections less than and greater than 2 weeks in duration.[38] Most of these were soft tissue infections.

Favorable results with leukocyte scanning also were obtained in a study of 50 patients with suspected low-grade or chronic osteomyelitis.[39] In this study, leukocyte scanning had a sensitivity of 83 percent and a specificity of 94 percent, compared to combined bone and gallium scanning, which had a sensitivity of 50 percent and a specificity of 78 percent. A study of 21 suspected subacute or chronic bone infections yielded similar results for leukocyte and combined bone and gallium scanning.[40] Both techniques had a sensitivity of 80 percent, whereas leukocyte scanning had a slightly lower specificity, 75 percent, compared to 83 percent for the combined method. One may conclude from these studies that ^{111}In-labeled leukocyte scanning is at least comparable to combined bone and gallium scanning in evaluating chronic osteomyelitis.

Advantages of leukocyte scanning are that imaging may be performed 4 hours after injection; however, imaging at 24 hours postinjection has been recommended because a 4 hour image may be falsely negative in the presence of osteomyelitis.[34] Poor spatial resolution is a major limitation of the method but may be overcome by comparison with the anatomic landmarks on a bone scan. Nevertheless, reliable separation of bone from soft tissue activity cannot always be accomplished. Another shortcoming of leukocyte scanning is that uptake by tumors, noninfectious arthritis, open fractures, and rapidly progressive neuroarthropathy may occur. Further drawbacks are the complex and time-consuming preparation required; the attention to proper imaging technique that is essential; the cost, which is two to three times that of a gallium study; and the relatively high radiation dose to the spleen.

In our experience, both ^{67}Ga and ^{111}In-labeled leukocyte imaging have significant limitations in the evaluation of chronic osteomyelitis, especially when superimposed on neuroarthropathy. Because it is less expensive and easier to perform, most centers rely on sequential bone and gallium imaging for the diagnosis of orthopedic infections.

COMPUTED TOMOGRAPHY AND MAGNETIC RESONANCE IMAGING

As already noted, foot disease constitutes one of the most serious long-term complications of diabetes mellitus and results from vascular compromise, peripheral neuropathy, or superimposed infection.[41,42] Fourteen percent of all diabetic patients are hospitalized annually for foot problems, with a mean in-patient hospital stay of 6 weeks per year.[43]

Infection is perhaps the most important manifestation of diabetic foot disease, owing to the potential for secondary osteomyelitis, suppurative arthritis, and generalized sepsis with endotoxic shock, the latter carrying a 40 to 90 percent mortality rate.[13,41,42,46,47] Infection of wounds occurs five times more frequently in diabetic than in nondiabetic patients, and once established, is more severe and more refractory to treatment.[48,49] Although conservative management with antibiotics and debridement may be successful for localized suppuration, extension to underlying bone or more proximal soft tissues, or both, via the plantar muscular compartments may require amputation.[41,50]

Soft Tissue Infection

Detection of early proximal soft tissue spread is essential if extensive pedal resections or even below the knee amputations are to be avoided.[51,52] Clinical techniques such as visual evaluation for persistent purulent discharge or edema of the malleolar area, wound probing, skin temperature measurement, and cut-down inspection of the retromalleolar tendon sheaths have been used previously to diagnose ascent of a known distal infection.[50,52,53] However, accurate assessment by such methods is often difficult owing to complicating vascular compromise and sensory neuropathy.[42]

Noninvasive imaging techniques, including contrast sinography, gallium 67 scintigraphy, and indium 111 leukocyte scanning, have also been advocated for determining the extent of inflammation in the diabetic foot.[21,42,54] None of these techniques is ideal; sinography may underestimate soft tissue involvement due to interference with contrast extravasation by granulation tissue, and experience with the latter two methods as applied to this clinical problem is limited.[42]

Furthermore, scan reliability may be altered in patients on prior antibiotic therapy, in whom leukocytes may fail to accumulate at a suppurative focus.[42] Positive gallium studies may be obtained in nonsuppurative inflammatory processes such as neuroarthropathy.[28]

Some investigators believe that the appropriate level for amputation in diabetic foot disease is best determined on the basis of the vascular status.[55,56] Segmental Doppler systolic pressures, arterial impedance plethysmography, photoplethysmography, noninvasive electromagnetic flowmetry, skin thermistor thermometry, three-phase skeletal scintigraphy, arteriography, and xenon 133 clearance studies have been used previously to assess soft tissue perfusion.[50,55–60] However, projectional overlap of skeletal structures is a problem in technetium 99m phosphate imaging, and the most accurate of the remaining techniques are invasive and have potential complications. Thus, it is apparent that an ideal preoperative means of facilitating the surgical goal of performing the most distal yet definitive amputation possible does not currently exist.

Once an infection has become established in a given compartment, progressive intracompartmental pressure elevation leads to extension into adjacent compartments, preferentially via musculotendinous transgressions of the intervening fascial septa. In the forefoot, where most diabetic foot infections begin, intermediate compartment disease chiefly spreads to the medial compartment along the adductor hallucis muscle and to the lateral compartment along the lumbrical and plantar interosseous muscles of the fifth toe; identical routes are employed for medial-to-intermediate and lateral-to-intermediate spread. Avenues of potential intercompartmental communication in the midfoot are of a lesser importance, since multicompartmental disease generally is present before the process has ascended to these levels. The predominant involvement of the intermediate compartment observed in patients with multicompartmental disease may reflect the fact that it contains the greatest amount of potential space.[6,61] Although dorsal extension has been documented by injection only from the lateral and intermediate compartments,[6,61] dorsal abnormalities in most patients suggest that it may occur from any plantar compartment. Furthermore, dorsal ascension may occur more readily than plantar, based on reported patterns of proximal extension. Similarly, the plantar fat may be involved by extension from any compartment, although it has been proved by injection only from the intermediate and lateral compartments.[6,61] Spread into the posterior compartment of the leg is a known potential consequence of intermediate compartment disease.[6,41,52,61]

The abnormal soft tissue densities seen on computed tomographic (CT) images in the diabetic foot may represent suppuration (Figs. 6-8 and 6-9), reactive granulation tissue, edema, or fibrosis, thus underscoring the limited contrast discrimination capability of this technique. Diabetic microangiopathy leads to thickening of the basement membrane of both capillaries and lymphatics, resulting in edema, which, if chronic, leads to irreversible fibrosis.[41] Although CT cannot reliably distinguish

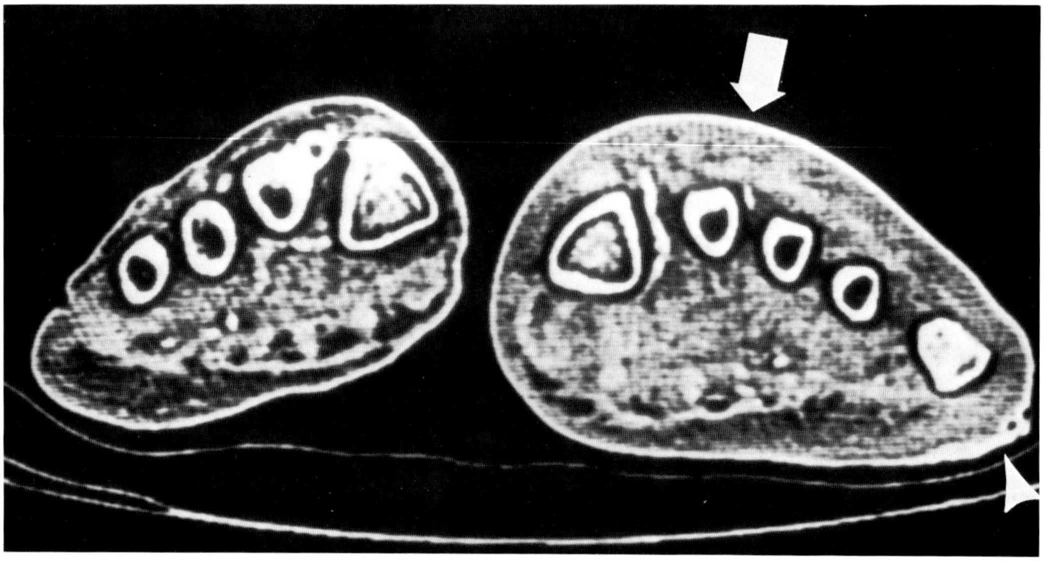

Fig. 6-8. CT scan of lateral compartment infection with dorsal extension. Soft tissue swelling and obliteration of fat planes are noted along the lateral aspect of the foot (arrowhead) as well as on the dorsum (arrow). In the contralateral foot, postoperative fibrosis is noted in the bed of the previous fifth ray resection. Vascular calcification is incidentally noted.

infection from soft tissue disease secondary to vascular compromise (Fig.6-10), the latter phenomenon may better determine the appropriate level for amputation.[55,56] Because most reported scans have not been performed with intravenous contrast material, further studies are required to evaluate its potential utility in this regard.

In general, areas of unequivocal soft tissue disease on CT images correlate well with the extent of infection as established by operative assessment,

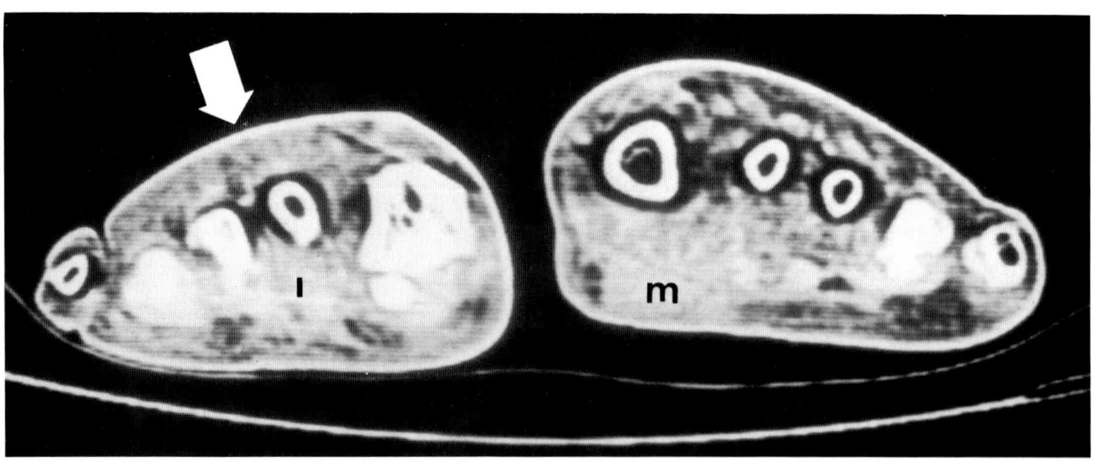

Fig. 6-9. CT scan of medial (M) and intermediate (I) compartment infections with dorsal extension on one side. Soft tissue swelling and obliteration of fat planes are noted in the affected compartments as well as along the dorsal aspect of one foot (arrow).

culture results, and ^{111}In-labeled leukocyte scanning. However, the presence of a transition zone extending over multiple levels lends a significant degree of subjectivity to prediction of the proximal margin of disease. Although imprecise, CT can contribute useful preoperative diagnostic information in the setting of diabetic foot infection.

Owing to its superior contrast discrimination capability, magnetic resonance imaging (MRI) may prove useful in distinguishing among the various types of abnormal soft tissue encountered in the diabetic foot. Diabetic patients with or without infections may have abnormal soft tissue signals and small joint effusions best shown on short-term inversion recovery (STIR) and T_2-weighted images (Fig. 6-11). The origin of this fluid is unknown. Ulcers usually form on the plantar aspect of the foot in diabetic patients as a result of the uneven distribution of body weight caused by peripheral neuropathy, similar to that of decubitus ulcer formation. The fluid accumulating in the soft tissues in the plantar aspect of the diabetic foot may result from the same mechanism of ulcer formation, with resultant stasis and fluid accumulation. Random traumas occurring as a consequence of the peripheral neuropathy—as opposed to the uneven weight distribution in the plantar aspect—may be responsible for the scattered pattern of the abnormal signal on the dorsal aspect of the foot. The frequently seen small joint effusion may also be related to peripheral neuropathy. Other possible causes of abnormal signal in the soft tissue include soft tissue infection and vascular insufficiency.[7]

MRI can distinguish lesions of the soft tissues from bone marrow disease and cellulitis from abscesses (Fig. 6-12).[7,62–64] In some diabetic patients, however, reduced contrast between the abscess and the abnormal soft tissue signal can cause diagnostic difficulty, especially for a small abscess in the plantar aspect of the foot. Although MRI is more sensitive than plain films and scintigraphy in detecting abscesses, reports have been shown that all three diagnostic techniques may fail to differentiate cellulitis from noninfectious edema.[7,62–64]

T_2-weighted images revealed abscesses better than STIR and T_1-weighted images. On STIR pulse

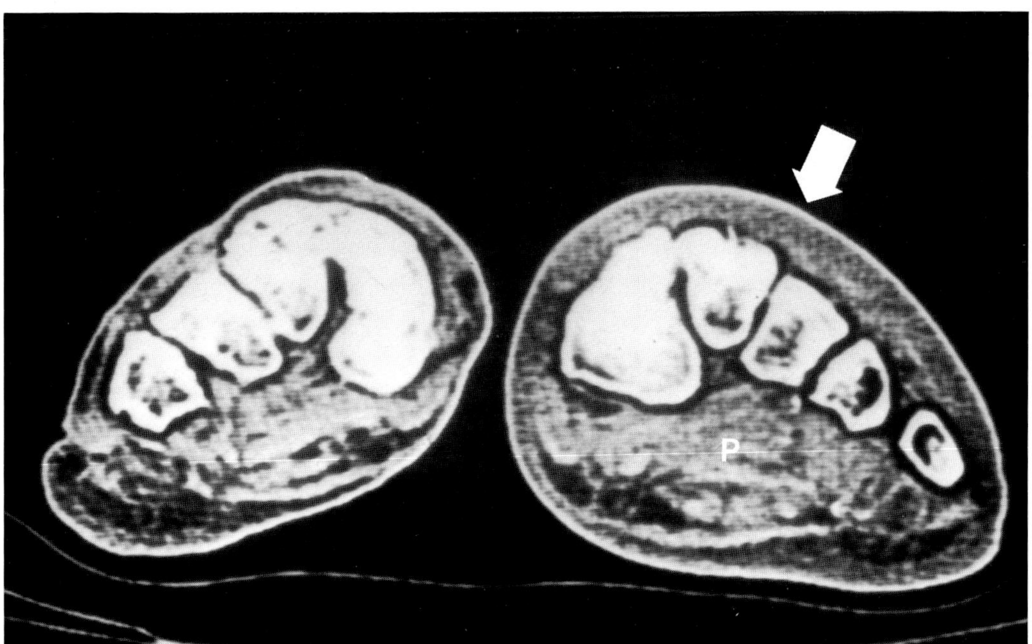

Fig. 6-10. CT depiction of diffuse edema in noninfected diabetic foot. Dorsal soft tissue swelling (arrow) and diffuse mild obliteration of intermuscular plantar fat planes (P) are noted; appearance is indistinguishable from infection. Incidentally evident is postsurgical absence of the fifth ray in the contralateral foot.

sequences, the abnormal soft tissue signal is so high in intensity it may obscure the abscess. T_1-weighted images also show very poor contrast between soft tissue and abscess. Postoperative fibrosis manifests relatively low signal intensity on all pulse sequences (Fig. 6-13). A head coil allows the entire foot to be examined easily and also significantly improves the resolution and signal-to-noise ratio.[7,61]

Osteomyelitis

Bone infections likewise can be detected accurately and sensitively with radionuclide studies, including ^{99m}Tc-MDP bone scintigraphy, ^{111}In-labeled leukocyte scanning, and ^{67}Ga-citrate studies.[7,13,17,21,65–68] Scintigraphic findings may be equivocal, however, owing to a lack of spatial resolution and an inability to visualize bone marrow

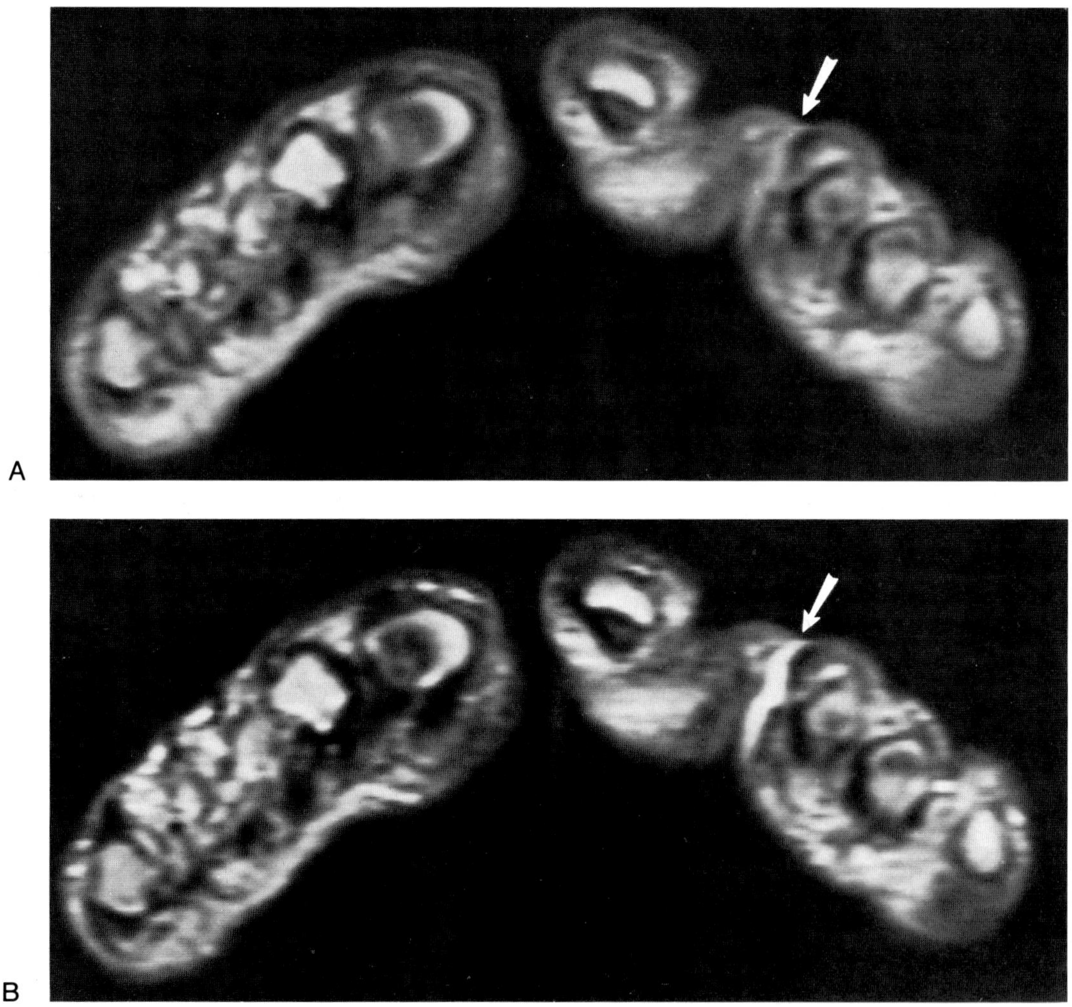

Fig. 6-11. Superficial soft tissue infection depicted by MRI. **(A)** On a proton density-weighted image, a curvilinear zone of intermediate signal intensity (arrow) is noted in the region of previous second ray resection. **(B)** On the corresponding T_2-weighted image, the area of abnormality brightens significantly (arrow).

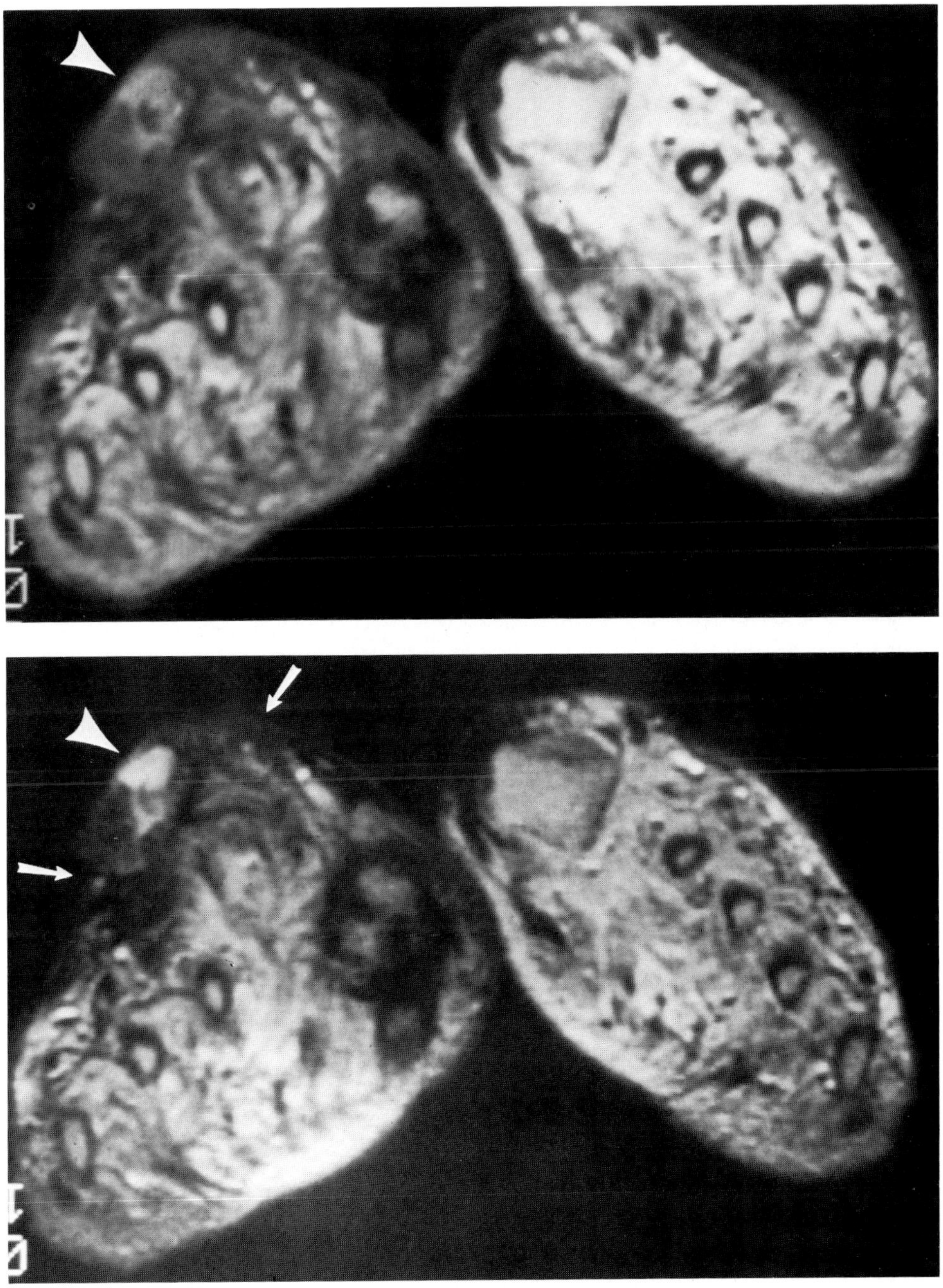

A

B

Fig. 6-12. MRI of abscess with surrounding granulation tissue and edema. (**A**) Proton density-weighted image in a patient with prior second ray resection reveals prominent soft tissue swelling along the dorsal aspect of the involved foot (arrowhead). The area of abnormality exhibits mixed signal intensity. (**B**) On a corresponding T_2-weighted image, a localized zone of increased signal intensity (arrowhead) is noted centrally within the soft tissue mass, indicative of active infection. The surrounding tissue remains low in signal intensity (arrows), and represents an area of combined edema and granulation tissue.

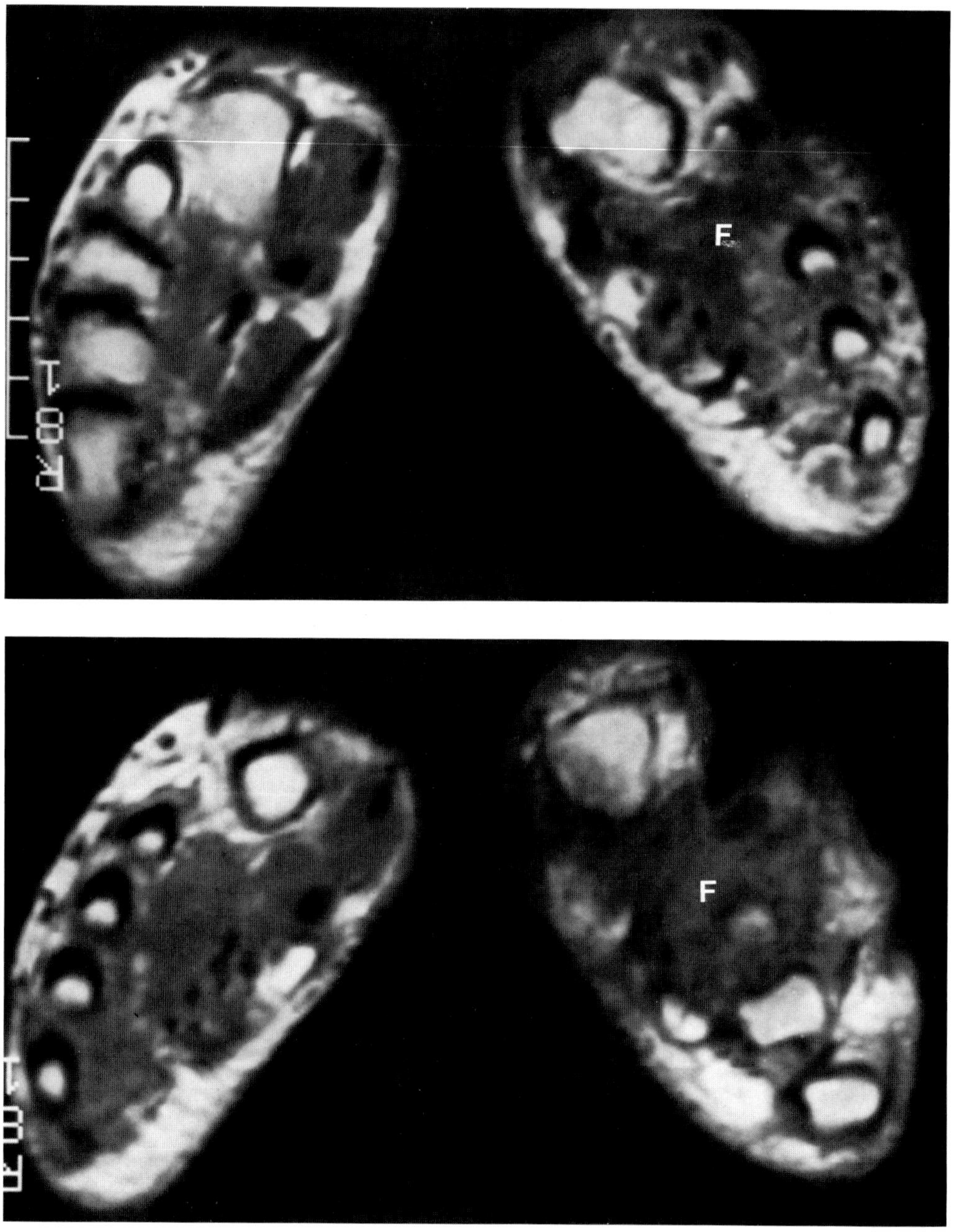

A

B

Fig. 6-13. (A & B) MRI of postoperative fibrosis. On sequential T_2-weighted images, the bed of the previous second ray resection exhibits uniformly intermediate signal intensity (F), with no apparent areas of brightening. This signal behavior is characteristic of postoperative fibrosis without superimposed active infection.

directly, leading to difficulty in differentiating soft tissue infections and osteomyelitis or in estimating the extent of involvement.[7,34,69-71] Scintigraphic results may not be reliable because of coexisting processes, such as diabetic neuroarthropathy or osteoarthropathy. Some authors[34,62] have reported significant false positive rates for scintigraphy in diabetic patients.

Preliminary results of comparisons between MRI and CT or ^{111}In-labeled leukocyte scans show that

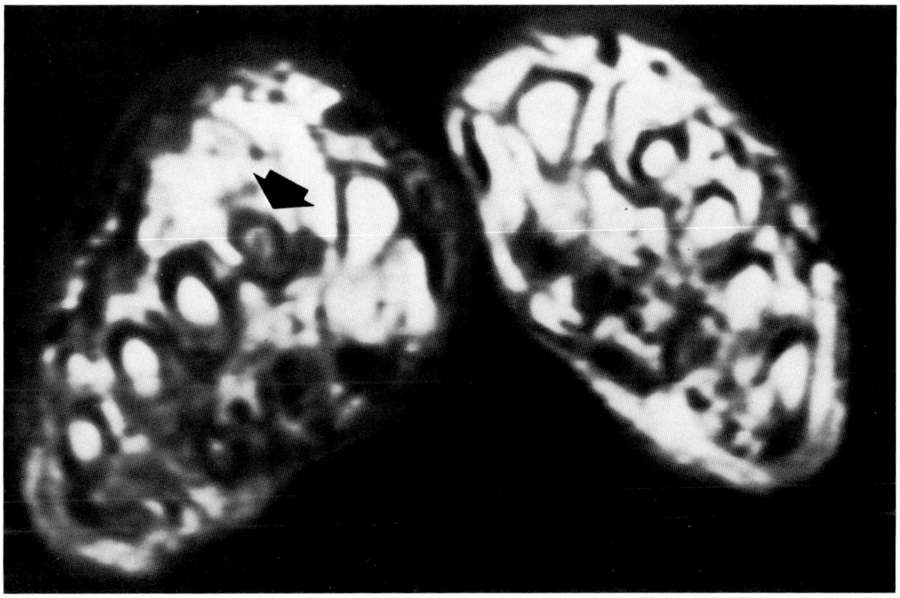

A

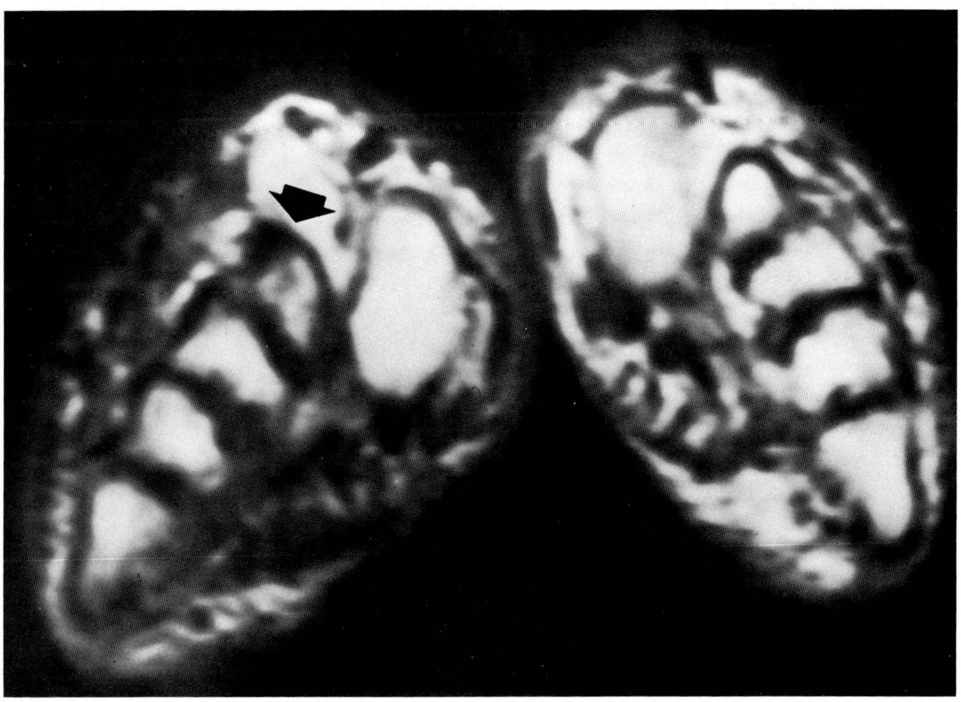

B

Fig. 6-14. MRI of osteomyelitis involving second metatarsal. T_1-weighted images in the shaft (**A**) and base (**B**) of the second metatarsal reveal localized decreased signal intensity within the marrow space (arrows). *(Figure continues.)*

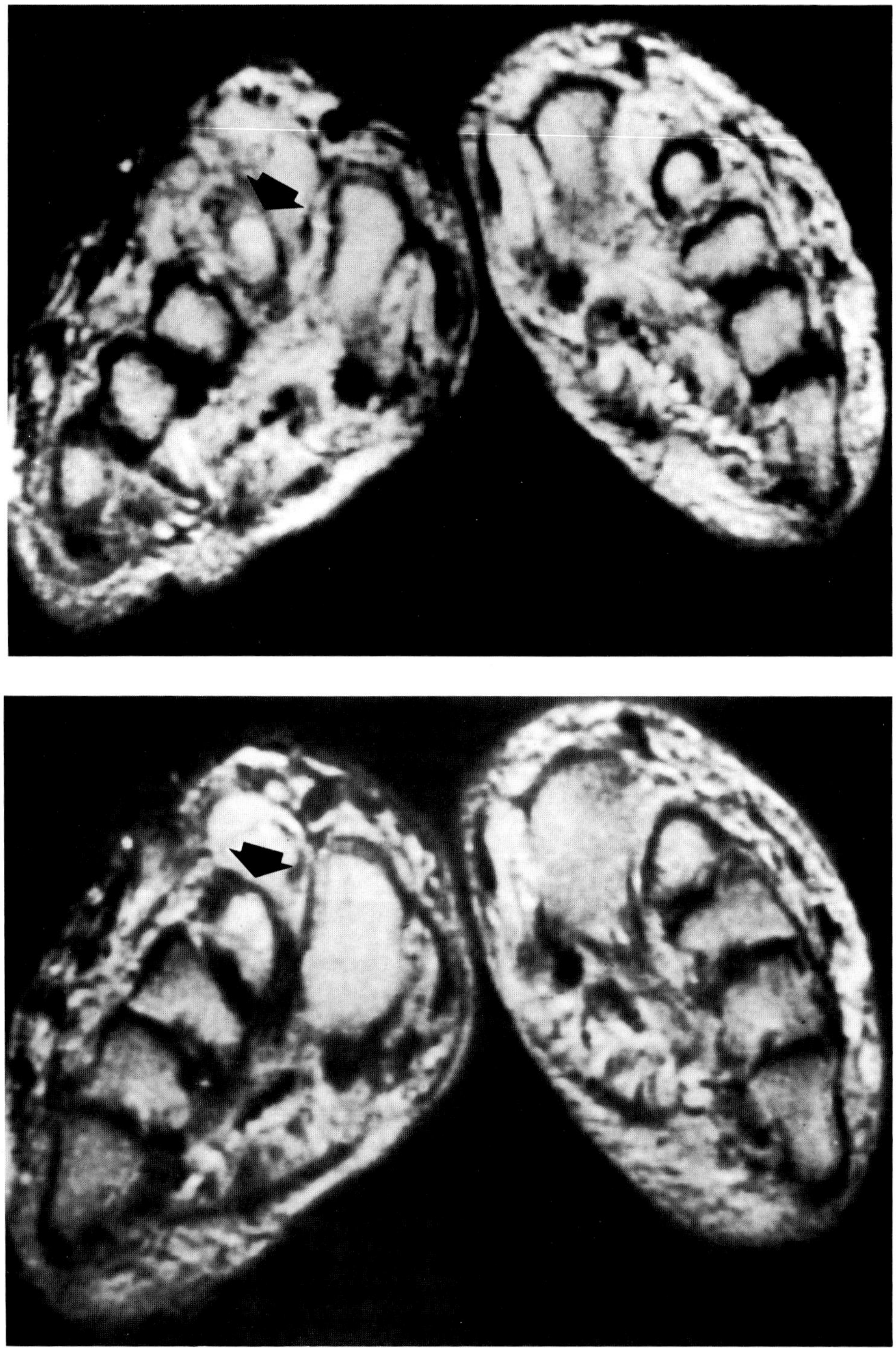

C

D

Fig. 6-14 (*Continued*). **(C & D)** On corresponding t_2-weighted images, the area of abnormality exhibits increased signal intensity (arrow).

MRI is more accurate than plain films and CT in detecting bone or soft tissue infections; moreover, it provides more detailed information on the extent of involvement than radionuclide studies. Although MRI does have a high sensitivity and specificity in detecting osteomyelitis,[7,62,72–77] it is less helpful than ^{111}In-labeled leukocyte scanning in evaluating patients postoperatively.[7,75]

Diagnosis of osteomyelitis of the foot in diabetic patients may be difficult because of the coexistence of chronic cellulitis, vascular insufficiency, and peripheral neuropathy. Yuh et al. have compared the diagnostic accuracies of plain films, bone scans, and MRI studies in diabetic patients.[7] Twenty-nine plain radiographs, 20 bone scans, and 30 MRI studies were obtained in 24 patients with suspected osteomyelitis of the foot. These patients had trauma, cellulitis, or unhealed ulcers. In contrast to previous reports, however, MRI had much higher sensitivity and specificity than bone scans in detecting osteomyelitis in diabetic patients. When 10 patients without pathologic proof of osteomyelitis (those who presumably had neuroarthropathy, vascular insufficiency, or cellulitis) were included, the sensitivity and specificity of all three techniques decreased.[7]

The foot infections of most of the patients in Yuh et al.'s study were serious and complicated, involving the bone and soft tissues, with coexistent bony changes caused by trauma or diabetic neuroarthropathy. This may have been partly responsible for the high sensitivity and specificity of MRI and the relatively high false positive rate of ^{99m}Tc-MDP bone imaging reported in this series.[7]

Of the three techniques compared in this series, MR had the lowest false positive rate. MRI can visualize bone marrow directly, which improves the sensitivity and specificity and therefore significantly reduces the false positive rate (Fig. 6-14). Osteomyelitis is best shown by T_1 and STIR imaging. As with plain film and CT, MRI cannot differentiate the abnormal signal caused by acute trauma from that of osteomyelitis. Although a significant change in the water content of bone marrow presumably is produced by both processes, chronic fractures do not reveal a significant increase in MRI signal intensity in the bone marrow. The most logical explanation for this is that the local edema produced during acute trauma has resolved. A similar mechanism may also account for the decrease of abnormal signal within the bone marrow seen in the follow-up examinations in patients with clinical evidence of improvement after intravenous antibiotic treatment.[7]

MR is thus an extremely useful technique for assessing osteomyelitis, particularly in the foot, in patients with diabetes mellitus. The ultimate role of MRI in the evaluation of osteomyelitis is not yet clear, however, and will require assessment of a larger number of diabetic patients.

REFERENCES

1. Faris I: The Management of the Diabetic Foot. Churchill Livingstone, New York, 1982
2. Pogonowska MJ, Collins LC, Dobson HL: Diabetic osteopathy. Radiology 89:265, 1967
3. Gondos B: The pointed tubular bone: its significance and pathogenesis. Radiology 105:541, 1972
4. Tawn DJ, O'Hare JP, O'Brien IAD et al: Bone scintigraphy and radiography in the early detection of diabetic foot osteopathy. Br J Radiol 61:273, 1988
5. Sartoris DJ, Devine S, Resnick D et al: Plantar compartmental infection in the diabetic foot: the role of computed tomography. Invest Radiol 20:772, 1985
6. Feingold ML, Resnick D, Niwayama G, Garetto L: The plantar compartments of the foot: a roentgen approach. I. Experimental observations. Invest Radiol 12:281, 1977
7. Yuh WTC, Corson JD, Baraniewski HM et al: Osteomyelitis of the foot in diabetic patients: evaluation with plain film, ^{99m}TC-MDP bone scintigraphy, and MR imaging. AJR 152:795, 1989
8. Boulton AJM, Scarpello JHB, Ward, JD: Venous oxygenation in the diabetic neuropathic foot: evidence of arteriovenous shunting. Diabetologia 22:6, 1982
9. Edmonds ME, Roberts VC, Watkins PJ: Blood flow in the diabetic foot. Diabetologia 22:9, 1982
10. Rayman G, Hassan A, Tooke JE: Blood flow in the skin of the foot related to posture in diabetes mellitus. Br Med J 292:87, 1986
11. Everhart JE, Pettitt DJ, Knowler WC et al: Medial arterial calcification and its association with mortality and complications of diabetes. Diabetologia 31:16, 1988
12. Maurer AH, Chen DCP, Camargo EE et al: Utility of three-phase skeletal scintigraphy in suspected osteomyelitis: concise communication. J Nucl Med 22:941, 1981

13. Park HM, Wheat LJ, Siddiqui AR et al: Scintigraphic evaluation of diabetic osteomyelitis: Concise communication. J Nucl Med 23:569, 1982
14. Rosenthall L, Lisbona R: p. 111. In: Skeletal Imaging. Appleton-Century-Crofts, Norwalk, CT, 1984
15. Alazraki N, Dries D, Datz F et al: Value of a 24-hour image (four-phase bone scan) in assessing osteomyelitis in patients with peripheral vascular disease. J Nucl Med 26:711, 1985
16. Israel O, Gips S, Jersuhalmi J et al: Osteomyelitis and soft-tissue infection: differential diagnosis with 24 hour/4 hour ratio of Tc-99m MDP uptake. Radiology 163:725, 1987
17. Seldin DW, Heiken JP, Feldman F et al: Effect of soft-tissue pathology on detection of pedal osteomyelitis in diabetics. J Nucl Med 26:988, 1985
18. Deutsch SD, Grandsman EJ, Spraragen SC: Quantitative regional blood flow anaylsis and its clinical application during routine bone scanning. J Bone Joint Surg 63A:295, 1981
19. Eymontt MJ, Alavi A, Dalinka MK et al: Bone scintigraphy in diabetic osteoarthropathy. Radiology 140:475, 1981
20. Hoffer P: Gallium and infection. J Nucl Med 21:484, 1980
21. Lisbona R, Rosenthall L: Observations on the sequential use of ^{99m}Tc-phosphate complex and ^{67}Ga imaging in osteomyelitis, cellulitis, and septic arthritis. Radiology 123:123, 1977
22. Staab EV, McCarney WH: Role of gallium 67 in inflammatory disease. Semin Nucl Med 8:219, 1978
23. Hoffer P: Gallium mechanisms. J Nucl Med 21:282, 1980
24. Tsan MF, Chen WY, Scheffel U et al: Studies on gallium accumulation in inflammatory lesions. I. Gallium uptake by human polymorphonuclear leukocytes. J Nucl Med 19:36, 1978
25. Weiner R, Hoffer PM, Thakur MI: Lactoferrin: Its role as a Ga-67 binding protein in polymorphonuclear leukocytes. J Nucl Med 22:32, 1981
26. Alazraki N, Fierer J, Resnick D: Chronic osteomyelitis: monitoring by ^{99m}Tc Phosphate and ^{67}Ga citrate imaging. AJR 145:767, 1985
27. Kolyvas E, Rosenthall L, Ahronhesum GA et al: Serial ^{67}Ga-citrate imaging during treatment of acute osteomyelitis in childhood. Clin Nucl Med 3:461, 1978
28. Glynn TP: Marked gallium accumulation in neurogenic arthropathy. J Nucl Med 22:1016, 1981
29. LaManna MM, Garbarino JL, Berman AT et al: An assessment of technetium and gallium scanning in the patient with painful total joint arthroplasty. Orthopedics 5:580, 1983
30. Reing CM, Richin PF, Kenmore PI: Differential bone scanning in the evaluation of a painful total joint replacement. J Bone Joint Surg 61A:933, 1979
31. Lawson JP, Hoffer PB: RSNA Refresher Course #211: Correlative nuclear bone imaging in benign disease. Presented at the 72nd annual meeting of the Radiological Society of North America, Chicago, IL, Nov. 31–Dec 5, 1986
32. Rosenthall L, Kloiber R, Damtew B et al: Sequential use of radiophosphate and radiogallium imaging in the differential diagnosis of bone, joint and soft tissue infection: quantitative analysis. Diagn Imaging 51:249, 1982
33. Gleason TJ, Seabold JE, Flickinger FW et al: Osteomyelitis in the presence of neuropathic osteoarthropathy: In-111 WBC/Tc-99m MDP bone and MR imaging. Presented at the 75th annual meeting of the Radiological Society of North America, Chicago, IL, Nov 26–Dec 1, 1989
34. Maurer AH, Millmond SH, Knight LC et al: Infection in diabetic osteoarthropathy: use of indium-labled leukocytes for diagnosis. Radiology 161:221, 1986
35. Schauwecker DS, Park HM, Burt RW et al: Combined bone scintigraphy and indium-111 leukocyte scans in neuropathic foot disease. J Nucl Med 29:1651, 1988
36. Splittgerber GF, Spiegelhoff DR, Buggy BP: Combined leukocyte and bone imaging used to evaluate diabetic osteoarthropathy and osteomyelitis. Clin Nucl Med 14:156, 1989
37. Sfakianakis GN, Al-Sheikh W, Heal A et al: Comparisons of scintigraphy with In-111 leukocytes and Ga-67 in the diagnosis of occult sepsis. J Nucl Med 23:618, 1982
38. Datz FL, Thorne DA: Effect of chronicity of infection on the sensitivity of the In-111-labeled leukocyte scan. AJR 147:809, 1986
39. Merkel KD, Brown ML, Dewanjee MK et al: Comparison of indium-labeled-leukocyte imaging with sequential technetium-gallium scanning in the diagnosis of low-grade musculoskeletal sepsis. J Bone Joint Surg 67A:465, 1985
40. Al-Sheikh W, Sfakianakis GN, Mnaymneh W et al: Subacute and chronic bone infections: diagnosis using In-111, Ga-67 and Tc-99m MDP bone scintigraphy, and radiography. Radiology 155:501, 1985
41. Arenson DJ, Sherwood CF, Wilson RC: Neuropathy, angiopathy, and sepsis in the diabetic foot. Part III: Sepsis. J Am Podiatry Assoc 72:35, 1982
42. Visser HJ, Jacobs AM, Oloff L, Drago JJ: The use of differential scintigraphy in the clinical

diagnosis of osseous and soft tissue changes affecting the diabetic foot. J Foot Surg 23:74, 1984

43. Kozak GP (ed.). Clinical Diabetes Mellitus. WB Saunders, Philadelphia, 1982, p. 215
44. Rubinstein A, Pierce CE Jr, Bloomgarden Z: Rapid healing of diabetic foot ulcers with continuous subcutaneous insulin infusion. Am J Med 75:161, 1983
45. Ellenberg M, Rifkin H. Diabetes Mellitus: Theory and Practice. McGraw-Hill, New York, 1970, p. 890
46. Joklik WK, Willett HP, Amos DB (eds): Zinsser Microbiology. 18th Ed. East Norwalk, CT, Appleton-Century-Crofts, 1984
47. O'Neal LW: Surgical pathology of the foot and clincopathological correlations. p. 108. In: Levin ME, O'Neal LW (eds): The Diabetic Foot. St Louis, MO, CV Mosby, 1977
48. Little JR, Kobayashi GE: Bateriology and infections in the diabetic foot. p. 97. In: Levin ME, O'Neal LW (eds): The Diabetic Foot. St Louis, MO, CV Mosby, 1977
49. Cruse PJE, Foord RA: Prospective study of 23,649 surgical wounds. Arch Surg 107:206, 1973
50. Kalker AJ, Kolodny HD, Cavuota JW: The evaluation and treatment of diabetic foot ulcers. J Am Podiatry Assoc 72:491, 1982
51. Jacobs RL, Karmody AM. Instructional Course Lectures. The American Academy of Orthopedic Surgeons. 28:118, 1979
52. Ger R: Newer concepts in the surgical management of lesions of the foot in patients with diabetes. Surg Gynecol Obstet 158:213, 1984
53. Ecker ML, Jacobs BS: Lower extremity amputation in diabetic patients. Diabetes 19:189, 1970
54. Alazraki N: Bone imaging by radionuclide techniques. p. 406. In: Resnick D, Niwayama G (eds): Diagnosis of Bone and Joint Disorders. 2nd Ed. Philadelphia, WB Saunders, 1988
55. Johnson RM: Considerations in the determination of the amputation level of the diabetic foot. J Am Podiatry Assoc 72:192, 1982
56. Lee BY, Trainor FS, Kavner D, McCann WJ, Madden JL: Noninvasive hemodynamic evaluation in selection of amputation level. Surg Gynecol Obstet 149:241, 1979
57. Moore WS, Henry RE, Malone JM et al: Prospective use of xenon Xe 133 clearance for amputation level selection. Arch Surg 116:86, 1981
58. Moore WS: Determination of amputation level: measurement of skin blood flow with xenon Xe 133. Arch Surg 107:798, 1973
59. Lawrence PF, Syverud JB, Disbro MA, Alazraki N: Evaluation of technetium-99m phosphate imaging for predicting skin ulcer healing. Am J Surg 146:746, 1983.
60. Greene G, Maurer AH, Malmud LS, Charles ND: "Cold spot" imaging with gas gangrene in three phase skeletal scintigraphy. Clin Nucl Med 8:410, 1983
61. Resnick D, Niwayama G: Osteomyelitis, septic arthritis and soft tissue infection: The mechanisms and situations. p. 2524. In: Resnick D, Niwayama G (eds): Diagnosis of Bone and Joint Disorders. 2nd Ed. WB Saunders, Philadelphia, 1988
62. Unger E, Moldofsky P, Gatenby R, Hartz W, Broder G: Diagnosis of osteomyelitis by MR imaging. AJR 150:605, 1988
63. Beltran J, Noto AM, McGhee RB et al: Infections of the musculosketal system: high field strength MR imaging. Radiology 164:449, 1987
64. Beltran J, McGhee RB, Shaffer PB et al: Experimental infections of the musculoskeletal system: evaluation with MR imaging and Tc-99m MDP and Ga-67 scintigraphy. Radiology 167:167, 1988
65. Gilday DL, Eng B, Paul DJ, Paterson J: Diagnosis of osteomyelitis in children by combined blood pool and bone imaging. Radiology 117:331, 1975
66. Duszynski DO, Kuhn JP, Afshani E, Riddlesberger MM Jr: Early radionuclide diagnosis of acute osteomyelitis. Radiology 117:337, 1975
67. Reba RC, Chandeysson PL: Imaging infection with indium 111-labeled leukocytes. p. 305. In: Takor ML (ed): Radiolabeled Cellular Blood Elements: Pathophysiology, Techniques, and Scintigraphic Applications. Plenum, New York, 1985
68. Sfakianakis GN, Al-Sheikh W, Heal A et al: Comparison of scintigraphy with in-111 leukocytes and Ga-67 in the diagnosis of occult sepsis. J Nucl Med 23:618, 1982
69. Gilday DL: Problems in the scintigraphic detection of osteomyelitis. Radiology 135:791, 1980
70. Garnett ES, Cockshott WP, Jacobs J: Classical acute osteomyelitis with a negative bone scan. Br J Radiol 50:757, 1977
71. Handmaker H: Acute hematogenous osteomyelitis: has the bone scan betrayed us? Radiology 135:787, 1980
72. Smith FW, Runge V, Permezel M, Smith CC: Nuclear magnetic resonance (NMR) imaging in the diagnosis of spinal osteomyelitis. Magn Reson Imaging 2:53, 1984
73. Fletcher BD, Scoles PV, Nelson AD: Osteomyelitis in children: detection by magnetic resonance. Radiology 150:57, 1984

74. Modic MT, Feiglin DH, Piraino DW et al: Vertebral osteomyelitis: assessment using MR. Radiology 157:157, 1985
75. Berquist TH, Brown ML, Fitzgerald RH Jr, May GR: Magnetic resonance imaging: application in musculoskeletal infection. Magn Reson Imaging 3:219, 1985
76. Tang JSH, Gold RH, Bassett LW, Seeger LL: Musculoskeletal infection of the extremities: evaluation with MR imaging. Radiology 166:205, 1988.
77. Quinn SF, Murray W, Clark RA, Cochran C: MR imaging of chronic osteomyelitis. J Comput Assist Tomogr 12:113, 1988

7

Environmental Stress and Tissue Breakdown

William M. Jenkin, D.P.M., D.A.B.P.S.
Steven J. Palladino, D.P.M., D.A.B.P.S.

Scientists and clinicians alike have been trying for ages to gain an understanding of the pathogenesis of ulceration in the diabetic patient. These efforts are not without clinical relevance. With an understanding of the process, effective intervention becomes possible at numerous levels. Treatment for ulcers could be specifically modified. Early warning signs could be identified so early treatment may be provided. Risk factors could be identified and patients stratified according to relative risk. Most importantly, preventative measures could be identified and instituted. It is clear that understanding the pathogenesis of ulceration is essential if one is to provide optimal care for diabetic patients.

It follows, then, that every effort should be made to enhance one's awareness of the pathogenic process. Then, with that knowledge, one should manipulate factors in favor of restoring and/or maintaining the intact state of the patient's foot. Unfortunately, all of the pieces to the puzzle are not in place yet, but a good conceptual understanding of the pathogenesis of ulceration is available. Furthermore, many specific risk factors and mechanisms, both intrinsic and extrinsic, have been identified. With these discoveries, interventional measures have been suggested. In all, the material presented here can serve to make the job of limb preservation in the diabetic patient much easier.

PATHOGENESIS CONCEPTUALIZED

Described in the most basic of terms, soft tissue failure occurs as the result of an abnormal interaction between an environmental stress and the soft tissues over a given period of time. In a foot with intact sensation, tissue disruption is most often encountered when it is subjected to an unavoidable, intense environmental stress, producing a defect such as a laceration or burn. The environmental stress is known at the time of injury. The temporal relationship is known and often instantaneous. The reason for soft tissue failure is easily explained.

In contrast, soft tissue breakdown in the insensate foot is often poorly explained. The patient presents to the physician one day with a pedal ulcer, not knowing how or why it developed. The environmental stress may not be recognized, and even if recognized, may not be considered unusual. The temporal relationship is often unknown. One might even be led to believe that there was some type of intrinsic soft tissue weakness that accounted for the ulcer, giving rise to the "trophic ulcer" concept. In fact, the soft tissues of an insensate individual may be no different than those in an individual with intact sensation, yet the soft tissues of the insensate individual are found to ulcerate. The key factor accounting for difference, then, must be the lack of protective sensation. The reason neuropathy can be such a critical factor may be found by re-examining the original statement that "soft tissue failure occurs as a result of an abnormal interaction between an environmental stress and the soft tissues over a given period of time." The duration of exposure of the soft tissues to the environmental stress is an integral part of soft tissue failure. Normally, when a stress-time relationship is perceived as noxious, there is a withdrawal response. Neuropathy robs the individual of the protective response, allowing the stress to act for a longer period of time, which may become deleterious to the soft tissues. By virtue of neuropathic loss of protective sensation, any environmental stress, even relatively normal ones, can produce soft tissue failure if given enough time. This is not to ignore the importance of the soft tissues' ability to withstand the deleterious effects of a given stress-time relationship. Nor is it to imply that under all circumstances, the soft tissues in diabetic patients remain as resistant to stress as healthy, nondiabetic soft tissues. In fact, diabetic soft tissues may become less resistant to failure. The ability of the soft tissues to resist failure must be considered a factor in ulcerogenesis. Nevertheless, the neuropathic loss of protective sensation is usually more influential in soft tissue failure than are changes to the soft tissues.

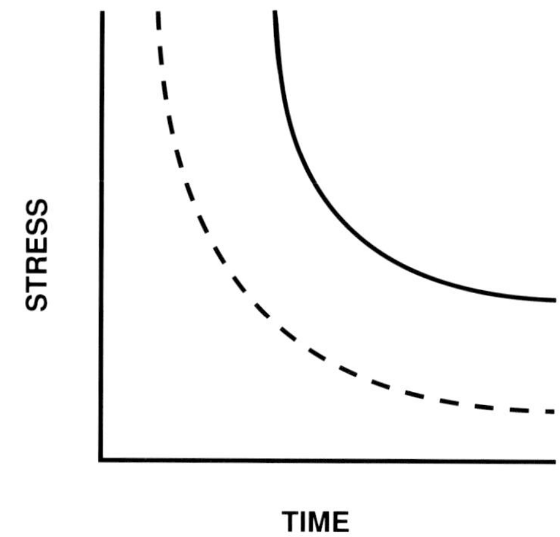

Fig. 7-1. Conceptual graphic demonstration of a stress-time relationship in normal human soft tissues. The broken line depicts the level at which any given stress-time relationship will be perceived as a noxious stimulus. This line constitutes the body's sensory protective threshold. The solid line depicts the level at which any given stress-time relationship will result in soft tissue breakdown. The line reflects the maximum ability of the soft tissues to resist breakdown. Note the implied safety zone between the lines.

To conceptualize the pathogenesis of ulceration in the diabetic patient then, the key factors include (1) the status of the sensory protective response, or protective threshold, (2) the type and magnitude of the applied stress, (3) the duration of stress application, and (4) the ability of the soft tissues to resist failure. With these factors in mind, a conceptual

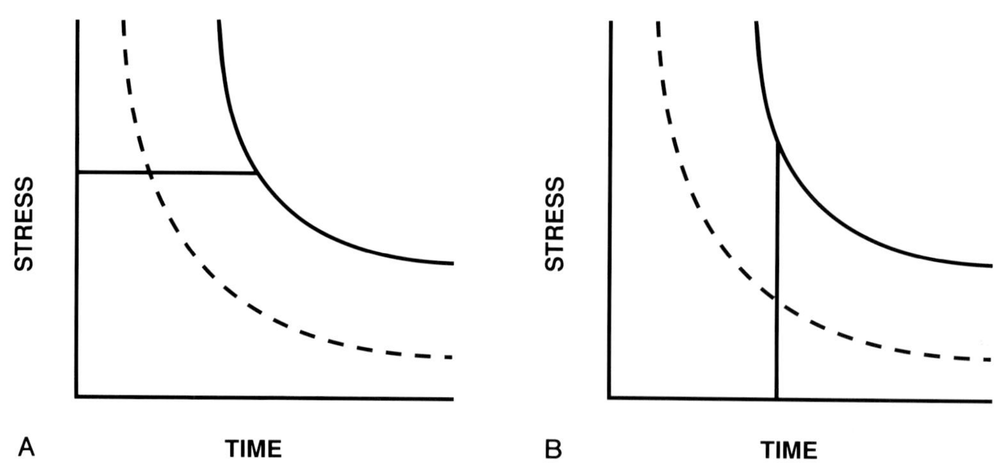

Fig. 7-2. Conceptual graphic demonstration of a stress-time relationship in normal human soft tissues. **(A)** For a given magnitude of applied stress, the stress will be perceived as noxious before soft tissue breakdown can occur, eliciting a withdrawal response. **(B)** For any given period of time, the magnitude of stress that would be perceived as a noxious stimulus is lower than that which would produce soft tissue breakdown.

model can be constructed, using a stress-time graph with two lines (Fig. 7-1). One line would represent points at which soft tissues fail, for any given stress-time relationship. The other line would represent the protective threshold, points where a stress-time relationship may begin to be perceived as a noxious stimulus. Thus, all key factors are represented. In a person without neuropathy, the line representing the protective threshold would lie much closer to the *x* and *y* axes than the line representing the soft tissue failure points. The arrangement as just described implies a margin of safety between protective threshold and soft tissue breakdown. For any given stress magnitude, the stress will be perceived as a noxious stimulus before acting long enough to produce a deleterious effect on the soft tissues (Fig. 7-2). Similarly, for any duration of stress application, a lower magnitude of stress is required to be perceived as a noxious stimulus than that required to produce tissue failure (Fig. 7-2).

The model can be used to demonstrate the effect of a progressive neuropathy, such as that seen with diabetes mellitus (Fig. 7-3). Starting with a normal relationship between the lines, one can expect that as the neuropathy progresses, the protective

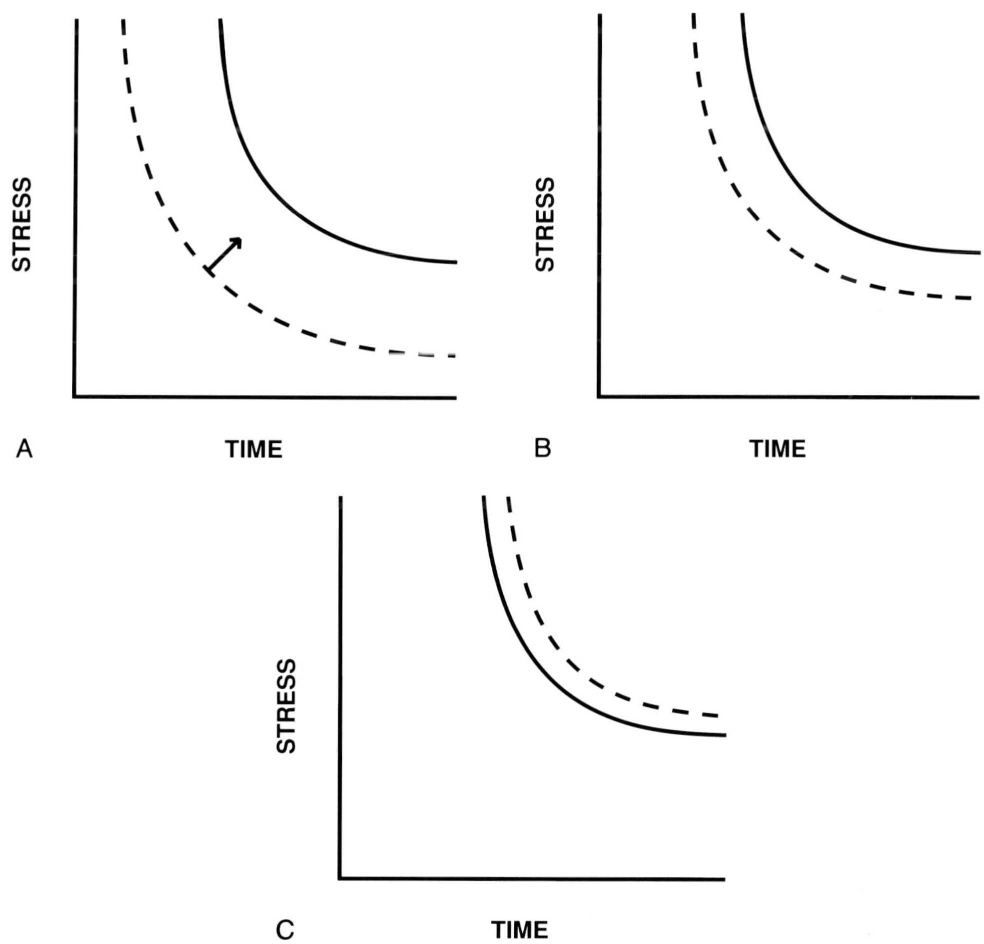

Fig. 7-3. Conceptual graphic demonstration of a stress-time relationship in the presence of a progressive neuropathy. (**A**) Starting with a normal relationship between the sensory protective threshold and the soft tissue breakdown point, neuropathy causes a shift (arrow) of the protective threshold. (**B**) The shift brings the protective threshold closer to the point of soft tissue breakdown. (**C**) At some point the shift in protective threshold progresses beyond a functional level, such that stress-time relationships will cause soft tissue breakdown before being perceived as noxious.

threshold line will shift toward the soft tissue failure line, which remains stationary. The person will retain protective sensory function as long as the protective threshold line remains closer to the x and y axes than the soft tissue failure line, although the margin of safety is reduced. Once the protective threshold line coincides with the soft tissue failure line or crosses it to become further from the x and y axes, the person becomes at risk for ulceration. In other words, soft tissue failure will occur before the withdrawal response can be initiated, for any given stress-time relationship.

Similarly, the model can be utilized to depict the effect of decreased capacity of soft tissues to resist failure (Fig. 7-4). In this case, the soft tissue failure line can be expected to shift gradually in the direction of the x and y axes, toward the protective threshold line, once again reducing the margin of

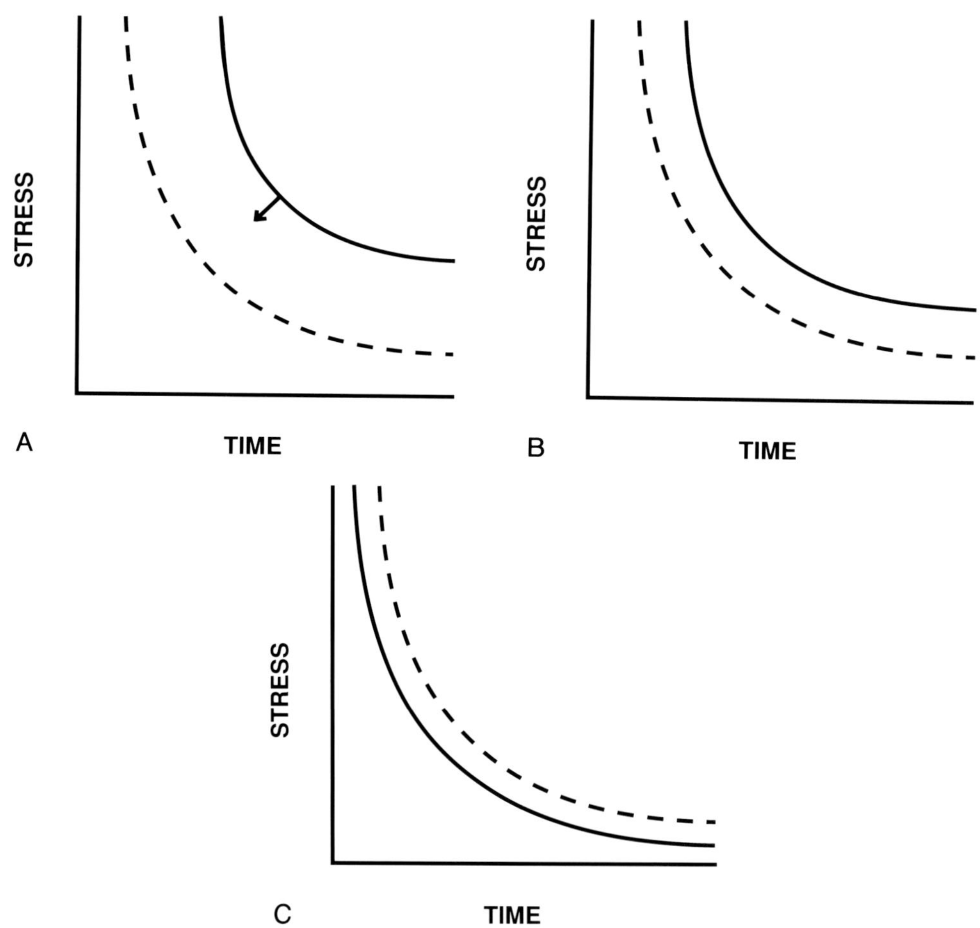

Fig. 7-4. Conceptual graphic demonstration of a stress-time relationship in which the soft tissues progressively become less resistant to breakdown. **(A)** Starting with a normal relationship between the sensory protective threshold and the soft tissue breakdown point, an aberrancy of the soft tissues causes a shift (arrow) of the soft tissue breakdown point. **(B)** The shift brings the soft tissue breakdown point toward the stress-time axes and thus closer to the protective threshold. **(C)** If the shift of the soft tissue breakdown point progresses further, indicating progressively less resistant soft tissues, the line may fall closer to the axes than the protective threshold. In such a situation, soft tissues readily break down before a stress-time relationship is perceived as noxious.

safety. Rarely does the soft tissue failure line shift so dramatically as to cross the stationary protective threshold line.

Finally, the model can be used to demonstrate what may actually occur in the diabetic state (Fig. 7-5). In diabetic patients, both lines may shift. The protective threshold line shifts away from the x and y axes. This certainly predominates. A smaller shift of the soft tissue failure line toward the x and y axes may also occur in some patients. Once the lines cross to assume a reversed relationship, the patient becomes at risk for ulceration.

In summary, conceptualization serves well to stimulate a general understanding of the process but falls short in describing more specific defects and mechanisms. The pathogenesis of diabetic ulceration is clearly multifactorial. Of the various factors discussed, sensory neuropathy is clearly the most important. When analyzing the major factors, one can begin to categorize them into those that are

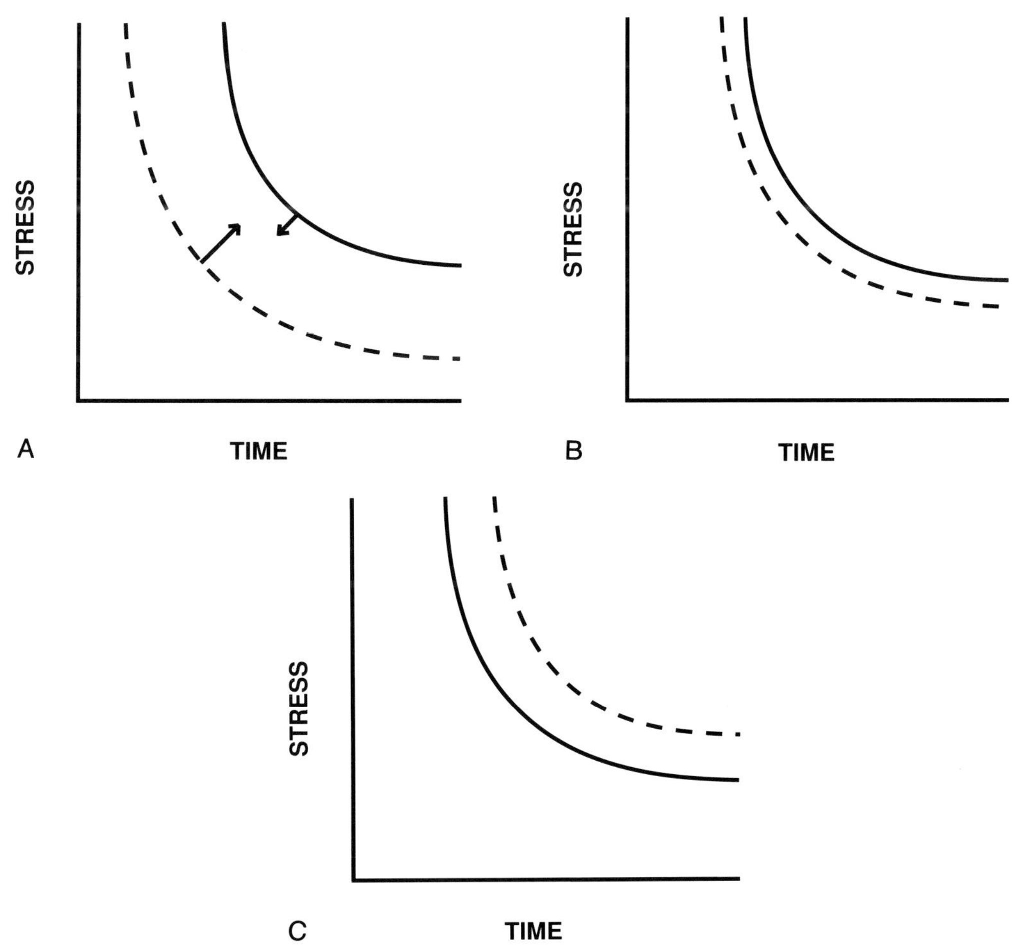

Fig. 7-5. Conceptual graphic demonstration of a stress-time relationship as it might occur in the actual diabetic state. **(A)** Starting with a normal relationship between the sensory protective threshold and the point of soft tissue breakdown, both lines may be seen to shift (arrows). **(B)** A more progressive shift away from the axes is seen with the sensory protective threshold, while some shift in the soft tissue's ability to resist breakdown might be seen, depicted as a shift toward the axes. The net result is that both lines shift toward each other, the sensory protective threshold being the one with the greater shift. **(C)** At some point, the lines cross and the subject becomes at risk for ulceration.

intrinsic factors, such as neuropathy and soft tissue resistance to failure, and those that are extrinsic factors, such as stress-time relationships. Categorization as such will serve to further the discussion in this chapter into more specific defects and mechanisms. Furthermore, the categorization may serve to focus interventional efforts and future research. With regard to preventive intervention, the most efficacious methods currently appear to be directed at the extrinsic factors, although some inroads are being made toward intrinsic factors, as will be discussed.

INTRINSIC FACTORS

Sensory Neuropathy

The most critical factor, intrinsic or extrinsic, in ulcerogenesis is sensory neuropathy. The conceptual model once again can serve to illustrate some important points regarding diabetic peripheral neuropathy as it applies to soft tissue breakdown. The first point to be made is that diabetic peripheral neuropathy, unfortunately, still remains a progressive disorder. The model demonstrates this by depicting the sensory protective level as a shifting line, where the shift is continually in the direction of decreased acuity and functional importance. A second point that can be made is that at some instant in time, sensation ceases to function in a protective manner. The model depicts this occurrence as that point where the protective sensory line crosses the soft tissue failure line. At that point, a "protective threshold" can be defined, where the patient becomes at risk for neuropathic ulceration. Implied is the potential to identify that protective threshold with some objective sensory screening. Third, all sensation is not lost at the protective threshold level. The protective sensory line isn't erased off the graph, but continues to drift further from the x and y axes, requiring progressively more intense stress-time stimuli to be perceived as noxious. Some sensation will still be perceived by patients that have lost their protective threshold, creating a diagnostic challenge.

The solution to the challenge is to identify and utilize an objective, reproducible, quantitative, sensitive, and specific test that can signal when a protective threshold is lost. The standard history and physical examination will just not suffice in identifying the protective threshold level. Subjectively, the neuropathy may have progressed so insidiously that the patient may have no awareness of sensory deficit and already have lost protective sensory function. By the time the patient may become aware of any sensory loss, 50 percent of the nerve endings in the skin may be lost and the protective threshold long since surpassed. When appropriately tested, patients with parasthesia or painful neuropathy quite frequently are found to still have functionally protective sensory level. Testing usually reveals a shift in the protective sensory level, consistent with neuropathy in these patients, but the subjective presence of paresthesia is not useful as a threshold indicator. Suprathreshold qualitative testing of sensory status may reveal "normal" findings in some cases. Clearly, the standard history and physical exam may be insufficient to detect a patient at risk.

In contrast, several methods have been devised that identify the protective threshold level and, thus, patients at risk. While all of the methods generally meet the desired features of a threshold-identifying test as previously described, some are, for a number of reasons, not best suited for large-scale clinical screening. At the Northern California Center for the Diabetic and Insensitive Foot, the method most frequently utilized for clinical screening of protective sensory levels involves the use of Semmes-Weinstein pressure aesthesiometry (Fig. 7-6). The Semmes-Weinstein pressure aesthesiometry device is handheld, with a single monofilament nylon probe attached at the end of the handle perpendicular to it. A series of devices are available, each with a monofilament calibrated to impart a different gradation of pressure. Research has indicated that the monofilament that imparts 5.07 log (0.1 mg) force coincides well with the threshold needed to protect against ulceration.

Because of its critical threshold-identifying capacity, the 5.07 monofilament is used for the clinical screening procedure. Patients are told that they will be touched with the device at various locations on their feet, and when they feel it, they are to

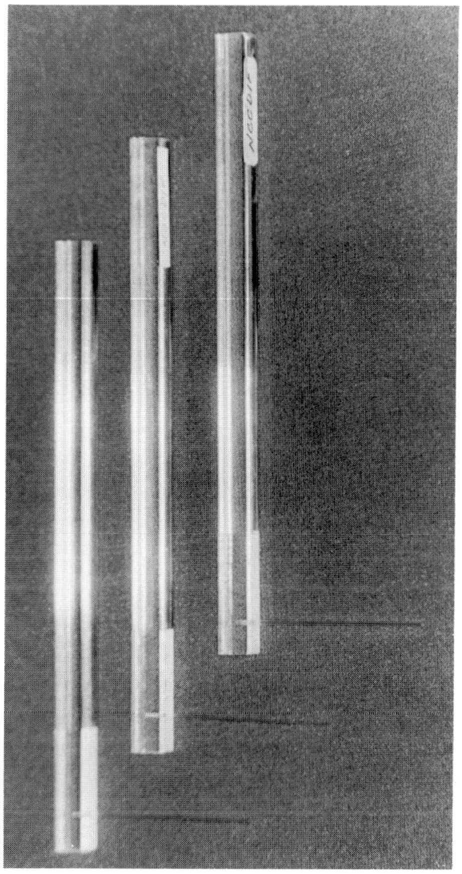

Fig. 7-6. Semmes-Weinstein pressure aesthesiometry devices. Each device has a nylon monofilament attached that has been calibrated to impart a different gradation of pressure. The monofilament that imparts 5.07 log (0.1 mg) force (the "5.07 monofilament") coincides well with the sensory protective threshold needed to protect against ulceration.

verbally identify where they felt it. Alternatively, patients could be told to point to the spot where they felt it. Patients are then asked to close their eyes for the test. The examiner then will apply the monofilament perpendicular to a test location until the monofilament subtlety bends, usually taking 1 to 2 seconds in the downward stroke and 1 to 2 seconds in the upward stroke. Without cueing the patient, the examiner waits for a localization response. A response in the near vicinity of the actual test location is considered correct. The examiner then proceeds to test multiple areas bilaterally, without verbal interaction with the patient. Areas commonly tested include the tips of the toes, the plantar aspect of the hallux interphalangeal joint, the plantar aspect of the ball of the foot, the medial aspect of the hallux and first metatarsal head, the dorsal first web space, the dorsal aspect of prominent toes, the lateral aspect of the fifth metatarsal head and fifth toe, the heel, and adjacent to any corn, callus, or erythematous area. It should be noted that the test is probably not valid across corns or calluses, so they must be either trimmed or tested on the periphery. Any test location that the patient consistently fails to localize is considered to have lost protective threshold function and is at risk for ulceration. Other methods using the Semmes-Weinstein monofilaments do exist, including the two-alternative, forced-choice method, but the method described has proved to be quick and effective for clinical screening. Therefore, with the 5.07 monofilament, a patient's sensory threshold status can be established during a clinical screening examination.

The next step is to utilize the information for optimal management of the patient. Patients found to have at risk areas can be placed on an intense program designed to prevent ulceration, which includes interventional measures and education that will be described later in this chapter. For patients with an intact sensory threshold, one cannot assume that they will remain so over time. Repeated testing at intervals not exceeding 6 months is recommended. In this manner, early detection of at risk areas is possible. Furthermore, the patient with intact protective sensation levels should be educated regarding the progressive nature of diabetic peripheral neuropathy, with emphasis on the importance of follow-up examinations and avoidance of neuropathic accelerating factors, such as poor blood glucose control and excessive alcohol consumption. Efforts to block the neuropathic process and/or restore nerve function have not met with clear success, as exemplified by studies involving aldose reductase inhibitors (ARI). Although there is hope for future progress in pharmacologic intervention in diabetic peripheral neuropathy, the best one can expect at this time is early detection of loss of sensory protection and activation of efforts to prevent resultant ulceration.

Soft Tissue Resistance to Ulceration

The human soft tissues, particularly those found in the foot, are amazingly resistant to failure under stress. For the soft tissues to successfully cope with stresses applied to them, there must be strategic structural and functional composition of those soft tissues. The soft tissues must disperse and/or dissipate forces applied to them. In the process, the soft tissues absorb energy. While some of the energy may be returned via elastic recoil, some may be converted to potentially deleterious heat, or even be found to create microscopic or macroscopic structural disruption. In essence, the absorbed energy may create an increased demand on the local circulation. Therefore, the strategy for coping with environmental stress requires a functionally effective soft tissue component, as well as a circulatory component.

The major feature of the human soft tissue that allows it to adapt so well to stresses applied to it is its *viscoelasticity*. The viscoelastic properties of the soft tissues are derived from the unique combination and organization of its components, including collagen, elastin, ground substance, subcutaneous fat, and fibrous septa within the subcutaneous fat. The advantages of viscoelasticity are implied in its name, specifically, both viscous and elastic characteristics. The viscous nature of soft tissues allows them to mold to the applied stress, increasing the surface area of contact, and thus decreasing the unit of force applied to any one given area. Furthermore, the stress will be decelerated by the viscous nature of the soft tissue. Therefore, the viscous aspect of soft tissue acts to both disperse and dissipate stresses applied to it. The elastic characteristic serves to absorb energy returning it to the environment via elastic recoil. Elasticity also serves to decelerate stresses. Therefore, the elastic characteristic of soft tissue acts to both dissipate stress as well as store and resolve energy. In concert as a viscoelastic substance, the soft tissues prove to be an effective means of coping with environmental stresses.

Viscoelasticity allows soft tissues to adapt to applied stresses in both space and time. The ability to adapt in space is afforded by moldability of the soft tissues. The ability to adapt in time is afforded by the thickness of the soft tissues. If any deleterious changes were to occur in either one of these two basic characteristics of soft tissue (moldability or thickness), then the viscoelastic function, and thus the resistance to breakdown, would be impaired. In diabetic patients, either moldability or thickness or both may become altered, increasing the risk for ulceration.

Plantar fat pad atrophy would certainly alter viscoelasticity. The fat pad can be found to atrophy in the elderly, patients on steroids after renal transplant, or patients in poor nutritional states or uremia. In fact, using ultrasonography, the plantar fat pads of diabetic patients with previous foot ulcers were found to be thinner than in diabetic patients without previous foot ulcer, who were in turn found to have thinner fat pads than normal subjects. Furthermore, the plantar fat pad thickness may also be compromised under the ball of the foot by distal displacement of the fat pad in association with the development of digital contractures attributed to motor neuropathy. The viscoelastic properties of the repair tissue of previous ulcerations and incisions is significantly inferior in both thickness and moldability. Longer standing, firmer types of edema will certainly alter moldability, and thus viscoelasticity. Sources of pedal edema in diabetic patients can be quite various but may be associated with hypertension, nephropathy, or the neuropathic edema created by the vasomotor effects of autonomic neuropathy, to mention a few. Autonomic neuropathy also has sudomotor effects, causing excessive dryness of the skin. Dry skin is not as moldable as hydrated skin, with resultant fissures clearly demonstrating the point. Nonenzymatic glycosylation of tissue proteins may also play a role in altering the moldability of the soft tissues. Glycosylation of hemoglobin serves as a prototype for the early steps of this process of nonenzymatic linkage of glucose, which can affect virtually any protein. Longer half-life proteins, such as collagen, undergo further linkages and changes to become advanced glycosylation end products (AGEs), which are highly cross linked and structurally altered. The net result over time is a clearly altered viscoelasticity of the soft tissues, which has been demonstrated to be quite extreme in some diabetic patients.

Intervention for patients who are at higher risk for ulceration because of impaired viscoelasticity has been and still remains to be through extrinsic alterations. The loss of viscoelasticity may be partially compensated with the addition of various insole materials of differing properties. Laminating materials may allow one to combine advantageous properties of various materials to arrive at a superior composite. Alternatively, a viscoelastic material is available for insole use. Of course, the addition of insole material to the inside of the shoe may necessitate an extra-depth shoe. Outersole materials, such as those used in the increasingly high-tech running shoe industry, may be manipulated in the patient's favor. Recently, encouraging results in the alteration of foot pressures with modified socks have been reported. Finally, artificially hydrating the skin with emollients is a mainstay in the treatment of patients with autonomic pedal xerosis.

In contrast, intervention through intrinsic alterations have been relatively unexplored. Augmentation of the soft tissues in diabetic patients with a history of ulceration by injection of collagen or silicone has been reported to be effective in reducing recurrences in small, isolated studies. When distinct mechanisms for viscoelastic deterioration can be implicated, certainly, specific preventive measures can be developed, such as maintenance of normoglycemia to avoid the development of collagen AGEs. Furthermore, the identification of specific mechanisms for viscoelastic deterioration may spur the development of applicable pharmaceuticals, such as aminoguanidine, which inhibits formation of AGEs, and ephedrine, which has been used to successfully treat neuropathic edema.

While deterioration of viscoelasticity may contribute to ulcer risk, so too can alteration of the circulatory status of the patient. Recall the supporting role of the vascular system in the overall resistance of the soft tissues to failure. In the diabetic patient, it is possible to have multifactorial derangement of the supportive nature of the vascular system. For purposes of discussion here, four categories of vascular derangement can exist: (1) atherosclerosis, or macroangiopathy; (2) basement membrane and capillary disorders, or microangiopathy; (3) hematologic abnormalities; and (4) vasomotor disturbances associated with autonomic neuropathy. While all of these types of derangement may produce deleterious effects on resistance to ulceration, grouping them for discussion purposes does not imply routine concurrence in patients.

Macroangiopathy can clearly and most severely impair the delivery of blood to the soft tissues. As adaptation to stresses by the soft tissues creates a demand for blood, the capacity to supply that blood can be exceeded. The first response is to withdraw from the stress. If the sensory protective threshold is not functional, exposure continues to the point of soft tissue failure. With macroangiopathy, the limitation in supply capacity may be such that little additional demand beyond baseline can be tolerated. Although most diabetic patients with neuropathic ulcerations do not have the severely advanced macroangiopathy just described, the process may remain a subtle factor.

The significance of microangiopathy in the development of foot ulcers remains disputed. There is no direct proof that microangiopathy is a causative factor in foot ulcers. However, microangiopathic changes have been demonstrated in the feet of diabetic patients. The condition is felt to derange transcapillary physiology. Therefore, it is hard to ignore the possibility that microangiopathy may be a factor. It is interesting to note that in patients with neuropathic ulcers, particularly those with advanced autonomic neuropathy, a high coincidence of retinopathy and nephropathy, both microangiopathic manifestations, can be found.

Numerous hematologic abnormalities have been identified in diabetic patients that may also compromise the function of the vascular system. Platelets are found to adhere to endothelial surfaces and aggregate more readily. Blood viscosity may be adversely affected. The deformability of red and white blood cells may become decreased. The net effect is altered hemorrheology of the arterioles and capillaries, and impaired delivery of blood. Furthermore, hemoglobin affinity for oxygen may increase as the hemoglobin becomes increasingly glycosylated, potentially impairing oxygen delivery at the tissue level.

Next to sensory neuropathy, the second most important factor for the development of neuropathic ulceration is autonomic neuropathy. The correlation of advanced autonomic neuropathy with neurotrophic ulceration has been repeatedly documented. While the correlation may be purely coincidental, it is likely that autonomic neuropathy produces a deleterious effect on the soft tissues through primarily vasomotor changes. Autonomic neuropathy mediated vasomotor and sudomotor changes that deteriorate viscoelasticity have already been discussed. Vasomotor disturbances probably also affect the blood delivery component of soft tissue resistance to failure. With autonomic vasomotor neuropathy, distal vessels, including precapillary physiologic arteriovenous anastomoses (AV shunts), become fully dilated. The patient's foot becomes hyperemic and warm. Pedal pulses are bounding when palpated. Dorsal veins become engorged and distended with highly oxygenated blood, shunted directly from the arterial side of the circulation through the wide-open AV shunts. With blood flowing through this new low resistance pathway, perfusion into the capillaries is reduced or bypassed completely. The result is a hyperperfused foot, with underperfused capillary beds. In addition, autonomic neuropathy may impair the hyperemic response to noxious stimuli. Still other mechanisms may be found for autonomic derangement of the delivery and reparative process in soft tissues.

Regardless of which of the identified various circulatory disturbances one speaks of, the effect is deleterious to the response of soft tissues to stress. Intervention can be directed at preventing the primary defect, or if already present, at reversing the deleterious effects of the defect. A preventative program would include avoidance of atherosclerotic risk factors and control of blood glucose to reduce microvascular, hematologic, and autonomic nerve derangement. Therapeutic intervention might include various forms of vascular surgery for macroangiopathies. Antiplatelet agents, such as aspirin and dipyridamole, as well as hemorrheologic agents, such as pentoxifylline, might be utilized when hematologic derangement of the delivery system is suspected. While ephedrine has been utilized to treat neuropathic edema, its effects on other autonomic vasomotor manifestations, particularly neuropathic ulcerations, have not been reported.

In summary, the soft tissue resistance to breakdown is a critical factor in ulcerogenesis. The ability of the soft tissues to cope with environmental stress is dependant upon a properly functioning viscoelastic soft tissue bed and a supportive vascular delivery system. Impairment of either component has a negative effect on soft tissue capacity to withstand environmental stress. Using the conceptual model again, impairment of either component will have the effect of shifting the soft tissue resistance line toward the x and y axes. Clearly, among all of the factors having an effect on the soft tissues, autonomic neuropathy appears to be critical, so much so that patients with autonomic neuropathy and sensory neuropathy are at significantly greater risk for ulceration, when compared to diabetic patients with sensory neuropathy alone. Further research is required to demonstrate the specific mechanism by with autonomic neuropathy exerts its deleterious effects on the soft tissues. In addition, it is hoped that a threshold test identifying an at risk status, similar to that which was described for sensory neuropathy, could be developed for autonomic neuropathy manifestations in the foot.

Intrinsic Stress Sources

One of the four factors described in the conceptual model was environmental stress. While environmental stress is considered an extrinsic factor, certain intrinsic alterations of the foot tend to heighten or focus the environmental stress. Although environmental stress will be addressed in more detail while discussing extrinsic factors, the intrinsic stress sources are more appropriately discussed here.

Bony prominences tend to focus stress onto a smaller area of distribution and, as such represent areas of risk. Certain prominences can occur in diabetic patients just as they do in nondiabetic patients, such as digital contractures, hallux valgus with bunion formation, tailor's bunions, and depressed metatarsals. Some of these prominences may demonstrate resultant corns or calluses, which additionally heighten and focus stress.

In diabetic patients, however, motor neuropathy can create additional problems. As paresis of the intrinsic musculature of the foot develops, the metatarsophalangeal joints are destabilized. As a result, digital contractures are allowed to develop and progress. The dorsal and distal aspects of all the toes, including the hallux, become areas of focused stress. Furthermore, the dorsal contracture of the toes at the metatarsophalangeal joints produces an increasing retrograde plantar-flexory force through the metatarsal heads. This accounts for the increased pressures often reported under the metatarsal heads of those diabetic patients with neuropathy and previous ulceration. The digital contractures also tend to displace the plantar fat pad distally, as previously discussed.

Subacute motor neuropathy can cause gradual weakness of the anterior muscle group of the leg, allowing the posterior group to gain mechanical advantage. A progressive limitation of ankle joint dorsiflexion can occur. As with equinus conditions, increased stress is transmitted to the plantar forefoot and across Lisfranc's as well as Chopart's joint.

Drop foot, sensory or motor ataxia, as well as common biomechanical problems create not only abnormal vertical stress under foot, but compounding shear stress as well.

Sensory neuropathy and autonomic neuropathy team up once again to allow the development of Charcot neuroarthropathy. The bony prominences created after subluxation are other areas of focused stress.

Joint immobility in the foot is poorly tolerated in the neuropathic individual, due to the focused stresses created. Hallux limitus is often associated with ulcers under the hallux interphalangeal joint. In other cases, collagen AGEs of joint capsule and/or tendon structures may be implicated. In fact, diabetic patients with a history of neuropathic ulceration have been found to have significantly less subtalar joint mobility than uncomplicated diabetic patients, who in turn had less subtalar mobility than healthy controls.

Finally, digital and ray resections can have the effect of focusing stress on an adjacent structure. Patients with hallux amputations tend to excessively load under the second metatarsal or the tip of the second toe. Of the isolated ray resections, the third and fifth tend to do best, with comparatively less stress transferred to adjacent metatarsals. Second and fourth ray resections tend to transfer more stress to adjacent areas, with first ray resections transferring the most stress. With multiple ray resections and isolated ray resections with a poor prognosis, one wonders if transmetatarsal amputation wouldn't be a superior choice.

Preventive intervention in situations such as those just discussed will be addressed in more detail in the next section on extrinsic factors. These situations also raise the question of whether to elect surgical intervention. Certainly, this avenue may be quite efficacious in reducing risk at a given site. A detailed discussion of surgical procedures, principles, and criteria is beyond the scope of this chapter but may be found elsewhere in this text, as well as other sources.

In summary, certain intrinsic alterations tend to focus or heighten stress in a given area. In the diabetic patient, motor neuropathy plays a dominant etiologic role in the development of these structural changes. Autonomic neuropathy, sensory neuropathy, and AGEs may also play important roles.

EXTRINSIC FACTORS

Returning to the conceptual model, the two important extrinsic factors are stress and time. Either magnitude of stress or duration of exposure can be modified, making these areas crucial in intervention. While an appreciation of the contributing intrinsic factors is important in the overall understanding of soft tissue failure, emphasis must be placed upon the extrinsic factors, which are, after all, the source of destruction, while at the same time, most easily modified in order to prevent damage. Protection of the limb becomes less difficult if both the health care provider and the patient know what to protect it from.

It must be emphasized that it is the inability of the diabetic subject to perceive pain at a level necessary to protect himself that sets the stage for ultimate tissue destruction by external factors. The subject must become aware of this lack of sensitivity and appreciate all of the external threats that are in his environment. Ultimately, the patient must assume responsibility for the care of his feet and begin to do consciously what he in the past did unconsciously—protect himself from harm.

An insensate, high risk foot may be damaged by stress of mechanical, thermal, or chemical origins while the subject functions in his "normal" environment. Each stress causes damage by a different method, depending upon different time and physical relationship.

Mechanical Stress

In mechanical terms "normal" stress applies to forces that are perpendicular to a surface and is expressed as pressure:

$$\text{Pressure} = \frac{\text{force}}{\text{area}}$$

Shear stresses result from forces placed parallel or oblique (tangential) to a surface. Damage occurs at a much lower level of pressure if an element of shear is introduced.

These extrinsic mechanical forces may effect their ultimate tissue destruction in one or several ways: (1) direct mechanical disruption, (2) tissue ischemia, or (3) inflammatory tissue autolysis (self-destruction).

Direct Mechanical Disruption

Direct mechanical disruption of tissue is caused by high pressures or a great force concentrated in a small area. Its mechanism of action is immediate by direct crushing, tearing, laceration, or penetration. This can occur when the entire weight of the body steps upon a sharp object such as a nail, thumbtack, piece of glass or a pointed stone. It takes a pressure of 1,300 (psi) or 100 kg/cm^2 (1 kg/cm^2 = 13 psi) to penetrate the intact tissue. The most common locations for this event to occur is on the plantar aspect of the foot, rarely involving other areas.

This external threat can for the most part be completely eliminated simply by never walking barefoot, inside or outside, and by avoiding sandals and instead wearing enclosed shoes. Inspecting the insides of the shoes for sharp objects before application will further prevent damage from direct mechanical destruction of tissue. Enclosed footgear suitable for use when bathing is available and is especially useful for streams or beaches.

Tissue Ischemia

Tissue destruction from ischemia is secondary to prolonged, continuous low pressure. Its mechanism of action is by tissue necrosis due to inadequate local blood perfusion. Pressures in the magnitude of 1 to 5 psi maintained for periods longer than 10 hours can create this type of damage. If vascular compromise is also present, then less time will be necessary to effect tissue breakdown. This is uncommon, but when it does occur, it is usually secondary to tight shoes, resulting in excessive pressure from circumferential tension. The pressure result of tension occurs only when the line of tension passes around a curve. This resultant pressure is inversely proportional to the radius of curvature (i.e., the smaller the curve, the greater the pressure):

$$\text{Pressure} = \frac{\text{tension}}{\text{radius}}$$

Consequently, areas such as the lateral aspect of the fifth metatarsal head, the styloid process, or the medial aspect of the first metatarsal head are subject to trauma from this process as are any other bony prominences such as a dorsal exostosis, hammer toe, claw toe, or mallet toe deformity (Fig. 7-7). The presence of a hallux abducto valgus bunion deformity creates curves in two planes, the transverse and longitudinal, making this area more susceptible to the effects of pressure from circumferential tension.

A postoperative dressing applied too tightly or utilizing a compressive type bandage may create pressure necrosis in the above areas. Furthermore, bulky dressings applied to a foot that is then placed back into a previously well-fitted shoe will result in areas of increased pressure.

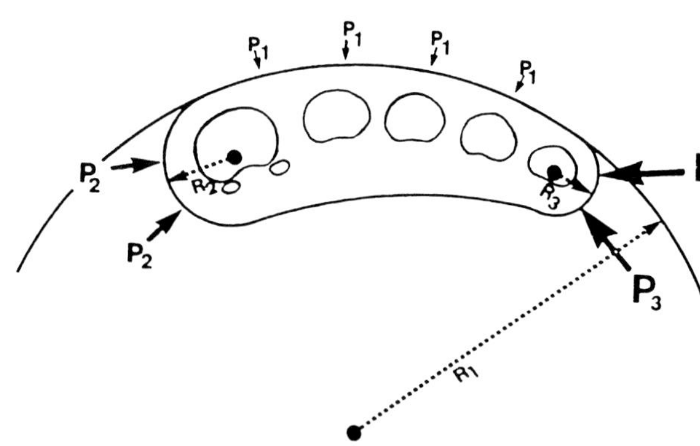

Fig. 7-7. Cross section of forefoot demonstrating pressure areas as a result of circumferential tension such as that applied by a shoe. When the line of tension passes around a curve, pressure results. The resultant pressure is inversely proportional to the radius of curvature. (From Brand PW: The insensitive foot (including leprosy). p. 1266. In Jahss MH (ed): Disorders of the Foot. WB Saunders, Philadelphia, 1982, with permission.)

An in-shoe object such as a marble, pebble, or improperly conceived device such as a metatarsal pad or an over-the-counter arch support will create areas of pressure. Devices that are not custom-molded to fit to the contours of the foot create localized areas of pressure on the foot as well as take up space within the shoe, making the shoe fit tightly.

Occasionally, tissue ischemia can occur interdigitally from the toes being squeezed too snugly by an ill-fitted, high-heeled, "pointed-toe" shoe, resulting in tissue necrosis and subsequent ulceration. This type of process can also occur when an edematous foot is placed in a previously well-fitted show.

Interdigital ulcerations may also be associated with prominent condyles or exostosis emanating from adjacent phalanges even if the foot is placed within a well-fitted shoe.

Prevention of damage from low pressure is accomplished simply by measuring and lessening the time it is applied and not so simply by attempting to accommodate or eliminate pressure points.

Proper shoe selection and establishing a breaking-in period is paramount. Shoes must be of the proper size, style, and fit. Insensate subjects unknowingly tend to fit themselves tight as they attempt to gain a feel of the shoe upon their foot, which should be avoided. On the other hand, at no time should the shoe be fitted loose as this will increase the amount of shear forces applied to the foot, especially the sides of the heel where irritation from the counter of the shoe occurs.

Shoes should be constructed of material that is "breathable" and capable of being and remaining stretched such as leather. Nonyielding, occlusive material with elastic memory such as plastics must be avoided.

According to Brand (1980), new shoes should be worn for no longer than 2 to 3 hours on the first day. Upon shoe removal, an inspection should be performed, looking for areas of excessive pressure on the foot as evidenced by localized redness, increased warmth, and possibly by the impression of the sock or hosiery upon the foot. If pressure points are discovered, the part of the shoe corresponding to the pressure point should be stretched. Repeating the above process, the shoe should then be worn again until it is broken in.

An extra-depth shoe is indicated if there are significant digital deformities that increase the vertical height of the toes or any time an insole or foot orthotic of greater than $\frac{1}{8}$ inch in depth is utilized.

If foot orthoses are employed, they should always be made from a mold of the foot. They should have as their primary goal to accommodate to the foot while increasing the weight-bearing surface of the sole. Consequently, they should be made of materials that mold to the foot such as various densities of Plastazote. Therefore, if the foot changes shape over time, so then will the device. The device will eventually bottom out necessitating that it be replaced. Boulton et al. (1987) demonstrated that during a 3-year study, significant alterations of loads under the foot may occur. This included both the appearance or disappearance of high pressure areas under the feet. Better the device flattening than the foot ulcerating from the use of a rigid support.

Brand (1980) established the three "5-hour" periods of shoe wearing per day cycle for the high risk foot. This involves keeping shoes at the workplace. These are exchanged at lunchtime with shoes that are worn to work. The second pair of shoes is then worn until evening; when at home this pair is exchanged for a third pair of shoes, which is worn until retiring. Consequently, each pair of shoes is worn for three periods, each approximately 5 hours in length, thereby lessening the potential for ulceration. This is based upon the knowledge that it is most unlikely that a person could physically place their foot into a shoe that would deliver more than 5 psi of pressure. This amount of pressure applied for 5 hours causes no damage in the foot with normal vascularity and contour. However, if maintained for 10 hours, gangrene will result. Peripheral vascular disease and skeletal deformities creating pressure points will lessen the above parameters and need to be addressed.

The foot with bulky dressings or the foot that is swollen should be placed into a specialized temporary type of shoe with adjustable closures. Constrictive or elastic dressings have no place in the management of the insensate foot. Furthermore, dressings saturated with solutions such as povidone iodine that harden and do not allow for swelling should be avoided, especially if they circumscribe digits.

In the appropriate candidate, serious consideration should be given to prophylactic surgery for such skeletal pathology as hallux abducto valgus with bunion, tailors' bunion, exostosis, or other digital deformities such as hammer toes, claw toes, or mallet toes. This will allow for better shoeing as well as eliminate potential pressure points.

Inflammatory Autolysis

Tissue destruction from inflammatory autolysis is secondary to repeated, intermittent, moderate stress in the range of 25 to 75 psi (1.5 to 5 kg/cm^2) applied to previously inflamed tissue. It is an insidious process occurring over time and is the most common cause of tissue ulceration in the high risk foot, especially upon its plantar aspect in the area of the forefoot. The sources of these pressures are from ground reactive forces that occur with normal daily walking in a regular shoe. These forces upon the foot are at their highest when the heel leaves the ground, and even in the sensate foot are painless unless repeated multiple times such as after taking a long brisk walk or jog. Following multiple repetitions, traumatic inflammation results as evidenced by localized tissue edema, redness, and increased temperature (hot spot). Brand (1977) states that these pressures are less than one-tenth of that which would cause direct mechanical disruption; nor, since the pressure is intermittent, would they cause ischemic tissue necrosis. Yet, in spite of this apparent 10 to 1 margin of safety and lack of ischemic threat, insensate feet commonly do break down and ulcerate even though enclosed, well-fitted shoes are worn. In a normal subject this process is perceived as painful and motivates the subject to alter the gait by limping or shortening the stride or resting the part, thereby altering the distribution or magnitude of forces until the pain subsides. At the most this process results in a blister formation. In the insensate high risk foot the subject proceeds to walk pain-free upon the damaged area without altering the gait and continues to traumatize the previously inflamed tissue, which subsequently ulcerates. The stress that eventually results in tissue breakdown is no more severe than that which was previously applied. What has changed is that it is now being applied to compromised, inflamed tissue that has not been allowed to rest in order to heal itself.

Stokes et al. (1975) demonstrated that diabetic subjects with plantar ulcers exerted maximum loads at the site of the ulcer as well as reduced toe loading. Ctercteko et al. (1981) confirmed these findings and also discovered that in addition to reduced toe loading there was a medial shift of maximum pressures under the metatarsal heads with the highest forces acting in the region of the first metatarsal head. It was concluded that the increased metatarsal head pressure at least in part was caused by altered toe loading. The altered toe loading is most likely due to a biomechanical fault, wherein the intrinsic muscles no longer stabilize the proximal phalanx onto the metatarsal and an imbalance between the flexor and extensor tendons develops. This process results in the so-called intrinsic minus foot (Lippmann et al., 1976; Brand 1977), leading to the formation of hammer toes and claw toes, which in turn place a retrograde plantar force onto the metatarsal head.

Prominent pressure points beneath metatarsal heads secondary to underlying skeletal deformities or biomechanical faults with resultant mechanically induced hyperkeratoses formation are especially prone to the above process. However, the absence of reactive hyperkeratosis does not necessarily mean that there are no abnormal forces being applied to an area. Boulton et al. (1987) demonstrated that abnormal toe loading resulting in increased metatarsal head pressure was also found to be present in diabetic subjects without any clinical signs of increased pressure or a clinically diagnosed neuropathy. They further state that the subjects in their study with abnormal pressures were significantly heavier than those with normal plantar pressures. This is most remarkable because foot pressures usually are not abnormal in heavier people because pressure is equal to force divided by area and heavier people tend to dissipate their weight over a larger area of the foot. Consequently, in the subject who has an insensate foot with abnormal plantar pressure, weight reduction becomes significant in lowering these forces.

Prevention of tissue damage from repetitive moderate stress requires increasing the weight-bearing surface area of the sole, specialized shoeing, modifying, and limiting the gait, and most importantly daily inspections of the foot for hot spots utilizing the hand or a skin thermometer. In resistant cases, occasionally surgical intervention must be employed.

Increasing the weight-bearing surface area of the sole is accomplished by utilizing a custom-molded accommodative orthotic made from a cast of the foot. It should be a composite device consisting of three layers. Next to the skin is a thin, antifriction-shear layer made of a material such as nylon, etc. Next is a middle accommodative layer consisting of a soft, yielding material such as a moderately dense closed-cell polyethylene foam. Finally, there is a bottom supportive layer consisting of a denser closed-cell polyethylene foam or similar material.

Extra-depth shoes must be employed when the above devices are utilized. Furthermore, if plantar forefoot ulcerations recur, the addition of a rigid shank from heel to toe along with a proper rocker sole design is indicated in order to lessen the forces on the forefoot when the heel leaves the ground.

Athletic-running shoes with removable Plastazote insoles have been demonstrated to reduce the size of plantar callus formation and when properly fitted, can be employed in the shoeing management of the diabetic foot.

Padded hosiery has been demonstrated to reduce dynamic foot pressures upon the high risk foot, but this is presently in its experimental phase. If or when employed, this should be used as an adjunct to the above shoeing management.

Custom-molded shoes made from a cast of the foot are indicated primarily in the severely deformed foot (i.e., postamputation or postneuroarthropathy). They should possess a rigid sole with a rocker design and a three-layered, accommodative, removable insole.

The gait should be modified by decreasing the length of stride as well as the number of steps per day, especially in the subject with a history of plantar ulcerations. A brisk, fast gait results in a greater length of stride as well as the amount of shear forces applied to the foot from the added acceleration and deceleration required. Jogging, brisk walking, and extended hikes might best be replaced by such activities as swimming or biking.

Shear Forces

As mentioned earlier shear forces compound the deleterious effects of the other forces. Unlike pressure, shear forces are extremely difficult to measure and little is really known about them. They are especially harmful to recently healed ulcerations, the reason being that the defect caused by the ulceration has been replaced by scar tissue, which due to the healing process is still inflamed, and it is also not as compliant as the surrounding tissue. Consequently, all of the shear forces are concentrated in this newly healed area, resulting in rapid tissue breakdown. According to Brand (1980), ulcer recurrence is most common within 1 month of healing. Appropriate shoeing with molded insoles must be available before a normal gait can be resumed. If not available, then a temporary healing shoe with a Plastazote insole must be utilized until the permanent shoes with insoles are ready. In any event the patient must be advised to lessen the amount of gait as well as the stride until the tissues have a chance to remodel and establish a plane of mobility between the skin and underlying skeleton. Holes cut out of various materials will relieve pressure from an area but will create a shear stress along the hole's margins at the point where the tissue bulges down into the hole. Because of shear stress, beveled margins without edges are to be employed in any type of "pressure-off" accommodation.

Thermal Stress

Guy et al. (1985) demonstrated that there was a striking loss of thermal sensitivity in diabetic subjects with neuropathic ulcerations and Charcot joints. In his study 50 percent of his subjects could detect an increase in temperature only when it reached a level equal to three times the limit found in normal subjects. Examination of the hand in the same group of subjects led to similar conclusions, although thermal sensitivity in the hands could be normal in the presence of abnormalities of the feet.

Sosenko et al. (1988) found that both warm and cold sensitivities were markedly impaired in diabetic patients. Even patients asymptomatic for neuropathy tended to have abnormal warm and cold sensitivities. In the diabetic subjects there was a greater insensitivity to warm than to cold and this increased with hyperglycemia.

The extremes of temperature, hot and cold, are a constant threat to the high risk foot. The mechanism of injury most often occurs immediately by direct tissue necrosis. The location of the injury depends upon the source of thermal energy. Simply stated, excessive heat in any form must be avoided. Before placing the foot in bath water or a soak, the water temperature should always be checked with a thermometer. Testing the temperature with the hand may be substituted in the event that there is no thermometer, providing the thermal sensation to the hand is intact. Annoying cold feet should be treated by such methods as wearing wool sock to bed at night. Heating pads and hot water bottles must never be applied to the legs or feet. Down comforters are recommended over electric heating blankets for total body warming. The subject must avoid placing the foot or any part of the leg upon a hot surface such as hot automobile floors occurring as a result of a long journey, radiant heaters, close to fires, or against the hot muffler of a motorcycle, lawnmower, etc. The patient must avoid walking barefoot around a swimming pool on hot cement, asphalt, or sand. Also, bathing in the sun for prolonged periods should be avoided to prevent sunburn.

Cold exposure must be avoided. Even moderately cold temperatures can institute vasospasms, which may slow the circulation to a part such as a toe, resulting in chilblains or pernio with subsequent ulceration. If this part is also at the same time receiving excessive, prolonged low pressure, then tissue necrosis resulting in ulceration will occur within less time than when the part had adequate vascularity. Extreme cold causes direct tissue destruction, resulting in frostbite and, if the temperature extreme is prolonged, gangrene. Nonconstricting, warm clothing must always be worn in cold environments. Extreme cold absolutely must be avoided.

Chemical Stress

Chemical injury to the foot is usually secondary to a corn, wart, or ingrown toenail remedy. Its mechanism or action is through a destructive chemical reaction. The location of this process is usually over a pressure point that has an associated mechanically induced hyperkeratosis that the patient has self-treated with a keratolytic preparation (i.e., a clavus on the dorsum of a hammer toe). These preparations destroy tissue nonselectively, meaning they will affect normal skin as well as the abnormal keratotic tissue. The topical keratolytic can erode completely through the skin if left in place long enough, resulting in an ulceration. The subject with a high risk foot can prevent this type of problem by never applying these preparations to the feet and always seeking professional care for problems with corns, calluses, warts, ingrown toenails, etc.

Chemical injury can occur at the workplace as a result of an accidental spill, which may go unnoticed by the subject with an insensate foot. Protective footgear should be worn, but if exposure is great a change in occupations is strongly advised.

CONCLUSION

The risk of a major amputation in diabetic subjects is 15 times higher than in nondiabetic subjects. More often than not, the process that led to this dreaded outcome began with a minor break in the integrity of the skin of the foot, which subsequently became infected. Loss of a limb does not necessarily have to be a "given" result of diabetes as this final tragedy is the end of a long chain of potentially preventable events.

In order to treat as well as prevent the initial break in the integrity of the skin, a thorough appreciation of the intrinsic as well as the extrinsic factors that contribute to the ultimate soft tissue breakdown must be attained. Once this knowledge is acquired, the goal of a successful outcome—*intact integument*—becomes simpler for both treatment and prevention.

SUGGESTED READINGS

Ahmed ME, Le Quesne LP: Quantitative sweat test in diabetics with neuropathic foot lesions. J Neurol Neurosurg Psychiatry 49:1059, 1986

Ahmed ME, Delbridge L, Le Quesne LP: The role of autonomic neuropathy in diabetic foot ulceration. J Neurol Neurosurg Psychiatry 49:1002, 1986

Ali A, Carroll M, Robertson KP, Fowler CJ: The extent of small fiber sensory neuropathy in diabetics with plantar foot ulceration. J Neurol Neurosurg Psychiatry 52:94, 1989

Anderson JG: Transverse metatarsal head resection—a radical approach to the problems of forefoot ulceration. Lepr Rev 46:191, 1975

Aronin N, Leeman SE, Clements RS: Diminished flare response in neuropathic diabetic patients: comparison of effects of substance P, histamine, and capsaicin. Diabetes 36:1139, 1987

Balkin SW: The fluid silicone prosthesis. Clin Podiatr 1:145, 1984

Banks AS, McGlamry ED: Charcot foot. J Am Podiatr Med Assoc 79:213, 1989

Barrett JP, Mooney V: Neuropathy and diabetic pressure lesions. Orthop Clin North Am 4:43, 1973

Bays HE, Pfeifer MA: Peripheral diabetic neuropathy. Med Clin North Am 72:1439, 1988

Bauman JH, Girling JP, Brand PW: Plantar pressures and trophic ulcerations. J Bone Joint Surg 45B:652, 1963

Beach RB, Thompson DE: Selected soft tissue research, an overview from Carville. Phys Ther 59:30, 1979

Bergtholdt HT, Brand PW: Thermography: an aid in the management of insensitive feet and stumps. Arch Phys Med Rehab 56:205, 1975

Bergtholdt HT, Brand PW: Temperature assessment and plantar inflammation. Lepr Rev 47:211, 1976

Bergthodlt HT: Temperature assessment of the insensitive foot. Phys Ther 59:18, 1979

Bern MM, Busick EJ: Disorders of the blood and diabetes. p. 748. In Marble A, Krall LP, Bradley RF et al (eds): Joslin's Diabetes Mellitus. 12th Ed. Lea & Febiger, Philadelphia, 1985

Bild DE, Selby JV, Pomeroy S et al: Lower extremity amputation in people with diabetes—epidemiology and prevention. Diabetes Care 12:24, 1989

Bojsen-Moeller F, Flagstad KE: Plantar aponeurosis and internal architecture of the ball of the foot. J Anat 121:599, 1976

Bojsen-Moller F: Anatomy of the forefoot, normal and pathologic. Clin Orthop 142:10, 1979

Borkowski M: An experimental study on the role of arteriovenous anastamoses in the pathogenesis of the trophic ulcer. Arch Immunol Ther Exp 21:363, 1973

Boulton AJM, Scarpello JHB, Ward JD: Venous oxygenation in the diabetic neuropathic foot: evidence of arteriovenous shunting? Diabetologia 122:6, 1982

Boulton AJM, Hardisty CA, Betts RP et al: Dynamic foot pressure and other studies as diagnostic and management aids in diabetic neuropathy. Diabetes Care 6:26, 1983

Boulton AJM, Franks CI, Betts RP et al: Reduction of abnormal foot pressures in diabetic neuropathy using a new polymer insole material. Diabetes Care 7:42, 1984

Boulton AJ, Kubrusly DB, Bowker JH et al: Impaired vibratory perception and diabetic foot ulceration. Diabetic Med 3:335, 1986

Boulton AJM, Betts RP, Newrick PG, Ward JD: Foot pressure abnormalities—a sensitive marker of early sensory neuropathy. Diabetes, suppl. 1, 35:12A, 1986

Boulton AJM, Kubrusly DB, Bowker JH et al: Impaired vibratory perception and diabetic foot ulceration. Diabetic Med 3:335, 1986

Boulton AJM, Betts RP, Franks CI et al: Abnormalities of foot pressure in early diabetic neuropathy. Diabetic Med 4:225, 1987

Boulton AJM: The importance of abnormal foot pressures and gait in the causation of foot ulcers. p. 11. In Connor H, Boulton AJM, Ward JD (eds): The Foot in Diabetes. John Wiley & Sons, New York, 1987

Boulton AJM, Betts RP, Franks CI et al: The natural history of foot pressure abnormalities in neuropathic diabetic subjects. Diabetes Res 5:73, 1987

Boulton AJM: The diabetic foot. Med Clin North Am 72:1513, 1988

Boulton AJM, Connor H: The diabetic foot 1988. Diabetes Med 5:796, 1988

Brand PW: Insensitive Feet: A Practical Handbook on Foot Problems in Leprosy. Leprosy Mission, London, 1977

Brand PW, Mooney V (eds): The effects of pressure on human tissues. Report III. Rehabilitation Services Administration, Washington, D.C., 1977

Brand PW: Pathomechanics of diabetic (neuropathic) ulcer and its conservative management. p. 117. In Bergan JJ, Yao JST (eds): Gangrene and Severe Ischemia of the Lower Extremities. Grune & Stratton, New York, 1978

Brand PW: Management of the insensitive limb. Phys Ther 59:8, 1979

Brand PW: Management of sensory loss in the extremities. p. 862. In Omer GE, Spinner M (eds): Management of Peripheral Nerve Problems. WB Saunders, Philadelphia, 1980

Brand PW: The insensitive foot (including leprosy). p. 1266. In Jahss M (ed): Disorders of the Foot. Vol. 2. WB Saunders, Philadelphia, 1982

Brand PW: the diabetic foot. p. 829. In Ellenberg M, Rifkin H (eds): Diabetes Mellitus: Theory and Practice. Medical Examination Publishing, New York, 1983

Brand PW: Other insensitive foot types similar to diabetes. p. 8. In Brenner MA (ed): Management of the Diabetic Foot. Williams & Wilkins, Baltimore, 1987

Brand PW: Repetitive stress in the development of diabetic foot ulcers. p. 83. In Levin ME, O'Neal LW (eds): The Diabetic Foot. CV Mosby, St. Louis, 1988

Brownlee M, Vlassara H, Cerami A: Nonenzymatic glycosylation and the pathogenesis of diabetic complications. Ann Intern Med 101:527, 1984

Brownlee M: Microvascular disease and related abnormalities: their relation to control of diabetes. p. 185. In Marble A, Krall LP, Bradley RF et al (eds): Joslin's Diabetes Mellitus. 12th Ed. Lea & Febiger, Philadelphia, 1985

Brownlee M, Cerami A, Vlassara H: Advanced glycosylation end products in tissue and the biochemical basis of diabetic complications. N Engl J Med 318:1315, 1988

Cerami A, Vlassara H, Brownlee M: Role of advanced glycosylation products in complications of diabetes. Diabetes Care , suppl. 1, 11:73, 1988

Chait A, Bierman E, Brunzell JD: Diabetic macroangiopathy. p. 323. In Alberti KGMM, Krall LP (eds): The Diabetes Annual. Elsevier Science Publishing, New York, 1985

Cohen, MP: Diabetes and protein glycosylation, measurement and biologic relevance. Springer-Verlag, New York, 1986

Cohen MP: The polyol paradigm and complications of diabetes. Springer-Verlag, New York, 1987

Coleman WC: Footware in a management program of injury prevention. p. 293. In Levin ME, O'Neal LW (eds): The Diabetic Foot. CV Mosby, St. Louis, 1988

Colwell JA, Lopes-Virella MF, Winocour PD, Halushka PV: New concepts about the pathogenesis of atherosclerosis in diabetes mellitus. p. 51. In Levin ME, O'Neal LW (eds): The Diabetic Foot. CV Mosby, St. Louis, 1988

Corbin, Doc, Young RJ, Morrison DC et al: Blood flow in the foot, polyneuropathy and foot ulceration in diabetes mellitus. Diabetologia 30:468, 1987

Crausaz FM, Clavel S, Liniger C et al: Additional factors associated with plantar ulcers in diabetic neuropathy. Diabetic Med 5:771, 1988

Ctercteko GC, Dhanendran M, Hutton, WC, Le Quesne LP: Vertical forces acting on the feet of diabetic patients with neuropathic ulceration. Br J Surg 68:608, 1981

Deanfield JE, Daggett PR, Harrison MJG: Role of autonomic neuropathy in diabetic foot ulceration. J Neurol Sci 47:203, 1980

Delbridge L, Appelberg M, Reeve TS: Factors associated with development of foot lesions in the diabetic. Surgery 93:78, 1983

Delbridge L, Ctercteko G, Fowler C et al: The aetiology of diabetic neuropathic foot ulceration. Br J Surg 72:1, 1985

Delbridge L, Perry P, Marr S et al: Limited joint mobility in the diabetic foot: relationship to neuropathic ulceration. Diabetic Med 5:333, 1988

Duckworth T, Betts RP, Franks CI, Burke J: The measurement of pressure under the foot. Foot Ankle 3:130, 1982

Duckworth T, Boulton AJM, Betts RP et al: Plantar pressure measurements and the prevention of ulceration in the diabetic foot. J Bone Joint Surg 67B:79, 1985

Duckworth T: Pedobarography. p. 108. in Helal B, Wilson D (eds): The Foot. Vol. 1. Churchill Livingstone, New York, 1988

Dyck PJ, Karnes J, O'Brien PC: Detection thresholds of cutaneous sensation. p. 107. In Dyck PJ, Thomas PK, Asbury AK et al (eds): Diabetic Neuropathy. WB Saunders, Philadelphia, 1987

Edmonds ME, Nicolaides K, Watkins PJ: The importance of autonomic neuropathy in the aetiology of diabetic neuropathic foot ulceration. Diabetologia 21:506, 1981

Edmonds ME, Roberts VC, Watkins PJ: Blood flow in the diabetic neuropathic foot. Diabetologia 22:9, 1982

Edmonds ME, Archer AG, Watkins PJ: Ephedrine: a new treatment for diabetic neuropathic oedema. Lancet 1:548, 1983

Edmonds ME: The diabetic foot: pathophysiology and treatment. Clin Endocrinol Metab 15:889, 1986

Edmonds ME: The neuropathic foot in diabetes. Part I: blood flow. Diabetic Med 3:111, 1986

Edmonds ME, Blundell MP, Morris ME et al: Improved survival of the diabetic foot: the role of a specialized foot clinic. Q J Med 60:763, 1986

Edmonds ME, Nicolaides K, Watkins PJ: Autonomic neuropathy and diabetic neuropathic foot ulceration. Diabetic Med 3:56, 1986

Edmonds ME: Experience in a multidisciplinary diabetic foot clinic. p. 121. In Connor H, Boulton AJM, Ward JD (eds): The Foot in Diabetes. John Wiley & Sons, New York, 1987

Edmonds ME, Watkins PJ: Management of the diabetic foot. p. 208. In Dyck PJ, Thomas PK, Asbury AK et al (eds): Diabetic Neuropathy. WB Saunders, Philadelphia, 1987

Ellenberg M: Diabetic neuropathic ulcer. J Mt Sinai Hosp 35:585, 1968

Ewing DJ, Clarke BF: Diabetic autonomic neuropathy: a clinical viewpoint. p. 66. In Dyck PJ, Thomas PK, Asbury AK et al (eds): Diabetic Neuropathy. WB Saunders, Philadelphia, 1987

Faris I: Small and large vessel disease in the development of foot lesions in diabetics. Diabetologia 11:249, 1975

Faris I, Duncan H: Vascular disease and vascular function in the lower limb in diabetes. Diabet Res 1:171, 1984

Ferrari E, Floravanti M, Patti AL, et al: Effects of long-term treatment (4 years) with pentoxifylline on haemorheological changes and vascular complications in diabetic patients. Phamatherapeutica 5:26, 1987

Frykberg RG: Podiatric problems in diabetes. p. 45. In Kozak GP, Hoar CS, Rowbotham JL et al (eds): Management of Diabetic Foot Problems. WB Saunders, Philadelphia, 1984

Gianfortune P, Pulla RJ, Sage R: Ray reactions in the insensitive or dysvascular foot: a critical review. J Foot Surg 24:103, 1985

Giurini JM, Habershaw GM, Chrzan JS: Panmetatarsal head resection in chronic neuropathic ulceration. J Foot Surg 26:249, 1987

Goodfield MJD, Millard LG: The skin in diabetes mellitus. Diabetologia 31:567, 1988

Gooding GAW, Stess RM, Graf PM et al: Sonography of the sole of the foot: evidence for loss of foot pad thickness in diabetes and its relationship to ulceration of the foot. Invest Radiol 21:45, 1986

Greene DA, Gregersen G, Zimmerman BR: Metabolic control. p. 177. In Dyck PJ, Thomas PK, Asbury AK et al (eds): Diabetic Neuropathy. WB Saunders, Philadelphia, 1987

Guy RJ, Clark CA, Malcolm PN, Watkins PJ: Evaluation of thermal and vibration sensation in diabetic neuropathy. Diabetologia 2:131, 1985

Habershaw G, Donovan JC: Biomechanical considerations of the diabetic foot. p. 32. In Kozak GP, Hoar SC, Robotham JL et al (eds): Management of Diabetic Foot Problems. WB Saunders, Philadelphia, 1984

Hall OC, Brand PW: The etiology of the neuropathic plantar ulcer. J Am Podiatr Assoc 69:173, 1979

Hampton GH: Therapeutic footwear for the insensitive foot. Phys Ther 59:23, 1979

Harati Y: Diabetic peripheral neuropathies. Ann Intern Med 107:546, 1987

Harkless LB, Dennis KJ: The role of the podiatrist. p. 249. In Levin ME, O'Neal LW (eds): The diabetic Foot. CV Mosby, St. Louis, 1988

Harrison MJG, Faris IB: The neuropathic factor in etiology of diabetic foot ulcers. J Neurol Sci 28:217, 1976

Hetherington VJ: The insensitive foot. p. 436. In McGlamry ED (ed): Fundamentals of Foot Surgery. Williams & Wilkins, Baltimore, 1987

Hoffman AF: Physiological considerations of the skin. p. 16. In McCarthy DJ, Montgomery R (eds): Podiatric Dermatology. Williams & Wilkins, Baltimore, 1986

Holewski JJ, Stess RM, Graf PM, Grunfeld C: Aesthesiometry: quantification of cutaneous pressure sensation in diabetic peripheral neuropathy. J Rehab Res Dev 25:1, 1988

Holewski JJ, Moss KM, Stess RM et al: Prevalence of foot pathology and lower extremity complications in a diabetic outpatient clinic. J Rehab Res Dev 26:35, 1989

Hultman JA. Mohr RN: Evaluation and treatment of diabetic foot problems. Mt. Sinai J Med 54:253, 1987

Huntley AC: Cutaneous manifestations in diabetes: general considerations. p. 23. In Jelinek JE (ed): The Skin in Diabetes. Lea & Febiger, Philadelphia, 1986

Jacobs RL: Hoffman procedure in the ulcerated diabetic neuropathic foot. Foot Ankle 3:142, 1982

Jelinek JE: Collagen disorders in which diabetes and cutaneous features coexist. p. 155. In Jelinek JE (ed): The Skin in Diabetes. Lea & Febiger, Philadelphia, 1986

Jennings PE, Barnett AH: New approaches to the pathogenesis and treatment of diabetic microangiopathy. Diabetic Med 5:111, 1988

Jones EW, McLain S, Jeffcoate WJ: Foot lesions in a diabetic clinic over a 32 month period. Diabetic Med 2:304A, 1985

Jones EW, Peacock I, McLain S et al: A clinico-pathological study of diabetic foot ulcers. Diabetic Med 4:475, 1987

Karat S: Trophic ulceration in the neuropathic foot in leprosy: lessons for diabetes. p. 109. In Connor H, Boulton AJM, Ward JD (eds): The Foot in Diabetes. John Wiley & Sons, New York, 1987

Kelly PJ, Coventry MB: Neurotrophic ulcers of the feet: a review of 47 cases. JAMA 168:388, 1958

Kosiak M: Etiology and pathology of ischemic ulcers. Arch Phys Med Rehab 40:62, 1959

Lang-Stevenson AI, Sharrard WJ, Betts RP, Duckworth T: Neuropathic ulcers of the foot. J Bone Joint Surg 67B:438, 1985

Larsen K, Holstein P: Abnormal extension of the big toe as a cause of ulceration in diabetic feet. Prosthet Orthot Int 11:31, 1987

Lepantalo M, Kangas T, Pietila J et al: Non-invasive characterization of angiopathy in the diabetic foot. Eur J Vasc Surg 2:41, 1988

Le Quesne LP: Surgical aspects of the diabetic foot. p. 69. In Connor H, Boulton AJM, Ward JD (eds): The Foot in Diabetes. John Wiley & Sons, New York, 1987

Le Quesne PM, Fowler CJ: A study of pain threshold in diabetics with neuropathic foot lesions. J Neurol Neurosurg Psychiatry 49:1191, 1986

Levin ME: The diabetic foot: pathophysiology, evaluation, and treatment. p. 1. In Levin ME, O'Neal LW (eds): The Diabetic Foot. CV Mosby, St. Louis, 1988

Levy DM, Abraham RR, Abraham RM: Small and large fiber involvement in early diabetic neuropathy: A study with a medial plantar response and sensory thresholds. Diabetes Care 10:441, 1987

Lippmann HI, Perotto A, Farrar R: The neuropathic foot of the diabetic. Bull N Y Acad Med 52:1159, 1976

Lippmann HI: Must loss of a limb be a consequence of diabetes mellitus? Diabetes Care 2:432, 1980

Logerfo FW, Coffman JD: Vascular and microvascular disease of the foot in diabetes. N Engl J Med 311:1615, 1984

Lorber D: Neuropathy and the diabetic foot. p. 18. In Brenner MA (ed): Management of the Diabetic Foot. Williams & Wilkins, Baltimore, 1987

Manley MT, Darby T: Repetitive mechanical stress and denervation in plantar ulcer pathogenesis in rate. Arch Phys Med Rehab 61:171, 1980

Martin MM: Neuropathic lesions of the feet in diabetes mellitus. Proc Roy Soc Med 47:139, 1954

Maser RE, Nielsen VK, Bass EB et al: Measuring diabetic neuropathy: assessment and comparison of clinical examination and quantative sensory testing. Diabetes Care 12:270, 1989

Masson EA, Hay EM, Stockley I et al: Abnormal foot pressure alone does not cause foot ulceration. Diabetic Med 6:424, 1989

McMillan DE: Pathophysiology of diabetic macro- and microvascular disease. p. 343. In Ellenberg M, Rifkin H (eds): Diabetes Mellitus, Theory and Practice. Medical Examination Publishing, New York, 1983

McMillan DE: The blood viscosity problem in diabetes. Clinical Diabetes 7:61, 1989

Most RS, Sinnock P: The epidemiology of lower extremity amputation in diabetic individuals. Diabetes Care 6:87, 1983

Mueller MJ, Diamond JE, Sinacore DR et al: Total contact casting in treatment of diabetic plantar ulcers—controlled clinical trials. Diabetes Care 12:384, 1989

Mulder GD, Jahnigen D, Vandepol CJ: The role of injectable collagen in the prevention of recurrent diabetic ulcers. J Am Podiatr Med Assoc 78:238, 1988

Nawoczenski DA, Birke JA, Coleman WC: Effect of rocker sole design on plantar forefoot pressures. J Am Podiatr Med Assoc 78:455, 1988

Neilubowocz J. Borkowski M, Baraniewski H: Opening of arteriovenous anastomoses and trophic ulcer formation after peripheral nerve injury. J Cardiovasc Surg 48:100, 1975

Newrick PG, Cochrane T, Betts RP et al: Reduced hyperaemic response under the diabetic neuropathic foot. Diabetic Med 5:570, 1988

Nielsen PE: Does diabetic microangiopathy cause the development of gangrene? Scand J Clin Lab Invest, suppl. 31, 128:229, 1973

Oakley W, Catterall RCF, Martin MM: Aetiology and management of lesions of the feet in diabetes. Br J Med 2:953, 1956

O'Hare JP, Morgan MH, Alden P, et al: Aldose reductase inhibition in diabetic neuropathy: clinical and neurophysiological studies of one year's treatment with sorbinil. Diabetic Med 5:537, 1988

O'Malley BC, Timperley WR, Ward JD, et al: Platelet abnormalities in diabetic neuropathy. Lancet 2:1274, 1975

O'Neal LW: Surgical pathology of the foot and clincopathologic correlations. p. 203. In Levin ME, O'Neal LW (eds): The Diabetic Foot. CV Mosby, St. Louis, 1988

Parkhouse N, Le Quesne PM: Impaired neurogenic vascular response in patients with diabetes and neuropathic foot lesions. N Engl J Med 318:1306, 1988

Partsch H: Neuropathien vom ulzero-mutilierenden Typ Klinik, Klassifikation, Durchblutungsmessungen. Vasa, suppl. 6:1, 1977

Pati L, Behera F: Metatarsal head pressure (MHP) sores in leprosy patients. Lepr India 53:588, 1981

Patil KM, Babu TS, Oommen PK, Srinivasan H: Foot pressure measurement in leprosy and footwear design. Indian J Lepr 58:357, 1986

Pollard JP, Le Quesne LP: Method of healing diabetic foot ulcers. Br Med J Clin Res 286:436, 1983

Rafferty P, Rodriques E, Fraser DM: Etiological factors in diabetic foot ulceration. Br J Clin Pract 40:11, 1986

Ross H, Bernstein G, Rifkin H: Relationship of metabolic control of diabetes mellitus to long-term complications. p. 907. In Ellenberg M, Rifkin H (eds): Diabetes Mellitus, Theory and Practice. Medical Examination Publishing, New York, 1983

Saboto S, Yosipovitch Z, Simkin A, Sheskin J: Plantar trophic ulcers in patients with leprosy. Int Orthop 6:203, 1982

Sargent WQ: Hemorheology. p. 71. In Levin ME, O'Neal LW (eds): The Diabetic Foot. CV Mosby, St. Louis, 1988

Schubotz R: Double-blind trial of pentoxifylline in diabetics with peripheral vascular disorders. Pharamatherapeutica 1:172, 1976

Schustek S, Jacobs AM: Diabetic autonomic neuropathy in the surgical management of the diabetic foot. J Foot Surg 21:16, 1982

Shipley DE: Clinical evaluation and care of the insensitive foot. Phys Ther 59:13, 1979

Simpson LO: Altered blood rheology in the pathogenesis of diabetic and other neuropathies. Muscle Nerve 11:725, 1988

Skorman SE: Use of injectable collagen to treat chronic diabetic foot ulcers. J Foot Surg 26:511, 1987

Slama G, Letanoux M, Thibult N et al: Quantification of early subclinical limited joint mobility in diabetes mellitus. Diabetes Care 8:329, 1985

Smith L, Plehwe W, Yue DK, Turtle JR: Electrodynogram in objective assessment of bearing pressures in the feet of diabetic patients. Diabetes Res Clin Pract, suppl. 1, 5:S312, 1988

Sosenko JM, Marta K, Soto RA et al: Specific assessments of warm and cool sensitivities in adult diabetic patients. Diabetes Care 11:481, 1988

Soulier SM: The use of running shoes in the prevention of plantar diabetic ulcers. J Am Podiatr Med Assoc 76:395, 1986

Soulier SM, Godsey C, Asay ED, Perotta DM: The prevention of plantar ulceration in the diabetic foot through the use of running shoes. Diabetes Educator 13:130, 1987

Spencer F, Sage R, Graner J: The incidence of foot pathology in a diabetic population. J Am Podiatr Med Assoc 75:590, 1985

Stess RP: New methods of evaluation and risk stratification of the diabetic insensate foot. J Foot Surg 25:503, 1986

Stess RM, Sisney PC, Moss KM et al: Use of liquid crystal thermography in the evaluation of the diabetic foot. Diabetes Care 9:267, 1986

Stokes IAF, Faris IB, Hutton WC: The neuropathic ulcer and loads on the foot in diabetic patients. Acta Orthop Scand 46:839, 1975

Stokes IAF, Hutton WC: The effect of the diabetic ulcer on the load bearing function of the foot. p. 245. In Kenedi RM, Cowden JM (eds): Bedsore Biomechanics. University Park Press, Baltimore, 1976

Thompson DE: the pathomechanics of soft tissue damage. p. 148. In Levin ME, O'Neal LW (eds): The Diabetic Foot. 3rd Ed. CV Mosby, St. Louis, 1983

Thompson DE: The effects of mechanical stress on soft tissue. p. 91. In Levin ME, O'Neal LW (eds): The Diabetic Foot. CV Mosby, St. Louis, 1988

Tilton RG, Faller AM, Burkhardt JK et al: Pericyte degeneration and acellular capillaries are increased in the feet of human diabetic patients. Diabetologia 28:895, 1985

Tooke JE, Rayman G, Boolell M: Blood flow abnormalities in the diabetic foot: diagnostic aid or research tool? p. 23. In Connor H, Boulton AJM, Ward JD (eds): The Foot in Diabetes. John Wiley & Sons, New York, 1987

Veves A, Masson EA, Fernando DJS, Boulton AJM: Use of experimental padded hosiery to reduce abnormal foot pressures in diabetic neuropathy. Diabetes Care 12:653, 1989

Walsh CH, Soler NG, Fitzgerald MG, Malins JM: Association of foot lesions with retinopathy in newly diagnosed diabetes mellitus. Lancet 1:878, 1975

Ward JD, Boulton AJM, Simms JM et al: Venous distension in the diabetic neuropathic foot. J Roy Soc Med 76:1011, 1983

Ward JD: Diabetic neuropathy. p. 28. In Alberti KGMM, Krall LP (eds): The Diabetes Annual. Elsevier Science Publishers, 1985

Ward JD, Boulton AJM: Peripheral vascular abnormalities and diabetic neuropathy. p. 89. In Dyck PJ, Thomas PK, Asbury AK et al (eds): Diabetic Neuropathy. WB Saunders, Philadelphia, 1987

Watkins PJ, Edmonds ME: Autonomic neuropathy: blood flow in the diabetic foot. p. 211. In Brostrom, Ljungstedt H (eds): Recent Trends in Diabetic Research. Almqvist and Wiksell International, Stockholm, 1982

Watkins PJ, Edmonds ME: Sympathetic nerve failure in diabetes. Diabetologia 25:73, 1983

Yamada H: Strength of biological materials. p. 224. Williams & Wilkins, Baltimore, 1970

Young RJ, Zhou YQ, Rodriguez E et al: Variable relationship between peripheral somatic and autonomic neuropathy in patients with different syndromes of diabetic polyneuropathy. Diabetes 35:192, 1986

Young RJ: Identification of the subject "at risk" of foot ulceration. p. 1. In Connor H, Boulton AJM, Ward JD (eds): The Foot in Diabetes. John Wiley & Sons, New York, 1987

8

Biomechanics of the Diabetic Foot

Harold D. Schoenhaus, D.P.M.
Elissa Wernick, D.P.M.
Ross S. Cohen

It has been known for quite some time that neurologic problems in the diabetic population are very common, particularly those of sensory deficiencies. However, sensory complications are only one part of the diabetic neurologic spectrum. Motor neuropathies are fairly common as well, and play a very significant role in altering diabetic gait parameters. In the past there has been some debate as to which is most important, sensory neuropathies[1] or motor neuropathies.[2] While there is some argument as to which type is most important, it is our belief that one is rarely seen without the other, and it is a combination of both types of neurologic deficits that will dictate the pathologic problems that occur in gait.

It is our opinion that gait adjustments made to accommodate for abnormal forces that produce foot lesions are not a function of pain perception. If they were, then an individual without any sensory loss would modify gait to accommodate for abnormal forces, and therefore we would not see the pathology that we do.

Moderate repetitive stress is thought by many to be the true etiology of mal perforans ulcers.[3] While this may not be true for ulcers on the dorsum of the foot, it is the etiology for ulcers on the plantar aspect of the foot. Forces greater than 10 kg/cm^2 acting on the foot during gait will contribute to ulcer formation on the plantar surface of the foot.[4] The development of a mal perforans ulcer is dependent on (1) the mechanical problems that preexist within the intrinsic foot type, (2) abnormal forces greater than 10 kg/cm^2,[4] (3) an atrophied plantar fat pad,[5] and (4) collagen glycosylation, which will decrease skin resiliency.[6] The specific location of the ulcer is determined by the mechanical pathology, and varies from patient to patient. Hence, it is faulty mechanics with dermopathy that creates the ulcer. The lack of pain perception becomes important when a mechanical problem acts to create an ulcer that the patient does not perceive and leaves unattended.

Although it is a combination of the two types of neuropathies that disrupt normal gait parameters, motor neuropathies have a more dramatic effect in altering gait than sensory. Motor neuropathies usually manifest themselves by the sixth decade of life and are most common in the lower extremities.[7,8] Motor paresis is a very common in the diabetic population and investigations have shown that 65 percent of diabetic patients with neuropathies have muscle weaknesses.[9] Motor neuropathies will manifest themselves as myopathic changes and are a result of demyelination, axonal swelling, endoneural edema, and fibrosis in the intramuscular nerve branches.[2] As a result of nerve degeneration, muscle atrophy will occur. Of course, specific muscle atrophy is a result of neuropathy of the nerve fibers supplying that muscle, and tends to affect all the muscles within selective compartments. Pathologic gait changes will result from these compartmental muscle weaknesses, and specific changes in the classic gait parameters are the result of the compartmental group atrophies that exist.

The first documented loss of a group of muscles in a diabetic patient was noted in 1882 by Bernard, when he noted neuropathy of the femoral nerve and atrophy of the anterior compartment of the thigh.[11] Since Bernard's time many other investigators have noted other muscle group losses in the diabetic patient. Intrinsic muscle atrophy in the foot and hand,[12] and anterior crural atrophy[11] are such examples. Although these group atrophies have been known for some time, very few investigators have applied this knowledge to pathologic developments in gait.

ANTERIOR CRURAL ATROPHY

Anterior group atrophy can occur for several reasons such as mononeuropathies involving the deep peroneal nerve and endoneural edema brought about because of poor diabetic control (Fig. 8-1). Regardless, anterior group atrophy is very common by the sixth decade of life. Its effect on the diabetic patient combined with existing skin problems, plantar fat pad degeneration, and sensory deficits is disastrous.

During the contact period of gait the anterior muscle group has two functions: deceleration of ankle plantar flexion, and smoothing the transition of forces from the lateral aspect of the foot to the medial side.[10] With the initiation of heel strike, ground reactive forces 10 to 15 percent greater than body weight are directed in a superior-posterior direction behind the ankle joint's axis of motion. These ground reactive forces are extremely powerful and create a strong plantar-flexory moment at the ankle joint. It is these ground reactive forces that plantar-flex the ankle and bring the forefoot to the supporting surface. Deceleration of ankle plantar flexion is needed to decrease the forces in which the forefoot encounters the supporting surface. Slowing down ankle plantar flexion is achieved through an eccentric contraction of the anterior group. If this is lost a foot slap will result along with an increase in load under the forefoot. This provides the proper environment for ulcer formation. Since not only is the force intensified under the metatarsal heads, it is produced earlier in the gait cycle and for a longer period of time than expected. Therefore, deceleration of ankle plantar flexion is one mechanism that the foot uses to absorb ground reactive forces, and its loss of function will encourage the formation of plantar mal perforans ulcers through additional trauma.

Smoothing ankle plantar flexion is not the only deceleration process occurring during contact phase (Fig. 8-2). When the heel strikes the supporting surface the subtalar joint is inverted 2°,

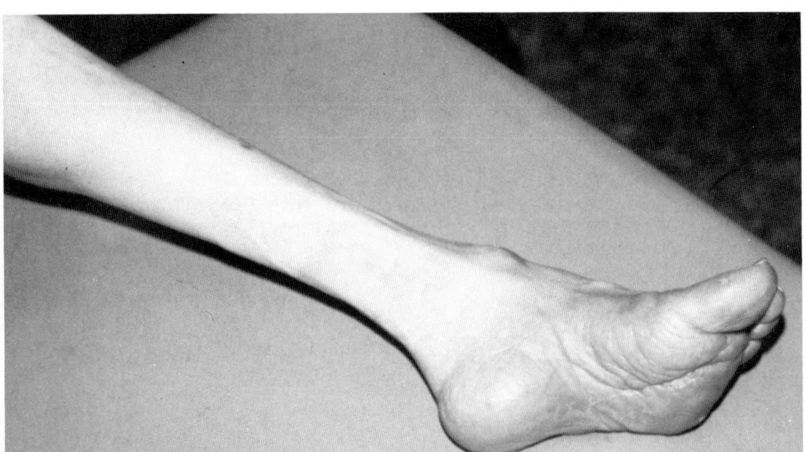

Fig. 8-1. Anterior group atrophy.

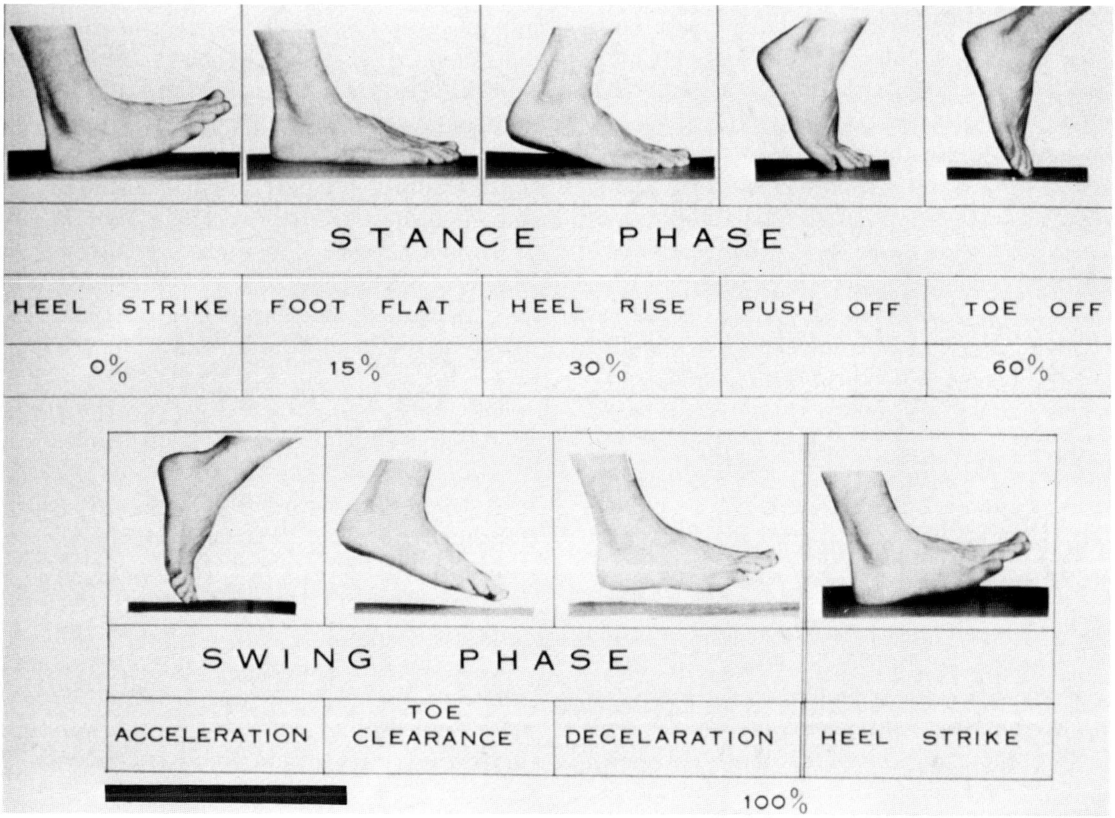

Fig. 8-2. Walking cycle.

and ground reactive forces are directed laterally to the subtalar joint axis. These forces are coming from the supporting surface, and must be buffered or pathology will develop in the foot, knee, or lower back. Buffering is achieved through contact phase pronation along with smooth ankle plantar flexion. At heel strike, because the ground reactive forces are directed laterally to the subtalar joint axis, the calcaneus will abduct and evert, and plantar flexion will occur; internal rotation of the leg will cause adduction of the talus. With this mechanism, forces are converted into transverse plane motion within the leg, and forces are transferred from the lateral border of the foot medially. Tibialis anterior and tibialis posterior will decelerate subtalar joint pronation and create a smooth loading of the forefoot from lateral to medial. The slowing down and smoothing out of forces encountered at the subtalar joint's end range of motion results in the direction of pronation, roughly 4° everted. Diabetic myopathy within the anterior compartment will decrease the leg's ability to smooth out contact phase pronation. In response to this, forces are transferred from lateral to medial much faster than should be, and as they progress medially they pick up more momentum than normal. Essentially, as the calcaneus everts, it does so with more momentum than normal. This means that as the subtalar joint everts to its end range of motion, it meets this point very abruptly and with more generated momentum than normal. Due to this abrupt stop jamming occurs at the subtalar joint's end range of motion. The jamming occurring within the subtalar joint is not recognized by the patient because of a lack in proprioception. Wolf's law will then work to remodel the subtalar joint. The result of this subtalar joint remodeling is a joint with a decreased range of motion.[13] When pathology progresses to this point neuropathic joint changes become obvious, and the mechanism of closed chain pronation is not as effective in absorbing ground forces. In addition, the range of subtalar motion usually decreases.

Under normal conditions a very delicate agonist-antagonist relationship exists between the anterior group muscles and the other two compartments of the leg, the posterior and lateral compartments. With anterior crural group atrophy there will usually be some posterior and lateral group weakness present as well, but the anterior atrophy is always greater. This places the posterior and lateral group muscles in a position of greater dominance and of greater mechanical advantage. Clinically, this will show up as a relative hypertrophy of the posterior compartment compared to the anterior compartment, with some very noteworthy changes that occur in gait.

The most significant change is that of an equinus deformity that results secondary to gastrocnemius-soleus overdominance. Since the antagonist function of the anterior muscle group is lost, there will be an increased plantar-flexory pull on the calcaneus. This situation creates severe pathomechanical sequelae, particularly in the diabetic patient. Investigators at the Veterans Affairs Medical Center, University of California, have shown that 63 percent of the 94 diabetic patients that they examined had limitation in dorsiflexion.[14]

When heel lift begins, at 67 percent of stance, body weight is shifted onto the metatarsal heads. With an equinus deformity, the midtarsal joint (MTJ) is unlocked creating hypermobility within the forefoot. Because the MTJ unlocks and allows for more movement around both the longitudinal and oblique MTJ axes, the foot does not have the intrinsic support it needs during propulsion, hence the hypermobility. With forefoot hypermobility during propulsion there is an increase in shear forces occurring under the metatarsal heads. A combination of shear forces under the metatarsal heads, decreased resiliency of the skin, and thinning of the plantar fat pad is very dangerous and will result in ulceration beneath one of the metatarsal heads. In addition, the patient may go into an "abductory twist" to try to compensate for the equinus, and create an ulcer on the medial aspect of the hallux.

Under normal conditions, near the end of propulsion, the tibialis anterior begins to contract and dorsiflexes the first ray. When the first metatarsal is up, the hallux is in a position slightly flexed on the first metatarsal. With the hallux flexed, it will assume a more stable position. The effect of this is a rigid beam for the extensor hallucis longus. With a stable hallux the extensor hallucis longus is in a position of greater mechanical advantage and will dorsiflex the foot at the ankle. Hence, in the diabetic patient with anterior group atrophy there is a problem with ankle dorsiflexion during swing phase.

Normally, the foot begins supinating in midstance and continues to supinate throughout propulsion. The supinated architecture provides intrinsic stability within the foot and, in addition, stabilizes the lateral column of the foot. Supination is dependent on internal rotation of the swinging limb, external rotation of the stance limb, and the muscles within the posterior compartment. In addition, lateral stability is further enhanced by soleus influence. The soleus stabilizes the lateral column of the foot against the ground, because of the direction its tendinous fibers run with respect to the subtalar joint and ankle joint. With the lateral column secure against the supporting surface, the peroneus longus is now in a position of mechanical advantage and can stabilize the first ray. With the first ray stable the first metatarsal head will glide over the sesamoid apparatus and allow for the 65° hallux dorsiflexion needed in propulsion. This mechanism relies on a securely fixed cuboid, positioned lower than the insertion of the peroneus longus on the medial cuneiform and base of the first metatarsal. Peroneus longus will then use the cuboid as a pulley and direct a substantial abductory posterior-plantar force on the first ray axis, stabilizing it against the ground. If this mechanism is not functioning properly, then the first ray is unstable and will not successfully glide over the sesamoid apparatus. The result of this is a hallux that does not achieve the 65° of dorsiflexion needed in propulsion and a hallux limitus will develop. The antagonist of peroneus longus is tibialis anterior; however, because of anterior group atrophy peroneus longus is relatively unopposed and its force will be very dominant. In the diabetic myopathic patient the tibialis anterior muscle does not function normally. In addition, the functioning of the forefoot is hypermobile and the peroneus longus loses its stable pulley because the cuboid is in the same plane as its insertion into the first metatarsal and medial cuneiform. In normal peroneus longus function it will influence the frontal and sagittal planes of the first ray axis equally with the same amount of motion in both planes. Because the forefoot is hypermobile and the cuboid is not the stable pulley that it should be, peroneus longus will acquire a pathomechanical influence around the first ray axis. Increased frontal plane motion with less sagittal plane motion will result. As a result of peroneus longus losing its sagittal plane influence at the first ray, it is no longer stable in the sagittal plane and ground reactive forces will dorsiflex the first ray. In addition, frontal plane motion is partially responsible for the shear forces that occur between the bones of the foot and the supporting surface and will produce keratomas underneath the metatarsal heads during stance. Therefore, these pathologic forces, combined with the existing problems in skin resiliency and plantar fat pad thinning, will cause an ulcer under the metatarsal heads.

INTRINSIC MUSCLE ATROPHY

Intrinsic muscle atrophy is a very common characteristic found in the diabetic neuropathic patient and will contribute to diabetic ulceration.[12] During propulsion the mechanical function of the digits must be as stable as a "rigid beam" or pathology will result. Digital stability is achieved through a very delicate balance between different muscle groups. When the lumbricales[15] and interossei contract, they create a flexion force at the metatarsophalangeal joint and an extension force at the proximal interphalangeal joint. The flexion force is antagonized by the muscles superior to the deep transverse metatarsal ligament, extensor digitorum brevis and the extensor digitorum longus. As is seen in other situations, there exists an agonist-antagonist relationship between the lumbricales and the muscles superior to the deep transverse metatarsal ligament. This relationship should be perfectly balanced so that no one group of muscles will dominate over the other. This allows the digits to be maintained parallel to the supporting surface with no extension or flexion seen at the metatarsophalangeal joints. As a result of an equal agonist-antagonist pull at the metatarsophalangeal joint, the digits will be maintained parallel to the supporting surface as the lesser metatarsal heads pivot over the plantar plates during propulsion. When the two agonist and antagonist muscle groups contract they will pull the proximal phalanx onto the metatarsal head; stability is a result of compression forces within the metatarsophalangeal joint. Extensor forces directed toward the proximal interphalangeal joint are produced by contraction of the lumbricales and extensor digitorum longus influence. Flexor digitorum brevis will antagonize these extension forces by directing flexion forces at the proximal interphalangeal joint, and should perfectly antagonize the extension forces.

Because these muscle forces are not producing motion in the sagittal plane, forces will then be directed toward creating compression between the proximal and middle phalanges and stability within the proximal and interphalangeal joints is achieved. With the proximal and middle phalanges stable and secure on the supporting surface, extensor digitorum longus will pull on the extensor hood. This force within the extensor hood will create the "rigid beam effect" by pulling the digit posteriorly onto the metatarsal head. Hence, through this mechanism of agonist-antagonist interaction, the rigid beam effect will occur and stability of the digits on the ground will result. Quadratus plantae also makes a contribution toward normal digit function. It originates on the posterior plantar surface of the calcaneus and inserts into the lateral side of the flexor digitorum longus tendon. When quadratus plantae contracts it will pull the tendons of flexor digitorum longus laterally. This will allow a better alignment of the long flexor tendons with respect to the digits. When the long flexors contract, they will pull straight on the digits. Without this straight alignment the long flexors would approach the digit at an angle and direct their force posterior medially instead of just posteriorly. Adducto varus deformities would then result due to the improper angulation of the long flexors.

Obviously, this stabilizing mechanism is very delicate and the loss of only this muscle group will result in pathology. In the diabetic patient with neuropathic sequelae the normal agonist-antagonist relationship is disrupted. Commonly, the diabetic neuropathic patient will have atrophy of all the intrinsics, as well as anterior crural atrophy. As a result there is a disruption of the delicate agonist-antagonist relationship and adductovarus claw toe deformities result (Fig. 8-3). Essentially, there is a loss of the rigid beam effect, and flexor digitorum longus will contract during the first half of propulsion relatively unopposed. In addition, due to atrophy of the quadratus plantae, flexor digitorum longus will pull on the digits in a posterior medial direction. Hence, adductovarus claw toes will result, with flexion of the metatarsophalangeal joints, and the interphalangeal joints and the toes will be in a varus position. Forces are no longer used to create compression within the metatarsophalangeal joints and interphalangeal joints, but instead are directed toward flexing these joints. With the adductovarus deformity retrograde forces are produced by the extensor digitorum longus contracting during the last half of propulsion. These retrograde forces are directed toward the metatarsal head in a posterior-plantar direction, and will increase the force under the metatarsal heads during propulsion. The retrograde force produced during the last half of propulsion is very powerful and will push the metatarsal heads against the supporting surface. When the metatarsal head pressure reaches 10 kg/cm^2 ulceration will occur under the metatarsal heads.[4] This is not only due to increased vertical forces on the metatarsal heads, but also to shear forces created by a hypermobile forefoot and

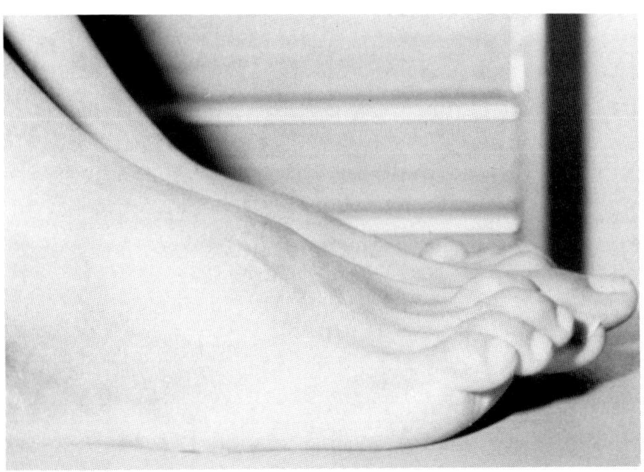

Fig. 8-3. Adductovarus claw toe deformities.

lack of skin resiliency. Additionally, we have demonstrated through electrodynographic studies that pressure under the forefoot occurs earlier than normal and therefore lasts longer than normal (Fig. 8-4). Hence it is a combination of the forefoot dealing with an increase in submetatarsal head pressure, shear forces, and being loaded for a long period of time that contribute to ulcer formation.

LOCATION OF PLANTAR MAL PERFORANS ULCERS

In the diabetic patient with myopathic pathology the specific location of the mal perforans ulcer is determined by the structural foot pathology present. Location of lesions such as tylomas and intractable plantar keratomas (IPKs) are always determined by the specific structural foot pathology in the nondiabetic individual. Essentially, it is the same mechanical factors that determine the location of plantar lesions in the nondiabetic individual that will dictate the location of plantar mal perforans ulcers in the diabetic patient. If one can identify any structural foot pathology that may be present, then a prediction can be made as to the specific location of the mal perforans ulcer before it occurs. Diabetic patients presenting with an uncompensated hindfoot varus deformity may expect to ulcerate beneath the fifth metatarsal head (Fig. 8-5). If a patient has a compensated hindfoot varus, then ulceration would occur under the second metatarsal head (Fig. 8-6).

A patient presenting with a partially compensated hindfoot varus may ulcerate under the fourth metatarsal head. Uncompensated forefoot varus deformities will usually cause ulceration under the fifth metatarsal head area, with compensate forefoot varus deformities creating ulceration under the second metatarsal head. Rigid forefoot valgus deformities will produce ulceration under the first metatarsal head, the fifth metatarsal head, or both the first and fifth metatarsal heads (Fig. 8-7). Therefore, if the structural foot pathology can be identified and controlled, then the plantar mal perforans ulcer may be prevented.

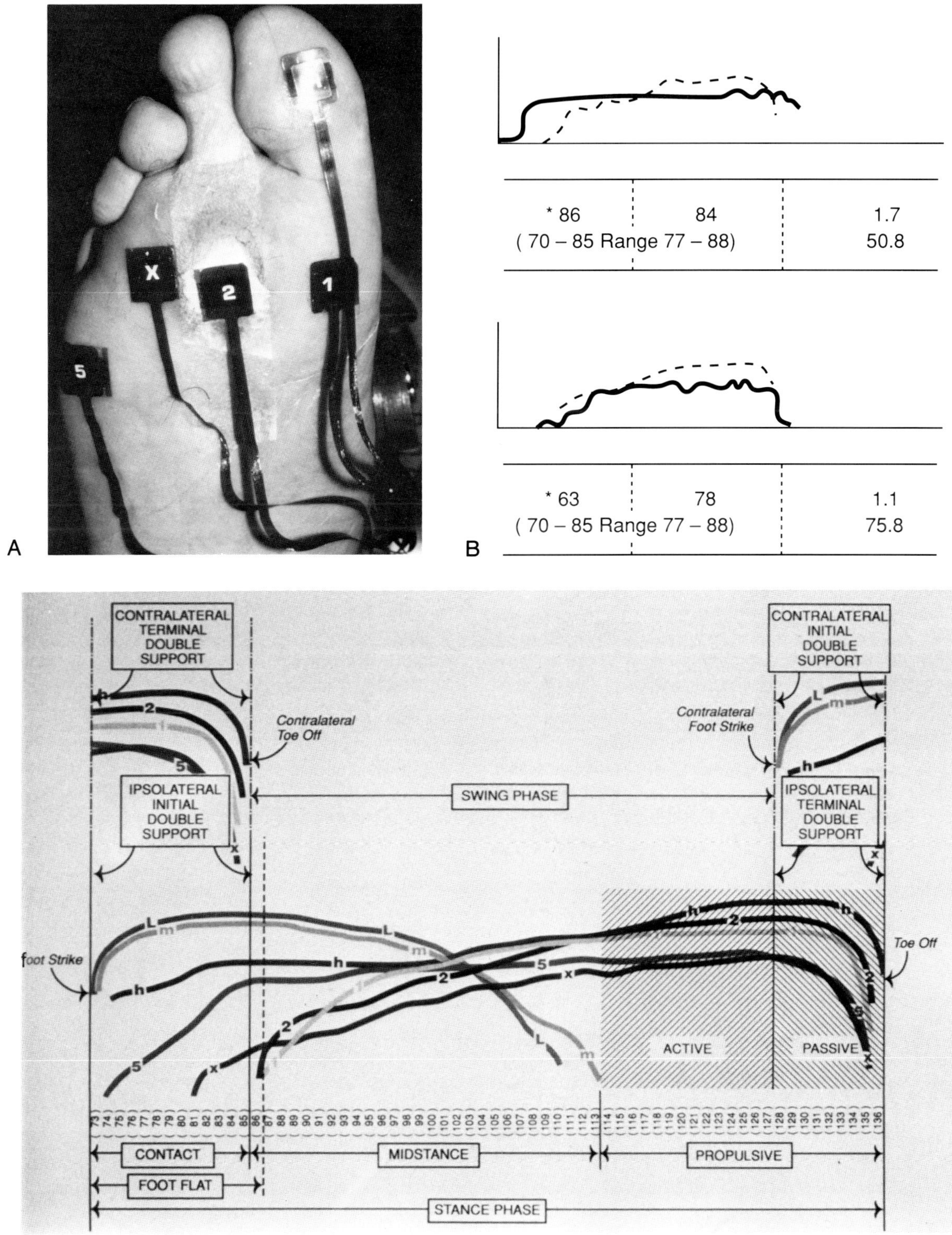

Fig. 8-4. Electrodynographic study. (**A**) Electrodynographic surface sensors located under the hallux and second metatarsal head over mal perforans ulcers. (**B**) Electrodynographic curves demonstrating early and prolonged pressure under the second metatarsal head as seen on the top curves. Note that the dotted line represents the normal. (**C**) Electrodynographic curves representing each sensor and its normal time curve during the stance phase of gait.

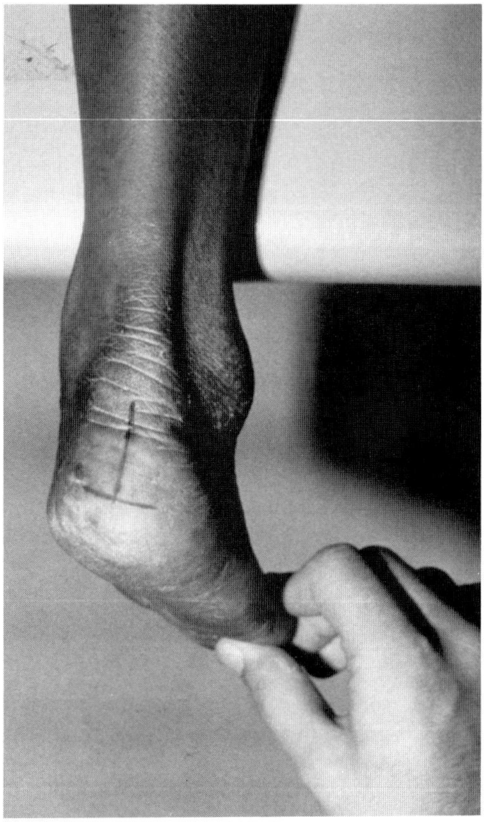

Fig. 8-5. Patient with an uncompensated hind foot varus deformity. A mal perforans ulceration may be expected to occur beneath the fifth metatarsal head.

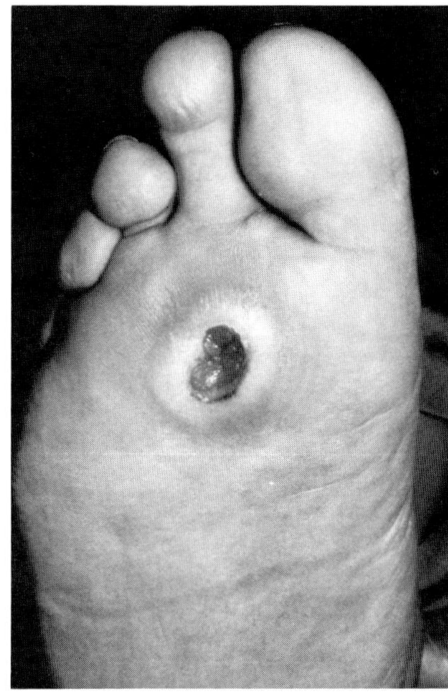

Fig. 8-6. Ulceration under the second metatarsal head.

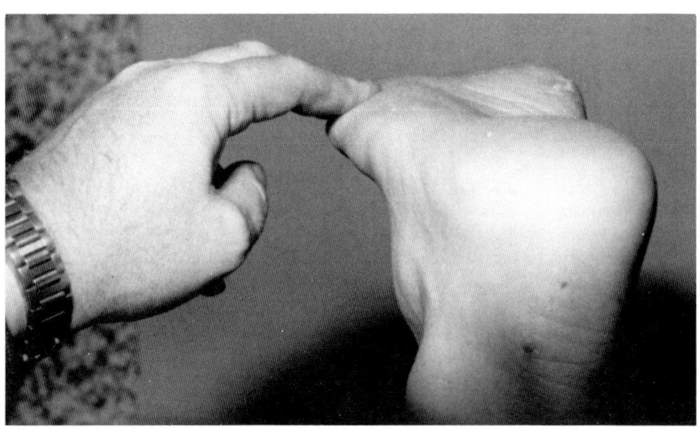

Fig. 8-7. Patient with rigid forefoot valgus deformity. Ulcerations may be expected under the first metatarsal head, the fifth metatarsal head, or both.

AMPUTATIONS IN THE FOOT

If severe enough, the consequences of ulceration often lead to amputation. Amputations in the foot can have a profound effect on altering the gait in individuals. These alterations, when occurring in the diabetic or high risk patient, often result in tissue damage, which, if severe enough, can result in subsequent amputation. In addition, alteration of normal foot mechanics can adversely influence the function of the ankle, knee, hip, and the back.

Understanding the normal and abnormal biomechanics associated with the loss of the particular body part is essential for proper care of the amputee and for prevention of future loss.

Hallux Amputation

The hallux is the pedal end organ responsible for transferring body weight in an efficient manner from one limb to another. Interruption in the normal function of this structure often creates compensations, the results of which can cause severe complications. The hallux is responsible for stabilizing the medial forefoot. When it is removed, the second toe attempts to take over this function; however, it does not have the osseous integrity or the muscular investments of the first toe. Ground reaction forces will buckle the digit, eventually forming a hammer toe. This deformity produces a retrograde force on the second metatarsal head, resulting in increased weight bearing, distal advancement of the plantar fat pad, callus formation,[16] and susceptibility to an ulcer or stress fracture.[17,18] Mann et al. reported an average of 15° more dorsiflexion in the second metatarsal phalangeal joint following hallux amputation.[17]

In addition, the hallux functions as a buttress for the rotation of the first metatarsal head. Once this loss has occurred, the medial column will advance distally, reducing the effectiveness of the first ray. Body weight will then transfer laterally onto the lesser metatarsals, increasing the potential for injury.

This lateral shift was demonstrated in a study by Mann et al., who found an increase in load, callus formation, and weight transfer under the second and third metatarsal heads.[17] Ianucci et al. reported the incidence of stress fracture under the second and third metatarsals following hallux amputation.[18]

During the operative procedure for removal of the hallux, no effort is made to secure the muscles that have been severed. As a result, proximal contraction of the tendons along with the sesamoid apparatus produces a plantarly directed first ray. This increased angulation of the metatarsal to the support surface results in weight bearing of a high amplitude over a prolonged period, the proper environment for ulcer formation.

Digital Amputation

Very commonly, individual digital resections are performed. Lesser toe amputations usually result in little functional disturbance in stance and gait.[19] In general, the function of the digits are to provide balance and proprioception.[20] The second digit also serves as the lateral buttress for the hallux.[21] As a word of caution when removing second digits, postoperative accommodation with a toe filler is mandatory to avoid a rapidly developing hallux valgus.

Lesser Ray Resections

Ray resections include removal of the phalanges, metatarsophalangeal joint, and the metatarsal shaft. They are in general unsuccessful procedures, often leading to transfer ulcerations of the remaining segment.[19] Gianfortune et al. reviewed 37 ray resections and found the highest success rate with third ray resections and the lowest with fifth ray resections.[22] This is understandable since the third metatarsal usually shares the load of the ground and body weight with the second and fourth rays and as such does not function independently as does the first and fifth rays. Hypermobility of the fifth ray often leads to callus formation under the fourth metatarsal head. A similar situation occurs with amputation of the fifth ray. The fourth metatarsal is now the lateralmost segment of the forefoot, subjected to protracted loads and potential breakdown. Furthermore, the removal of the fifth metatarsal can result in a varus attitude of the foot. The peroneus brevis has its insertion on the base of the fifth metatarsal and is the primary muscle responsible for pronation of the subtalar joint. Therefore, its removal by ray resection results in unopposed function of the posterior tibial and soleus muscles. These muscles, no longer antagonized by the pull of the peroneus brevis, will result in a supinated foot.[15]

First Ray Resections

One of the functions of the first ray during the stance phase of gait is to help resist pronation of the hindfoot. With removal of this segment, body weight rapidly shifts medially. The second metatarsal, now functioning as the medialmost segment in the forefoot, is subjected to a heightened load and eventual ulcer formation. In addition, this medial weight shift, along with loss of the plantar fascia and intrinsics to the hallux, collapses the medial architecture and eventually sets up navicular ptosis and ulcer formation.[17] Therefore, removal of the first ray and hallux has a high incidence of subsequent ulcer formation at adjacent locations on the foot.

Transmetatarsal Amputations

The indications for transmetatarsal amputations are gangrene of one or more toes, osteomyelitis of one or more toes, or an open infected lesion in a neurotrophic foot.[23] Because the transmetatarsal amputation is deemed functionally successful with a high probability to primarily heal, many surgeons will utilize it as opposed to ray and digital resections. Most of the research that has been done on the transmetatarsal amputation relates to its ability to primarily heal from the surgical perspective. Little has been done in the way of long-term follow-up functionally. Although a useful amputation, it is not without complications and is particularly susceptible to reamputation in the diabetic population.[20]

The osseous component that is removed during a transmetatarsal amputation includes all the digits, the metatarsophalangeal joints, and the metatarsal heads. How much of the metatarsal shafts should remain depends on the clinical situation. Three levels of transmetatarsal amputations are performed: the distal amputation, whereby the metatarsals are transected at the metatarsal necks; the midshaft amputation; and the proximal amputation. In midshaft and proximal amputations, only the bases of the metatarsals remain. This is clinically significant as to the functional outcome of the procedure in that the more distal amputations provide for better structural integrity. The greater the forefoot length, the better the mechanical function of the foot. The metatarsal length provides two functions. First, it allows for increased stability during midstance[24] and provides a greater lever arm for propulsion. Second, the increased length allows extrinsic muscle function to be maximized due to the increased lever arm around which they function. As shown by Green et al., patients with transmetatarsal amputations have far less disability since the length of the forefoot remains greater than that of the hindfoot.[24]

The metatarsophalangeal joints function as the terminal hinge in the stance phase of gait, allowing adequate plantar flexion (30°) and knee flexion (45°) to occur during propulsion. They also serve via dorsiflexion of the toes to tighten the plantar skin, which resists the anterior/posterior shear forces that accumulate and transfers them to the osseous structures below, which is more equipped to handle them than the soft tissue.[25] Removal of the metatarsophalangeal joints causes the distal hinge to move more proximally. The distalmost aspect of the foot, the remaining metatarsal shafts, then acts as the terminal interface over which the body must pass in the final stages of gait, which is still intact in the transmetatarsal amputation, albeit reduced.[20]

Because of the removal of the joints, this distal segment cannot function as the metatarsophalangeal joints would, and is unsuccessful in dissipating the shear forces that are now concentrated at the distal aspect of the stump. Without restricting passive movement and tightening the framework, these forces will eventually break down the tissue, resulting in distal plantar breakdown, which is the most common complication of this amputation.[26]

Surgical removal of the anterior muscle group insertions leaves most of the dorsiflexors functionless. Mild equinus deformities with reduction in the swing and contact phases of gait[20] will occur as a result of the loss of the antagonist function of the long extensors of the foot. The anterior muscle group functions just prior to heel contact to decelerate pronation and ankle plantar flexion.[15] Although the tibialis anterior is intact, it is not powerful enough to overcome the posterior muscle group. It is really the extensor hallucis longus, by virtue of its long lever arm, that is the most powerful dorsiflexor of the foot. With it removed, there results an increase in rapid ankle plantar flexion, early forefoot loading, a decrease in contact, and an increase in the midstance phase of gait.

Removal of the plantar flexors along with the plantar aponeurosis reduces the ability of the forefoot to resist flattening of the foot. Eventual lowering of the longitudinal arch will occur, despite the fact that the foot is shortened.

Despite this, the transmetatarsal amputation is a useful procedure, with far less complications than are seen in the most proximal amputations; therefore, it is still a viable alternative to the Syme or below knee amputation. Its success is largely due to the fact that (1) it maintains a foot lever arm, (2) it preserves all gait parameters with the exception of part of heel off and toe off, and (3) it lowers energy expenditure by smoothing the path of the center of gravity during walking.[20]

Lisfranc and Chopart Amputations

When gangrene or osteomyelitis extends beyond the metatarsophalangeal joints, a transmetatarsal amputation will no longer suffice. More proximal levels such as the Lisfranc and Chopart amputations have long been regarded as useless and thus many surgeons have chosen to bypass these procedures, utilizing the Syme or below knee.[27,28] The reasoning behind the surgeons' opting for more proximal amputations than that of Lisfranc or Chopart are the complications involved in function. These complications are manifested in significant equinovarus deformities of the remaining stump as well as unsatisfactory prosthetic fitting.

Chopart and Lisfranc amputations have frequently been associated with severe pathologic equinus. The reason for this is twofold. First and most obvious, the only remaining pedal musculature is that of the gastrocnemius-soleus complex. Second, as relates to foot structure, when an amputation takes place in the midfoot, the calcaneal inclination is reduced. The normal clacaneal inclination angle of 18° to 22° is dependent on a 15° metatarsal declination. With the distal segment removed, the calcaneus becomes more parallel with the weight-bearing surface, thus decreasing the distance between origin and insertion of the gastrocnemius-soleus complex, resulting in an equinus deformity of the stump.

Gait Parameters

No discussion of pedal amputation is complete without regard to how the foot functions in gait. Certain generalities can be drawn with respect to all amputations, particularly all unilateral pedal amputations. The gait patterns of these amputees have wide ranging effects on the entire musculoskeletal system. In general, it has been observed that the more proximal the amputation, the shorter the swing phase will be on the affected side. Also, a longer midstance period is noted with a greater degree of knee extension as well as a greater amount of pelvic drop. These parameters of gait are also greatly affected by the ratio of length of forefoot to hindfoot.[24] In a normal foot, the required ankle plantar flexion seen at propulsion assists the leg in maintaining its functional length following knee flexion. With full forefoot length, we would not expect to see a visible drop in the pelvis. But in a foot with a tarsal amputation, one can clearly visualize the pelvic drop since this extremity is functionally shortened.

The effects on gait after transmetatarsal amputation was studied by Friedman et al., who utilized the electrodynogram system to show the dynamics of force distribution after transmetatarsal amputation. They concluded that not only was there an increased load taken up by the distal metatarsal shafts, but that it also occurred for a longer duration of time.[20]

CONCLUSION

Distal segmental amputation can be successful and rewarding. However, a thorough understanding of consequent alteration of function is essential. Thus, in order for an amputation to be considered successful, several criteria must be satisfied:

1. It must have the ability to primarily heal without contracture.
2. It must provide walking and standing patterns that approach normal ambulation.
3. There must be effective and pain-free transfer of body weight.
4. It must have the ability to evenly distribute body weight and pressure.
5. It must maintain gait parameters as close to normal as possible.
6. There must be optional alignment of the remaining segment with a forefoot to rearfoot length relationship of at least 1:1.
7. It must preserve muscle function.[29]

Since there is a high degree of mortality and morbidity associated with proximal amputations,[30,31] the use of partial pedal amputation can greatly enhance the quality of life when indicated. As stated by Rubin and Cohen, "Mobility is often the key to survival."[32]

REFERENCES

1. Holewski JJ, Stess RM, Graf PM, Grunfeld C: Aesthesiometry: quantification of cutaneous pressure sensation in diabetic peripheral neuropathy. J Rehabil Res Dev 25:1, 1988
2. Chokroverty S, Reyes MG, Tonaki H: The syndrome of diabetic amyotrophy. Ann Neurol 2:181, 1977
3. Hall OC, Brand PW: The etiology of the neuropathic plantar ulcer. J Am Podiatr Med Assoc 69:173, 1979
4. Duckworth T, Boulton AJM, Betts RR, Franks CI, Ward JD: Plantar pressure measurements and the prevention of ulceration in the diabetic foot. J Bone Joint Surg [Br] 67B:79, 1985
5. Lippmann HI, Perotto A, Farrar R: The neuropathic foot of the diabetic. Bull NY Acad Med 52:1159, 1976
6. Hamlin CR, Kohn RR, Luschin JH: Apparent accelerated aging of human collagen in diabetic mellitus. Diabetes 24:902, 1975
7. Ellenberg M: Diabetic neuropathy of the upper extremities. Journal of Mount Sinai Hospital 35:134, 1968
8. Ellenberg M: Diabetic neuropathy, p. 822. In Ellenberg M, Rifkin H (eds): Diabetes Mellitus: Theory and Practice. McGraw-Hill, New York, 1970
9. Bischoff A: Die diabetische Neuropathie. p. 415. In von Oberdisse K (ed): Diabetes Mellitus. Springer Verlag, Berlin, 1977
10. Basmajian JV: Muscles Alive: Their Functions Revealed by Electromyography. 3rd Ed. Williams & Wilkins, Baltimore, 1974
11. Byrnes CM: Anterior crural neuritis. J Nerv Ment Dis 40:758, 1913
12. Ellenberg M: Diabetic neuropathic ulcer. Journal of Mount Sinai Hospital 35:585, 1968
13. Delbridge L, Perry P, Marr S et al: Limited joint mobility in the diabetic foot: relationship to neuropathic ulceration. Diabetic Medicine 5:333, 1988
14. Holewski JJ, Moss KM, Stess RM et al: Prevalence of foot pathology and lower extremity complications in a diabetic outpatient clinic. J Rehabil Res Dev 26:35, 1989
15. Root ML, Orien WP, Weed JH: Normal and Abnormal Function of the Foot. Clinical biomechanical Corporation, Los Angeles, 1977
16. Hlavac H, Schoenhaus H: The plantar fat pad and some related problems. J Am Podiatr Med Assoc 151, 1970
17. Mann R, Poppen N, O'Konski M: Amputation of the great toe: a clinical and biomechanical study. Clin Orthop 226:197, 1988
18. Ianucci A, Lai King P, Channell R, Farrell D: Spontaneous fractures of the lesser metatarsals secondary to an amputated hallux and peripheral neuropathy. J Foot Surg 26:66, 1987
19. Sanders L: Amputations in the diabetic foot. Clin Podiatr Med Surg 4:481, 1987
20. Friedman L, Padula P, Root B et al: Studies on the survival of transmetatarsal amputation stumps. Vas Surg 23:34, 1989
21. Seligman R, Trepal M, Gioregini R: Hallux valgus secondary to amputation of the second toe. J Am Podiatr Med Assoc 76:89, 1986
22. Gianfortune P, Pulla RJ, Sage: Ray resections in the insensitive or dysvascular foot: a critical review. J Foot Surg 24:103, 1985
23. McKittrick LS, McKittrick JB, Risley TS: Transmetatarsal amputation for infection or gangrene in pa-

tients with diabetes mellitus. Ann Surg 130:826, 1949
24. Green W, Cary J: Partial foot amputation in children: a comparison of the several types with the Symes amputation. J Bone Joint Surg 64A:3, 1982
25. Bollsen-Moller F, Lamoreux L: Significance of free dorsiflexion of the toes in walking. Act Orthop Scand 50:471, 1979
26. Swindt C, Lulloff R, Rogers S: Transmetatarsal amputations. Orthop Clin North Am 4:31, 1973
27. Parziale J, Hahn K: Functional considerations in partial foot amputations. Orthop Rev 12:3, 1988
28. Millstein S, McCowan S, Hunter G: Traumatic partial foot amputations in adult: a long-term review. J Bone Joint Surg 70B:251, 1988
29. Summers G, Morrison J, Cochrane G: Foot loading characteristics of amputees and normal subjects. Prosthet Orthot Int 11:33, 1987
30. Scarlet J, Blais M: Statistics on the diabetic foot. J Am Podiatr Med Assoc 79:306, 1989
31. Duggan G, DeAndrade J, Gregts D: Time line for the diabetic foot in reconstructive surgery of the foot and leg, update 1988. Doctors Hospital Podiatry Education and Research 105, 1988
32. Rubin G, Cohen E: Prostheses and orthoses for the foot and ankle. Clin Podiatr Med Surg 5:695, 1988

9

Pressure Assessment Methods in the Foot

Ewan A. Masson, M.B., M.R.C.P.
A.J.M. Boulton, M.D., M.R.C.P.

There has been increasing interest in the biomechanical aspects of the diabetic foot in recent years, in particular the relationships between stress patterns and the development of plantar ulcers. It is generally accepted that abnormalities of the distribution of pressure under the feet have a contributory role in the ulcerative process.[1] Many groups have provided evidence that in the context of an insensitive foot, the site of ulceration will almost invariably correspond to a site of high pressure.[2,3] High pressure per se however, does not appear to cause plantar ulceration in the absence of significant sensory neuropathy.[4] It is at present uncertain whether the development of high plantar pressure in the diabetic foot is the direct result of nerve dysfunction or whether it coexists in those patients who develop neuropathy. Some authors have reported that abnormalities of dynamic foot pressure recordings may be an early indicator of neuropathy,[5] although soft tissue factors and foot deformity also play a role that may be independent.[6]

It is undoubtedly true that treatments which traditionally have been based on empirical principles aiming to reduce stress on the feet (for example, casting techniques and special shoes) are successful in healing ulcers. There have been many attempts to study the distribution of pressure under the feet, with techniques ranging from simple devices to highly sophisticated computerized assessments. Several broad conclusions can be drawn from these studies, for example, that sites of abnormal pressure can predict the site of ulceration in susceptible individuals, and that the various techniques employed to modify the pressure distribution have a role in the healing and secondary prevention of ulceration in patients who present with diabetic foot ulcers.

What is not clear, however, is the exact significance of high plantar pressure in the diabetic patient who has not demonstrated a susceptibility to ulceration, although some consider that all diabetic patients with such pressure abnormalities should be considered to be at risk.

When considering the technical specifications and spatial resolution of the various devices available to measure plantar pressure, it is important to remember the basic fact that the pressure is defined as force per area. Thus, the "ideal" device would measure force accurately and have a high spatial resolution. It would also be capable of rapid assessments of change so that meaningful dynamic studies during a footstep are possible. The measurement techniques available to look at the foot-floor interface approach these problems in different ways, which are discussed below. Measurements of pressure acting on the foot within shoes have almost exclusively employed different sorts of discrete transducers attached to the plantar surface of the foot. By their very presence they modify the pressure distribution under the foot by their effect as foreign bodies, and are subject to considerable technical problems of calibration, placement, and performance. To date most workers have studied principally vertical pressure, which is stress in only a single plane relating to a three-dimensional structure. In reality, shear forces act on every surface of the foot, and it has been hypothesized that they are important in the etiology of ulcers. However, although there have been some attempts to develop a way of measuring these stresses, to date no ideal technology exists.

METHODS OF ASSESSING FOOT PRESSURE AT THE FOOT-FLOOR INTERFACE

Although many methods for the assessment of plantar pressure have been described over the last century, until fairly recently they were at best semiquantitative and shared the flaw of providing a deformable surface for contact with the foot, which will inevitably affect the observed pressure distribution. An early attempt to examine pressure distribution was described last century in which the subject stepped on a bag filled with clay or plaster in order to leave an imprint.[7] Although a deep imprint could reflect a high pressure area, it could also be due to an abnormality of the shape of the foot.

In the early part of this century a variety of techniques using different types of rubber matting were described. This early work provided the principle of some of the most sophisticated devices described below, and one technique in particular, the Harris mat, is still used today.

The kinetograph developed by Morton consisted of a rubber mat with a flat upper surface and longitudinal ridges on the underside, which was laid on an ink fabric over a piece of paper.[8] Standing on this would deform the ridges, producing a denser inked imprint at sites of higher pressure. A similar device was described by Elftman, where a mat with pyramidal projections was placed on an illuminated glass plate suspended on a supporting frame[9] (Fig. 9-1). Deformation of the projections could be observed from below, and cine photography could be

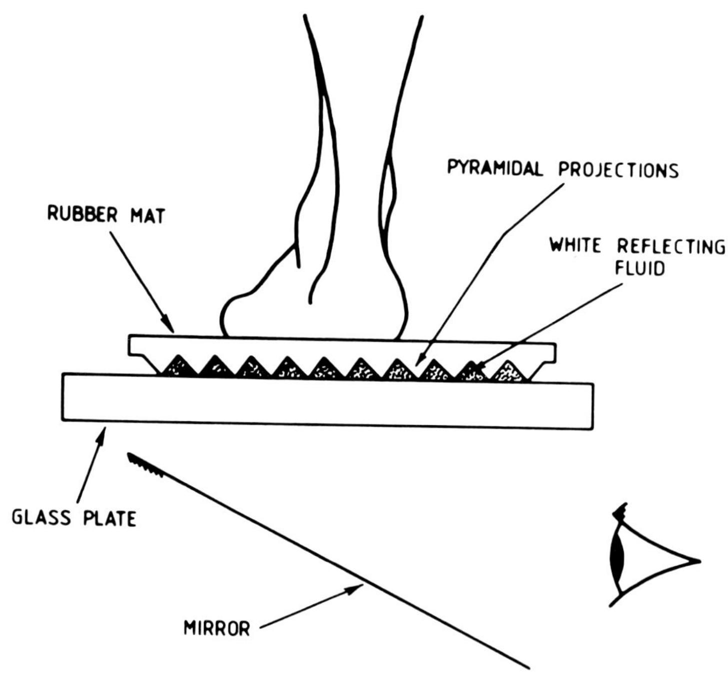

Fig. 9-1. A diagram of Elftman's optical principle. As the foot exerts pressure on the rubber mat, the projections are compressed, and the pressure pattern can be observed from the underside of the glass plate.

used to record a footstep. The Harris mat is a development of the deformable mat printing principle, where a square grid of projections is subdivided twice into smaller squares with progressively smaller ridges.[10] Thus when pressure increases, the grid pattern printed becomes denser as the smaller ridges are brought into contact with the printing surface (Fig. 9-2). Although this is a semiquantitative technique, the pressures at which maximal printing occurs are within the normal range of observed pressures; thus it may be useful for identifying sites of relatively greater pressure without giving information on their magnitude.

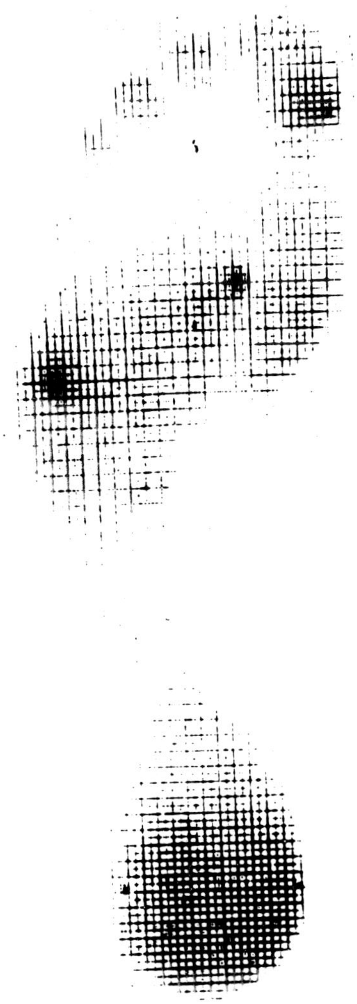

Fig. 9-2. An example of a printed image produced by the Harris mat. The denser printed patterns with finer grid markings indicate the high pressure areas.

A rather different technique was reported in 1954 by Barnett.[11] His "plastic pedograph" consisted of an array of plastic rods mounted vertically on a thick slab of foam rubber. Horizontal lines drawn on the rods at different levels for each row could be observed from the side as they were moved by applied pressure. Thus a three-dimensional image of plantar pressure could be obtained; however, although the rods could be calibrated for force applied, the spatial resolution is limited by the size of the rods. The other weakness of this device was that it still depended on substantial deformation of the surface to indicate applied pressure, which, as discussed above, will modify the results obtained. The footstep could be recorded on film, but such a system would be likely to have high hysteresis, which restricts the information usefully obtainable from high frequency dynamic studies.

The next technological advance was the assembly of a series of beams supported on load cells that were incorporated into a walkway, producing an assembly that did not deform significantly, but could measure load sequences during a footstep.[12] The apparatus suffered from the limitations of small size, so that the load distribution for a whole footstep could only be built up from several parts; in addition the composite beam assembly had to be turned through 90° and the data gathering process repeated in order to measure transverse as well as longitudinal distributions of load. However, this report represented an important advance in that high frequency electronic data gathering was employed in a system that, although of low resolution, also had low hysteresis. A development of this principle employing transparent beams and video camera recording of both the lateral aspect of the foot during the footstep and the plantar surface has also been reported.[13]

The most advanced systems described to date are based on computer analysis and imaging of electronically gathered data. Essentially two techniques have gained popularity for this purpose. One, the Sheffield optical pedobarograph, uses a modification of the optical principle mentioned above and is illustrated in Figure 9-3.[14] A glass plate is illuminated at two opposing edges by strip lights and is covered by a thin film of opaque white material on which the patient stands or walks. Light

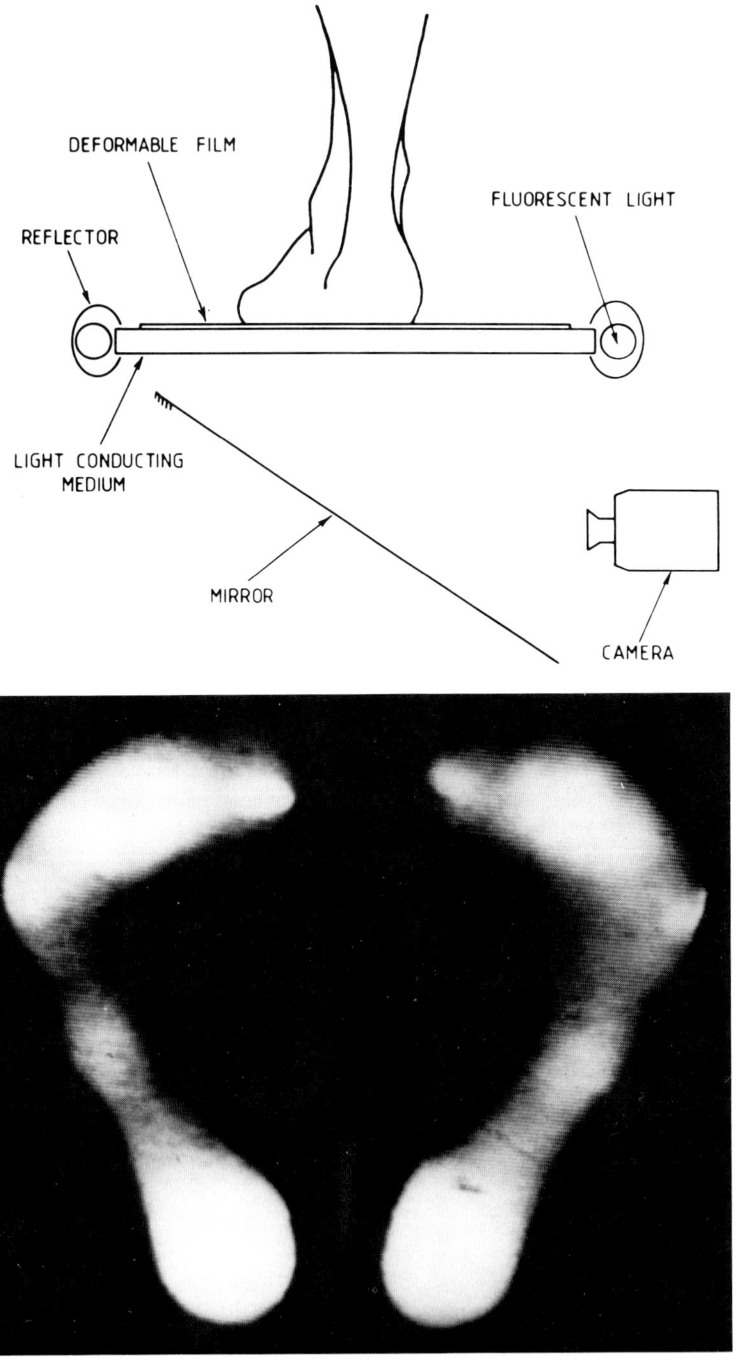

A

B

Fig. 9-3. **(A)** The Sheffield optical pedobarograph. The apparatus consists of a glass plate illuminated from the sides, producing total internal reflection. A thin plastic material, which at the microscopic level has projections like that shown in Fig. 9-1, covers the plate. Where pressure is applied, light is scattered and refracted out of the glass. As more pressure is exerted, more light is scattered, which produces a gray scale image picked up by the video camera. An electronic interface produces a digital representation of this data for computer analysis. Simultaneous recording of force transducer output (on which the glass plate is mounted) enables accurate frame by frame calibration. (See Franks et al.[15]) **(B)** The gray scale pressure pattern as seen by the video camera.

is totally internally reflected within the glass plate except at points where the film is pressed against the glass. At these points, light is refracted out of the plate, and because the film used has microscopic irregularities that are increasingly brought into contact with the glass as pressure is increased, the higher the applied pressure, the higher the intensity of the light scattered. This image is picked up by a video camera and can either be viewed directly or the image digitized for later analysis and storage. Modifications of the system originally described led to the incorporation of the pressure plate into a walk path (Fig. 9-4), and a microprocessor control system allows dynamic data capture at up to 25 Hz. Mounting the glass plate on force transducers allows individual calibration of each frame of digitized information.[15] These can then be superimposed on each other to allow areas of interest to be identified, which can then be further analyzed to produce time-pressure plots for each area, and the integral under the curve to be calculated. Examples of the output of the system on a graph plotter are shown in Figure 9-5. A commercial version of this device is available (Biokinetics, Bethesda, MD). The spatial resolution of this system is very high (pixel size, approximately 1 × 1.5 mm), and the material currently used for covering the glass plate allows pressures of up to 30 kg/cm^2 (approximately 2.9 MPa) to be measured accurately. Hysteresis is low, and efficient and accurate data capture is possible at high frequency. The visual identification of areas of interest for analysis may reduce standardization between footsteps, but in practise this has not proved to be a problem, even in the presence of foot deformity.

The alternative approach to data processing is to use an array of load cells or to generate a matrix of pressure-sensitive elements by a series of longitudinal and transverse overlapping strips, separated by a thin film. When pressure is applied, the capacitance of each element changes, and data sampling can be undertaken at high frequency. This is the principle of the commercially available EMED system (Novel USA, Minneapolis, MN). These devices can be used to generate elegant three-dimensional pressure distribution displays, or plots similar to

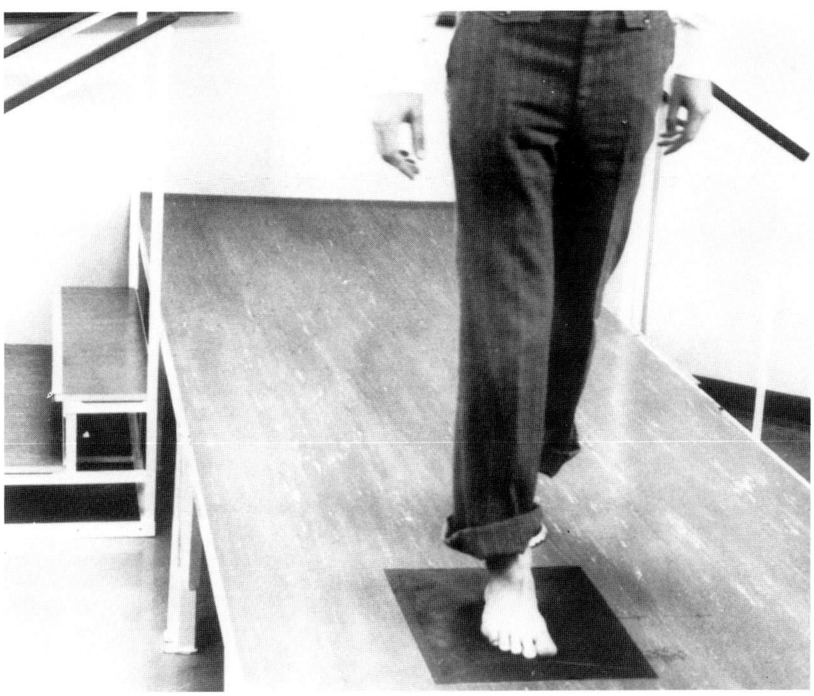

Fig. 9-4. The pedobarograph walkway: the patient has stood on the pressure sensitive area, and data are being recorded on disc for offline analysis.

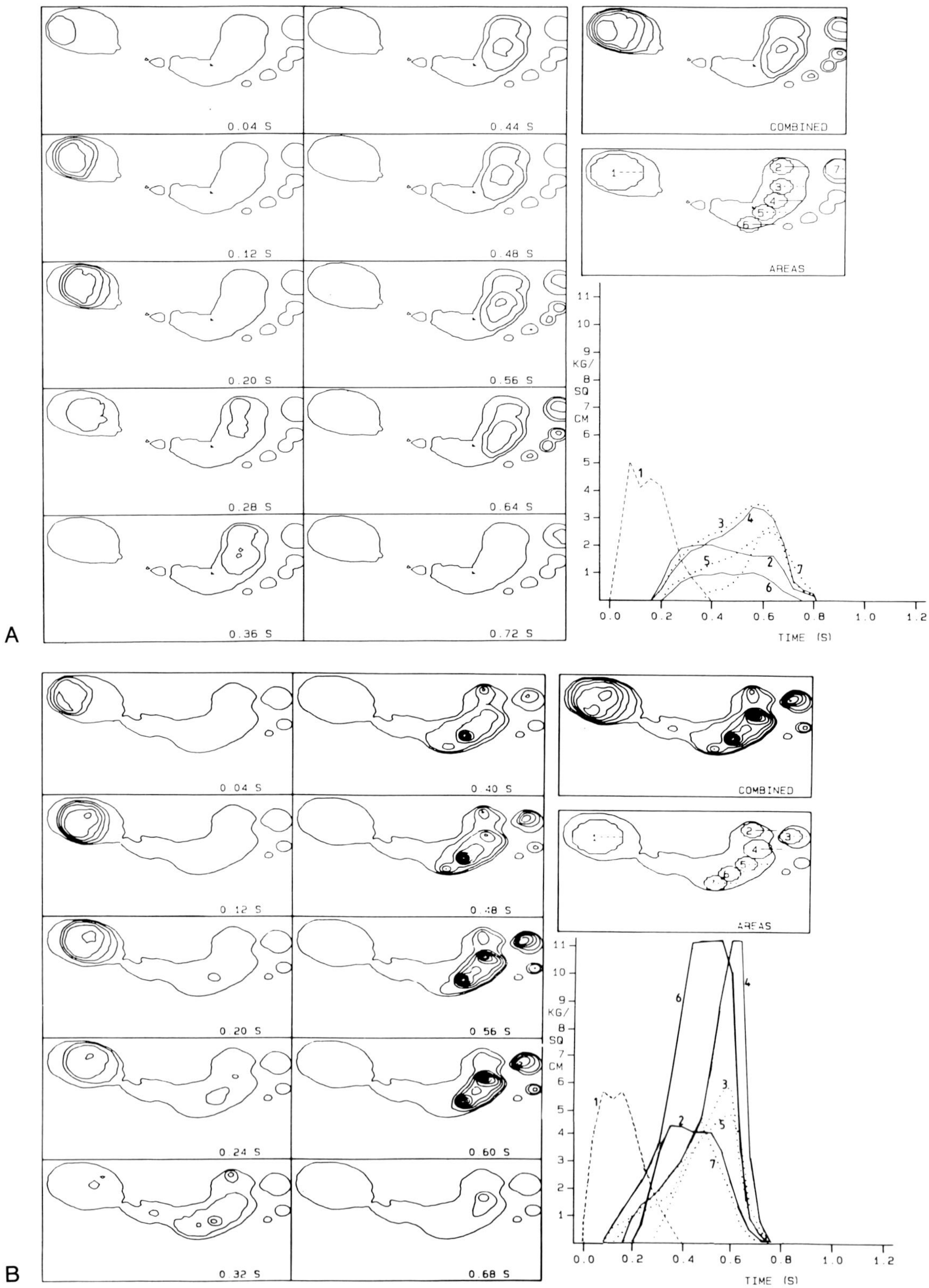

Fig. 9-5. One of the alternative data displays for the pedobarograph is the isopressure contour plot. **(A)** Contour plot of a normal footstep. Ten sample frames are shown on the left, with the time from heel strike (top left) to toe off (bottom middle). On the top right are the superimposed frames' "combined" plot, and the selected areas of interest for analysis below it. The graph shows the time-pressure plot for each area of interest selected. **(B)** The pedobarograph plotter output from a diabetic patient with a history of foot ulceration. Note the high pressure areas under the second and fourth metatarsal heads (numbered 4 and 6).

those described in Figure 9-5. However, this approach does not allow the degree of accuracy possible with the optical systems because the spatial resolution is limited to the size of the individual elements, thus pressure measured is "averaged" from the total force applied to the element divided by its area.

A similar but distinct approach was described by Hennig and colleagues using an array of piezoelectric devices.[16] Although more complex to construct, this approach has mechanical and electronic advantages comprehensively discussed by its developers. It is capable of a high degree of accuracy, with less "cross-talk" or electronic interference between the load-sensitive elements. The data generated are, as with the devices described above, digitized and computer-processed for display and analysis purposes.

PRESSURE MEASUREMENTS WITHIN SHOES

Pressure measurements within shoes is much more difficult technically. Early attempts to assess pressure patterns in insensitive extremities were described by Brand.[17] He described the use of microcapsules filled with dye (the principle used in pressure-sensitive copy paper) incorporated into gloves or slippers in order to find areas of high stress. At points of stress the microcapsules would rupture, thus staining the area and marking it for attention. This approach, however, does not give quantitative or immediate information, although it could highlight problems away from the plantar surface of the foot.

The other methods of in-shoe pressure measurements that have been described can broadly be split into two categories, one using a small number of discrete transducers of various designs that are attached to areas of interest under the foot,[17,18,19,20] and the other using an array of transducers of the piezoelectric type[16] or a matrix of elements similar to that described above that are incorporated into an insole.[21] None is perfect. The discrete transducers have the difficulty that they may not be positioned under the precise area of anatomic interest. They are of finite thickness, and if not rigid they may respond to bending as well as loading. The presence of such devices can alter pressure distribution and even gait pattern by their presence as foreign bodies. They are subject to the difficulties of low spatial resolution described above, which will make them relatively insensitive to small areas of greatly elevated pressure, even if positioned correctly. One system is currently available commercially (Electrodynogram, Langer Electronics Group, Deer Park, NY). However, the accuracy and reliability of the sensors used have been questioned.[22]

The latter approach using arrays of sensors is very much more appealing, but not without technical limitations. There will still be a foreign body effect that will influence the pressure distribution, and spatial resolution is still limited. Reliability is made more difficult to achieve because in-shoe devices need to have considerable thermal and mechanical stability compared to those that can be built into a walkway. A commercial insole containing a matrix of sensors is available (EMED, Novel USA, Minneapolis, MN).

ALTERNATIVE APPROACHES TO STRESS ASSESSMENT

One group has approached the problem of shear forces acting on the foot during walking. Shear transducers were developed that were approximately 16 mm in diameter and 2 mm thick.[23] Six of these transducers were attached to the plantar surface of the foot and measurements reported when subjects wore different sorts of footwear.[24] Clearly the relatively large size of these transducers makes data interpretation difficult for reasons already discussed. Development work is currently in progress in an attempt to produce very much smaller transducers, (P. Laing, personal communication), but test information is not yet available.

Another way of looking at the results of stress on body surfaces is to measure the temperature changes caused by pressure or inflammation. Various techniques for thermography have been described, mainly by using infrared detectors that give a Gray scale "map" of surface body temperature,[25,26] or by the use of liquid crystal devices that give a colour contour image of temperature differences across the surface tested.[27] These have been used to show that inflammation resulting from ulceration not surprisingly produces a local rise in temperature, and the adequate relief of pressure (whether sustained or from repeated minor stress) reduces this warming. Indeed it has been clearly demonstrated that pressure on body surfaces will produce a local increase in temperature probably due to arteriolar dilatation.[25] Infrared thermography has been used to follow the progress of lesions on insensitive feet and to give an indication that protective strategies intended to promote healing have indeed been effective.[26,28] A study of 65 patients divided into 3 groups (control, diabetic patients, and diabetic patients with a history of foot ulceration) apparently showed that patients who had proved their susceptibility to foot ulceration had higher temperatures on the soles of the feet than those who had not.[27] This may reflect increased blood flow in the extremities of such patients, due to arteriovenous shunting as a result of sympathetic nerve dysfunction.[29] However, the differences between the groups were not large, and the technique probably will not give a better indication of risk than clinical assessment. Recent work in progress has reported a correlation between the results of thermographic assessment of diabetic feet and pressure studies using the electrodynogram, which has been described above.[30]

CLINICAL STUDIES OF FOOT PRESSURE IN THE DIABETIC FOOT AND APPLICATIONS OF FOOT PRESSURE MEASUREMENT

Because of the different methodologies described for the assessment of plantar pressure, direct comparison of data from different institutes is not possible. For example, using optical devices of very high spatial resolution, small areas of very high pressures (> 30 kg/cm^2)[31] have been recorded in the diabetic foot, which have not been approached using less sensitive methodologies.

One of the earliest systematic studies of pressure relating to the development of neuropathic ulceration was published by Barrett and Mooney.[32] They studied 25 consecutive diabetic patients with neuropathy, using both the Harris mat and the Brand slipper sock as described above. Harris mat testing showed that ulcers often occurred at sites of high loading, and that in patients without ulceration high pressure areas could be seen that were taken to be points of high risk. Testing with the slipper sock demonstrated that there was excessive loading under the metatarsal area in the neuropathic patients when walking, which was interpreted as evidence of high shear forces, and it was noted that walking with ordinary shoes caused considerably more staining in some patients than walking barefoot. The authors assessed these shoes and found that they were of inappropriate design, with rigid soles and stiff uppers; furthermore, they were invariably too small in these patients.

An early quantitative study of loading related to foot ulceration in diabetes was reported by Stokes et al. in 1975.[2] This study used the device consisting of a series of beams mounted on force transducers, incorporated into a walkway, as described above. Three groups of patients were studied; these were taken to represent a varying degree of susceptibility to ulceration. The first group comprised 6 feet with active or healed ulceration; the second, 13 feet that were not ulcerated in patients who had a history of contralateral ulceration or local surgery (ray or digital amputation); and the third, 18 feet with callosity, but no ulceration. Data from these groups were compared with that from 60 normal subjects. The authors concluded that ulceration occurred at sites of maximum load, that toe loading was reduced in all the diabetic groups, and that increased loads seen in the ulcer groups were associated with higher body weight. While this latter conclusion may appear to be intuitively reasonable, it is not supported by more recent work. Callosity did not correspond directly with sites of maximum loading in nonulcerated feet, and no differences were seen between the maximum loading of ulcerated feet and contralateral feet. A later, larger study using an array of load cells came to broadly similar conclusions, this time after studying 24 patients with ulceration, 21 neuropathic patients without ulceration, and 47 control subjects.[33] All ulcer sites corresponded with sites of maximal loading, but ulcerated feet did not have higher loading than the contralateral foot. However, the nonulcerated group had lower loading, although there was overlap between the groups.

Boulton et al. reported a study of 82 diabetic patients divided into neuropathic and nonneuropathic groups, and 41 age-matched controls.[3] Foot pressure was measured with the computerized optical pedobarograph, and various other measures of nerve function and sensory perception were undertaken in order to define risk-associated factors for ulceration. The high resolution system demonstrated that all 22 of the ulcerated feet in the neuropathic group had a peak pressure greater than 11.4 kg/cm². Of the nonulcerated neuropathic patients, 31 percent also had elevated plantar pressure, and although elevation of vibration perception threshold was the best measure other than foot pressure to correlate with ulceration, 10 of the 28 neuropathic nonulcer patients also had such elevation. Thus it seems clear that although neuropathy and high pressures are probably contributory to, and the former permissive of, ulcer formation, it is not inevitable that patients deemed to be susceptible by these criteria will develop ulcers.

Our own recent work would tend to confirm this view. A comparative study of high pressure feet, some due to arthritic foot deformity and the other group due to diabetes, demonstrated that ulceration does not occur in high pressure feet in the absence of neuropathy.[4] Peak plantar pressures were greatly elevated in both groups.

Although elevation of plantar pressure frequently coexists with neuropathy in diabetic patients, the exact pathogenesis of the pressure abnormality in diabetes remains to be elucidated. It has been reported that plantar pressure abnormality may be observed in very mild diabetic neuropathy,[5] and the speculation has been made that this is a cause and effect relationship. Certainly reduced toe function and clawing of the toes are frequently observed in neuropathic patients with elevation of plantar pressure, but these deformities can also be seen in the normal population, and it is likely that foot deformity is an important factor in the genesis of elevated plantar pressure irrespective of its etiology. Our recent studies of joint mobility and foot function suggest that the most important determinant of peak plantar pressure in neuropathic and nonneuropathic diabetic patients may be alterations in joint mobility rather than the degree of nerve dysfunction.[6]

Despite the varying results obtained by the different systems used to measure plantar pressure, and the uncertainty about the exact meaning of the results obtained, the measurement of such pressure has clinical relevance. Whether or not the presence of high plantar pressure can be viewed as an independent risk factor for diabetic foot ulcers, it is undoubtedly true that in a patient who is susceptible to ulceration, sites of particular risk can be identified by pressure analysis. It has been demonstrated that static studies may not reveal all areas vulnerable to abnormal stress and that studies during walking should be carried out for a comprehensive assessment.[34] This has important implications for the orthotist who may be asked to provide footwear to offload certain high pressure areas. Conventional standing assessments are likely to be inadequate, and high pressure areas do not always declare themselves clinically by developing callus or thick, hard skin. It is also important to note that the only follow-up study so far reported suggests that there may be substantial changes to the pressure distribution under the diabetic foot over time[35]; thus, the provision of different types of footwear and orthoses may need to be reviewed on a regular basis in patients selected for such treatment.

The measurement of plantar pressure has also been used in order to optimize the design of specialist footwear, with the demonstration that changing the type of rocker sole can significantly influence the in-shoe loading of the foot.[20] Measurements made with in-shoe transducer arrays have been used to confirm that padded insoles influence the pressure distribution and have suggested that certain types of shoe can increase the pressure demonstrated by barefoot studies,[21] confirming the early observations made by qualitative methods.[32] This report may provide a clue to the lack of correspondence of clinical pressure areas with obvious callus with those measured by barefoot studies on walkways. The reduction of pressure using insole materials has also been reported using the optical pedobarograph, this time measuring pressures at the insole-walkway interface,[31] and on the basis of present evidence it seems likely that measurements of this type have clinical validity. We have also recently reported that the use of padded hosiery specially designed to redistribute pressure can provide significant pressure reductions in high pressure diabetic feet that are not seen in association with conventional hosiery.[36]

Most of the studies discussed thus far have measured vertical stress, which as previously mentioned is unlikely to be the only important component of tissue damage leading to ulceration.[37] However, no satisfactory technology exists to measure shear stresses, but one of the only studies to address this problem reported that different shoe designs (and plaster casts) had a major influence on the shear stress experienced by their wearers.[24] This is clearly an important factor that will require careful evaluation in the future as techniques for its assessment improve.

CONCLUSIONS

At the present time, plantar foot pressure measurement does not have an essential place in the routine assessment of the diabetic patient. Although many cross-sectional studies have linked high plantar pressure to the sites of ulcers in neuropathic patients, high pressure alone does not, however, seem to cause ulcers.[4] Even in the presence of sensory dysfunction, ulceration does not always occur when definitely elevated pressure can be demonstrated. This last point emphasizes that the development of ulceration in the diabetic foot is a multifactorial process (discussed in detail in Ch. 10). For this reason, and because high plantar pressure occurs in the absence of significant neuropathy in diabetic patients,[5] the demonstration of elevated pressure cannot be assumed to be evidence of risk in itself. However, in patients with other risk factors, or those who have demonstrated their susceptibility to ulceration, the demonstration of pressure patterns can be an aid to the design of appropriate footwear[20] and insoles designed to offload pressure areas.

Pressure measurements in the research context can be used to investigate the relationships of biomechanics to the development of clinical problems. In addition they have been used to validate empirical methods of pressure distribution such as the use of padded insole materials[21,31] and padded hosiery.[36]

The demonstration of abnormal pressure patterns can also be used to help educate patients with insensitive feet as to the presence of risk and to its site. Education will remain the most important factor in preventing the recurrence of ulceration, but it is essential that attention be paid to the feet by health care professionals, an important area of neglect in the past. Indirect stress assessment methods such as thermography have been used to monitor progress and compliance with treatment.

In the present state of understanding of the biomechanics of the diabetic foot and the etiology of ulcers in diabetic patients, the experienced clinical eye remains the best instrument for the assessment of risk. However, quantitative assessments are essential for the testing of hypotheses relating to mechanisms of tissue damage and to pressure redistribution treatments.

REFERENCES

1. Boulton AJM: The diabetic foot. Med Clin North Am 72:1513, 1988
2. Stokes IAS, Faris IB, Hutton WC: The neuropathic ulcer and loads on the foot in diabetic patients. Acta Orthop Scand 46:839, 1975
3. Boulton AJM, Hardisty CA, Betts RP et al: Dynamic foot pressure and other studies as diagnostic and management aids in diabetic neuropathy. Diabetes Care 6:26, 1983
4. Masson EA, Hay EM, Stockley I et al: Abnormal pressure alone does not cause foot ulceration. Diabetic Med 6:426, 1989
5. Boulton AJM, Betts RP, Franks CI et al: Abnormal foot pressure in early diabetic neuropathy. Diabetic Med 4:225, 1987
6. Fernando DJS, Masson EA, Veves A, Boulton AJM: Are abnormal foot pressures caused by limited joint mobility? (abstracted) Diabetic Med (in press)
7. Beely F: Zur mechanik des stehens. Uder die bedentung des fussgewolbes beim stehen. Langenbecks Archiv fur klinische Chirurgie 27:457, 1882
8. Morton DJ: The Human Foot. Columbia University Press, New York, 1935
9. Elftman H: A cinematic study of the distribution of pressure in the human foot. Anat Rec 59:481, 1934
10. Harris RI, Beath T: Army foot survey—an investi-

gation of foot ailments in Canadian soldiers. National Research Council of Canada, NRC, No. 1574, Ottawa, 1947
11. Barnett CH: A Plastic Pedograph. Lancet 2:273, 1954
12. Hutton WC, Drabble GE: An apparatus to give the distribution of vertical load under the foot. Rheum Phys Med 11:313, 1972
13. Dall G: Dynamic assessment of the load distribution on the plantar surface of the foot using the University of Cape Town walkway and its clinical application. Foot Ankle 4:286, 1984
14. Betts RP, Franks CI, Duckworth T: Analysis of pressures and loads under the foot. Part 1: Quantification of the static distribution using the PET computer. Part 2: Quantification of the dynamic distribution. Clin Phys Physiol Meas 1:101, 1980
15. Franks CI, Betts RP, Duckworth T: A microprocessor-based image processing system for dynamic foot pressure studies. Med Biol Eng Comput 21:566, 1983
16. Hennig EM, Cavanagh PR, Albert HT, Macmillan NH: A piezoelectric method of measuring the vertical contact stress beneath the human foot. J Biomed Eng 4:213, 1982
17. Brand PW, Ebner JD: Pressure sensitive devices for denervated hands and feet. J Bone Joint Surg 51A:109, 1969
18. Bauman JH, Brand PW: Measurement of pressure between foot and shoe. Lancet 1:629, 1963
19. Stott JRR, Soames RW: A method for recording the instantaneous pressure distribution under the feet during walking. J Anat 132:472, 1981
20. Coleman WC: The relief of pressures using outer shoe sole modifications. Proceedings of the International Conference on Biomechanics and Clinical Kinesiology of the Hand and Foot. Indian Institute of Technology, Madras, 29, 1985
21. Schaff P, Kirsch D, Hauser W, Mehnert H: Eine Gerateentwicklung zur messung der druckverteilung unter der Fu sohle im schuh und deren anwendbarkeit in der diabetologie. Akt Endokr Stoffw 7:129, 1986
22. Cavanagh PR, Ulbrecht JS: Plantar pressure in the diabetic foot. In Sammarco GJ (ed): The Diabetic Foot (1990, in press)
23. Tappin JW, Pollard JP, Beckett EA: Method of measuring shear forces on the sole of the foot. Clin Physics Physiol Meas 1:83, 1980
24. Pollard JP, Le Quesne LP, Tappin JW: Forces under the foot. J Biomed Eng 5:37, 1983
25. Goller H, Lewis DW, McLaughlin RE: Thermographic studies of human skin subjected to localised pressure. AJR 113:749, 1971
26. Bergtholdt HT: Temperature assessment of the insensitive foot. Phys Ther 59:18, 1975
27. Stess RM, Sisney PC, Moss KM et al: Use of liquid crystal thermography in the evaluation of the diabetic foot. Diabetes Care 9:267, 1986
28. Bergtholdt HT, Brand PW: Thermography: an aid in the management of insensitive feet and stumps. Arch Phys Med Rehabil 56:205, 1975
29. Boulton AJM, Scarpello JHB, Ward JD: Venous oxygenation in the diabetic neuropathic foot: evidence of arterio-venous shunting? Diabetologia 22:6, 1982
30. Evans A, Bowen K: Thermographic findings in a diabetic podiatry clinic—preventative screening potential? A preliminary report. Diab Res Clin Prac, suppl. 1, 5:S310, 1988
31. Boulton AJM, Franks CI, Betts RP et al: Reduction of abnormal foot pressures in diabetic neuropathy using a new polymer insole material. Diabetes Care 7:42, 1984
32. Barrett JP, Mooney V: Neuropathy and diabetic pressure lesions. Orthop Clin North Am 4:43, 1973
33. Ctercteko GC, Dhanendran M, Hutton WC, Le Quesne LP: Vertical forces acting on the feet of diabetic patients with neuropathic ulceration. Br Med J 68:608, 1981
34. Duckworth T, Boulton AJM, Betts RP et al. Plantar pressure measurements and the prevention of ulceration in the diabetic foot. J Bone Joint Surg 67B:79, 1985
35. Boulton AJM, Betts RP, Franks CI et al: The natural history of foot pressure abnormalities in neuropathic diabetic subjects. Diabetes Res 5:73, 1987
36. Veves A, Masson EA, Fernando DJS, Boulton AJM: The use of experimental padded hosiery to reduce abnormal foot pressures in diabetic neuropathy. Diabetes Care 12:653, 1989
37. Brand PW: Repetitive stress in the development of diabetic foot ulcers. p. 83. In Levin ME, O'Neal LW (eds): The Diabetic Foot. CV Mosby, St. Louis, 1988

10

Diabetic Foot Ulcerations

Robert G. Frykberg, D.P.M., F.A.C.F.S.

Perhaps the most prevalent of all characteristic diabetic foot lesions is the ulceration, often termed the *mal perforans ulcer*. Whether of neuropathic or ischemic origin, the ulcer per se is not always a serious lesion. However, its presence places the diabetic foot at high risk for progressing to the more serious complications of infection and gangrene with subsequent amputation. The ultimate outcome is therefore dependent upon multiple factors, all of which directly relate to the appropriateness of therapy and the time at which it was instituted.

Foot ulceration and infection are leading causes of hospitalization for patients with diabetes mellitus in both the United States and Britain.[1–3] The medical, social, and economic impact of these disorders is enormous, with attendant costs of hospitalization alone running into hundreds of millions of dollars annually.[4] Approximately two-thirds of all nontraumatic amputations performed in the United States (50,000 per year) are done on diabetic patients whose foot lesions have progressed from simple ulceration or infection to gangrene.[4–6] Following one lower extremity amputation, there is a 50 percent incidence of serious contralateral foot lesion within 2 years and a 51 percent incidence of contralateral amputation within 5 years.[7,8] Furthermore, the 3-year survival rate for a diabetic amputee only approximates 50 percent.[9] This fell to a level of 31 percent after 5 years in a study combining both diabetic and nondiabetic amputees.[10] Considering that diabetic patients already have a 15 times greater risk of amputation than their nondiabetic counterparts, these statistics vividly illustrate the potential consequences of the neglected or inappropriately treated foot ulcer.[11]

Major lower extremity amputation resulting from a nonhealing lesion of the foot should be considered a failure in management of the underlying disease processes. This does not imply, however, that such amputations should not take place or necessarily constitute a breach in care. To the contrary, these procedures are often life saving in the presence of fulminating infection, extensive gangrene, or following unsuccessful attempts at limb salvage.[12] The failure often results from a delay in treatment due to the "willful self-neglect" of the patient who does not seek early medical attention for a newly discovered foot lesion.[13] Early detection of such lesions by the physician can only take place if both shoes and stockings are routinely removed at each office or clinic visit.[14] The failure to promptly and aggressively institute the proper care for diabetic foot ulcers can often lead to an exacerbation of the problem with subsequent need for amputation of a toe, ray, foot, or leg. The aim of therapy, therefore, should be early intervention to allow prompt healing of the lesion, and once healed, to prevent its recurrence. As will be discussed in the following pages, optimal care for such lesions depends upon the treating physicians' understanding of the pathophysiology involved in the etiology of ulceration, a basic knowledge of the principles of treatment, and the conviction that a coordinated multidisciplinary team approach will best accomplish the goal of limb salvage. Above all else, *prevention* of foot lesions should be the ultimate goal.[2,15] The prerequisite for prevention is always education of the patient in proper foot care.

This has consistently been shown to reduce both the incidence of foot ulceration as well as the number of amputations in the diabetic population.[16–19]

ETIOLOGY OF ULCERATION

Diabetic foot ulceration is a multifactorial process involving various intrinsic complications of diabetes mellitus as well as external forces or events which directly cause injury to the foot at risk.[2,16,20–22] Diabetic neuropathy, vascular disease, and susceptibility to infection are the three undisputed factors which predispose the diabetic foot to ulceration. This triad, however, rarely results in a foot lesion without concomitant trauma or injury. The external force causing injury may be as trivial as a tight or wrinkled stocking. The significance lies in the fact that a blister or pressure lesion thus created on an insensate or ischemic foot serves as a portal of entry for bacterial pathogens. The progression or resolution of this lesion therefore depends upon the metabolic status of the patient, the patient's ability to sense and protect from further injury, adequacy of circulation, and subsequent treatment of the lesion. Figure 10-1 details the interactions between the major contributory factors and trauma (physical stress) in the pathogenesis of diabetic foot ulceration.

Young[20] and Boulton[23,24] further discuss the identification of patients at risk for developing foot ulceration. Such identification is of course dependent upon a basic understanding of the causation of the lesions. Additional factors to be considered must include social, occupational, and level of diabetic foot care education, as well as prior history of ulceration.[16,20] These extrinsic variables are illustrated by Rosenqvist, who found that two-thirds of a large diabetic population had moderate or severe foot disease.[25] Despite this, only 54 percent with severe disease sought professional attention for their foot care. Table 10-1 lists these and additional risk factors that must be considered when attempting to identify those patients most susceptible to foot ulceration.

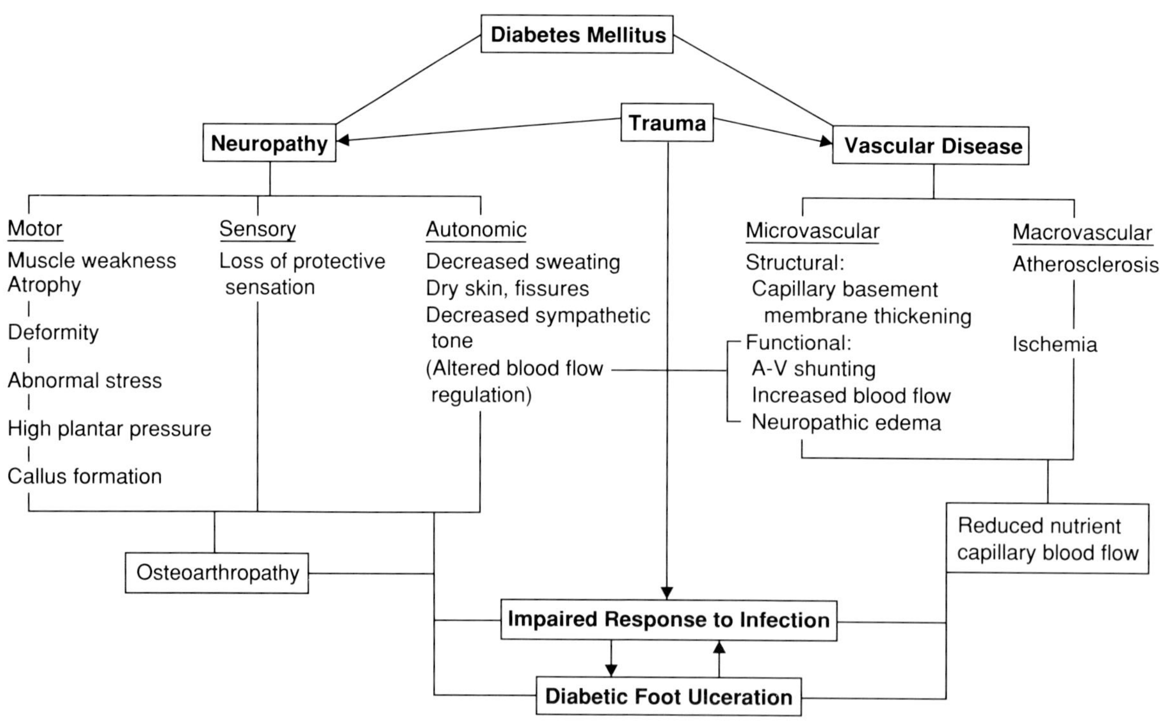

Fig. 10-1. Interactions between major contributory factors in the etiology of diabetic ulceration. (Modified from Boulton,[23] with permission.)

Table 10-1. Risk Factors for Diabetic Foot Ulceration

Peripheral neuropathy—somatic sensorimotor, autonomic
Peripheral vascular disease—impaired flow regulation
Susceptibility to infection—immunopathy
Foot deformities and high plantar pressures—hammertoes, hallux valgus, Charcot deformities, callus formation
Previous history of ulceration
Blindness, decreased visual acuity, retinopathy
Nephropathy
Duration of diabetes
Age
Weight
Cigarette smoking
High alcohol consumption
Level of foot care education, diabetes education
Occupations requiring standing and walking
Nonenzymatic glycosylation of proteins
Limited joint mobility

Each intrinsic contributory factor will be discussed individually in terms of its general pathophysiology in diabetes mellitus and its role in the etiology of ulcer formation. Extrinsic and physical or environmental components are equally important and are discussed in terms of their potential effect on the high risk foot.

Peripheral Neuropathy

Peripheral neuropathy is an extremely common complication of diabetes mellitus, apparently related to both the intensity (degree of hyperglycemia) and duration of the disease. In a major longitudinal study of over 4,000 diabetic patients, Pirart found the prevalence of neuropathy to be 8 percent at the time of diagnosis of diabetes and increasing to 50 percent after a duration of 25 years.[26] More recent studies report the incidence of polyneuropathy in 39 percent of their patients and additionally, a strong correlation with age and the male gender as well as with duration of disease.[27,28]

Specifically, distal symmetric polyneuropathy involving sensory, motor, and autonomic fibers is the major underlying factor in the development of diabetic foot ulcers.[23,29–31] Although not all patients with clinically demonstrable neuropathy develop ulceration, those diabetic patients with such lesions in the absence of discernible arterial disease are consistently found to have evidence of both somatic (sensorimotor) and autonomic nerve dysfunction.[2,14,29,31–33] Conversely, patients with significant ischemia who develop foot ulceration, which is characteristically painful, may also have coexisting neuropathy that renders their ischemic lesions painless. Other syndromes of diabetic neuropathy include focal neuropathies such as cranial, radiculopathy, plexopathy, and the mononeuropathies, as well as cardiovascular, gastrointestinal, and genitourinary autonomic dysfunction.[34] These disorders, however, do not play a direct role in the pathogenesis of foot lesions.

The etiology of diabetic neuropathy is fully discussed elsewhere in this text. Briefly, it is multifactorial in the sense that it involves multiple sites within the nerves themselves and in the microvasculature. Axon degeneration, alterations in axon transport mechanisms, paranodal swelling, segmental demyelination, axoglial disjunction, nonenzymatic glycosylation of neural and microvascular tissues, and ischemic mechanisms have been implicated as neuropathologic etiologies for the nerve dysfunction.[35–40] A unifying concept of the biochemical basis for these changes and the attendant electrophysiologic abnormalities revolves around the effects of chronic hyperglycemia and activation of the polyol pathway. The enzyme aldose reductase permits the conversion of glucose to sorbitol, which accumulates within the nerve and Schwann cell. Intracellular accumulation of sorbitol results in a depletion of myoinositol and subsequent altered phosphoinositide metabolism. This in turn interferes with sodium-potassium ATPase activity, resulting in altered nerve impulse conduction.[40] These physiologic abnormalities are rapidly reversible upon correction of hyperglycemia. However, long-standing diabetes results in the structural changes noted above due to the persistence of intracellular sorbitol and the direct effects of chronic hyperglycemia.[37]

Somatic sensorimotor neuropathy is the most common and recognizable type of nerve disorder affecting diabetic patients. It is typically symmetrical bilaterally in a "glove and stocking" distribution with both a sensory and motor component. Sensory involvement of small fibers leads to a loss of pain and thermal sensation, while that of large fibers leads to a reduction in vibration perception thresholds and light touch sensation. Usually, a mixed fiber neuropathy ensues, involving both large and small myelinated fibers. In addition to the above findings, these patients also lose proprioceptive sensation and knee and ankle reflexes. Presenting complaints range from numbness, hypoesthesia, pins and needles, burning pains, coldness, itching, heaviness, and tingling, to complete anesthesia.[2,41,42] Frequently, these patients are assymptomatic and quite unaware of their neuropathy until they develop a neuropathic foot lesion. Electrophysiologic testing of nerve function in neuropathic patients invariably shows abnormalities of vibration and thermal perception, with the most severe findings occurring in those neuropathic patients with a history of foot ulceration.[20,33,43,44]

Motor neuropathy is frequently a counterpart of the mixed fiber symmetrical sensory neuropathy. Motor fibers to the intrinsic muscles of the feet are involved and demonstrate slowed motor conduction velocities or absent action potentials.[2] Typically, the foot assumes a characteristic appearance wherein there is atrophy and wasting of the intrinsic musculature. Their ineffective stabilizing function at the level of the metatarsal-phalangeal and interphalangeal joints allows the dynamic contracture of the long flexors and extensors. Subsequently, hammertoes and clawtoes develop, which lead to prominence of the metatarsal heads and abnormal weight distribution on the foot. The contractures of the toes often result in ulceration due to shoe irritation dorsally or excessive pressures on the tips of the toes as they attempt to stabilize the foot in propulsion. Boulton et al. have demonstrated the increased pressures under the metatarsal heads of neuropathic patients as compared to nondiabetic controls and nonneuropathic diabetic subjects.[43] Those patients with a prior history of neuropathic ulceration had abnormally high pressure in every case under the sites of previous ulcers. Accordingly, primary and recurrent ulceration can be directly attributed to the effects of chronic sensorimotor neuropathy on the structure of the foot and the associated abnormal pressures encountered in the presence of insensitivity.

Painful neuropathy is a less common but more disabling type of diabetic neuropathy.[42] Although pain is characteristic of the focal mononeuropathies, it can also be a very distressing symptom of sensory polyneuropathy, lasting from months to years and very prone to nocturnal exacerbation.[41] Small myelinated and unmyelinated fibers, which also carry sympathetic fibers, are affected, thereby resulting not only in pain and thermal disturbances, but in sympathetic dysfunction as well. These patients bear a remarkable resemblance to those suffering from causalgic syndromes.[45] Young et al. have demonstrated that those patients with painful neuropathy have a higher ratio of small fiber to large fiber damage, whereas those patients developing neuropathic ulcers are typified by more severe large fiber disease.[33] Putatively, the hyperesthesia, lesser degree of large fiber involvement, and characteristically good vascular perfusion of the feet render these patients less susceptible to ulceration. However, there are patients with symptoms of pain or dysesthesias who also demonstrate marked loss of external pain and perception. Ward has termed this the *painful-painless* leg.[46] Such patients therefore live in constant discomfort in addition to the ever present risk of unsensed injury.

Autonomic neuropathy is present in the great majority of patients with peripheral sensory neuropathy.[32,33,47,48] Furthermore, autonomic dysfunction has been strongly associated with the incidence of neuropathic ulceration.[31,49] Although there is conflicting evidence regarding the comparative severity of involvement between nonulcerating and ulcerating neuropathic patients, all studies show a significant degree of autonomic abnormalities in these two sets of patients when compared to diabetics without neuropathy and in normal controls.[32,33,43–45,48] Defective sudomotor and vasomotor function are the two parameters most commonly evident in the diabetic foot.[50] Impaired sweat production is very prevalent in these patients and is usually associated with abnormal autonomic cardiovascular reflexes.[47] Clinically, this anhydrosis is manifested by dry, cracking skin that is predisposed to fissuring, callous formation, and subsequent ulceration. Vasomotor disturbances resulting from sympathetic nerve failure are very prevalent in all neuropathic patients and have even been detected in diabetic patients thought to be unaffected by neuropathy.[45,48,50] Sympathetic dysfunction results in a loss of vasomotor tone with a substantial increase of peripheral blood flow reported to be as high as five times normal.[45] The increased perfusion is mediated by the opening of arteriovenous shunts resulting in distension of dorsal veins, increased warmth, and raised venous PO_2 levels approaching almost arterial levels.[52,53] This increased skin blood flow is nonnutritive, however, since arteriovenous shunting may reduce nutrient capillary blood flow and thereby predispose to ulceration.[2] Other attendant effects of sympathetic denervation are loss of the venivasomotor reflex, neuropathic edema, postural hypotension, impaired maximum perfusion, and increased bone blood flow with associated demineralization.[54,55] Newrick et al. have found a deficient hyperemic response to pressure under the feet of neuropathic patients due to an altered autoregulatory mechanism associated with autonomic dysfunction.[56] In concert with a pre-existing impairment of nutritive capillary blood flow and neuropathic edema, this further reduction of normal flow in response to the relative ischemia of standing could augment the inherent tendency of the neuropathic foot to ulcerate.

Peripheral Vascular Disease

Abnormal peripheral blood flow is the second major element involved in the etiology of diabetic foot lesions. Although ischemia frequently plays a role in the pathogenesis of foot ulceration, it must not be considered a universal finding in all patients with such lesions. On the contrary, ulcerations of predominantly neuropathic origin are usually associated with a state of relative hyperperfusion due to abnormalities of the microcirculation.[48,57] Customarily, diabetic vascular disease is categorized into large vessel atherosclerotic disease (macroangiopathy) and that affecting the capillaries (microangiopathy). The term *small vessel disease,* referring to a variant of macroangiopathy involving the small arteries and arterioles in the feet, is a point of considerable controversy and should probably be abandoned.[57,58]

Ischemia is the result of atherosclerotic occlusive disease of large arteries from the aorta to the distal leg. Although histologically the macrovascular disease is identical to that in nondiabetic persons, it occurs at an earlier age and with greater severity in patients with diabetes.[59,60] The distribution of lesions is different in that there is a strong propensity to involve the infrapopliteal tibial and peroneal vessels in addition to the superficial femoral artery while sparing the arteries of the foot.[61] The hemodynamic significance of the occlusive arterial disease is usually quantified by assessment of segmental Doppler systolic pressures and the corresponding ankle-brachial pressure index as discussed by Yao et al.[62] Ankle pressures below 70 mmHg and ankle-brachial ratios below 0.45 in the diabetic patient are usually regarded to be the minimal criteria for healing foot lesions and local amputations.[63]

There has been a persistent misconception regarding the presence of arteriolar occlusive disease in the foot and its relevance to ischemic lesions in feet with palpable pedal pulses.[64] Logerfo and Coffman have refuted the validity of the "small vessel disease" hypothesis by citing subsequent light microscopy, arterial casting, and physiologic studies that failed to confirm the incidence of occlusive microvascular disease.[65–67] Medial arterial calcification, also known as Monckeberg's medial sclerosis, is a fairly common radiographic finding in the feet and legs of diabetic patients but does not contribute to intravascular occlusion or the atherogenic process.[68] To the contrary, blood flow at rest has been found to be increased in these patients.[69] Strongly associated with neuropathy, calcification of the tunica media follows the smooth muscle atrophy attendant with long-term sympathetic denervation.[70] Medial calcification typically results in falsely high segmental arterial pressures and ankle-brachial systolic pressure indices.[71–73] In such cases, these measurements of distal arterial perfusion can become very inaccurate prognosticators of the healing of foot lesions.[72,74] A recent study infers that the prevalence of abnormally elevated pressure indices associated with calcification is significantly higher in insulin-dependent diabetics and is related more to the duration of diabetes than to age.[75]

Microangiopathy consists of both structural and functional abnormalities of the microcirculation. The hallmark of diabetic microangiopathy is a thickening of muscle capillary basement membrane and is most likely a consequence of chronically impaired glucose tolerance, nonenzymatic glycosylation of collagen and proteoglycans, and genetic susceptibility.[76] Although the altered basement membrane may explain the increased transcapillary leakage of large proteins (albumin) and may interfere with leukocyte migration, there is apparently no interference with oxygen diffusion.[58] Aside from altered hemorrheologic properties, endothelial cell dysfunction, and platelet disturbances, the major functional effect of diabetes on the microcirculation is a distinct alteration in blood flow. As previously discussed, the increase in blood flow mediated by early sympathetic failure in neuropathic patients averages five times greater than that in nondiabetic subjects.[77] Measurements of transcutaneous oxygen tension ($tcPO_2$) on the feet and legs of neuropathic patients yield significantly higher levels than in nonneuropathic and nondiabetic controls. This study correlates well with laser Doppler flowmetry results indicating increased resting blood flow in similar groups of patients.[55] Higher skin temperatures, venous distension on the dorsum of the foot, arterialization of venous blood, neuropathic edema, and loss of the normal venoarteriolar reflex upon standing are additional findings in diabetic neuropathic patients and are presumably due to widespread arteriovenous shunting.[45,57] Impaired vascular reactivity to ischemia and increased temperatures have been demonstrated by both $tcPO_2$ and laser Doppler flux measurements.[56,78–81] A reduction in maximum hyperemic response to ischemia, standing, and heating is found in diabetic patients with and without neuropathy as compared to normal controls. Additionally, Parkhouse and co-workers have demonstrated a reduced or absent axon reflex flare due to impairment of nociceptive C fiber function in patients with progressive degrees of insensitivity.[82,83] The diminished neurogenic inflammatory response to noxious stimuli and concomitant loss of pain perception highlight the significance of nociceptive fiber dysfunction in the development of neuropathic plantar ulcers. In concert with each other, these abnormalities of the microcirculation render the diabetic foot extremely susceptible to injury and inadequately prepared to respond to such insult through impairment of normal autoregulatory function.

Infection

Infection is not usually the direct cause of an ulceration; however, it is certainly a major determinant of both treatment and prognosis for any foot lesion. In 1965, Pratt reported that approximately 25 percent of all diabetes-related hospital admissions were for the treatment of infected foot lesions and gangrene.[84] Even today, such foot disorders account for more in-hospital days than any other complication of diabetes.[1] It is widely accepted that foot infections are a frequent and serious problem for these patients, although there is an apparent lack of documentation as to whether or not infections in general occur with increased frequency in diabetes.[85]

The inherent susceptibility of the diabetic foot to infection is directly attributable to neuropathy or vascular disease acting alone or in combination. Additionally, certain defects in leukocyte function and wound repair have been identified that contribute to the altered host response to injury seen in patients with diabetes.[86] Bagdade et al. found that leukocyte phagocytosis was significantly reduced in patients with poorly controlled diabetes and that with correction of hyperglycemia the microbiocidal rates were improved, although less than normal.[87] Neutrophil dysfunction was corroborated by Tan et al., who also reported impaired intracellular bacterial killing that was unaffected by blood glucose levels.[88] Defects in chemotaxis and phagocytosis that impair the inflammatory phase of wound healing appear to be insulin-sensitive and may play a vital role in subsequent wound repair.[86]

Diabetic patients tolerate infection poorly, infection adversely affects diabetes control, and uncontrolled diabetes adversely affects the infection.[89] Because systemic signs of serious infection are frequently absent or occur late in these patients, all infections must be aggressively treated to prevent proximal extension, gangrene, and septicemia. When present, fever and leukocytosis indicate persistent infection that negatively impacts upon successful local treatment.[90] Goodman et al. have found that these parameters are very strongly correlated with operative success rates when local definitive procedures are indicated.[91] Another recent study indicated that the majority of diabetic patients with serious pedal infections were in poor glycemic control, had elevated sedimentation rates, white blood cell counts within the normal range, and 62 percent had evidence of zinc deficiency.[92]

It is universally accepted that diabetic foot infections tend to be polymicrobial in nature and frequently harbor anaerobic organisms synergistically with the usual aerobes.[1,92–101] On the average, three to five bacterial isolates can be recovered from each patient. The most common organisms encountered are the aerobic gram-positive cocci, including *Staphylococcus aureus*, coagulase-negative *Staphylococcus*, *Streptococcus* species, and enterococci. Gram-negative pathogens frequently cultured include *Proteus* species, *Escherichia coli*, and other various species of Enterobacteriaceae. *Pseudomonas aeruginosa*, interestingly enough, is encountered much less often than these other gram-negative bacilli. Several studies that have quantified the types of organisms found in diabetic foot infections confirm that this often feared organism is present in approximately 10 to 20 percent of the cultures taken, whereas *Proteus* species may account for 26 to as high as 55 percent of the infections.[1,96–98,102,103] Anaerobes, although rarely occurring in pure culture, can be recovered in over 80 percent of these patients and will often exhibit heavier growth than the accompanying aerobic pathogens.[96] *Bacteroides* species are the most important organisms of this group and have been the only anaerobes cultured from the blood in diabetic patients developing bacteremia subsequent to foot infections.[104] Bacterial synergism may play a role in its pathogenicity since *B. fragilis* has been shown to have increased pathogenic activity in the presence of enterococci.[105] Table 10-2 is a composite listing of the bacterial isolates and their frequencies as found in diabetic foot infections by various investigators.[106]

The unreliability of sinus tract cultures and superficial swab cultures of ulcers is well known and has been investigated by numerous authors.[1,94,96–98,107] Whenever possible, deep tissue specimens should be obtained by avoiding draining sinuses to provide reliable cultures indicative of the true underlying pathogens. Empiric antibiotic selection should be based upon the severity of infection, status of the patient, and the knowledge that these infections are polymicrobial in over 70 percent of the patients cultured.[97,103] Additional treatment is always required, including rest, elevation, surgical drainage and debridement, and dressings. Hospitalization and parenteral antibiotics are necessary for moderate or severe infections involving deeper structures, when there are systemic signs of toxicity or fever, or when the infection progresses despite appropriate out-patient therapy.[108] Vascular reconstruction, when indicated, is usually performed following initial drainage procedures when the infection has been brought under control.[89] Definitive procedures, including minor (local) or major amputation, and corrective and prophylactic foot surgery can then be safely performed, resulting in a reported limb salvage rate of 73 percent.[90] Even so, Kucan and Robson reported in their series that nearly one-half of the patients with severe foot infections developed contralateral limb–threatening infections within 18 months.[109] Therefore, follow-up care *must* include a program of spe-

Table 10-2. Frequency (%) of Selected Bacterial Isolates from Diabetic Foot Infections

	Investigator (no. patients)					
Organism	*Louie*[93] (20)	*Sapico*[96] (32)	*Gibbons*[1] (100)	*Wheat*[97] (54)	*Calhoun*[103] (850)	*Scher*[98] (65)
Staph. aureus	35	25.0	54	37	45.9	35.4
Staph. epidermidis (coagulase neg.)	30	9.3	32	32	22.6	27.7
Enterococcus	45	40.6	32	27	28.7	N/A
Proteus mirablis	55	28.1	22	17	26.1	55.8
Pseudomonas aeruginosa	20	15.6	14	7	15.9	23.1
Bacteroides sp.	85	67.0	67	33	15.6	84.6

(Modified from Tan and File,[106] with permission.)

cial footwear and patient education aimed at prevention. Out-patient management of less severe foot infections can be accomplished only through close observation and cooperation of the patient with the physician.[110,111] Accordingly, the patient must clearly understand that hospitalization might indeed be required for more intensive treatment as dictated by the course of the infection. The various types of infections prevalent in the diabetic foot, their respective treatments, and antibiotic therapies are presented in other chapters within this text. Figure 10-2, however, illustrates an algorithm useful in the management of the infected diabetic foot.

Pathogenesis of Ulceration

Trauma of some type when applied to the neuropathic or ischemic extremity is capable of producing ulceration and subsequent infection. On occasion, however, ulceration can follow infection in patients with these same predisposing factors. An apparently innocuous interdigital fissure or corn can lead to a massive plantar space infection and necrotizing fasciitis in the compromised host.[112] Ulcer formation will commence when the soft tissue infection breaks to the surface by way of draining sinuses and necrotic bullae. The vast majority of ulcers, however, are primarily due to traumatic origin, whether found in an ischemic or an insensitive foot, or in the high risk foot with both ischemia and neuropathy. Traumatic injuries can be subdivided into mechanical, thermal, and chemical components. Although mechanical trauma is the most significant of the three, too many limbs have been lost to the catastrophic consequences of any type of injury to the diabetic foot.

Mechanical forces are the major threat to the integrity of the high risk foot and seemingly dominate the history of an ulceration from inception to healing to subsequent recurrence.[113] These forces can be subdivided into parallel or oblique components, commonly termed *shearing forces*, and vertical or perpendicular components. Shear stress tends to slide superficial tissues (skin) over deeper tissues or vice versa when the weight of the body firmly plants the sole of the foot on the ground. If it were not for the presence of bursae and tendon sheaths to allow for this sliding, the tissues would be torn apart from the shearing during locomotion. When ulceration occurs and subsequently heals, this sliding mechanism is lost due to scarring; shear forces do indeed traumatize deeper tissues, and ulcer recurrence frequently ensues.[113] Pollard and LeQuesne have analyzed two types of shear, longitudinal and transverse, and have reported that neurotrophic ulcers occur not only at the expected sites of maximum vertical force but concurrently at the site of maximal horizontal shear.[114]

The significance of high vertical forces and maximum loading in the etiopathogenesis of ulcerations has been extensively investigated and reported by numerous researchers.[31,41,113–124] Structural deformities induced by neuropathy such as hammertoes, prominent metatarsal heads, and Charcot joints are common sites of peak pressures and concomitant ulceration. A recent study confirms the abnormally high forefoot pressures associated with reduced toe loading secondary to clawtoe deformities in both diabetic and rheumatoid patients.[117] The integral role of sensory loss in the etiopathogenesis of ulceration was also confirmed in that only those diabetic patients with significant neurologic deficits *and* high pressures developed ulcers. The excessive pressures are manifested by the plantar callosities that develop under these sites. Neglected calluses become thickened in time, hemorrhage underneath, eventually ulcerate, and frequently progress to deep abscess formation if the accumulated fluid is not drained early.[31] Such lesions have been labeled *preulcerative* and are considered to be the most frequent cause of mechanically induced ulcerations.[2,125] Surprisingly, it seems that callus formation on the toes is a more frequent precursor of ulceration than plantar metatarsal head lesions, since three large studies indicate that over 50 percent of the ulcers treated were on the digits.[29,103,126] Consequently, tight-fitting shoes can be implicated as the most frequent precipitating factor of ulceration, whether ischemic or neuropathic in origin.[29] In the neuropathic foot, poorly fitting shoes press on contracted hammertoes causing areas of hyperkeratosis dorsally and distally that will eventually ulcerate. Off-loading of the toes (reduced toe purchase and weight transmission) results in higher than normal pressures being borne by the metatarsal heads, which are

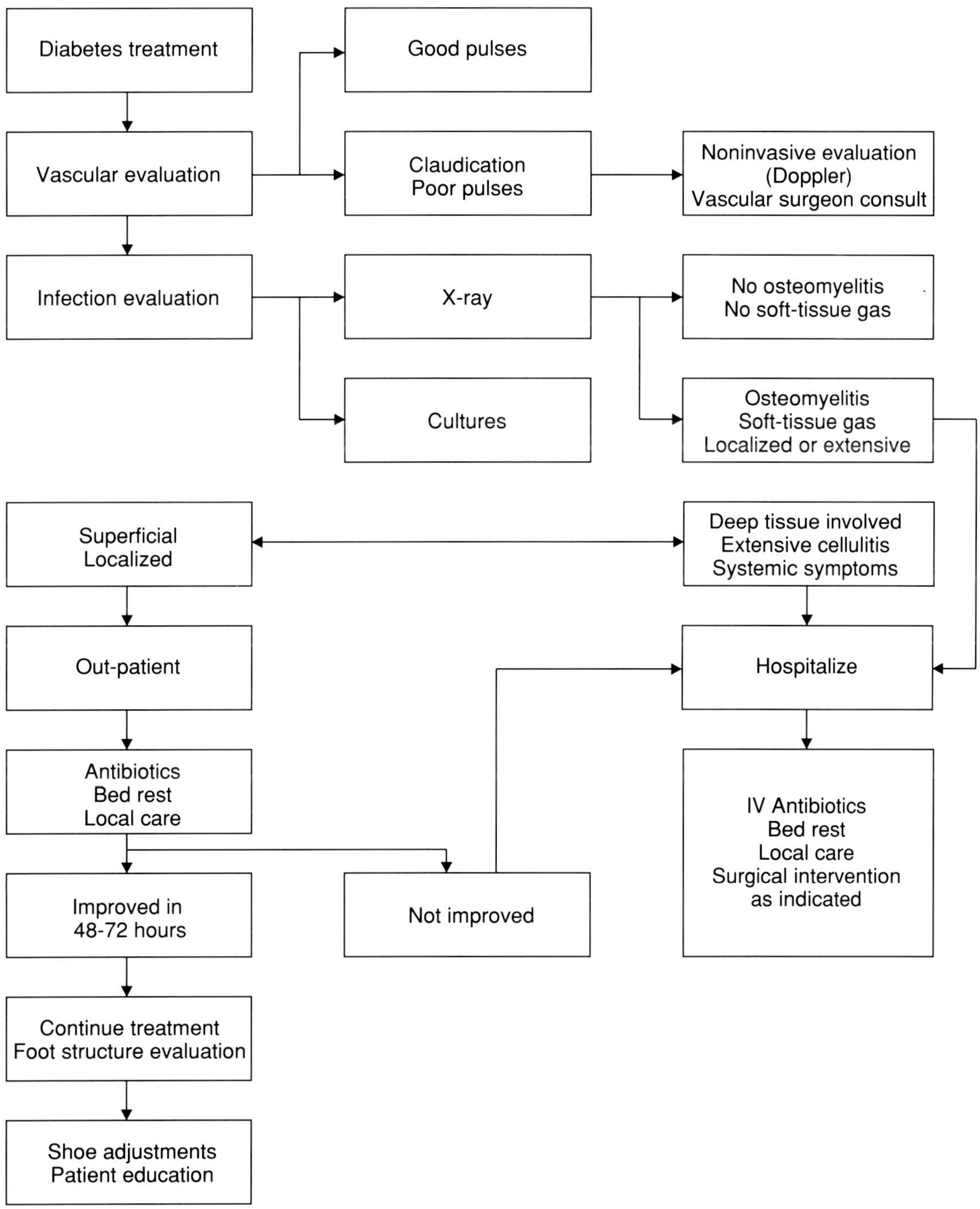

Fig. 10-2. Algorithm for management of diabetic foot infections. (From Bessman and Kasim,[111] with permission.)

then predisposed to callus formation and subsequent ulceration (Fig. 10-3).[13] In the ischemic foot, there is less of a tendency to cause keratosis as an initial response to injury.[127] Instead, localized pressure from shoes tends to have a blistering effect with subsequent tissue necrosis, commonly affecting the medial and lateral borders of the foot as well as the apex of the hammertoe deformity.[29]

Brand describes four ways that mechanical forces can seriously injure the high risk foot.[128,129] A sharp impact on a small object will result in a very high localized force that will penetrate the skin. This occurs when one steps on a nail or thumbtack. Light pressure sustained for a long period of time will cause ischemic necrosis, such as when a snug shoe is worn all day long. Moderate, normal stresses repeated many times without rest will create an inflammatory autolysis and eventual necrosis. This is perhaps the most frequent mechanism of ulceration in the neuropathic patient, since the warning sense of pain is lost.[2,23] Lastly, walking on infected tissues spreads the infection into deeper or more proximal planes, creating further injury. Insensitivity to pain permits these injuries to go undetected for long periods prior to ulcer formation in the patient with neuropathy. Additionally, these patients do not limp as a normal person would do, and therefore weight is periodically borne on the wound, creating further injury.[129] The hypersensitive ischemic foot will not tolerate continued weight bearing once injury has occurred, but it is unable to heal the wound created. The ischemic neuropathic foot is in double jeopardy since mechanical stress continues as the ulcer or infection progresses in the inattentive patient who does not have the physiologic means to adequately resolve the foot lesion.

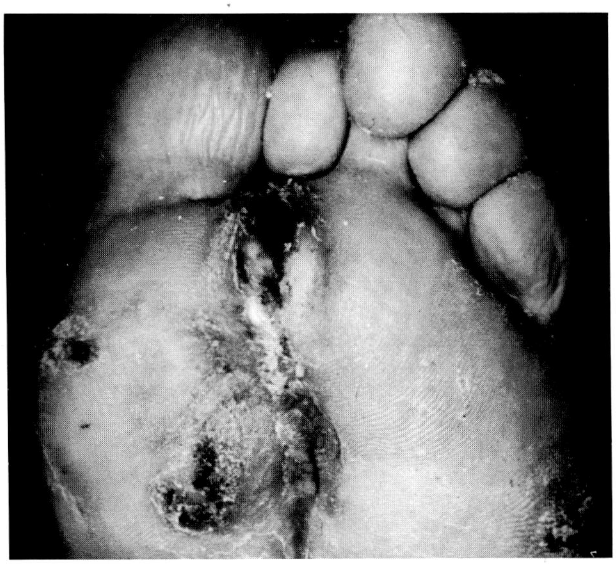

Fig. 10-3. Subkeratotic ulceration under second metatarsal head due to off-loading of the associated hammertoe.

Thermal and chemical trauma are not frequent causes of diabetic foot ulcers, but when such trauma does occur the results are equally as significant. Thermal injuries directly cause trauma to the epithelium and deeper tissues dependent upon the degree of heat or cold applied to the foot and the duration of exposure. Most commonly, heat is involved and usually in the form of extremely hot foot soaks. Other thermal injuries might include lesions resulting from walking barefoot on a hot sandy beach or pavement, from putting one's feet too close to a fire or heater, or from frostbite due to inadequate footwear in cold weather (Fig. 10-4). The latter circumstance also includes the secretary who wears nothing on her feet but nylons and dress pumps when she walks the city streets on her commute to and from work. Chemical injuries most frequently are caused by keratolytic agents.[2] These "corn cures" contain salicylic acid in varying strengths, all of which can be disastrous to the high risk foot. Over-the-counter availability of these and other caustic chemicals should be condemned by all.

Other Risk Factors

There are still additional risk factors that ostensibly predispose the diabetic patient with neuropathy or ischemia to ulceration, as previously indicated in Table 10-1.[130] Increasing age, duration and control of diabetes, body weight, social and employment circumstances, level of education and understanding of diabetes, frequency of podiatric care, denial, reduced visual acuity, and cigarette smoking have all been associated with the development of foot lesions.[4,13,16,25,26,29,115] Structural deformities such as hammertoes, bunions, and metatarsal head protrusions can be congenital or acquired. Often the result of chronic sensorimotor neuropathy and intrinsic muscle atrophy, these de-

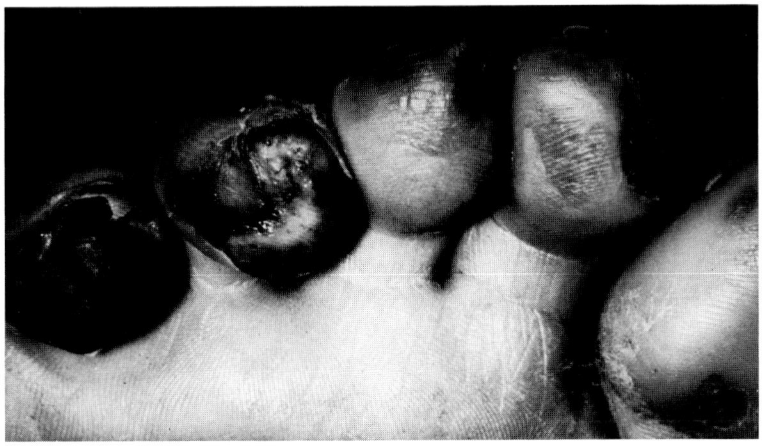

Fig. 10-4. Thermal necrosis on tips of digits caused by patient resting his feet on the walls of a sauna.

formities alter the normal weight-bearing distributions within the foot and result in abnormally high pressures concentrated under the metatarsal heads during stance and gait.[122] Excessive pressures borne by the plantar surface as well as on the lateral and dorsal surfaces by shoe impingement will obviously predispose the insensate or ischemic foot to eventual ulceration. Correspondingly, abnormal biomechanical function will have the same result. Feet that have previously undergone amputation of any part or even those having had corrective surgery will have a commensurate alteration in biomechanical function and attendant pressure distribution. The intimate association between structural and biomechanical changes and their role in the pathogenesis of ulceration are more fully discussed in Chapters 7 and 8.

Alteration of the structure and function of proteins seems to be omnipresent in patients with diabetes mellitus and may be responsible for many of the chronic complications of the disease.[31] In the presence of prolonged hyperglycemia, nonenzymatic glycosylation of proteins occurs as free glucose spontaneously attaches to protein molecules.[131–135] In time, this results in an irreversible glycosylated end product with altered physical and chemical properties. Just as this process occurs on the hemoglobin molecule, in the lens, in myelin, and in capillary basement membranes, it also takes place on the structural proteins collagen and keratin.[31,134,136,137] In collagen, intermolecular cross-linking is increased by such glycosylation much the same as is seen in the normal aging process.[132] This is most pronounced in the collagen from younger adult diabetic patients, whereas samples from older diabetics seem to have values within the normal range of age-matched nondiabetic subjects.[131] Essentially, an accelerated aging process of collagen is evident by its stiffening, insolubility, and resistance to digestion by collagenase. Skin thickness, primarily a function of collagen content, has recently been shown to be increased in patients with insulin-dependent diabetes mellitus and was correlated with both duration of diabetes and glycemic control.[135] Similarly, glycosylation of keratin produces a tissue that is also more rigid than normal and more prone to develop thick, hard calluses in response to pressure and surrounding mal perforans ulcerations.[31,130,137] Putatively then, the thickening and rigidity of the skin and subcutaneous tissues of the sole of the foot predispose them to ulceration through an inadequate dissipation of the vertical and shear stresses encountered during locomotion.

Limited joint mobility (LJM) is another fairly common, but often overlooked, finding in diabetic patients characteristically affecting the small joints of the hands.[138–144] Initially reported in studies of adolescent patients with long-standing diabetes, it has subsequently been found to effect 43 percent of insulin-dependent patients with duration of diabetes ranging from 3 to 53 years.[140] Presumably a consequence of nonenzymatic glycosylation of periarticular connective tissue, limited joint mobility has also been correlated with an increased risk for microvascular complications.[141] Others consider it to be another chronic complication of diabetes that develops in tandem with other age- and duration-related manifestations of the disease.[140] As one might expect, LJM also is seen involving both large and small joints of the foot.[138,145–147] Delbridge and associates reported that in addition to limited mobility in the hands there was a significant reduction in subtalar joint and hallux range of motion in patients with neuropathic ulcers as compared to uncomplicated diabetics and nondiabetic controls.[138] Furthermore, subtalar range of motion was most reduced in those feet with ulcers in contrast to the paired nonulcerated feet. Mueller et al., who also noted significantly less ankle dorsiflexion, confirmed these findings in ulcerated patients and correlated the severity of limitation with the severity of insensitivity as measured by Semmes-Weinstein monofilaments.[147] Since a major function of the ankle and subtalar joints is to provide shock absorption during locomotion, any restriction of motion of these joints can lead to inadequate dissipation of vertical and shear forces. As indicated by these studies, the limitation of motion evident in the significantly neuropathic patient may therefore be a contributory factor in the pathogenesis of ulceration by increasing mechanical stress on the plantar surface of the foot. Additionally, Crausaz et al. found that decreased visual acuity frequently accompanied reduced joint mobility in ulcerated neuropathic patients as compared to uncomplicated neuropathic and nonneuropathic diabetic patients.[146] Since 71 percent of their ulcerated patients had insufficient vision to adequately inspect their feet and joint flexibility was significantly reduced, these patients were physically incapable of self-examination and foot care. Therefore, they recommend that these two parameters be assessed routinely in all footcare education programs and that patients demonstrating decreased visual acuity, LJM, and neuropathy be considered at risk for future ulceration.

Ulcer Classification

Although a multitude of factors are presumably implicated, foot lesions in the diabetic patient can be generally attributed to neuropathy, ischemia, or infection. Frequently, more than one element of this diabetic foot triad are present prior to ulceration and predispose the foot to ulceration when it is subjected to trauma. Once present, classification of the lesion facilitates a rational approach to treatment as well as the prediction of its healing potential.[103,126] Calhoun et al. found that classification of foot lesions not only enabled them to institute proper treatment regimens, but additionally, when such protocols were followed, the treatment outcomes were significantly more successful than when protocol was not followed.[103] A variety of wound classification systems have been offered based upon such parameters as extent of infection, extent of tissue loss, location, and the degree of ischemia contrasted to the role of neuropathy.[1,126,127,148–150]

Williams et al. in 1974 assessed the temperature of the involved foot to categorize necrotic lesions in such a way as to indicate relative perfusion and establish a general course of therapy.[150] Necrosis in a cold foot indicated gangrene in an ischemic foot that required vascular surgery to heal. Since distal reconstructive procedures had not yet been perfected, patients in this category were usually relegated to major amputations. Necrosis in a hot foot depicted an infected foot with abundant circulation, typical of the very common neuropathic mal perforans ulcer. Adequate drainage, excision of necrotic tissue, and local amputations when required would generally provide a successful outcome. Necrosis in a warm foot indicated infrapopliteal disease with good collateral circulation. Perfusion to the foot was marginal, but local procedures would be attempted in an effort to salvage the limb. Once again, neither tibial nor pedal bypasses were successful at that time. Hence, loss of the limb would occur in approximately 50 percent of the patients where local procedures failed.

Others have evaluated diabetic foot lesions based primarily upon a neuropathic nonischemic versus ischemic origin.[2,127] Obviously, there is frequently an overlapping between these two parameters. In such instances the ischemic neurotrophic ulcer must be treated in the same manner as a purely ischemic lesion since the loss of adequate tissue perfusion is the greatest single impediment to healing. Edmonds and associates, finding this system most useful, report that the neuropathic ulcer is a much more frequent complication than

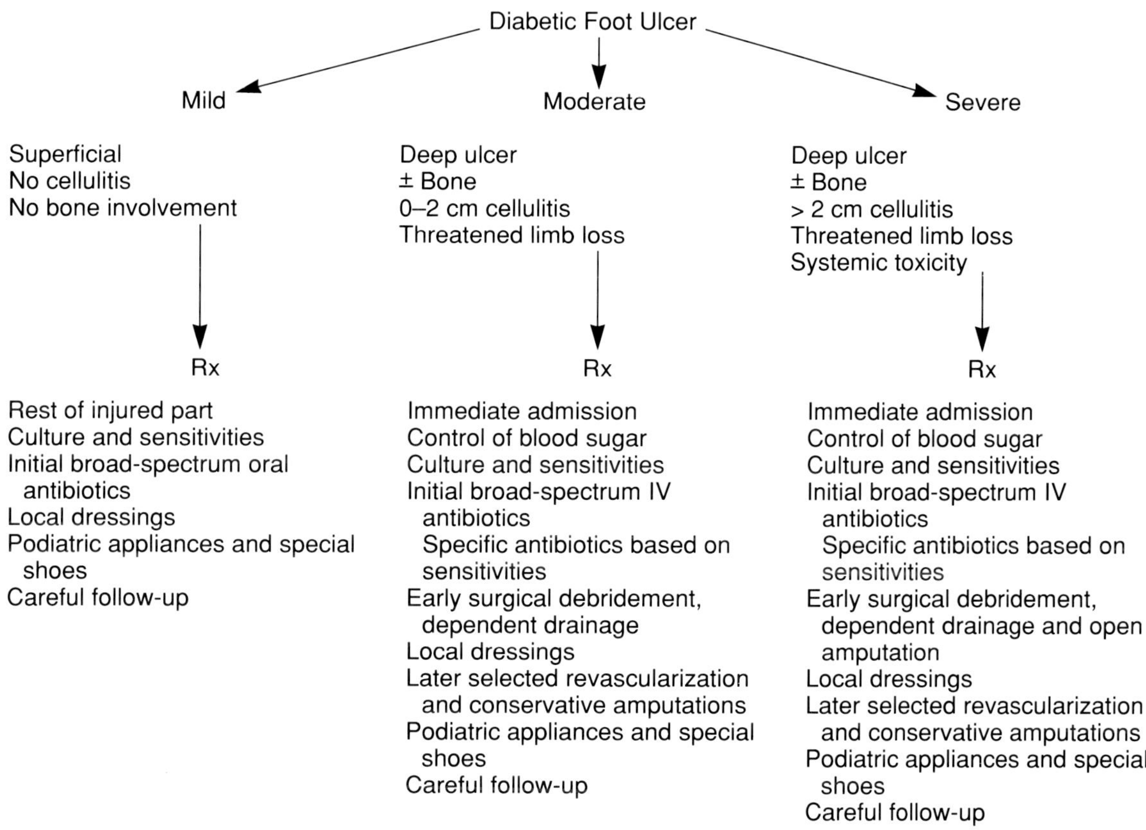

Fig. 10-5. Gibbons classification system based on severity of infection. (From Gibbons and Eliopoulos,[1] with permission.)

the ischemic lesion and is almost universally associated with callous formation.[2,29] Conversely, ischemic lesions are often painful and typified by the absence of callus. In a large study of ulcerated patients, 62 percent of the lesions were classified as purely neuropathic as opposed to the 38 percent of ischemic lesions, some of which also had evidence of neuropathy.[29] Tight-fitting shoes were the most common precipitating factor of ulceration in both groups. Whereas the neurotrophic lesions were preceded by hyperkeratosis, the ischemic ulcers were often the direct result of epithelial damage, blistering, and tissue necrosis. Assigning the lesions to one of these two groups and instituting the appropriate treatment resulted in an 86 percent healing rate for the neuropathic ulcers and 72 percent for ischemic ulcers.

Gibbons and Eliopoulos in 1984 reported a categorization of foot lesions into three groups on the basis of severity of infection.[1] The mild group (I) consisted of stable, superficial, and relatively uncomplicated ulcers with no cellulitis. Even in this

Table 10-3. Wagner Grading System for Diabetic Foot Lesions

Grade	*Lesion*
Grade 0	No open lesions; may have deformity or cellulitis
Grade 1	Superficial ulcer
Grade 2	Deep ulcer to tendon, capsule, or bone
Grade 3	Deep ulcer with abscess, osteomyelitis, or joint sepsis
Grade 4	Localized gangrene — forefoot or heel
Grade 5	Gangrene of entire foot

group there was an average of three bacterial isolates found per ulcer comprised of gram-positive and gram-negative aerobes as well as anaerobes. Moderately infected ulcers (group II) were deep, often penetrating to bone, and had up to 2 cm of cellulitis. Although systemic signs of toxicity were frequently lacking, threatened limb loss in the majority of patients often required multiple operations including drainage, amputations, and arterial revascularization to salvage the extremity. Group III comprised severely infected ulcers or gangrene with cellulitis extending beyond 2 cm. These patients were ill, with fever, and demonstrated a marked loss of glycemic control. Amputation was usually required in this group, with two-thirds having successful forefoot amputations and one-third of the patients losing their limbs to major amputations. The majority of patients studied fell into the moderate and severe categories, as would be expected in a tertiary care center. Interestingly, however, these infections also averaged three bacterial isolates per culture with enterococci, *Proteus*, and *Pseudomonas* species predominating. This classification scheme is commonly employed at the New England Deaconess Hospital and Joslin Diabetes Center. When matched with appropriate treatment regimens involving a multidisciplinary team, a high success rate for primary ulcer healing or limb salvage can be anticipated (Fig. 10-5).

The most widely accepted classification system for diabetic foot ulcers and lesions is the one proposed by Wagner that is based upon the depth of penetration and extent of tissue necrosis.[151-153] As with other methods of assessing such lesions, the Wagner classification appropriately directs treatment in accordance with the severity of the problem, and by doing so favorably affects the treatment outcome.[103,151] In this system, the various lesions found in the diabetic foot are separated into six categories or grades (Table 10-3). The *grade 0* foot is one that has no open lesions and intact skin. There may, however, be potential sites of ulceration such as hammertoes, bunions, prominent metatarsal heads, or Charcot deformities (Fig. 10-6). Hyperkeratotic lesions indicate areas of increased pressures and should be considered as preulcerative in neuropathic patients.[125] *Grade 1* lesions are superficial ulcers penetrating through the skin but not below the subcutaneous adipose layer (Fig. 10-7). Superficial infection with cellulitis may be present. A *grade 2* ulcer is deep and penetrates through the fat to tendon, capsule, or bone without deep abscess formation or osteomyelitis (Fig. 10-8). Once the ulcer penetrates into the

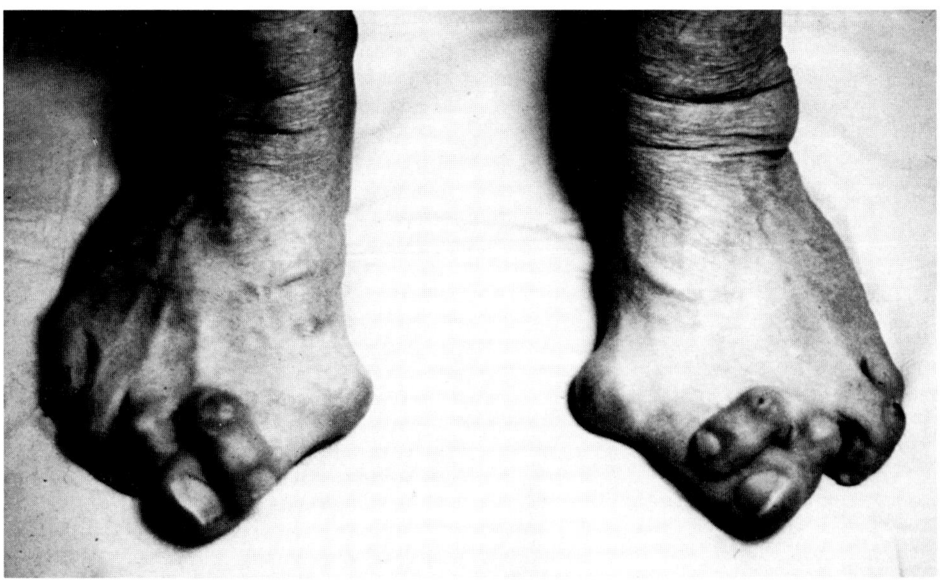

Fig. 10-6. Grade 0 foot. No open lesions but hammertoes and bunions are obvious potential sites for ulceration.

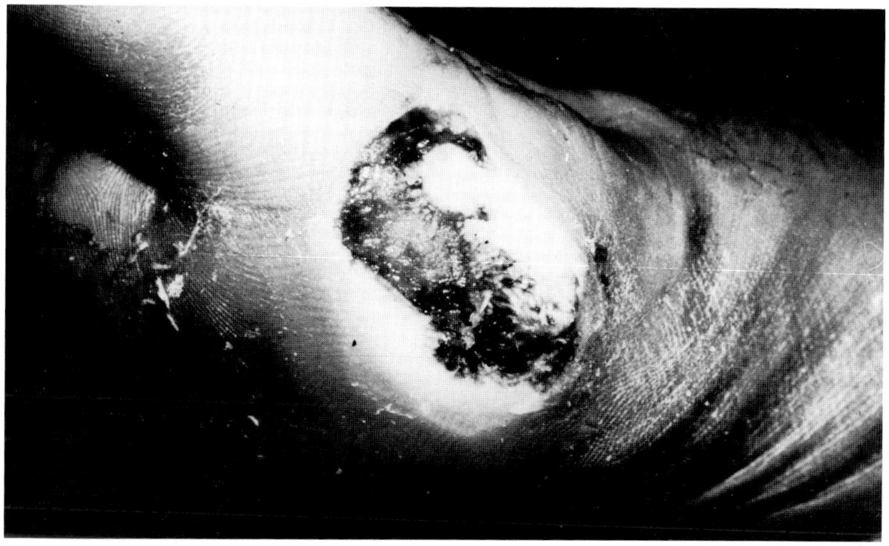

Fig. 10-7. Grade 1 ulcer. Superficial lesion caused from shoe pressure against underlying bunion deformity.

joint, forms a deep abscess, or osteomyelitis ensues, it must be considered as a *grade 3* lesion (Fig. 10-9). Plantar compartment abscesses, tendon sheath infections, and necrotizing fasciitis without digital gangrene also fall into this category.[100,101,112,148] These are limb-threatening lesions that require hospitalization and surgical intervention for adequate treatment. *Grade 4* implies that some part of the foot is gangrenous, usually the toes, forefoot, or even the heel. Most of the foot, however, is intact and salvageable if there is adequate perfusion or if vascular reconstruction is feasible (Fig. 10-10). A *grade 5* foot has extensive gangrene or necrosis to the point that it is entirely

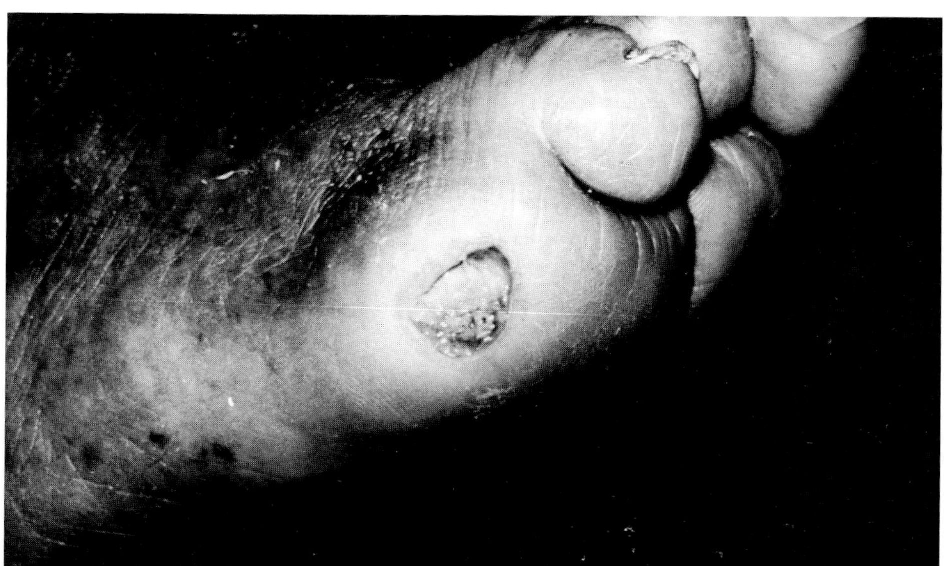

Fig. 10-8. Grade 2 ulcer. Deep through fat extending to capsule of fifth metatarsophalangeal joint. This was caused from a tight cast.

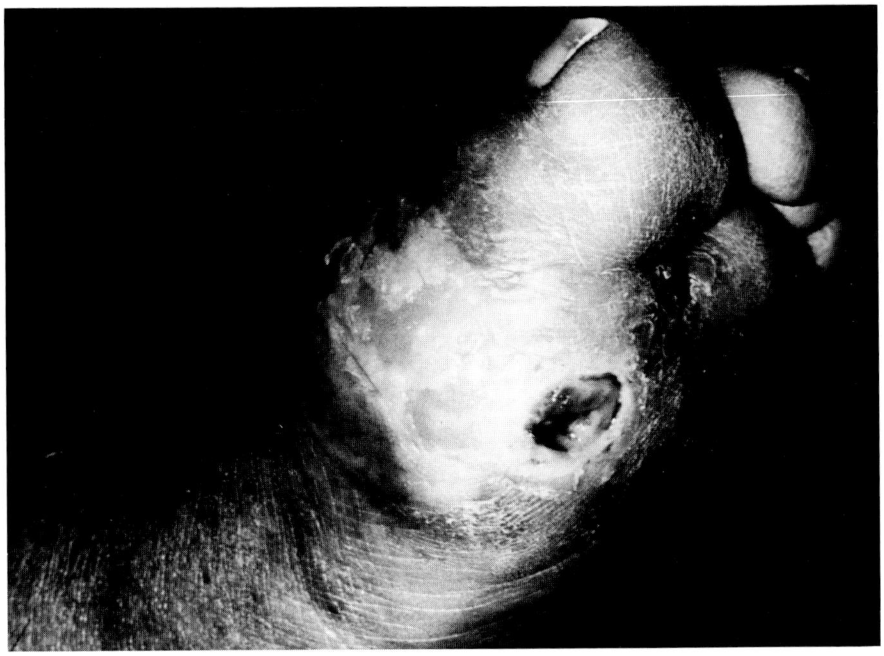

Fig. 10-9. Grade 3 ulcer. Probes into first metatarsophangeal joint with deep abscess and cellulitis.

beyond salvage and major amputation is required (Fig. 10-11).

There is an obvious progression in severity with each subsequent grade of foot lesion. Accordingly, a grade 0 foot can progress to a grade 4 or 5 foot if it is neglected or inadequately treated. Hence, it is important to also match each lesion with the requisite treatment program. Furthermore, the vascularity of the foot must be evaluated to determine the prognosis for healing as well as course of therapy. Doppler segmental pressures are used to calculate the "ischemic index" or ankle-brachial

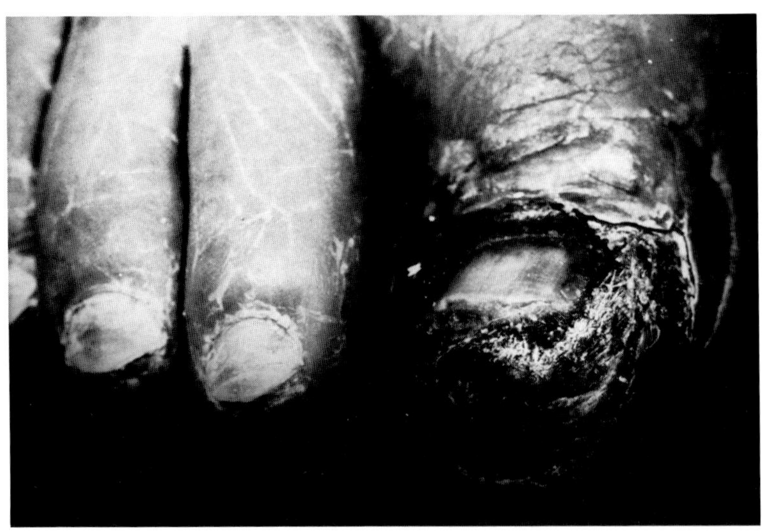

Fig. 10-10. Grade 4 foot. Gangrenous hallux with cellulitis.

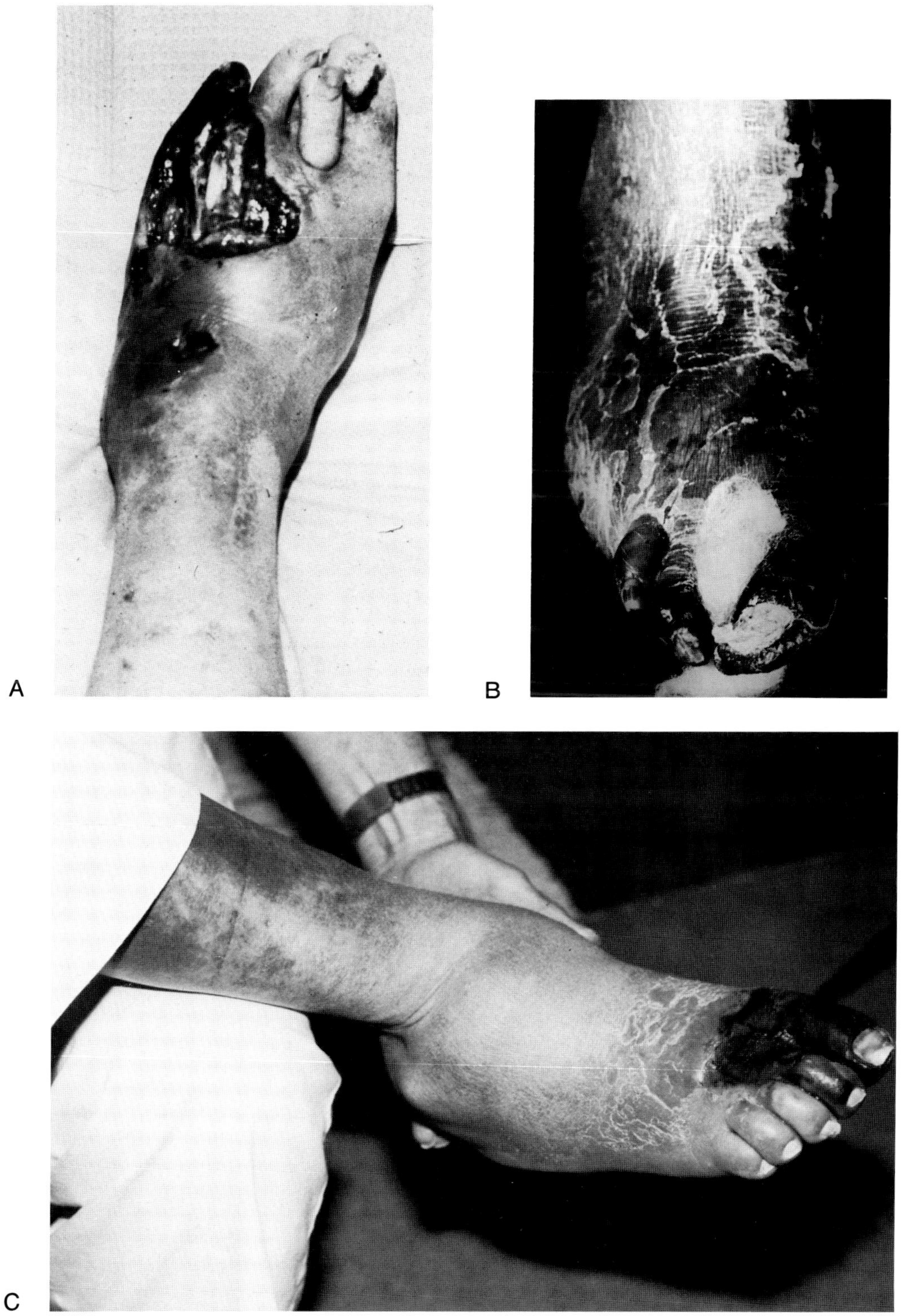

Fig. 10-11. Grade 5 feet. (A) Entire Charcot foot is involved with infection and necrosis. Below knee amputation was required. (B) Ischemic foot with extensive gangrene. (C) Severe Charcot ankle with gangrenous forefoot and cellulitis.

ratios.[63,151,153] Wagner reports that healing in the diabetic foot can be achieved with a 90 percent success rate when the ankle-brachial index is above 0.45 and when the grading system is used to properly direct treatment.[151] Elaborate algorithms have been devised to aid in the formulation of various treatment plans for each type of lesion with consideration given to ischemic versus well perfused feet, the presence of systemic toxicity, osteomyelitis, etc.[152] Although general principles of ulcer treatment will be discussed in the following section, Table 10-4 provides an overview of the treatment protocol for each foot grade.

Site of ulceration has not been found to be a useful determinant factor in prediction of outcome or in the development of treatment programs.[29,103,126] Apelqvist et al. recently reported that there was no appreciable difference in primary healing rates between the various sites of ulceration studied.[126] In contrast, there was clearly such a difference when the wounds were classified according to type and severity as used in the Wagner system. As a matter of interest, however, it is useful to document the distribution of diabetic foot lesions concomitantly with their wound classification. This same study revealed that the most common site of ulceration was on the digits (51 percent) with the great toe affected in 28 percent of the patients. Calhoun et al., in a study of 850 lesions, also found that 51 percent involved the phalanges, while the incidence of metatarsal lesions was 38 percent.[103] Although Ctercteko et al.[115] noted that most ulcers in their small series were located under the metatarsal heads, Edmonds et al. presented a review of 386 ulcers wherein most lesions of either neuropathic or ischemic etiologies were situated on the toes.[29] The location of the lesions are, however, helpful in ascertaining the direct cause of ulceration and accordingly, in their treatment and prevention. For example, a lesion on the dorsal apex of a hammertoe deformity is obviously a result of shoe pressure on the contracted digit (Fig. 10-12). Any treatment plan must therefore include eventual correction of the deformity or modification of footwear to provide more room in the toebox. If such preventive measures are not taken, the lesion will certainly recur.

TREATMENT

The treatment of diabetic foot ulcerations whether of neuropathic or ischemic origin need not be considered a complex undertaking. Each lesion must be individually assessed as to its etiology, vascularity, depth of penetration, extent of infection, and degree of neuropathy present using any classification system desired. Once these parameters are known, the subsequent treatment follows a

Table 10-4. Wagner Classification Treatment Protocol[a]

Grade 0	*Grade 1*	*Grade 2*	*Grade 3*	*Grade 4*	*Grade 5*
Proper shoes Education Podiatric care Prevention Self foot care Prophylactic surgery Antibiotics for cellulitis	Culture-directed antibiotics Wound care Radiographs Restrict or modify weight bearing (casting, healing sandals, padding, etc.) Bone resections p.r.n. Diabetes control	Same as grade 1 Assess soft tissue and bone thoroughly Probe for sinus tracts Deep debridement	Hospitalize I.V. antibiotics Deep I & D with debridement Metabolic control Scintigraphy Osteomyelitis Rx Joint and bone resections Plastic surgical closure p.r.n.	Same as grade 3 except for need of local amputation (determined by tissue viability and vascularity)	Major amputation required

[a] In each grade appropriate radiographic, clinical laboratory, and vascular assessment must be made. Vascular reconstruction should be performed as indicated in concert with the given treatment protocol. The goal of each grade (except 5) is to convert the foot to grade 0.

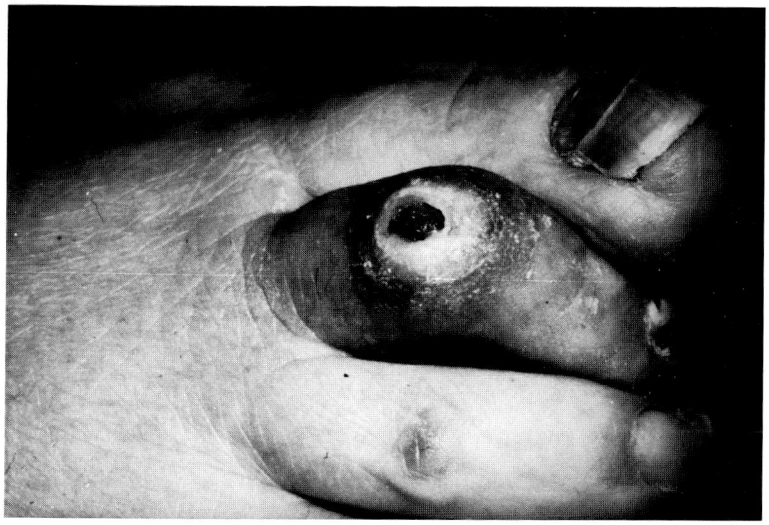

Fig. 10-12. Dorsal ulceration due to shoe pressure on the hammertoe.

logical progression aimed at promoting healing of the lesion through avoidance of further trauma or weight bearing, appropriate wound care, and control of infection and ischemia. Control of concurrent metabolic perturbations including hyperglycemia, renal failure and nutritional deficiencies are also paramount in the overall management of these patients.[148,154,155]

As mentioned earlier, neuropathic ulcers are typified by the presence of callus over and around the periphery of the lesion. In fact, ulcerations often underlie the thickened hyperkeratotic tissues that seemingly appear to be only discolored callosities. Only upon debridement and unroofing of the lesions can their true extent be determined. Ischemic ulcers by contrast are rather atrophic in appearance and do not generally exhibit callus formation. In both types there is a full thickness loss of epithelium down to a base of either a necrotic, fibrous appearance or one of abundant granulations. Every ulcer must be probed to ascertain the depths to which it penetrates (tendon, bone, joint, etc.), the extent of its borders, and to explore for hidden sinus tracts and abscess cavities (Fig. 10-13). All callous, necrotic, and devitalized tissue must be sharply debrided back to healthy, bleeding borders and all abscesses must be thoroughly drained. Removal of all eschar and the promotion of free drainage are of absolute necessity. Keratolytic and enzymatic debriding agents are of questionable value in this regard and should rarely, if ever, be used. Ulcers should never be soaked since this can macerate or even burn the compromised tissues and may even result in spreading the deep tissue bacteria.[89]

The severity of infection and extent of tissue necrosis are the two parameters working in conjunction with each other that most determine the exigency of the problem and need for hospitalization. If the infection is relatively mild and the ulcer is superficial, patients can be managed as out-patients provided they are compliant and have the visual acuity and family support to care for their foot lesion.[89] Aerobic and anaerobic cultures should be taken and the patient should be started on broad spectrum oral antibiotics. First-generation cephalosporins, antistaphylococcal penicillins, clindamycin, ciprofloxacin, and amoxicillin/clavulanate are reasonable choices to initiate therapy.[156–158] *Staphylococcus aureus, Staph. epidermidis,* enterococci, gram-negative enteric bacilli, and *Bacteroides fragilis* must always be the suspected pathogens.[96,156] The antibiotic agent should then be adjusted according to the culture and sensitivity results and the progress of the wound. It remains unclear as to the necessity for systemic antibiotic therapy for those stable, noncellulitic ulcers showing no sign of frank infec-

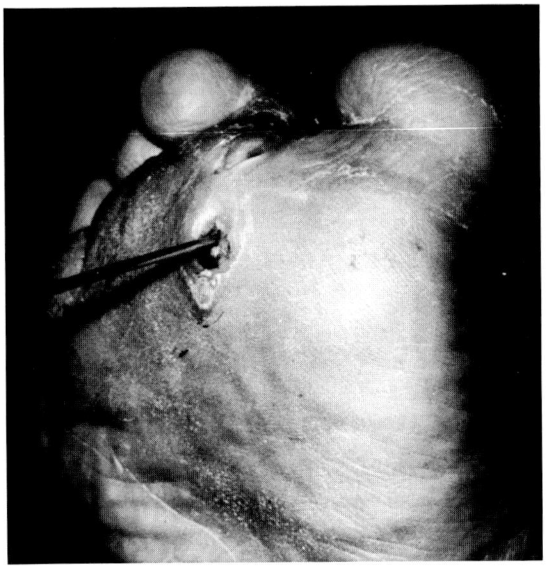

Fig. 10-13. Ulcer is probed to ascertain the proper depth and to detect sinus tracts. This 2-mm ulcer probed into the second metatarsophangeal joint.

tion.[156,159,160] Local wound care at this point should be directed at protecting it from further trauma and contamination, to contain wound drainage, and to provide topical antibacterial coverage that also serves to clean and debride the ulcer.[159,161] Recommended topical medications include one-quarter strength povidone-iodine solution or silver sulfadiazine cream. When applied once or twice daily and covered with a dry gauze pad, these agents are bactericidal and do not harm the healing tissues. Gentle mechanical debridement of surface eschar is also accomplished with each dressing change. For crusted lesions requiring frequent debridement, one-quarter strength Dakins solution might be employed since it is bactericidal and also aids in loosening necrotic debris.[161] Table 10-5 lists a variety of topical medications and special dressings that can be utilized in the management of these lesions.

Moderate or severely infected lesions probing to bone or joint (grade 3 and higher) frequently, although not always, demonstrate systemic signs of toxicity such as fever, malaise, loss of glucose control, and leukocytosis.[92] Immediate hospitalization for surgical debridement and drainage in addition to parenteral administration of antibiotics is required for these patients. Aggressive surgical therapy, including primary digital or forefoot amputations performed as drainage procedures will often lead to successful limb salvage even in patients with moderate ischemia.[90,98,162–164] Since approximately 70 percent of these infections are polymicrobial, antibiotic coverage should be quite broad initially to effectively treat the most common aerobic and anaerobic pathogens. Combination therapy is usually indicated since no agent can universally cover all species of *Pseudomonas, Proteus, Serratia,* enterococci, coagulase-positive and negative staphylococci, methicillin-resistant staphylococci, *Bacteroides* species, the anaerobic gram-positive cocci, etc. Although triple therapy including ampicillin, clindamycin, and gentamicin was once popular, there is a current consensus that aminoglycosides should be avoided to prevent renal toxicity in these susceptible patients.[156] Empiric therapy with newer agents such as ampicillin/sulbactam, ticarcillin/clavulanate, imipenem, or third-generation cephalosporins usually provide adequate initial coverage that should then be modified appropriately pending reliable culture and sensitivities.[97] The principles, rationale, and types of antibiotic therapy are fully discussed in Chapter 11.

A major determinant of the final outcome of the foot lesion is the degree of vascularity present in the involved extremity. Hence, vascular assessment plays a critical role in the overall management

Table 10-5. Topical Medications and Special Dressings

Topical medications
1/4-strength 1% povidone-iodine solution
1% silver sulfadiazene cream
Garramycin cream, bacitracin ointment, triple antibiotic ointment
1/4-strength Dakin's solution
Hydrogen peroxide
Special dressings
Occlusive hydrocolloids—Duoderm (ConvaTec), Tegasorb (3M)
Semiocclusive hydrogels—Spenco Secondskin (Spenco)
Semipermeable films—Op Site (Smith & Nephew), Bioclusive (Johnson & Johnson), Tegaderm (3M)
Nonadherent gauze—Adaptic (Johnson & Johnson), Telfa (Kendall)

of any diabetic foot lesion.[165] Each patient must be examined to ascertain the presence or absence of peripheral pulses, dependent rubor, delayed venous filling time, and temperature changes indicative of ischemia. If abnormalities are found, appropriate vascular diagnostic studies should be performed. The value of noninvasive vascular testing in the prediction of healing of foot lesions is well documented, ranging from Doppler-assisted segmental leg, ankle, and toe pressures, to duplex and color Doppler imaging, and to measurements of transcutaneous oxygen tension and laser Doppler flow.[166–176] A recent report by Apelqvist and colleagues indicates that the combined use of ankle and toe systolic pressure measurements is quite useful in this regard.[177] Although there was no upper limit of ankle pressure that would ensure primary healing (due to medial arterial calcification and incompressibility), no lesions healed primarily where ankle pressures fell below 40 mmHg. Conversely, there was no lower limit of toe blood pressure that could predict failure. However, 85 percent of their patients healed their ulcers primarily when systolic toe pressures exceeded 45 mmHg. Therefore, these two easily obtained parameters can be used together with a fairly high degree of confidence in determining the prognosis for healing of foot ulcers.

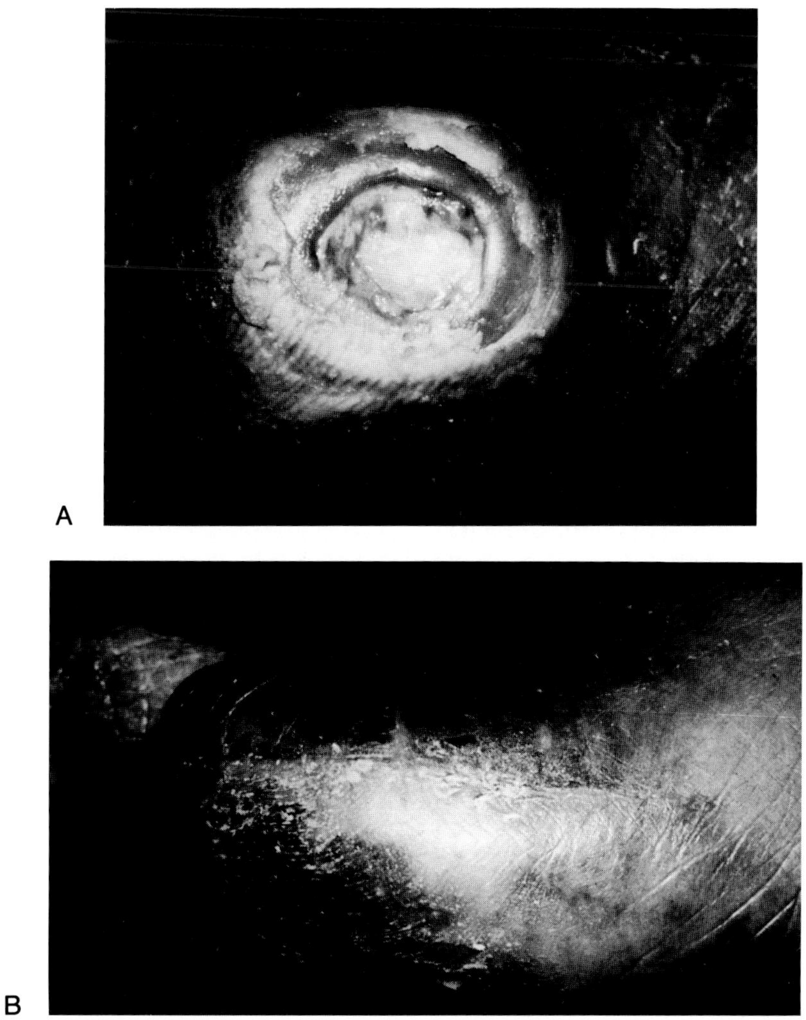

Fig. 10-14. (**A**) Nonhealing grade 2 ischemic ulcer. (**B**) After popliteal-dorsalis pedis bypass grafting the ulcer was successfully excised along with the underlying first metatarsal head.

When noninvasive arterial studies reveal inadequate perfusion to the foot, vascular surgery consultation is warranted to assess the need for angiography and subsequent arterial reconstruction. With improved operative techniques, greater experience, and widespread success with distal arterial reconstruction to the tibial, peroneal, and pedal vessels, the limb salvage rates in diabetic patients with threatened limb loss have ranged from 59 to 90 percent.[90,178–181] Successful antecedent bypass grafting not only minimizes subsequent levels of amputation in the gangrenous forefoot but also provides a restitution of perfusion to the foot adequate enough to allow local bone resections and podiatric reconstructive procedures[182] (Fig. 10-14).

Radiographic evaluation is, of course, a requisite part of treatment, which commences upon initial encounter with the patient. Both plain and magnification radiographs will reveal signs of cortical erosion indicative of osteomyelitis as well as areas of gas formation from undrained abscesses.[183,184] Cortical erosions and joint lesions must also be distinguished from diabetic osteolysis in the tubular bones of the forefoot and hypertrophic forms of osteoarthropathy found in the midfoot and solid bones of the rear foot.[185,186] Where the clinical history and findings are suggestive of either an infectious process or neuroarthropathy or both, scintigraphic studies are indicated. Contrasting the use of both three-phase bone scans and indium 111-labeled leukocyte scans in this situation, various researchers have found that leukocyte imaging has a significantly higher specificity for osteomyelitis.[187–190] Furthermore, uninfected osteoarthropathy does not accumulate the labeled white blood cells. Gallium imaging, although sensitive in areas of infection, also can be positive in Charcot joints and does not have the specificity of indium scanning.[188,189] Magnetic resonance imaging and computed tomography scans are also useful in the diagnosis of osteomyelitis and help differentiate infections of soft tissue only from those additionally involving bone.[191]

Once the infection is under control and adequacy of circulation has been established, definitive surgical treatment is required in those lesions with associated osteomyelitis, joint sepsis, gangrene, and extensive tissue loss. In grade 3 lesions with clinically apparent osteomyelitis or joint sepsis, joint resection is necessary to remove all infected bone and cartilage. In the first metatarsophalangeal joint the sesamoids should also be removed for this same reason. Conservative procedures such as this, including interphalangeal joint resections, can usually be successfully accomplished without the traditional need for digital, ray, or transmetatarsal amputations[192] (Fig. 10-15). A dorsal approach can be employed and closed primarily as long as the plantar ulcer is fully debrided and provides adequate drainage.[193] Prompt healing of the ulcer will usually ensue with local wound care consisting of light packing and topical antibacterial agents of choice. Persistent wound drainage and positive cultures portend an inadequate debridement of infected tissue, necessitating a repeat operation. When negative cultures are obtained, the systemic antibiotics can safely be discontinued.

An alternative method is to fully excise the ulcer and underlying bone through the same incision, which is then packed open and allowed to heal by secondary intention or delayed primary closure. Occasionally, primary closure of the excised ulcer may be employed where there is a minimum of drainage and necrosis in the well-vascularized foot. However, this wound must be monitored closely and opened promptly if drainage and cellulitis develop. In recent years this method has been combined with the temporary insertion of antibiotic-impregnated polymethylmethacrylate beads for both septic joints and osteomyelitis.[194–198] The beads are packed into the fully debrided cavity in close proximity to the infected bone. Since the wound is closed primarily, a very high bactericidal concentration of the antibiotic (usually gentamicin) is attained locally as it diffuses from the beads into the surrounding hematoma. After 1 to 2 weeks the beads are removed and the wound is once again sutured. Success is heralded by abundant granulations around the beads, a minimum of drainage, and sterile cultures. As necessary, the procedure may be repeated, the antibiotic changed, or augmented with other appropriate techniques.

Traditional treatment of osteomyelitis consists of a coordinated surgical and medical approach, with great emphasis placed on thorough debridement of necrotic bone and sequestra.[197,198] Aerobic and anaerobic bone cultures are mandatory to elucidate

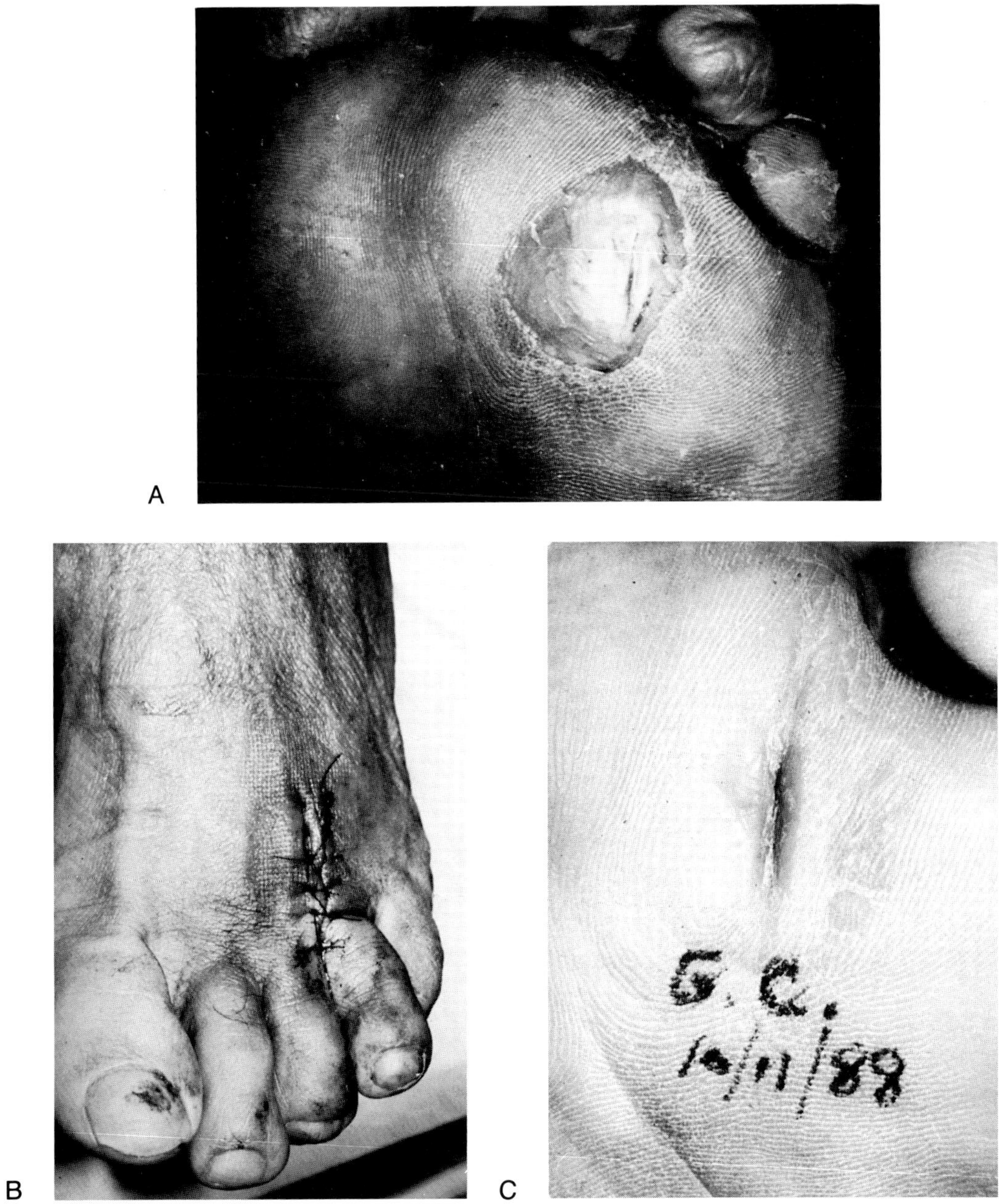

Fig. 10-15. (A) Chronic draining plantar ulcer probing into third and fourth metatarsophalangeal joints. (B) Resection of third and fourth metatarsophalangeal joints was performed through a dorsal incision. (C) Ulcer healed at one month with inverted scar.

the true underlying pathogens, since sinus tract cultures are known to be extremely unreliable.[107] Following adequate debridement, drainage, packing of cavities, and appropriate wound closure, culture directed parenteral antibiotic therapy is continued for 4 to 6 weeks. When infected bone is completely excised, as in the case of a metatarsal head, therapy may be ceased upon eradication of remaining soft tissue infection. Recent reports indicate that oral therapy alone or in addition to short-term intravenous antibiotic administration can be effective in treating osteomyelitis in the feet of diabetic patients.[197,199,200] Oral ciprofloxacin therapy has enjoyed a 60 to 76 percent success rate when administered for 3 months at high doses after conservative debridement of necrotic tissue.[158,201] When necessary, anaerobic coverage can be provided by adding oral metronidazole twice daily to this regimen. Although still under investigation, oral therapy has great potential benefit for improving the final outcome as well as decreasing both the stress and cost of treating patients with osteomyelitis.[158,197]

When the ulcers or soft tissue defects are either large or slow to heal, split thickness skin grafting can be utilized provided the bacterial counts are below 10^5 per gram of tissue.[159,160,202] Local muscle transpositions have been found helpful in providing a good base upon which to graft, even when performed primarily with the bone or joint resections[192,203,204] In ischemic extremities, such lesions can successfully be managed by combining distal revascularization with microvascular free muscle transfer and subsequent skin grafting.[205-207] This has been particularly useful for treating large defects of the ankle and heel with chronic osteomyelitis and exposure of bone and tendon. Relying on these reconstructive techniques rather than primary ablative surgery in the viable foot, major limb amputations and even minor amputations can be avoided in the majority of patients.[192,205]

For chronic or recurrent neuropathic ulcerations of the forefoot without osteomyelitis or joint infection, metatarsal osteotomies can often be successfully employed.[125,182,208] By elevating one that is plantarflexed or by shortening a long metatarsal, an osteotomy has the effect of reducing excessive pressures borne on the sole of the foot during ambulation (Fig. 10-16). Since sites of abnormally high pressures have been shown to correlate with ulcer formation,[43,115-116] reduction of these forces through the use of osteotomies can also promote healing of chronic ulcers as well as prevent their recurrence. Single or panmetatarsal head resections will have the same end result and often are performed when a simple osteotomy proves unsuccessful in healing a plantar lesion.[193,209,210] When transfer lesions develop secondary to prior surgery on a single metatarsal or when recurrent ulcerations develop despite conservative care, Giurini et al. have found that panmetatarsal head resections have an extremely favorable long-term success rate in preventing further ulceration.[209] For pressure lesions occurring in other sites, such as under Charcot deformities of the midfoot, simple excision of the bony prominence should be contemplated in the well-perfused foot[153,211-213] (Fig. 10-17).

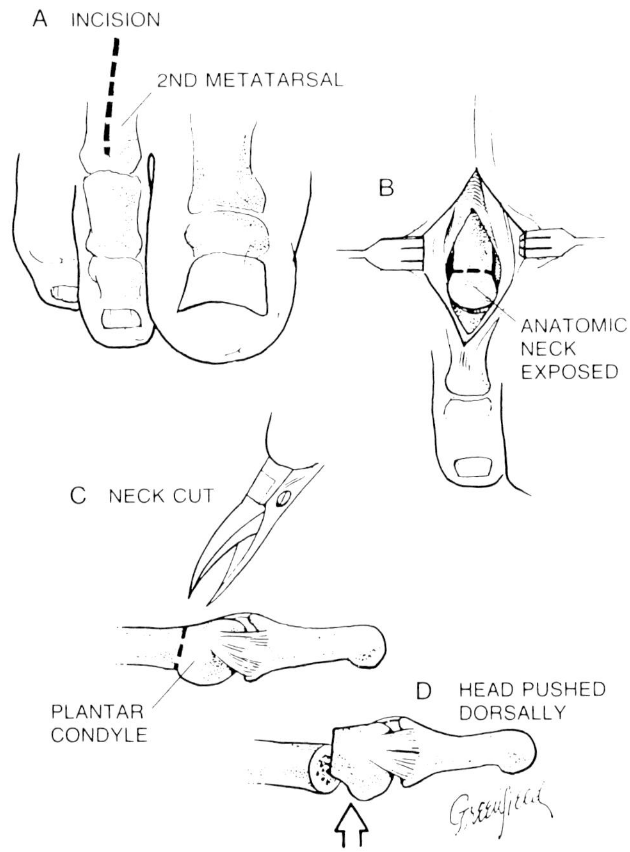

Fig. 10-16. Second metatarsal osteotomy. **(A)** Dorsal incision placed over the head and neck of the metatarsal. **(B)** Longitudinal capsulotomy exposes the anatomical neck. Dotted line represents the location of the transverse osteotomy. **(C)** Osteotomy must be performed proximal to the plantar condyles. **(D)** The head is pushed dorsally to reduce the plantarflexed position. (From Frykberg,[182] with permission.)

Digital amputations for localized gangrene of the lesser toe(s) with or without ischemia will often permit a fairly rapid recovery with minimal alterations in foot mechanics and a good long-term

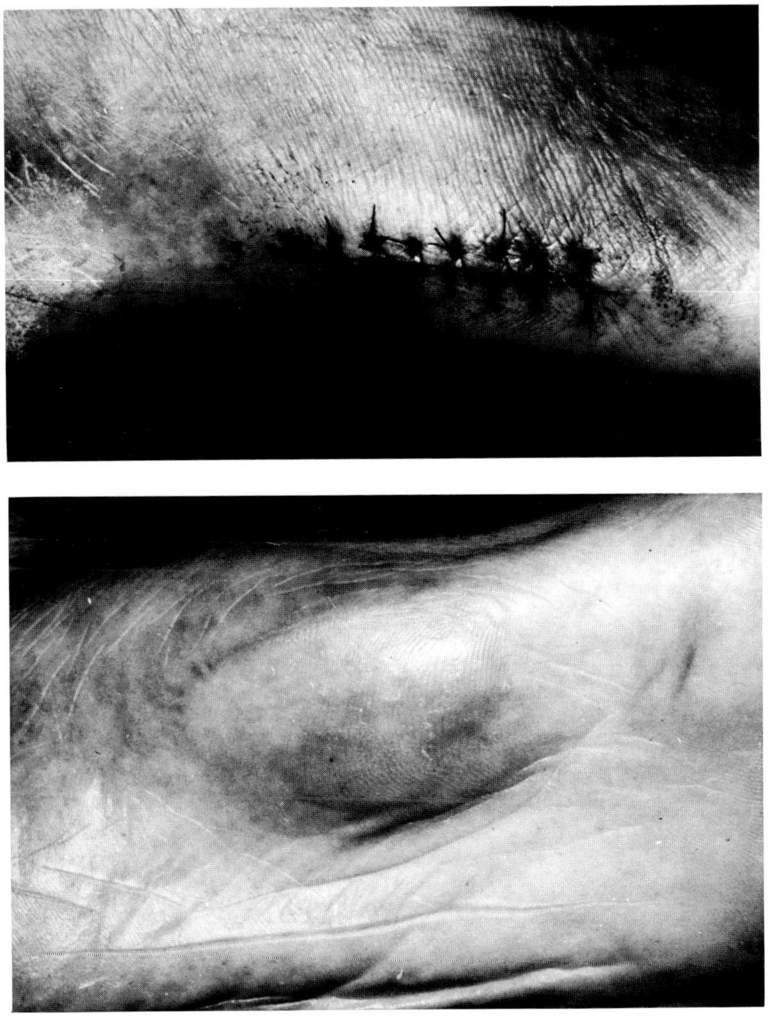

Fig. 10-17. (A) One-week post excision Charcot navicular exostosis for recurrent ulceration. (B) At 2-year follow-up there was no recurrence.

prognosis.[127,214–217] In their large series, Sizer and Wheelock reported only a 2.2 percent failure rate when pedal pulses were present as opposed to an 11 percent failure rate in the absence of palpable pedal pulses.[214] Hodge and associates in 1989 also report favorable results for distal amputation even in the presence of ischemia and make a plea for conservatism in this regard as related to limb salvage.[216] If the ulcer only involves part of the toe such as the interphalangeal joint, a resection arthroplasty can usually be performed that will save the toe from needless amputation (Fig. 10-18). Success depends not only upon the vascularity of the toe but also upon removing all cartilage from both sides of the joint, which may harbor bacteria.

Hallux amputations can result in more significant biomechanical alterations and should be avoided when not necessitated by gangrene or ischemia. Ulceration commonly affects the great toe and has frequently been attributed to hallux limitus.[218–219] Such lesions have been quite effectively managed by resection of the base of the proximal hallucal phalanx, thereby providing an increased amount of available dorsiflexion to the great toe.[220–221] When the metatarsophalangeal joint is directly involved

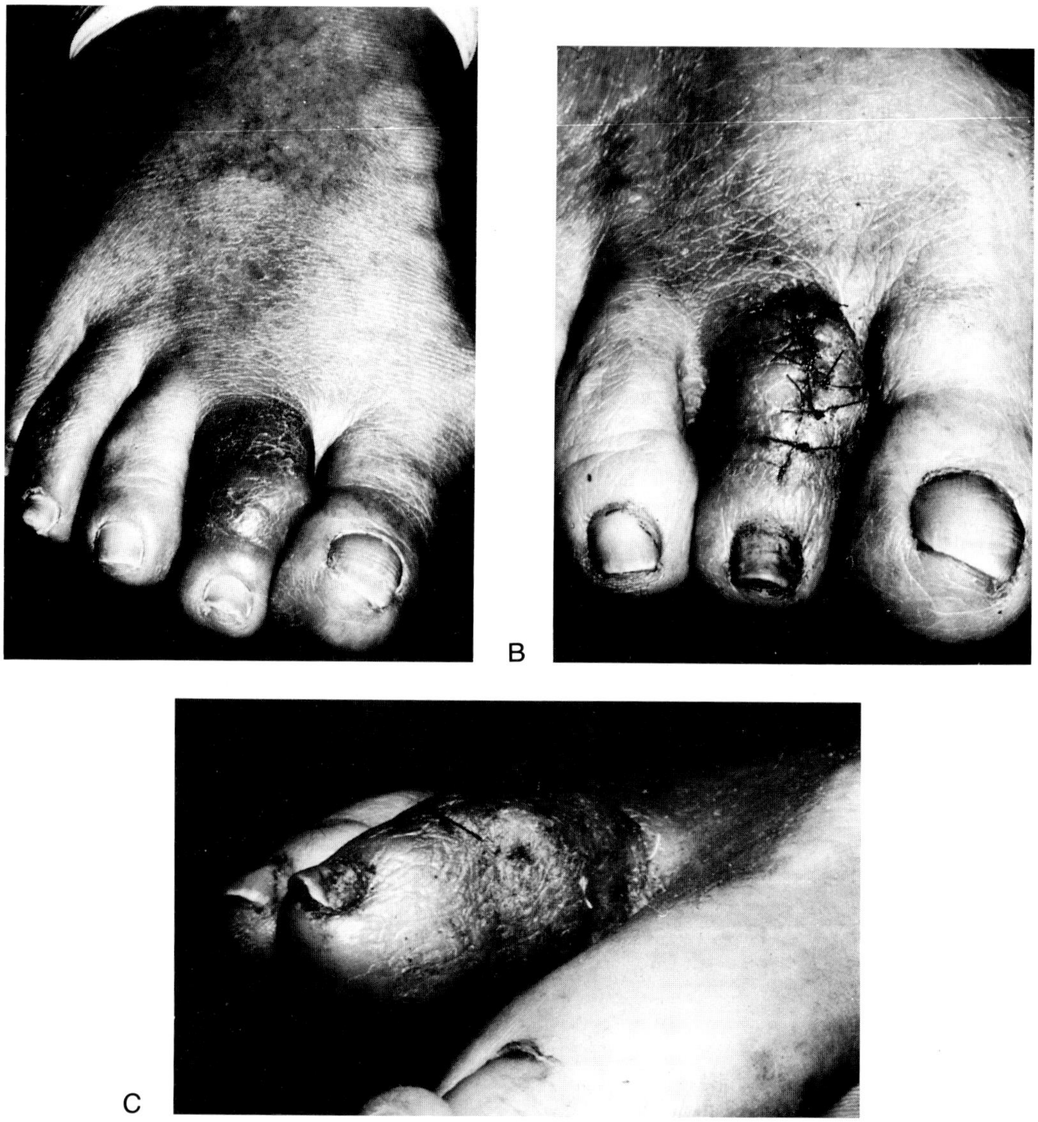

A B C

Fig. 10-18. (**A**) Cellulitis of second toe with recurrent medial ulcer involving the proximal interphalangeal joint. Culture was positive for *Staph. epidermidis.* (**B**) Interphalangeal joint resection under local anesthesia obviated the need for toe amputation. (**C**) Drainage ceased and ulcer closed within two weeks.

with the ulceration, the Keller arthroplasty should be combined with a first metatarsal head resection and removal of both sesamoids (Fig. 10-19). Nonhealing lesions directly plantar to the first metatarsal head usually respond well to excision only of the underlying sesamoid bone as long as there is no joint sepsis present.

Amputation of any part of the foot or extremity is one of the most feared consequences of diabetes. As the patient sees it, the loss of one digit or part of a foot will eventually lead to amputation more proximally or contralaterally. Unfortunately, this has indeed been the case in diabetic patients. Klamer et al. determined that 34 percent of diabetic patients who develop foot lesions will require a major amputation.[222] Moreover, their re-

A B C

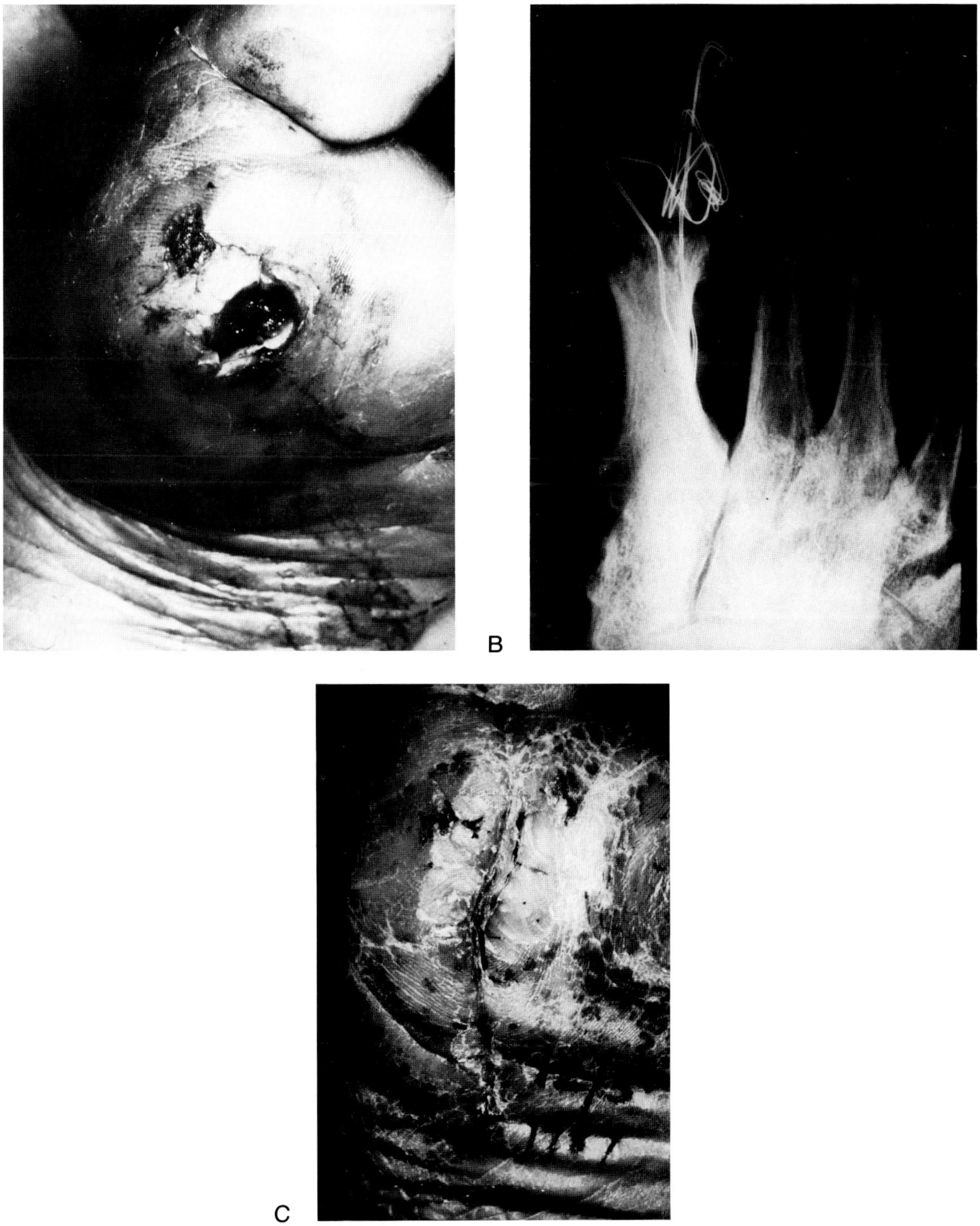

Fig. 10-19. (**A**) Grade 3 ulcer with infected first metatarsophalangeal joint. (**B**) Radiograph demonstrating resection of base of phalanx, first metatarsal head, and sesamoids with implantation of gentamicin beads. Lesser rays had previously been amputated. (**C**) Healed plantar incision.

sults corroborate the findings of Kucan and Robson in that approximately 50 percent of the patients with foot lesions will develop lesions of the other foot as well.[109] Fortunately, the management of diabetic foot lesions in recent years has focused on *limb preservation* through distal revascularization, early control of sepsis, conservative distal amputations, reconstructive foot surgery, and prevention.[90,159,178–179,192,200,216] Prediction of healing of foot lesions as well as amputation levels has been greatly augmented by the use of transcutaneous oxygen tension measurements and laser Doppler velocimetry in addition to standard measurements of segmental systolic pressures down to the toes.[172,175–177,223] Trials of hyperbaric oxygen therapy for the treatment of diabetic foot lesions have given conflicting results to date and the role of this modality is still a matter of debate.[224–228] Apparently, however, there is a consensus that topical oxygen therapy is of little value in the realm of limb salvage and that only systemic hyperbaric oxygen therapy will be efficacious in this regard.

Although the number of major amputations should continue to decline in future years, it is unfortunate that there will still be a need for partial foot amputation in the scheme of high risk foot management and limb salvage. The various types of amputations performed on the diabetic lower extremity, their indications, and techniques are fully discussed in Chapter 17.

Conservative Management and Footwear Considerations

Any type of ulceration must, above all else, be treated with rest and avoidance of pressure.[182] All treatment methods that allow ambulation on the affected foot must therefore be considered only second best to complete non-weight-bearing. In today's society, however, long periods of bed rest or hospitalization are generally unacceptable to both patients and third-party payors alike. Consequently, ambulatory treatment methods for diabetic foot ulcers must be considered an integral part of the overall care given to such lesions.

Since most neuropathic lesions are the result of chronic repetitive stress sustained during ambulation, some accommodation must be made to the footwear or insole or both.[129] For dorsal or lateral lesions of the toes and forefoot, a simple hole cut out of the shoe over the affected site can often expedite healing. As discussed in Chapters 23 and 24, a variety of pressure attenuation methods can be employed to redistribute the weight-bearing forces across the plantar surface of the foot in an attempt to "off-load" the site of ulceration. Such devices as rocker bottom shoes, metatarsal bars, accommodative insoles in extra-depth shoes, and a variety of foot orthoses are frequently successful in this regard. Brenner reported favorable results with the use of a platform shoe that extends the heel anteriorly to just behind the metatarsal heads.[229–230] However, it is frequently necessary to fabricate temporary healing sandals to promote healing of the lesion.[182] These sandals are easily fabricated in the office from a heat-molded total contact Plastazote insert placed in a postoperative surgical shoe (Figs. 10-20 and 10-21). They provide accommodation of the pressure lesions, an even redistribution of pressure across the entire plantar surface of the foot, and force the patient to take shorter, nonpropulsive steps with a subsequent reduction in shear and vertical forces. The sole of the foot is protected plantarly and the toes are free from pressure dorsally. Once healing has occurred, the inserts can be modified and transferred into extra-depth shoes for continued protection and support.[63] Commercially available healing shoes can be dispensed in place of the custom-made healing sandal when appropriate and can be retained as slippers or house shoes for long-term protection (Fig. 10-22). Running shoes have also been found to be efficacious in the reduction of excessive callus formation and putatively are effective in the prevention of primary and recurrent ulcerations that might result from these hyperkeratotic pressure lesions.[231,232] When severe foot deformity precludes the use of regular footwear or

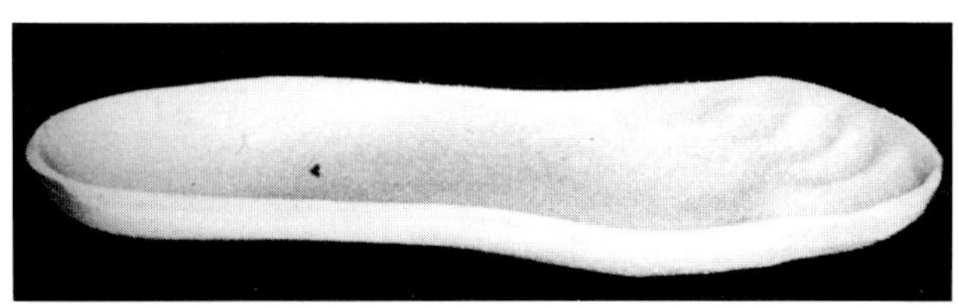

Fig. 10-20. Heat-molded Plastazote insert.

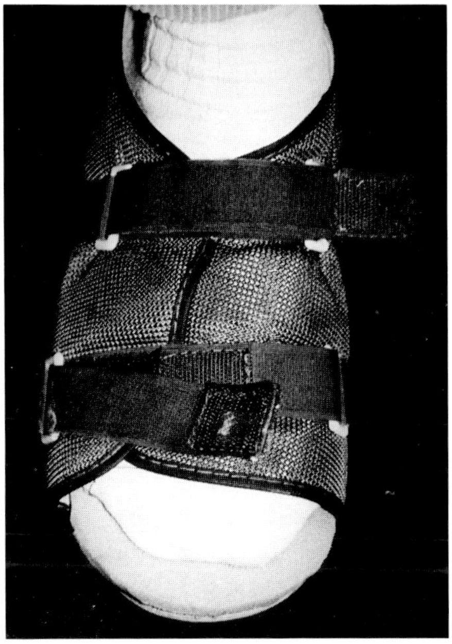

Fig. 10-21. Healing sandal. Plastazote insert placed into a Darco postoperative shoe.

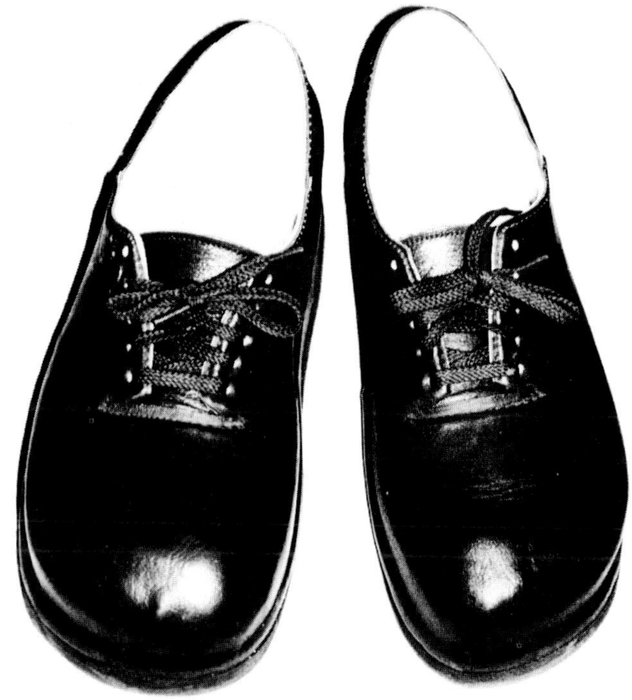

Fig. 10-23. Custom-made "molded" shoes.

when the aforementioned shoe modifications prove ineffective, custom-made "molded" shoes are indicated to prevent ulcer recurrence (Fig. 10-23).

On occasion, accommodative aperture pads may be used in lieu of healing sandals or special insoles to disperse the pressure to surrounding tissues.[182,233] An adhesive foam pad ⅛ to ¼ inch in thickness with a central aperture is secured around the ulcer with paper tape (Fig. 10-24). A topical

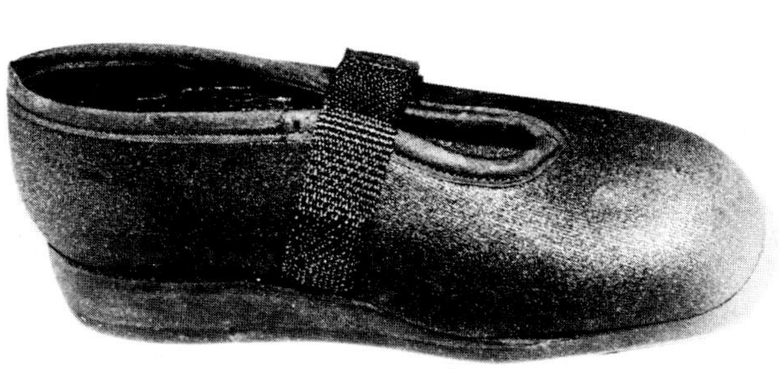

Fig. 10-22. Commercially available healing shoes used during ulcer treatment can later be used as house shoes or slippers.

antibacterial agent is applied to the ulcer and a sterile gauze pad is then taped in place over the ulcer and pad. The patient cares for the lesion daily and changes only the overlying gauze pad. The foam pad is then changed by the treating physician weekly during visits for debridement and evaluation until the ulcer has healed.

Total contact casting has gained widespread popularity and success in the management of neuropathic ulcerations, especially for those on the forefoot.[63,113,129,153,234-235] Average duration of casting until healing is usually reported in the range of 4 to 6 weeks regardless of ulcer duration prior to cast therapy.[234,236-239] The basic premise behind casting is that when immobilized with this specific technique, there is a significant reduction in both shear and vertical force to the site(s) of high pressure, a rapid reduction of edema, and an even redistribution of forces across the sole of the foot.[63,114,239-241] While remaining ambulatory, patients with uncomplicated ulcerations can therefore heal their lesions fairly rapidly and with a minimum of care at home. Total contact casting is not,

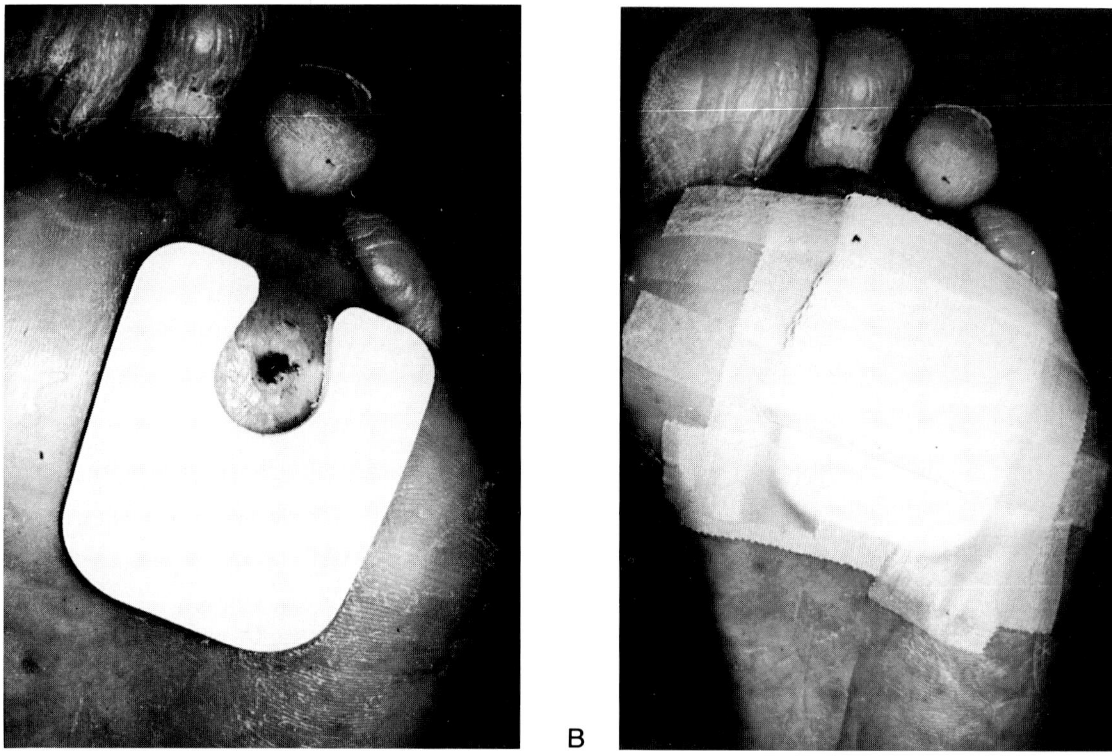

A B

Fig. 10-24. (**A**) Aperture pad surrounding an ulcer disperses weight away from the lesion. (**B**) Gauze pad taped in place over the aperture pad is changed daily.

however, without certain inherent dangers and must be utilized with caution as well as expertise. The technique of cast application, its indications, contraindications, and complications are fully discussed in Chapter 22.

Variations of total contact casting have been utilized with generally good results. Diamond and associates have successfully employed a molded double-rocker plaster shoe in a patient for whom below knee contact casting was contraindicated due to fragile skin of the lower leg.[242] The technique differs from the traditional cast in that it extends only to the level of the ankle. Along the same lines, Burden et al. have described their favorable experience with the "Scotchcast boot." [243,244] This consists of a lightly padded boot enclosed by a shell of fiberglass casting tape with a window cut out over the ulcer to facilitate dressing changes. The ankle is not enclosed by the fiberglass so that ambulation can be accomplished with the use of a surgical shoe or rocker-bottom shoe.

Another casting variation not previously described is this author's technique utilizing an Unna boot in combination with a single roll of fiberglass casting tape (Fig. 10-25). The uncomplicated plantar ulcer is thoroughly debrided and silver sulfadiazine cream is applied topically. After protecting the toes with lambswool interdigitally, a small sheet of ⅛-inch pink plastazote is folded loosely over them to provide dorsal, distal, and plantar protection. The zinc oxide – impregnated bandage is rolled lightly over the entire foot and ankle, directly covering the ulcer and completely enclosing the toes. Extra reinforcement is given to the heel and forefoot areas. Next, a 3- or 4-inch stockinette is pulled over the Unna boot underlayer. A single roll of 4-inch fiberglass casting tape is then applied from the toes to just below the malleoli, firmly but not snugly, giving reinforcement also to the plantar aspect of the heel and forefoot. For large feet or heavier patients an additional roll might be required. Once set, the fiberglass is trimmed at the

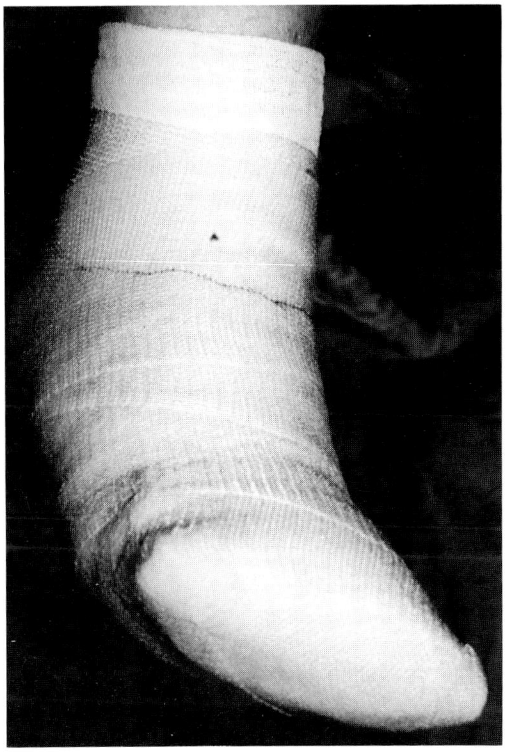

Fig. 10-25. Unna/fiberglass boot prior to trimming around ankle. See text for fabrication details.

ankle so that the malleoli and immediate dorsum of the foot are covered only by the Unna boot and stockinette. The rough edges should be covered with elastoplast tape. This cast will allow motion at the ankle and permit the patient to ambulate in a surgical shoe within 30 minutes. It should be changed weekly since the single layer of fiberglass will not withstand long periods of use. Patients find this boot cosmetically acceptable, relatively lightweight, and rather easy to walk upon as compared to other types of casts. The results obtained are similar to those of the Scotchcast boot with an additional benefit of excellent hydration of the skin due to the direct application of the zinc oxide bandage. As with any casting method, caution must be exercised to prevent iatrogenic pressure lesions due to pistoning or from wrapping the layers too tightly. Furthermore, its use cannot be recommended on ischemic feet.

Prefabricated walking casts have become commercially available from various manufacturers. Initially intended for post-traumatic or postoperative use, they can be used for treating neuropathic ulcers and osteoarthropathy as well. The Aircast (Aircast Incorporated, Summit, NJ) is one such example that has been used quite effectively for the former conditions.[245] Its use in the diabetic neuropathic foot has met with limited success (unpublished data). The primary advantage of prefabricated casts aside from the obvious benefit of easy application is that they are removable. Hence, the foot and wound can be inspected and cared for daily by the patient. Since this type of device is not custom-made, one must be quite certain that it is wide enough so as not to cause impingement on either the medial or lateral border of the affected foot. Additional padding on the foot plate is usually required to provide adequate cushioning and total contact weight dispersion as in the healing sandal.

PREVENTION

Prevention *must* be considered the key element in effecting a reduction in the incidence of recurrent or primary diabetic foot lesions, and consequently, in the number of lower extremity amputations. This consists not only of comprehensive regular foot care and examinations but also of patient education, professional education, and specialized shoes or footwear modifications.[2,4,15–19,29,246–250]

The role of a specialized foot clinic and accordingly, podiatric care, in the preservation of the diabetic foot has been well established by Edmonds[2,29,249] and others.[4,18,19] At the Diabetic Foot Clinic of the King's College Hospital, a systematic and coordinated approach to foot lesions resulted in the healing of 86 percent of neuropathic ulcers and 72 percent of ischemic ulcers.[249] Intensive podiatric care was an essential part of both treatment and prevention. The recurrence of ulceration was significantly reduced by the use of special footwear. The rate of recidivism was 83 percent in those patients insistent on wearing their own shoes, while it was only 26 percent for those patients who agreed to wear specially constructed or modified shoes. Furthermore, the number of amputations performed annually was reduced by more than 50 percent within 3 years after the initiation of this program. Davidson reported similar results at the Grady Memorial Hospital in Atlanta after instituting both comprehensive podiatry services as well as an extensive patient education program.[18] Finding that foot care saved more limbs than vascular surgery, Lippman recounted that no amputations occurred in his elderly population following the introduction of a foot care program.[19] The previous yearly amputation rate had been 8 to 15 percent. Figure 10-26 depicts the suggested composition of a comprehensive diabetic foot service that should be considered only one facet of an overall management program for diabetic patients. Table 10-6 lists the essential components of a prevention-oriented foot care program embraced by the diabetic foot service.

Patient education is also an essential element in the prevention and treatment of foot lesions. As part of the Memphis Diabetes Continuing Care Program, patient education coupled with other prevention-oriented strategies resulted in a 67 percent reduction in hospitalization for lower extremity amputation.[251] Assal et al., studying the impact of diabetes patient education on therapy and complications, found that an *85 percent reduction* in below knee amputations was achieved at the University Hospital of Geneva due to a specific foot care teaching program.[252] Conversely, Rosenqvist determined that two-thirds of a randomized sample of diabetic patients living in Stockholm County had moderate or severe foot disease.[25] However, only 54 percent with severe foot disease sought professional foot care by a podiatrist, physician, or nurse despite the fact that 72 percent of these same patients found it difficult to take care of their own feet. These statistics imply a failure to educate the very patients who need it most and who are at the greatest risk for lower extremity amputation. Delbridge et al. have shown that patients who developed foot lesions had significantly less knowledge of their diabetes and its complications as well as a lack of understanding of proper foot care.[16] Diabetic patients without a history of foot disease understood more about diabetes, its management,

Table 10-6. Essential Elements of a Prevention-Oriented Foot Care Program

Initial foot screening history and examination
Determination of risk status
Regular podiatric examinations and prophylactic care
Patient education on foot care techniques, daily inspection, potential problems, and need for early intervention
Consultation with specialty services and laboratory testing as needed
Use of modified footwear, orthoses, or custom shoes

(Modified from Bild et al,[4] with permission.)

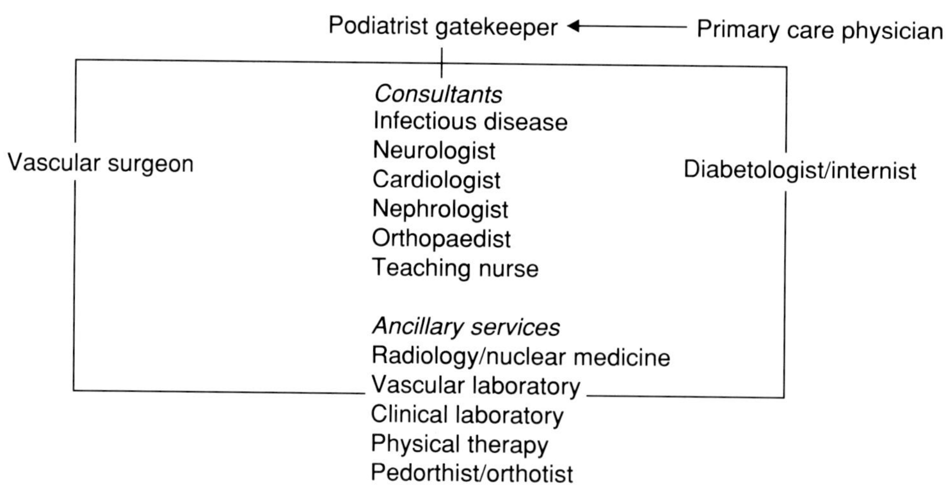

Fig. 10-26. Suggested scheme for the composition of a coordinated diabetic foot service.

and the care of their feet than those persons with active or prior foot lesions. In addition to the suggested protective effect of patient education in avoiding foot lesions, they also correctly give credence to the psychological denial of such lesions, termed *willful self-neglect* by Walsh et al.[13] Recognizing the importance of foot care education, the Committee on Practice of the American Diabetes Association has recommended that all patients with evidence of sensory neuropathy (or other risk factors) should be educated about the risk and prevention of foot problems.[253]

Physician education and the education of all staff concerned with the management of patients with diabetes are also important factors in the degree of prevention exercised in practice. Bailey and coworkers studied the patterns and incidence of foot examination in a diabetes clinic.[254] They found that in a one-day study of 65 patients, only 12.3 percent had their feet examined, whereas the prevalence of foot examination in the previous year was 49.2 percent. The most significant determinants for foot examination were physician variability, clinic protocol, and patient recall of foot education regarding prevention. Cohen, in another study of physicians' foot examination habits, reported that such an examination took place for only 60 percent of the patients.[14] When the patients presented with bare feet they were examined from 65 to 72 percent of the time. When they presented to the physician with shoes and socks on, however, the incidence of foot examination was only 15 to 19 percent. In yet a more recent retrospective study of diabetic patients, only 55 percent of the patients had a recorded foot examination including that subset who were referred to the podiatry clinic.[255] These researchers found, as the others had before them, that preventive care and examinations were underutilized and not a part of routine primary care encounters with diabetic patients. Since approximately 50 percent of lower extremity amputations can be avoided by effective, prevention-oriented foot care, it is critical that all health care providers be educated in this regard. At the very least, all diabetic patients should be instructed to remove both shoes and stockings at each physician visit. This can be reinforced by instituting a clinic or office protocol requiring the same for each patient encounter.[14]

FOOT SCREENING

An essential part of the prevention program for diabetic patients should be the foot screening examination.[23,130] Foot screenings should be performed for every newly diagnosed patient with diabetes, and at least annually thereafter for those patients who do not regularly see a podiatrist. While not intended to supplant the necessity for foot examination at every visit with the physician, the comprehensive foot evaluation is designed to ascertain the condition of the foot and assess its risk status. Once a level of risk for foot injury or ulceration has been determined, appropriate management schemes including footwear recommendations can be followed to prevent such lesions (see Chapter 24).

Aside from the obvious visual inspection of the foot necessary to detect present or impending lesions and structural deformities, the screening examination should also consist of in-depth neurologic and vascular assessment (Table 10-7). The role of impaired vibratory perception in the etiology of foot ulceration has been well documented.[256] Accordingly, objective testing of this sensory parameter with a biothesiometer (Biomedical Instruments, Newburg, OH) has been found useful in identifying those patients at risk of foot ulceration.[43,117,256,257] Recent reports suggest that measurements of current perception thresholds (CPT) may be equally effective in this regard.[258,259] Others propose that testing cutaneous pressure sensation (aesthesiometry) with Semmes-Weinstein monofilaments is the easiest and most discriminating method of detecting patients in danger of neuropathic ulceration.[130,248,260] Holewski et al. have determined that the inability to detect a monofilament of 5.07 log (0.1 mg) force, equal to 10 g of linear pressure, implies a loss of protective sensation and is considered the risk discriminator level.[260] Thermal sensitivity testing, electrodiagnostic studies, and a variety of tests of autonomic nerve function have also been recommended by the panelist of the San Antonio Conference on Diabetic Neuropathy[28] and others[47,130,261–262] to quantitatively evaluate the status of peripheral nerve function in these patients.

Vascular evaluation should consist not only of

Table 10-7. The Foot Screening Examination

Parameter	*Clinical Examination*	*Objective Testing*
Skin	Visual inspection: lesions, scars, calluses, interdigital maceration paronychia, fungal nails	C&S, fungal cultures
Sensory	Pinprick sensation Light touch Vibration Proprioception	Biothesiometry Semmes-Weinstein monofilaments Thermal discrimination test
Motor	Wasting, weakness, foot drop, limp Absent tendon reflexes	Electrophysiologic testing
Autonomic	Absent sweating Dryness, fissuring Distended dorsal veins	Quantitative sweat test Transcutaneous oximetry Laser Doppler velocimetry
Vascular	Leg and foot pulses Rubor/pallor Venous/capillary filling Skin temperature	Noninvasive Doppler studies Photoplethysmography Thermography Infrared thermometry
Deformity	Hammertoes, hallux valgus Prominent metatarsal heads Charcot deformity	Radiographs Scintigraphy Plantar pressure assessment

(Modified from Boulton,[23] with permission.)

venous and capillary filling times, tests for dependent rubor, and the status of pedal and leg pulses, but when diminished, should also include noninvasive arterial Doppler testing. In addition to the standard appraisal of the ankle-brachial systolic pressure index (ABI) wherein normal values equal 1.0 to 1.1, various researchers have also found systolic toe pressures to be useful in determining adequacy of distal perfusion.[70,168,171,172,177] Falsely elevated ABIs occur in diabetic patients due to medial calcification, perhaps more so in those patients treated with insulin.[263] Therefore, arterial wall stiffness may mask underlying peripheral vascular disease in these patients. To avoid misinterpretation of vascular laboratory results, one must always reconcile these with the corresponding clinical and radiographic findings. Thermography has been reported useful in determining temperature variations within the feet.[264,265] Stess and co-workers demonstrated significantly increased skin temperatures and identifiable thermographic emission patterns in neuropathic diabetic patients with active or past histories of ulceration.[264] Putatively, this modality can therefore be useful in screening for those diabetic patients at risk of ulceration.

Increased pressure, both vertical and shear, is a major factor in the causation of ulceration when coexistent with neuropathy and/or other risk factors.[16,31,43,115] Measurements of plantar pressures have been rather consistent in the feet of diabetic patients with neuropathy and previous history of ulceration wherein significantly higher pressures are found than in the feet of nondiabetic controls and diabetic patients without neuropathy.[43,115–117,122,266] Accordingly, evaluation of plantar pressures in both static and dynamic phases of gait should be a recommended part of the screening examination to identify those patients in a high risk category.[235] The Harris and Beath footprinting mat is an inexpensive method of documenting areas of excessive pressures and can easily be done in the office.[267] More sophisticated computerized systems include the Pedobarograph (Biokinetics, Bethesda, MD), the EMED system (Novel Electronics, Inc., Minneapolis, MN), and the Electrodynogram (Langer Biomechanics, Deer Park,

NY). A complete discussion of the various pressure assessment methods can be found in Chapter 9.

RISK ASSESSMENT

Once evaluated, the patient should be assigned into a foot risk status or category. Such a categorization enables the treating physician to appropriately develop a treatment, education, and prevention program for the patient according to level of risk and need. The simplest approach is to identify those patients with any previously mentioned risk factor (neuropathy, ischemia, deformity, decreased visual acuity, etc.) and assign them to an "at risk" category.[23] This group of patients requires regular podiatric care for reasons of prophylaxis as well as early detection and treatment of complications attendant with the high risk diabetic foot. Continual education in all aspects of the diabetic foot with emphasis on prevention must be considered an essential part of their care. Patients with apparently healthy feet are placed into a normal or "not at risk" category with the understanding that periodic examinations are necessary to detect any changes in their status. These patients should receive general advice on foot care and be educated in the importance of such care as it relates to prevention and the early recognition of impending problems.

Others have proposed more detailed foot risk classification systems according to the presence of insensitivity, deformity, previous ulceration, active bone destruction, or high plantar pressures.[130,235,268] However, these authors did not also address the significant risk factor of ischemia in their categorizations. Taking all these factors into consideration, a suggested risk status classification is listed in Table 10-8. Since diabetes mellitus alone is a potential risk factor, diabetic patients with healthy feet and no deformity should be assigned to risk status 1. Patients with normal sensation who also have deformity (hammertoes, bunions, etc.) or high plantar pressures (often manifesting as callosities) are put into risk category 2 due to the potential for future ulceration. Documentation of sensory neuropathy as previously described without deformity or high plantar pressures would place the patient into risk status 3. Patients in risk category 4 have ischemia as the primary finding without evidence of insensitivity or deformity. Those patients with a combination of risk factors including neuropathy, ischemia, deformity, or high plantar pressures are most at risk and are assigned a risk status of 5. Also included in this category are patients with a prior history of ulceration, ipsilateral or contralateral amputation, and those with active or quiescent neuroarthropathy.

Table 10-8. Risk Status Classification

1. Normal sensation with no deformity
2. Normal sensation with deformity (or high plantar pressures)
3. Insensitivity without deformity
4. Ischemia without deformity
5. Complicated
    - Combination insensitivity, ischemia, and/or deformity
    - Prior history of ulceration
    - Charcot deformity

Obviously, patients with more significant levels of risk will require more frequent and comprehensive care. Whereas patients in risk category 1 might require examination only once or twice per year (in addition to foot care instructions and preventive education), patients with the highest risk feet require routine visits and podiatric care every 4 to 8 weeks as individual circumstances warrant. Great emphasis must also be placed on preventive education, recognizing the prevalence of denial in these patients and the difficulties encountered when one attempts to change their behavioral patterns.[23] Patient education in foot care can be considered the single most important element in preventing diabetic foot lesions and subsequent amputation.[248] Hence, foot care guidelines such as those listed in Table 10-9 should be given to each patient and more importantly, should be discussed at each encounter.

Special attention to footwear has been identified as a major factor in the prevention of recurrent ulceration.[29] For those patients with minimal deformity, a running shoe or similar type of footwear might be suggested since these have been found to measurably reduce the size of plantar calluses in a diabetic patient population.[231,232] Additionally,

Table 10-9. Foot Care Guidelines

1. Inspect your feet daily for blisters, bleeding, and lesions between toes. Use a mirror to see the bottom of the foot and the heel.
2. Have a family member or friend check them if you are unable to.
3. Have regular foot examinations by your podiatrist or physician.
4. Always remove both shoes and stockings when visiting your doctor.
5. Always wear well-fitted stockings or socks with your shoes. Padded hosiery may reduce pressure and be more protective.
6. Inspect the soles and inside your shoes for foreign objects before putting them on.
7. Shoes should be properly measured, comfortable, and easy to put on at the time of purchase. There should be no "break-in" period.
8. Wear leather shoes with adequate room for the toes. Running or athletic shoes are best for recreational walking.
9. Change shoes every 4 to 6 hours.
10. In cold weather wear insulated boots or heavier socks. Be sure the shoes allow enough room to allow for heavier socks.
11. Do not walk barefooted in the house, outside, or at the beach. This also includes steam rooms and saunas.
12. Do not use hot water bottles or heating pads to warm your feet. Use warm socks instead.
13. Do not soak your feet.
14. Do not use acids or chemical corn removers.
15. Do not perform "bathroom surgery" on corns, calluses, or ingrown toenails.
16. Wash feet daily and be sure to dry well between the toes. Apply moisturizing cream liberally, but avoid between toes.
17. Test the temperature of your bathwater with your elbow or a thermometer. Do not let hot water drip on toes.
18. Trim your nails straight across and file them gently. Have a podiatrist treat you regularly if you cannot do this yourself.
19. Call your podiatrist or physician immediately if you detect a new lesion or if your foot becomes swollen, red, or painful. Stay off your foot until you see your doctor.
20. Learn all you can about your diabetes and how it can affect your feet.
21. Maintain good diabetes control and do not smoke.

such footwear is often wide and deep enough to allow a very comfortable fit without excessive pressure dorsally and laterally. Many athletic or walking shoes are now furnished with removable insoles that can be replaced with custom-made orthoses or a variety of particularly suitable insole materials.[269,270] In addition to the very popular and easy to work with Plastazote (Alimed Inc., Dedham, MA), PPT (Langer Biomechanics Group, Deer Park, NY), Spenco (Spenco Medical Corp., Waco, TX), and Sorbothane (Sorbothane, Inc., Kent, OH) insoles have been found quite effective in attenuating high pressures under the foot.[119,266,270,271] Furthermore, a new type of padded hosiery, ThorLo (Thorneburg, Statesville, NC), has demonstrated a 26 percent reduction in peak forefoot pressure under the foot whereas there was none when patients wore their own hosiery.[118,121] The potential benefits of wearing these socks are quite obvious, especially when worn in combination with protective insoles and proper shoes.

Extra-depth shoes with or without modification should be used for patients with deformities preventing them from wearing the aforementioned type of footwear. Patients with hallux valgus, bunions, hammertoes, and mild Charcot deformities are best treated with extra-depth shoes and appropriate orthoses or insoles. Custom-molded shoes of various designs are indicated in those patients with severe deformity or for whom depth inlay shoes with inserts have not proven effective. In an effort to determine the cost effectiveness of therapeutic shoes in the diabetic population at risk, the congressionally mandated Medicare Therapeutic Shoe Demonstration began in 1989.[272] Presumably, appropriate use of depth inlay shoes with inserts or custom-molded shoes will prove to be clinically effective in reducing the incidence of diabetic foot complications. If this indeed does result, such a policy will become a permanent part of the Medicare program providing reimbursement for and, hopefully, increased utilization of therapeutic footwear in the diabetic patient population.

CONCLUSION

Ulceration in the diabetic foot is a multifaceted problem primarily due to underlying neuropathy, ischemia, or infection. Each of these factors, acting alone or in concert, predispose the foot to ulceration when subjected to mechanical, thermal, or chemical trauma. Although infection usually follows ulceration or injury to the neuropathic or ischemic foot, it can also secondarily lead to ulceration and gangrene. Uncontrolled infection is a major cause of tissue necrosis and hospitalization for diabetic patients. Infection superimposed on an ischemic limb constitutes a medical emergency threatening both limb and life.

Gangrene and the loss of a limb are perhaps the most feared complications of diabetes. Since these are very frequently preceded by ulceration, it behooves both the patient and physician to guard vigilantly against its development and once encountered, to treat aggressively and prevent its recurrence. Treatment must be based on a thorough understanding of the pathogenesis of these lesions as well as specific knowledge of the principles of ulcer care and the varieties of treatments available. Of paramount importance, a multidisciplinary approach to diabetic foot lesions must be embraced if we are to successfully accomplish the goal of a 50 percent reduction in lower extremity amputation rates.

Limb salvage and, by extension, reduction in the incidence of foot ulceration, are greatly dependent upon prevention. Preventive programs must rely heavily on patient education, physician and professional staff education, regular foot examinations, proper footwear, and good diabetic control. When necessary, regular podiatric care should be a part of this program, augmenting the daily foot care and inspection as practiced by the patient or family members. While not all infections, ulcerations, and amputations can be prevented, there can and should be a significant improvement in their incidence and overall morbidity through a cohesive effort on the part of all those concerned with managing the high risk foot in patients with diabetes mellitus.

REFERENCES

1. Gibbons GW, Eliopoulos GM: Infection of the diabetic foot. p. 97. In Kozak GP, Hoar CS, Rowbotham JL et al (eds): Management of Diabetic Foot Problems. WB Saunders, Philadelphia, 1984
2. Edmonds ME: The diabetic foot: pathophysiology and treatment. Clin Endocrinol Metab 15:889, 1986
3. Boulton AJM, Bowker JH: The diabetic foot. p. 225. In Olefsky JM, Sherwin R (eds): Diabetes Mellitus: Management and Complications. Churchill Livingstone, New York, 1985
4. Bild DE, Selby JV, Sinnock P et al: Lower extremity amputation in people with diabetes: epidemiology and prevention. Diabetes Care, 12:24,1989
5. Brand PW: The diabetic foot. p. 829. In Ellenberg M, Rifkin H (eds): Diabetes Mellitus: Theory and Practice. 3rd Ed. Medical Examination Publishers, New York, 1983
6. West KM: Specific morbid effects (complications). p. 331. In: Epidemiology of Diabetes and Its Vascular Lesions. Elsevier, New York, 1978
7. Goldner MG: The fate of the second leg in the diabetic amputee. Diabetes 9:100, 1960
8. Silbert S: Amputation of the lower extremity in diabetes mellitus. Diabetes 1:297, 1952
9. Palumbo PJ, Melton LJ: Peripheral vascular disease and diabetes. p. 1. In: Diabetes in America: Diabetes Data Compiled 1984. (NIH publ. no. 85–1468). US Government Printing Office, Washington, DC, 1985
10. Couch NP, David JK, Tilney NL, Crane C: Natural history of the leg amputee. Am J Surg 133:469, 1977
11. Most RS, Sinnock P: The epidemiology of lower extremity amputations in diabetic individuals. Diabetes Care, 6:87, 1983
12. Kahn O, Wagner W, Bessman AN: Mortality of diabetic patients treated surgically for lower limb infection and/or gangrene. Diabetes 23:287, 1974
13. Walsh CH, Fitzgerald MG, Soler NG, Malins JM: Association of foot lesions with retinopathy in pa-

tients with newly diagnosed diabetes. Lancet 1:878, 1975
14. Cohen SJ: Potential barriers to diabetes care. Diabetes Care 6:499, 1983
15. Davidson MB: Diabetic foot ulcers: protective primary care. Geriatrics 40:15, 1985
16. Delbridge L, Appleberg M, Reeve TS: Factors associated with the development of foot lesions in the diabetic. Surgery 93:78, 1983
17. Assal JP, Gfeller R, Ekoe JM: Patient education in diabetes. p. 276. In Bostrum H, Ljungstedt N (eds): Recent Trends in Diabetes Research. Almqvist and Wiksell International, Stockholm, 1981
18. Davidson JK, Alogna M, Goldsmith M, Borden J: Assessment of program effectiveness at Grady Memorial Hospital—Atlanta. p. 329. In Steiner G, Lawrence PA (eds): Educating Diabetic Patients. Springer Verlag, New York, 1981
19. Lippman HI: Must loss of limb be a consequence of diabetes mellitus? Diabetes Care, 2:432, 1979
20. Young RJ: Identification of the subject "at risk" of foot ulceration. p. 1. In Connor H, Boulton AJM, Ward JD (eds): The Foot in Diabetes. John Wiley & Sons, Chichester, 1987
21. Shenaq SM, Dinh TA: Diabetic foot ulcers: what can be done to prevent and control them. Postgrad Med, 85:323, 1989
22. Levin ME: The diabetic foot: pathophysiology, evaluation, and treatment. p. 1. In Levin ME, O'Neal LW (eds): The Diabetic Foot. CV Mosby, St. Louis, 1988
23. Boulton AJM: The diabetic foot. Med Clin North Am 72:1513, 1988
24. Boulton AJM: The diabetic foot 1988. Diabetic Med 5:1, 1988
25. Rosenqvist U: An epidemiologic survey of diabetic foot problems in the Stockholm County 1982. Acta Med Scand, suppl. 687:55, 1984
26. Pirart J: Diabetes mellitus and its degenerative complications: a prospective study of 4,400 patients observed between 1947 and 1973. Diabetes Care 1:168, 1978
27. DCCT Research Group: Factors in development of diabetic neuropathy. Diabetes, 37:476, 1988
28. American Diabetes Association: Report and recommendations of the San Antonio conference on diabetic neuropathy (Consensus statement). Diabetes Care 11:592, 1988
29. Edmonds ME, Blundell MP, Morris ME et al: Improved survival of the diabetic foot: the role of a specialised foot clinic. Q J Med 232:763, 1986
30. Oakley W, Catterall RCF, Mencer Martin M: Aetiology and management of lesions of the feet in diabetes. Br Med J 2:953, 1956
31. Delbridge L, Ctercteko G, Fowler C, Reeve TS, Le Quesne LP: The aetiology of diabetic neuropathic ulceration of the foot. Br J Surg 72:1, 1985
32. Ahmed ME, Delbridge L, LeQuesne LP: The role of autonomic neuropathy in diabetic foot ulceration. J. Neurol Neurosurg Psychiatry 49:100, 1986
33. Young RJ, Yue QZ, Rodriquez E et al: Variable relationship between peripheral somatic and autonomic neuropathy in patients with different syndromes of diabetic polyneuropathy. Diabetes 35:192, 1986
34. Greene DA: Neuropathy in the diabetic foot: new concepts in etiology and treatment. p. 76. In Levin ME, O'Neal LW (eds): The Diabetic Foot. CV Mosby, St Louis, 1988
35. Clements RS: Diabetic Neuropathy—new concepts of its etiology. Diabetes 28:604, 1979
36. Dyck PJ, Zimmerman BR, Vilen TH et al: Nerve glucose, fructose, sorbitol, myo-inositol, and fiber degeneration and regeneration in diabetic neuropathy. N Engl J Med 319:542, 1988
37. Greene D: The pathogenesis and prevention of diabetic neuropathy and nephropathy. Metabolism, suppl. 1, 37:25, 1988
38. Sima AAF, Bril V, Nathaniel V et al: Regeneration and repair of myelinated fibers in sural–nerve biopsy specimens from patients with diabetic neuropathy treated with sorbinil. N Engl J Med 319:548, 1988
39. Greene DA, Lattimer SA, Sima AAF: Are disturbances of sorbitol, phosphoinositide, and Na^+-K^+-ATPase regulation involved in the pathogenesis of diabetic neuropathy? Diabetes 37:688, 1988
40. Asbury A: Understanding diabetic neuropathy. N Engl J Med 319:577, 1988
41. Boulton AJM, Ward JD: Diabetic neuropathies and pain. Clin Endocrinol Metab 15:917, 1986
42. Watkins PJ: Diabetic neuropathy—I. Br Med J 285:493, 1982
43. Boulton AJM, Hardisty CA, Betts RP et al: Dynamic foot pressure and other studies as diagnostic and management aids in diabetic neuropathy. Diabetes Care 6:26, 1983
44. Newrick PG, Boulton AJM, Ward JD: The distribution of diabetic neuropathy in a British clinic population. Diabetes Research, 2:263, 1986
45. Watkins PJ, Edmonds ME: Sympathetic nerve failure in diabetes. Diabetologia 25:73, 1983
46. Ward JD: The diabetic leg. Diabetologia 22:141, 1982
47. Ahmed ME, LeQuesne PM: Quantitative sweat test in diabetics with neuropathic foot lesions. J Neurol Neurosurg Psychiatry 49:1059, 1986

48. Corbin DOC, Young RJ, Morrison DC et al: Blood flow in the foot, polyneuropathy and foot ulceration in diabetes mellitus. Diabetologia 30:468, 1987
49. Deanfield JE, Daggett PR, Harrison MJG: The role of autonomic neuropathy in diabetic foot ulceration. J Neurol Sci 47:203, 1980
50. Ewing DJ, Clarke BF: Diabetic autonomic neuropathy: present insights and future prospects. Diabetes Care 9:648, 1986
51. Fagius J: Microneurographic findings in diabetic polyneuropathy with special reference to sympathetic nerve activity. Diabetologia 23:415, 1982
52. Watkins PJ: Foot blood flow in diabetic neuropathy. J Roy Soc Med 76:996, 1983
53. Ward JD, Simms JM, Knight G et al: Venous distension in the diabetic neuropathic foot (physical sign of arteriovenous shunting). J R Soc Med 76:1011, 1983
54. Tooke JE, Rayman G, Boolel M: Blood flow abnormalities in the diabetic foot: diagnostic aid or research tool? p. 23. In Connor H, Boulton AJM, Ward JD (eds): The Foot in Diabetes. John Wiley & Sons, Chichester, 1987
55. Rayman G, Hassan A, Tooke JE: Blood flow in the skin of the foot related to posture in diabetes mellitus. Br Med J 292:87, 1986
56. Newrick PG, Cochrane T, Betts RP et al: Reduced hyperaemic response under the diabetic neuropathic foot. Diabetic Med 5:570, 1988
57. Irwin ST, Gilmore J, McGrann S et al: Blood flow in diabetics with foot lesions due to "small vessel disease." Br J Surg 75:1201, 1988
58. Logerfo FW: Vascular disease, matrix abnormalities, and neuropathy: implications for limb salvage in diabetes mellitus. J Vasc Surg 5:793, 1987
59. Ganda Om P: Pathogenesis of macrovascular disease in the human diabetic. Diabetes 29:931, 1980
60. Colwell JA, Lopes-Virella M, Halushka PV: Pathogenesis of atherosclerosis in diabetes mellitus. Diabetes Care 4:121, 1981
61. Logerfo FW, Gibbons GW: Ischemia in the diabetic foot: modern concepts and management. Clin Diabetes 7:72, 1989
62. Yao ST, Hobbs JT, Irvine WT: Ankle systolic pressure measurements in arterial disease affecting the lower extremities. Br J Surg 56:676, 1969
63. Mooney V, Wagner FW: Neurocirculatory disorders of the foot. Clin Orth 122:53, 1977
64. Goldenberg S, Alex M, Joshi RA et al: Nonatheromatous peripheral vascular disease of the lower extremity in diabetes mellitus. Diabetes 8:261, 1959
65. Logerfo FW, Coffman JD: Vascular and microvascular disease of the foot in diabetes. N Engl J Med, 311:1615, 1984
66. Strandness DE, Priest RE, Gibbons GE: Combined clinical and pathologic study of diabetic and nondiabetic peripheral arterial disease. Diabetes 13:366, 1964
67. Conrad MC: Large and small artery occlusion in diabetics and nondiabetics with severe vascular disease. Circulation 36:83, 1967
68. Picus D, Staple TW, Gilula LA, Hardy DC: Radiographic imaging and treatment of vascular disease in the diabetic patient. p. 182. In Levin ME, O'Neal LW (eds): The Diabetic Foot. CV Mosby, St. Louis, 1988
69. Gilbey SC, Walters H, Edmonds ME et al: Vascular calcification, autonomic neuropathy, and peripheral blood flow in patients with diabetic nephropathy. Diabetic Med 6:37, 1989
70. Edmonds ME, Morrison M, Laws JW, Watkins PJ: Medial arterial calcification and diabetic neuropathy. Br Med J, 284:928, 1982
71. Raines JK, Darling RC, Buth J et al:Vascular laboratory criteria for the management of peripheral vascular disease of the lower extremities. Surgery 79:21, 1976
72. Gibbons GW, Wheelock FC, Siembeda C et al: Noninvasive prediction of amputation level in diabetic patients. Arch Surg 114:1253, 1979
73. Carter SA: The relationship of distal systolic pressures to healing of skin lesions in limbs with arterial occlusive disease, with special reference to diabetes mellitus. Scand J Clin Lab Invest, suppl 128, 31:239, 1973
74. Emanuele MA, Buchanan BJ, Abraira C: Elevated leg systolic pressures and arterial calcification in diabetic occlusive vascular disease. Diabetes Care 4:289, 1981
75. Goss DE, De Trafford J, Flynn MD: The prevalence of raised ankle/brachial pressure index in diabetics referred for the assessment of arterial disease, abstracted. Diabetic Med, suppl 5, 5:31, 1988
76. Jennings PE, Barnett AH: New approaches to the pathogenesis and treatment of diabetic microangiopathy. Diabetic Med 5:111, 1988
77. Archer AG, Roberts VC, Watkins PJ: Blood flow patterns in painful diabetic neuropathy. Diabetologia 27:563, 1984
78. Gaylarde PM, Fonseca VA, Llewellyn G et al: Transcutaneous oxygen tension in legs and feet of diabetic patients. Diabetes 37:714, 1988
79. Haitas B, Barnes A, Shogry MEC et al: Delayed vascular reactivity to ischemia in diabetic microangiopathy. Diabetes Care 7:47, 1984

80. Wilson S, Belch JJF, Jennings PE: Laser Doppler assessment of early microvascular impairment in Type I diabetic patients, abstracted. Diabetic Med suppl. 1, 6:A16, 1989
81. Boulton AJM, Newrick PG, Cochrane T, Betts RP: Reduced hyperaemic response under the diabetic foot: additional aetiological mechanism for ulceration, abstracted. Diabetologia, 30:502A, 1987
82. Parkhouse N, LeQuesne PM, Scurr JH: Reduced axon reflex flare in diabetics with neuropathic foot lesions, abstracted. Br J Surg 6:534, 1987
83. Parkhouse N, LeQuesne PM: Impaired neurogenic vascular response in patients with diabetes and neuropathic foot lesions. N Eng J Med 318:1306, 1988
84. Pratt, TC: Gangrene and infection in the diabetic. Med Clin North Am, 49:987, 1965
85. Wheat LJ: Infection and diabetes mellitus. Diabetes Care 3:187, 1980
86. McIntyre KE: Control of infection in the diabetic foot: the role of microbiology, immunopathy, antibiotics, and guillotine amputation. J Vasc Surg 5:787, 1987
87. Bagdade JD, Root RK, Bulger RJ: Impaired leukocyte function in patients with poorly controlled diabetes. Diabetes 23:9, 1974
88. Tan JS, Anderson JL, Watanakunakorn C, Phair JP: Neutrophil dysfunction in diabetes mellitus. J Lab Clin Med 85:26, 1975
89. Gibbons GW: The diabetic foot: Amputations and drainage of infection. J Vasc Surg 5:791, 1987
90. Taylor LM, Porter JM: The clinical course of diabetics who require emergent foot surgery because of infection or ischemia. J Vasc Surg 6:454, 1987
91. Goodman J, Bessman AN, Teget B, Wagner W: Risk factors in local surgical procedures for diabetic gangrene. Surg Gynecol Obstet, 143:587, 1976
92. Leichter SB, Allweiss P, Harley J et al: Clinical characteristics of diabetic patients with serious pedal infections. Metabolism suppl 37:22, 1988
93. Louie TS, Bartlett JG, Tally FP, Gorbach SL: Aerobic and anaerobic bacteria in diabetic foot ulcers. Ann Int Med 85:461, 1976
94. Sharp CS, Bessman AN, Wagner FW et al: Microbiology of superficial and deep tissues in infected diabetic gangrene. Surg Gynecol Obstet 149:217, 1979
95. Fierer J, Daniel D, Davis C: The fetid foot: lower extremity infections in patients with diabetes mellitus. Rev Infect Dis 1:210, 1979
96. Sapico FL, Witte JL, Canawati HN et al: The infected foot of the diabetic patient: quantitative microbiology and analysis of clinical features. Rev Infect Dis, suppl. 1, 6:S171, 1984
97. Wheat LJ, Allen SD, Henry M et al: Diabetic foot infections: bacteriologic analysis. Arch Int Med 146:1935, 1986
98. Scher KS, Steele FJ: The septic foot in patients with diabetes. Surgery 104:661, 1988
99. Jones EW, Edwards R, Finch R, Jeffcoate WJ: A microbiological study of diabetic foot lesions. Diabetic Med 2:213, 1985
100. DeValentine S, Fredenburg M, Loretz L: Infections of the diabetic foot. Clin Pod Med Surg 4:395, 1987
101. Livingstone R, Jacobs R, Karmody A: Plantar abscess in the diabetic patient. Foot Ankle 5:205, 1985
102. Goldberg D, Neu HC: Infectious diseases of the diabetic foot. p. 98. In Brenner MA (ed): Management of the Diabetic Foot. Williams & Wilkins, Baltimore, 1987
103. Calhoun JH, Cantrell J, Cobos J et al: Treatment of diabetic foot infections: Wagner classification, therapy, and outcome. Foot Ankle, 9:101, 1988
104. Sapico FL, Bessman AN, Canawati HN: Bacteremia in diabetic patients with infected lower extremities. Diabetes Care 5:101, 1982
105. Bessman AN, Sapico FL, Tabatabai M, Montgomerie JZ: Persistence of polymicrobial abscesses in the poorly controlled diabetic host. Diabetes 35:448, 1986
106. Tan JS, File TM: Diagnosis and treatment of diabetic foot infections. Comp Ther 14:57, 1988
107. Mackowiak PA, Jones SR, Smith JW: Diagnostic value of sinus-tract cultures in chronic osteomyelitis. J Am Med Assoc 239:2772, 1978
108. Tan JS, Flanagan PJ, Donovan DL, File TM: Team approach in the management of diabetic foot infections. J Foot Surg, suppl. 1, 26:S12, 1987
109. Kucan JO, Robson MC: Diabetic foot infections: Fate of the contralateral foot. Plast Reconstr Surg 17:439, 1986
110. Gleckman RA, Roth RM: Diabetic foot infections —Prevention and treatment. West J Med 142:263, 1985
111. Bessman AN, Kasim S: Managing foot infections in the older diabetic patient. Geriatrics 40:54, 1985
112. Sabacinski KA, Tillo TH, Giurini JM et al: Necrotizing fasciitis. J Foot Surg 28:106, 1989
113. Bauman JH, Brand PW: Plantar pressures and trophic ulceration. J Bone Joint Surg (Br) 45:652, 1963
114. Pollard JP, LeQuesne LP: Method of healing diabetic forefoot ulcers. Br Med J 286:436, 1983
115. Ctercteko GC, Dhanendran M, Hutton WC, LeQuesne LP: Vertical forces acting on the feet of diabetic patients. Br J Surg 68:608, 1981

116. Duckworth T, Boulton AJM, Betts RP et al: Plantar pressure measurements and the prevention of ulceration in the diabetic foot. J Bone Joint Surg (Br) 67:79, 1985
117. Masson EA, Hay EM, Stockley I et al: Abnormal foot pressures alone may not cause ulceration. Diabetic Med 6:426, 1989
118. Masson EA, Veves A, Fernando D, Boulton AJM: A new method of reducing plantar pressures in diabetic patients with and without foot ulceration, abstracted. Diabetic Med, suppl. 1, 6:A29, 1989
119. Boulton AJM, Franks CI, Betts RP et al: Reduction of abnormal foot pressures in diabetic neuropathy using a new polymer insole material. Diabetes Care 7:42, 1984
120. Boulton AJM, Betts RP, Franks CI et al: The natural history of foot pressure abnormalities in neuropathic diabetic subjects. Diabetes Res 5:73, 1987
121. Veves A, Masson EA, Fernando DJS, Boulton AJM: Use of experimental padded hosiery to reduce abnormal foot pressures in diabetic neuropathy. Diabetes Care 12:653, 1989
122. Boulton AJM: The importance of abnormal foot pressures and gait in the causation of foot ulcers. p. 11. In Connor H, Boulton AJM, Ward JD (eds): The Foot in Diabetes. John Wiley & Sons, Chichester, 1987
123. Thompson DE: The effects of mechanical stress on soft tissue. p. 91. In Levin ME, O'Neal LW (eds): The Diabetic Foot. CV Mosby, St. Louis, 1988
124. Barrett JP, Mooney V: Neuropathy and diabetic pressure lesions. Orthop Clin North Am 4:43, 1973
125. Dannels EG: A preventive metatarsal osteotomy for healing pre-ulcers in American Indian diabetics. J Am Pod Med Assoc 76:33, 1986
126. Apelqvist J, Castenfors J, Larsson J et al: Wound classification is more important than site of ulceration in the outcome of diabetic foot ulcers. Diabetic Med 6:526, 1989
127. Sage R, Doyle D: Surgical treatment of diabetic foot ulcers: A review of forty-eight cases. J Foot Surg 23:102, 1984
128. Brand PW: Repetitive stress in the development of diabetic foot ulcers. p. 83. In Levin ME, O'Neal LW (eds): The Diabetic Foot. CV Mosby, St. Louis, 1988
129. Brand PW: Other insensitive foot types similar to diabetes. p. 8. In Brenner MA (ed): Management of the Diabetic Foot. Williams & Wilkins, Baltimore, 1987
130. Sims DS, Cavanagh PR, Ulbrecht JS: Risk factors in the diabetic foot. Phys Ther, 68:1887, 1988
131. Kohn RR, Schnider SL: Glucosylation of human collagen. Diabetes, suppl. 3, 31:47, 1982
132. Brownlee M, Vlassara H, Cerami A: Non-enzymatic glycosylation and the pathogenesis of diabetic complications. Ann Int Med 101:527, 1984
133. Kennedy L, Baynes JW: Non-enzymatic glycosylation and the chronic complications of diabetes: an overview. Diabetologia 26:93, 1984
134. Monnier VM, Cerami A: Non-enzymatic glycosylation and browning of proteins in diabetes. Clin Endocrinol Metab 11:431, 1982
135. Collier A, Patrick AW, Bell D et al: Relationship of skin thickness to duration of diabetes, glycemic control, and diabetic complications in male IDDM patients. Diabetes Care 12:309, 1989
136. Schnider SL, Kohn RR: Glucosylation of human collagen in aging and diabetes mellitus. J Clin Invest 66:1179, 1980
137. Delbridge L, Ellis CS, LeQuesne LP: Non-enzymatic glycosylation of keratin from the diabetic foot. Br J Surg 70:305, 1983
138. Delbridge L, Perry P, Marrs S et al: Limited joint mobility in the diabetic foot: relationship to neuropathic ulceration. Diabetic Med 5:333, 1988
139. Slama G, Letanoux M, Thibult N et al: Quantification of early subclinical limited joint mobility in diabetes mellitus. Diabetes Care 8:329, 1985
140. Beacom R, Gillespie EL, Middleton D et al: Limited joint mobility in insulin-dependent diabetes: relationship to retinopathy, peripheral nerve function and HLA status. J Med 219:337, 1985
141. Rosenbloom A, Silverstein JH, Lezotte DC et al: Limited joint mobility in childhood diabetes mellitus indicates increased risk for microvascular disease. N. Engl J Med 305:191, 1981
142. Rosenbloom A, Silverstein JH, Riley WJ, Maclaren NK: Limited joint mobility in childhood diabetes: family studies. Diabetes Care 6:370, 1983
143. Shinabarger NI: Limited joint mobility in adults with diabetes mellitus. Phys Ther 67:215, 1987
144. Rosenbloom A: Limitation of finger joint mobility in diabetes mellitus. J Diabetic Complic 3:77, 1989
145. Clavel S, Crausaz FM, Liniger C, Assal JP: Unsuspected risk factors for perforating plantar ulcers in diabetic neuropathy. Diabetologia 30:508A, 1987
146. Crausaz FM, Clavel S, Liniger C et al: Additional factors associated with plantar ulcers in diabetic neuropathy. Diabetic Med 5:771, 1988
147. Mueller MJ, Diamond J, Delitto A, Sinacore DR: Insensitivity, limited joint mobility, and plantar ulcers in patients with diabetes mellitus. Phys Ther 69:453, 1989

148. Sage RA: Diabetic ulcers: Evaluation and management. Clin Pod Med Surg 4:383, 1987
149. Kalker AJ, Kolodny HD, Cavuoto JW: The evaluation and treatment of diabetic foot ulcers. J Am Pod Assoc 72:491, 1982
150. Williams H, Hutchinson K, Brown G: Gangrene of the feet in diabetics. Arch Surg 108:609, 1974
151. Wagner FW: Transcutaneous Doppler ultrasound in the prediction of healing and the selection of surgical level for dysvascular lesions of the toes and forefoot. Clin Orthop 142:110, 1979
152. Wagner FW: The dysvascular foot: a system for diagnosis and treatment. Foot Ankle 2:64, 1981
153. Wagner FW: Treatment of the diabetic foot. Compr Ther 10:29, 1984
154. Skyler JS: Complications of diabetes mellitus: relationship to metabolic dysfunction. Diabetes Care 2:499, 1979
155. Dickhaut SC, DeLee JC, Page CP: Nutritional status: importance in predicting wound-healing after amputation. J Bone Joint Surg 66A:71, 1984
156. Sapico FL: Foot infection in patients with diabetes mellitus. J Am Pod Med Assoc 79:482, 1989
157. LeFrock JL: Use of Ciprofloxacin in podiatric medicine. J Am Pod Med Assoc 79:497, 1989
158. Peterson LR, Lissack LM, Canter K et al: Therapy of lower extremity infections with Ciprofloxacin in patients with diabetes mellitus, peripheral vascular disease, or both. Am J Med 86:801, 1989
159. Robson MC, Edstrom LE: The diabetic foot: an alternative approach to major amputation. Surg Clin North Am 57:1089, 1977
160. Towne JB: Management of foot lesions in the diabetic patient. p. 661. In Rutherford RB (ed): Vascular Surgery. WB Saunders, Philadelphia, 1984
161. Rowbotham JL, Gibbons GW, Gray M, Frasca J: Local treatment of the diabetic foot. p. 113. In Kozak GP, Hoar CS, Rowbotham JL et al (eds): Management of Diabetic Foot Problems. WB Saunders, Philadelphia, 1984
162. Pinzur MJ, Sage R, Abraham M, Ostermn H: Limb salvage in lower extremity gangrene. Foot Ankle 8:212, 1988
163. Pinzur MJ, Kaminsky M, Sage R et al: Amputations at the middle level of the foot. J Bone Joint Surg 68A:1061, 1986
164. Robson MC, Edstrom LE: Conservative management of the ulcerated diabetic foot. Plast Reconstr Surg 59:551, 1977
165. Kwasnik EM: Limb salvage in diabetics: challenges and solutions. Surg Clin North Am 66:305, 1986
166. Yao JT: Noninvasive techniques of measuring lower limb arterial pressures. p. 83. In Bernstein EF (ed): Noninvasive Diagnostic Techniques in Vascular Disease. CV Mosby, St. Louis, 1985
167. Carter SA: Role of pressure measurements in vascular disease. p. 513. In Bernstein EF (ed): Noninvasive diagnostic techniques in vascular disease. CV Mosby, St. Louis, 1985
168. Kirby KA, Arkin DB, Laine W: Digital systolic pressure determination in the foot. J Am Pod Med Assoc 77:340, 1987
169. Holstein P: The distal blood pressure predicts healing of amputations of the feet. Acta Orthop Scand 55:227, 1984
170. Faris I, Duncan H: Skin perfusion pressure in the prediction of healing in diabetic patients with ulcers or gangrene of the foot. J Vasc Surg, 2:536, 1985
171. Holstein P, Lassen NA: Healing of ulcers on the feet correlated with distal blood pressure measurements in occlusive arterial disease. Acta Orthop Scand 51:995, 1980
172. Bone GE, Pomajzl MJ: Toe blood pressure by photoplethysmography: an index of healing in forefoot amputation. Surgery 89:569, 1981
173. Lewis BD, James EM, Welch TJ: Current applications of duplex and color Doppler ultrasound imaging: carotid and peripheral vascular system. Mayo Clin Proc 64:1147, 1989
174. Niehaus LP, Kallibjian A: Application of transcutaneous oxygen measurement in podiatric surgery. J Foot Surg 28:124, 1989
175. Wyss CR, Matsen FA, Simmons CW, Burgess EM: Transcutaneous oxygen tension measurements on limbs of diabetic and nondiabetic patients with peripheral vascular disease. Surgery 95:339, 1984
176. Karanfilian RG, Lynch TG, Zirul VT et al: The value of laser Doppler velocimetry and transcutaneous oxygen tension determination in predicting healing of ischemic forefoot ulcerations and amputations in diabetic and nondiabetic patients. J Vasc Surg 4:511, 1986
177. Apelqvist J, Castenfors J, Larsson J et al: Prognostic value of systolic ankle and toe blood pressure levels in outcome of diabetic foot ulcers. Diabetes Care 12:373, 1989
178. Bloom RJ, Stevick CA: Amputation level and distal bypass salvage of the limb. Surg Gynecol Obstet 166:1, 1988
179. Andros G, Harris RW, Salles-Cunha SX et al: Lateral plantar artery bypass grafting: Defining limits of foot revascularization. J Vasc Surg 10:511, 1989
180. Hurley JJ, Auer AI, Hershey FB et al: Distal arterial reconstruction: patency and limb salvage in diabetics. J Vasc Surg 5:796, 1987

181. Andros G, Harris RW, Salles-Cunha SX et al: Bypass grafts to the ankle and foot. J Vasc Surg 7:785, 1988
182. Frykberg RG: Podiatric problems in diabetes. p. 45. In Kozak GP, Hoar CS, Rowbotham J et al (eds): Management of Diabetic Foot Problems. WB Saunders, Philadelphia, 1984
183. Hardy DC, Staple TW, Picus D, Gilula LA: Imaging of the diabetic foot. p. 131. In Levin ME, O'Neal LW (eds): The Diabetic Foot. CV Mosby, St. Louis, 1988
184. Gventer M: Radiological evaluation of the diabetic foot. p. 48. In Brenner MA (ed): Management of the Diabetic Foot. Williams & Wilkins, Baltimore, 1987
185. Zlatkin MB, Pathria M, Sartoris DJ, Resnick D: The diabetic foot. Radiol Clin North Am 25:1095, 1987
186. Frykberg RG, Kozak GP: The diabetic Charcot foot. p. 103. In Kozak GP, Hoar CS, Rowbotham J et al (eds): Management of Diabetic Foot Problems. WB Saunders, Philadelphia, 1984
187. Maurer AH, Millmond SH, Knight LC et al: Infection in diabetic osteoarthropathy: use of indium-labeled leukocytes for diagnosis. Radiology 161:221, 1986
188. Schauwecker DS, Park HM, Burt RW et al: Combined bone scintigraphy and indium-111 leukocyte scans in neuropathic foot disease. J Nucl Med 29:1651, 1988
189. Keenan AM, Tindel NL, Alavi A: Diagnosis of pedal osteomyelitis in diabetic patients using current scintigraphic techniques. Arch Int Med, 149:2262, 1989
190. Techner LM, Eiser CA, Laine W: Indium-111 imaging in osteomyelitis and neuroarthropathy. J Am Pod Med Assoc 76:23, 1986
191. Sartoris D, Resnick D: Magnetic resonance imaging of the diabetic foot. J Foot Surg 28:485, 1989
192. Ger R: Prevention of major amputations in the diabetic patient. Arch Surg 120:1317, 1985
193. Singer A: Surgical treatment of mal perforans. Arch Surg 111:964, 1976
194. Walenkamp GHIM: Gentamicin-PMMA beads: A clinical, pharmacokinetic, and toxicological study. Drukkerij Cliteur, Amsterdam, 1987
195. Schein CS, Black JR: Implanted gentamicin beads in the treatment of osteomyelitis. J Am Pod Med Assoc 77:563, 1987
196. Marcinko DE: Gentamicin-impregnated beads: an introduction and review. J Foot Surg, 24:116, 1985
197. Mader JT, Calhoun JH: Long bone osteomyelitis. J Am Pod Med Assoc 79:476, 1989
198. Waldvogel FA, Vasey H: Osteomyelitis: The past decade. N Engl J Med 303:360, 1980
199. Wilson KH, Kauffman CA: Oral antibiotic therapy for osteomyelitis of the foot in diabetic patients. South Med J 78:223, 1985
200. Bamberger DM, Daus GP, Gerding DN: Osteomyelitis in the feet of diabetic patients. Am J Med 83:653, 1987
201. Slama TG, Misinski J, Sklar S: Ciprofloxacin therapy of osteomyelitis. Contemp Orthop 16:1, 1988
202. Masson EA, Cooper MAC, Boulton AJM: Split-skin grafting in the management of extensive neuropathic ulceration. Diabetic Med 6:171, 1989
203. Ger R: Muscle transposition in the management of perforating ulcers of the forefoot. Clin Orthop 175:186, 1983
204. Ger R: Newer concepts in the surgical management of lesions of the foot in the patient with diabetes. Surg Gynecol Obstet, 158:213, 1984
205. Cronenwett JL, McDanile MD, Zwolak RM et al: Limb salvage despite extensive tissue loss. Arch Surg 124:609, 1989
206. Colen LB: Limb salvage in the patient with severe peripheral vascular disease: the role of microsurgical free-tissue transfer. Plast Reconstr Surg 78:389, 1987
207. May JW, Gallico GG, Lucash FN: Microvascular transfer of free tissue for closure of bone wounds of the distal lower extremity. N Engl J Med 306:253, 1982
208. Gudas CJ: Prophylactic surgery in the diabetic foot. Clin Pod Med Surg 4:445, 1987
209. Giurini JM, Habershaw GH, Chrzan JS: Panmetatarsal head resection in chronic neuropathic ulceration. J Foot Surg 26:249, 1987
210. Harkless LB, Dennis KJ: The role of the podiatrist. p. 249. In Levin ME, O'Neal LW (eds): The Diabetic Foot., CV Mosby, St. Louis, 1988
211. Frykberg, RG: Diabetic osteoarthropathy. p. 75. In Brenner MA (ed): Management of the Diabetic Foot. Williams & Wilkins, Baltimore, 1987
212. Banks AS, McGlamry ED: Charcot foot. J Am Pod Med Assoc 79:213, 1989
213. Lesko P, Maurer RC: Talonavicular dislocations and midfoot arthropathy in neuropathic diabetic feet. Clin Orthop 240:226, 1989
214. Sizer JS, Wheelock FC: Digital amputations in diabetic patients. Surgery 72:980, 1972
215. Benton GS, Kerstein MD: Cost effectiveness of early digit amputation in the patient with diabetes. Surg Gynecol Obstet 161:523, 1985

216. Hodge MJ, Peters TG, Efird WG: Amputation of the distal portion of the foot. South Med J 82:1138, 1989
217. Sanders LJ: Amputations in the diabetic foot. Clin Pod Med Surg 4:481, 1987
218. Larsen K, Holstein P: Abnormal extension of the big toe as a cause of ulceration in diabetic feet. Prosthet Orthot Int 11:31, 1987
219. Birke JA, Cornwall MW, Jackson M: Relationship between hallux limitus and ulceration of the great toe. J Orthop Sport Phys Ther 10:172, 1988
220. Downs DM, Jacobs RL: Treatment of resistant ulcers on the plantar surface of the great toe in diabetics. J Bone Joint Surg 64A:930, 1982
221. Dannels E: Neuropathic foot ulcer prevention in diabetic American Indians with hallux limitus. J Am Pod Med Assoc 79:447, 1989
222. Klamer TW, Towne JB, Bandyk DF, Bonner MJ: The influence of sepsis and ischemia on the natural history of the diabetic foot. Am Surg 53:490, 1987
223. Rhodes GR, Skudder P: Salvage of ischemic diabetic feet: role of transcutaneous oxygen mapping and multiple configurations of in situ bypass. Am J Surg 152:165, 1986
224. Baroni G, Porro T, Faglia E et al: Hyperbaric oxygen in diabetic gangrene therapy. Diabetes Care 10:81, 1987
225. Leslie CA, Sapico FL, Ginunas VJ, Adkins RH: Randomized controlled trial of topical hyperbaric oxygen for treatment of diabetic foot ulcers. Diabetes Care 11:111, 1988
226. Gorman DF, Harding PE, Roberts AP et al: Topical hyperbaric oxygen for treatment of diabetic foot ulcers. Diabetes Care 11:819, 1988
227. Davis JC: The use of adjuvant hyperbaric oxygen in treatment of the diabetic foot. Clin Pod Med Surg 4:429, 1987
228. Hill RK: Clearing an oxygen confusion. Diabetes Care 12:661, 1989
229. Brenner MA: An ambulatory approach to neuropathic ulceration. J Am Pod Med Assoc 64:862, 1974
230. Brenner MA: Debridement, local care, and management of diabetic lesions. p. 110. In Brenner MA (ed): Management of the Diabetic Foot. Williams & Wilkins, Baltimore, 1987
231. Soulier SM: The use of running shoes in the prevention of plantar diabetic ulcers. J Am Pod Med Assoc 76:395, 1986
232. Soulier SM, Godsey C, Asay ED, Perrotta DM: The prevention of plantar ulceration in the diabetic foot through the use of running shoes. Diabetes Educator 13:130, 1987
233. Frykberg RG: Podiatric problems in diabetes. p. 426. In Kozak GP (ed): Clinical Diabetes Mellitus. WB Saunders, Philadelphia, 1982
234. Walker SC, Helm PA, Pulliam G: Total contact casting and chronic diabetic neuropathic foot ulcerations: healing rates by wound location. Arch Phys Med Rehabil 68:217, 1987
235. Stess RM, Hetherington VJ: The diabetic and insensitive foot. p. 523. In Levy LA, Hetherington VJ (eds): Principles and Practice of Podiatric Medicine. Churchill Livingstone, New York, 1989
236. Helm PA, Walker SC, Pullium G: Total contact casting in diabetic patients with neuropathic foot ulcerations. Arch Phys Med Rehabil, 65:691, 1984
237. Boulton AJM, Bowker JH, Gadia M et al: Use of plaster casts in the management of diabetic neuropathic foot ulcers. Diabetes Care 9:149, 1986
238. Mueller MJ, Diamond JE, Sinacore DR et al: Total contact casting in treatment of diabetic plantar ulcers. Diabetes Care 12:384, 1989
239. Sinacore DR, Mueller MJ, Diamond JE et al: Diabetic plantar ulcers treated by total contact casting. Phys Ther 67:1543, 1987
240. Burnett O: Total Contact Cast. Clin Pod Med Surg 4:471, 1987
241. Coleman WC, Brand PW, Birke JA: The total contact cast, a therapy for plantar ulceration on insensitive feet. J Am Pod Med Assoc 74:548, 1984
242. Diamond JE, Sinacore DR, Mueller MJ: Molded double-rocker plaster shoe for healing a diabetic plantar ulcer. Phys Ther 67:1550, 1987
243. Burden AC, Jones GR, Jones R, Blandford RL: Use of the "Scotchcast boot" in treating diabetic foot ulcers. Br Med J 286:1555, 1983
244. Burden AC, Beshya SA, Jones R, Curryer G: Modifications to the "Scotchcast boot". Diabetic Med, suppl. 5, 5:30, 1988
245. Kalish SR, Pelcovitz N, Zawada S et al: The Aircast Walking Brace versus conventional casting methods. J Am Pod Med Assoc 77:589, 1987
246. Shuman CR: Foot disorders in diabetics: source of serious morbidity. Postgrad Med, 74:109, 1983
247. Rausher H, Rausher SR, Friedman EA: Preserving feet in the uremic diabetic: the physicians role. J Diabetes Complic 2:145, 1988
248. Levin ME: On the evaluation, prevention, and treatment of diabetic foot lesions. J Diabetes Complic, 3:211, 1989
249. Edmonds ME: Experience in a multidisciplinary diabetic foot clinic. p. 121. In Connor H, Boulton AJM, Ward JD (eds): The Foot in Diabetes. John Wiley & Sons, Chichester, 1987
250. Ward JD: Essential requirements for diabetic foot

care. p. 151. In Connor H, Boulton AJM, Ward JD (eds): The Foot in Diabetes. John Wiley & Sons, Chichester, 1987

251. Runyan JW, VanderZwaag R, Joyner MB, Miller ST: The Memphis diabetes continuing care program. Diabetes Care 3:382, 1980
252. Assal JP, Muhlhauser I, Pernet A et al: Patient education as the basis for diabetes care in clinical practice and research. Diabetologia 28:602, 1985
253. American Diabetes Association: Position statement on standards of medical care for patients with diabetes mellitus. Diabetes Care 12:365, 1989
254. Bailey TS, Yu H, Rayfield EJ: Patterns of foot examination in a diabetes clinic. Am J Med 78:371, 1985
255. Payne TH, Gabella BA, Michael SL et al: Preventive care in diabetes mellitus. Current practice in urban health-care system. Diabetes Care 12:745, 1989
256. Boulton AJM, Kubrusly DB, Bowker JH et al: Impaired vibratory perception and diabetic foot ulceration. Diabetic Med 3:335, 1986
257. Jennings M, Newrick PG, Knight G et al: The use of biothesiometry to detect patients at risk of diabetic neuropathic ulceration. Diabetologia 29:553A, 1986
258. Masson EA, Veves A, Fernando D, Boulton AJM: Evaluation of a new device for measurement of peripheral nerve function in diabetes. Diabetic Med, suppl. 1, 6:A29, 1989
259. Rendell MS, Dovgan DJ, Bergman TF et al: Mapping diabetic sensory neuropathy by current perception threshold testing. Diabetes Care 12:636, 1989
260. Holewski JJ, Stess RM, Graf PM, Grunfeld C: Aesthesiometry: Quantification of cutaneous pressure sensation in diabetic peripheral neuropathy. J Rehabil Res Dev 25:1, 1988
261. Guy RJC, Clark CA, Malcolm PN, Watkin PJ: Evaluation of thermal and vibration sensation in diabetic neuropathy. Diabetologia 28:131, 1985
262. Wieman TJ, Huang KC, Tsueda K et al: Peripheral somatic sensory neuropathy and skin galvanic response in the feet of patients with diabetes. Surg Gynecol Obstet, 168:501, 1989
263. Goss DE, Trafford J de, Roberts VC et al: Raised ankle/brachial pressure index in insulin-treated diabetic patients. Diabetic Med, 6:576, 1989
264. Stess RM, Sisney PC, Moss KM et al: Use of liquid crystal thermography in the evaluation of the diabetic foot. Diabetes Care 9:267, 1986
265. Baer MS, Hetherington VJ, Lockyer JE, Long DH: Preliminary report on the use of liquid crystal thermography in podiatry. J Foot Surg 27:398, 1988
266. Smith L, Plehwe W, McGill M et al: Foot bearing pressure in patients with unilateral diabetic foot ulcers. Diabetic Med 6:573, 1989
267. Silvino N, Evanski PM, Waugh TR: The Harris and Beath footprinting mat: Diagnostic validity and clinical use. Clin Orthop 151:265, 1980
268. Birke JA, Sims DS: The insensitive foot. p. 133. In Hunt GC (ed): Physical Therapy of the Foot and Ankle. Churchill Livingstone, New York, 1988
269. Donovan JC, Scardina RJ, Frykberg RG et al: New England Deaconess Hospital Podiatry Service sport orthotic device. J Am Pod Med Assoc 69:571, 1979
270. Brodsky JW, Kourosh S, Stills M, Mooney V: Objective evaluation of insert material for diabetic and athletic footwear. Foot Ankle, 9:111, 1988
271. Leber C, Evanski PM: A comparison of shoe insole materials in plantar pressure relief. Prosthet Orthot Int, 10:135, 1986
272. Wooldridge J, Handwerger S: The benefits of prevention: The Medicare therapeutic shoe demonstration. Diabetes Spectrum 2:390, 1989

11

Diabetic Foot Infections

Francisco L. Sapico, M.D., F.A.C.P.
Alice N. Bessman, M.D.

TYPES, CHARACTERISTICS, AND MANIFESTATIONS

The feet are one of the most used parts of the body, are necessary for daily activities pertaining to locomotion, and are therefore subject to repetitive trauma. Trauma, in turn, may lead to open lesions that allow ingress of pathogenic microbes. In the diabetic person, the pathogenesis of foot infections is multifaceted. Vascular insufficiency, neuropathy, and decreased resistance to infection, possibly from metabolic imbalance, have all been implicated. In the individual patient, the relative contribution of each of these factors can vary. The presence of peripheral neuropathy can lead to an insensate foot, to impaired ability of the foot to sweat, in turn leading to drying, fissuring, and cracking, and to deformities arising from poorly perceived microfractures. These changes, in the presence of the diabetic state, with or without significant vascular impairment, can set the stage for the entry of bacterial pathogens and the progression of the infectious process.

It has been a commonly held belief that infections, in general, occur more frequently or are more severe in diabetic as compared to nondiabetic individuals. This concept, however, has been challenged by others. In his review of the medical literature dealing with this problem, Wheat concluded that only bacteriuria in adult women has been statistically documented to be more prevalent in diabetic patients.[1] However, even though prospective controlled studies are sadly lacking in this regard, we believe that the medical literature convincingly demonstrates that diabetic patients are overrepresented in certain severe and life-threatening infections such as invasive external otitis, mucormycosis, emphysematous cholecystitis, and pyelonephritis, as well as renal papillary necrosis and perinephric abscesses.[2–8] Diabetic patients also represent around 60 percent of nontraumatic foot or leg amputations, the majority of which are secondary to infectious complications.[9]

Defects in immune function have been described as occurring in diabetics. White cell dysfunction in diapedesis, adherence, chemotaxis, phagocytosis, and killing ability has been described in diabetic patients.[10–14] In general, these defects are aggravated by poor glucose control. Poor granuloma formation and poor healing have also been seen in diabetic mice.[15]

Salvapandian reviewed the different types of foot infections and their characteristics in 1982.[16] These infections can occur in nondiabetic as well as diabetic persons, although the presence of the diabetic state can aggravate the risks and the morbidity associated with these infections. Foot infections can occur in the wake of acute or chronic trauma. These post-traumatic foot infections can be classified as follows:

Infected blister. This is usually secondary to improperly fitting footwear, which causes separation of the superficial layers of the epidermis from the deeper layers, with resultant accumulation of clear fluid. Skin breakdown leading to communication with the outside can allow bacterial infection to supervene (Fig. 11-1).

Infected abrasion. This follows the traumatic removal of the horny layer of the skin, leaving the deeper layers open to the elements.

Infected ulcer. This is usually an extension of a previous abrasion and is usually due to pressure from the outside. These lesions generally occur over a bony prominence, such as a metatarsal head (mal perforans).

Puncture wounds. These usually result from inadvertent, and frequently unperceived, stepping on sharp objects such as nails and tacks. The association between *Psuedomonas aeruginosa* infections and the wearing of rubber sneakers at the time of a puncture injury has been emphasized in the past.[17-19]

Infected calluses. These are usually a result of repeated intermittent pressure due to poorly fitting footwear and/or bony prominences and foot deformities as an end result of diabetic neuropathy and osteoarthropathy. These calluses may develop an open area secondary to trauma or from overzealous attempts by the patient to remove the callus, thus allowing ingress of bacteria.

Infected corns. These are conical wedges of keratinized tissue with the apices pointing inward. These usually occur on the heel or under metatarsal heads, and the pathogenesis is similar to the callus.

Infections following severe mechanical trauma such as in crush injuries or degloving injuries. Degloving injury usually follows accidents wherein heavy objects run over parts of the body, with resultant extensive loss of skin.

Infections can also follow the development of open areas in the skin such as the development of fissures. These fissures commonly occur between the toes or in the flexor creases of the toes. These may be associated with dry hyperkeratotic skin or may occur in areas where the skin is moist, especially in the presence of deformities of the toes. Bacterial infections can also be superimposed on chronic infectious processes in the feet such as those associated with dermatophytic fungi, other fungi such as *Candida, Coccidioides, Blastomyces, Cryptococcus,* or more unusual bacterial pathogens

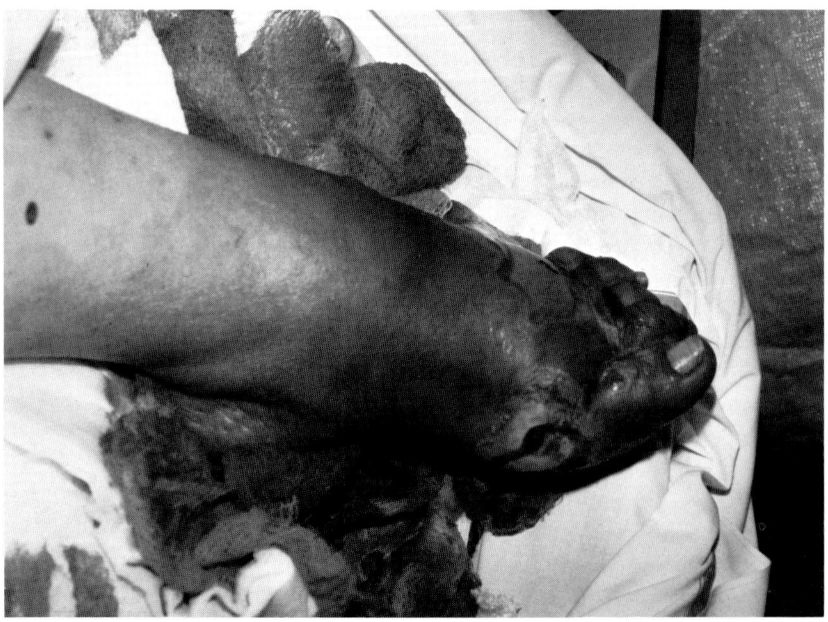

Fig. 11-1. A typical infected, insensate foot in a diabetic patient. Poorly fitting footwear resulted in an ulcerative lesion on the medial aspect of the foot, over the metatarsal head prominence. The open lesion, in turn, allowed ingress of bacterial pathogens and subsequent infection.

such as *Nocardia, Actinomyces,* or *mycobacteria.* These infections can be part of disseminated mycoses with metastatic infection to the feet.

Depending on the severity of the illness and the extent of tissue involvement, these infections can vary in their clinical manifestations. Chronic, poorly healing ulcers may be minimally symptomatic, but associated cellulitis may result in fever, pain, tenderness in the involved area, and peripheral leukocytosis. The elderly diabetic patient may sometimes manifest no systemic symptoms. Crepitant anaerobic cellulitis is a disease entity that often results from mixed anaerobic and aerobic superinfection of a long-standing diabetic foot ulcer. The infection gives rise to extensive gas formation that dissects underneath the skin, thus giving rise to crepitus on palpation. Patients usually demonstrate fever and leukocytosis. With appropriate management, this infection can usually be easily controlled.

Once pyogenic infections occur in the diabetic foot, they may ascend up the leg and sometimes progress to a necrotizing soft tissue infection. These infections are frequently caused by synergistic interaction of multiple bacteria, including anaerobes, aerobes, and microaerophilic bacteria. Included in these severe and life-threatening infections are synergistic necrotizing fasciitis and nonclostridial anaerobic myonecrosis (erstwhile erroneously called synergistic necrotizing cellulitis). Necrotizing fasciitis is manifested by a rapidly spreading infection that dissects along the path of the superficial fascia, causing necrosis and purulence. Perforating arteries supplying the skin may be involved as the infection spreads, giving rise to ischemic and gangrenous changes on the skin surface. Nonclostridial anaerobic myonecrosis, on the other hand, involves muscle and is therefore a deeper process. The latter process is located underneath the deep enveloping fascia. Occasionally, this process can be caused solely by anaerobic streptococci and has therefore been referred to as anaerobic streptococcal myonecrosis. The classic "gas gangrene," or clostridial myonecrosis, does not appear to be any more common in the diabetic population. All these disease processes can be distinguished from one another at surgical exploration. Patients with synergistic necrotizing soft tissue infections are generally toxic and highly febrile. These conditions can be associated with high mortality (20 to 50 percent). These processes have been discussed in depth in recent publications.[20,21]

Necrotizing fasciitis and nonclostridial anaerobic myonecrosis are generaly considered to be "synergistic" infections because of the commonly held belief that the multiple bacteria involved (frequently anaerobes and aerobes) enhance one another's growth. In a genetically diabetic mouse model, Bessman and colleagues indeed demonstrated that *Bacteroides fragilis* and enterococci enhance each other's capacity to produce subcutaneous abscesses.[22]

MICROBIOLOGY

The polymicrobial nature of diabetic foot gangrene and nonhealing chronic diabetic foot ulcers has been known for at least half a century. In his classic paper in 1939, Zierold emphasized the role of anaerobic bacteria such as the Welch bacillus (now known as *Clostridium perfringens*) as well as anaerobic streptococci in diabetic gangrene.[23] In 1943, Weiss isolated *Proteus* sp., an aerobic β-hemolytic streptococcus, an anaerobic diphtheroid, and *B. melaninogenicus* from the infected amputation stump of a 72-year-old diabetic patient.[24] Ziment et al., in 1969, reported on the microbiology of bone and joint infections in 8 patients, 7 of whom were diabetic.[25] The most commonly isolated microorganisms were *B. fragilis, B. melaninogenicus,* anaerobic streptococcus, *Fusobacterium* spp., *Proteus* spp., *Staphylococcus aureus,* and *Streptococcus* spp. In 1976, Louie et al. studied the microbiology of the foot ulcers of 20 diabetic patients, using culture specimens obtained with a dermal curette after inital debridement of the base of the ulcer to remove overlying necrotic and presumably superficially colonized tissue.[26] Again, these lesions were shown to have polymicrobial flora, with an average of 5.8 bacterial species (3.2 aerobes and 2.6 anaerobes) per specimen. *Peptococcus* spp. was the most frequent isolate. Other frequently isolated microorganisms were *P. mirabilis, B. fragilis, Enterococcus* spp., *S. aureus, B. melaninogenicus, Clostridium* spp., and *Escherichia coli.*

In 1978 and 1979, Sharp et al. compared the concordance between deep tissue swab cultures obtained at surgery with swab culture of drainage from superficial ulcers in 52 diabetic patiens.[27,28] Poor concordance was obtained between the two modalities of culture collection. The deep tissue culture showed an average of 2.3 microorganisms per specimen, but only 27 percent yielded anaerobes (*B. fragilis* being the most common anaerobic isolate). This study confirmed previous suspicions that superficial serial cultures may not always reveal the true microbiology present in deep tissue. Other authors had questioned the reliability of surface cultures, such as those obtained from sinus tracts, in predicting the underlying microbiology in deeper tissues, such as in osteomyelitis.[29] The fewer number of microorganisms per specimen and the relative scarcity of anaerobes seen in Sharp et al.'s study can be attributed to the suboptimal anaerobic microbiology techniques employed in the study.

In 1979 Fierer et al. studied the microbiology obtained at surgery from 30 infected diabetic feet and again showed a mixture of aerobes and anaerobes in 17 of the 30 specimens.[30] *Peptococcus* spp., *B. fragilis, Proteus* spp., *E. coli, Enterococcus* spp., and *S. aureus* were the most frequent isolates.

In 1980 and 1984 Sapico and colleagues methodically studied the quantitative deep tissue microbiology of amputated diabetic feet of 32 patients and compared the concordance of superficial swab cultures, curettage of the ulcer base, and needle aspiration after saline injection with the results of deep tissue cultures.[31,32] In this study, specimens were obtained immediately after surgical amputation, and deep tissue cultures were obtained after dissection through disinfected, intact skin, away from open ulcers that could be superficially colonized with microorganisms. Anaerobic transport media were used, and the specimens were immediately transferred to the anaerobic glove box, where tissue grinding, dilutions, and plating were performed. This study revealed an average of 4.8 microorganisms per specimen, with a very impressive heavy growth on quantitative cultures (Table 11-1). Twenty-five specimens yielded both aerobes as well as anaerobes, 6 yielded a pure culture of aerobes, and 1 yielded only anaerobes. When present, the anaerobes were isolated in heavier density than aerobes. The most frequently isolated species of microorganisms in this study are shown in Table 11-2. Also in this study ulcer concordance was examined between the commonly used modalities of culture collection (swab of ulcer, needle aspiration after saline injection, and curettage of the ulcer base) and the deep tissue culture results; better results were obtained from the curettage cultures. Swab cultures of the ulcer had a tendency to isolate microorganisms not present in the deep tissue. On the other hand, needle aspiration had a tendency to miss microorganisms that were actually seen in the deep tissue. It is very probable that

Table 11-1. Number of Isolates per Specimen and Growth Density of Microorganisms Recovered from 32 Deep Tissue Specimens from Infected Diabetic Feet

	Aerobes	*Anaerobes*	*Combined*
Number of isolates per specimen	2.8	2.0	4.8
Growth density (Log_{10}/g)	6.0	7.5	6.6

Table 11-2. The Most Frequently Isolated Microorganisms from the Deep Tissue in 32 Diabetic Patients with Infected Feet (Percentage of Patients Studied)

Microorganism	*Percentage*
Aerobes	
Gram-negative bacilli	
P. mirabilis	28
E. coli	16
P. aeruginosa	16
E. Aerogenes	12
Gram-positive cocci	
Enterococcus sp.	41
S. aureus	25
Group B streptococcus	16
Anaerobes	
Gram-negative bacilli	
B. fragilis	19
B. ovatus	9
B. ureolyticus	9
Gram-positive bacilli	
P. magnus	28
P. anaerobius	19
Gram-positive bacilli	
C. bifermentans	9

the curettage cultures yielded better results because the overlying superficial necrotic tissue at the base of the ulcer was debrided before cultures were taken, thus removing the majority of surface colonizers that are not present in deep tissue.

In 1986 Wheat et al. compared the agreement between "reliable" cultures and "unreliable" cultures (where contact with an open ulcer or openly draining lesions could not be avoided) and found complete agreement in only 27 percent of the 26 diabetic patients where simultaneous reliable and unreliable cultures were obtained.[33] These infections were again found to be polymicrobial (at least 4 microorganisms per patient), and anaerobes were isolated in 83 percent of the cases.

In a recent study of 65 diabetic patients who underwent amputation for infected feet, cultures were obtained by aspiration of bullae or abscesses, or by biopsy of soft tissue or bone.[34] The most commonly isolated microorganisms in this study were *Bacteroides* spp. (85 percent), *Peptococcus* spp.(80 percent), *Proteus mirabilis* (56 percent), groups A and D streptococci (45 percent), other *Proteus* spp. (37 percent), *S. aureus* (35 percent), *Clostridium* spp. (35 percent), *Propionibacterium* spp. (31 percent), *E. coli* (29 percent), *S. epidermidis* (28 percent), *Pseudomonas* spp. (23 percent), and *Klebsiella* spp.(15 percent). There was an average of 5.8 isolates per patient (2.3 anaerobes and 3.5 aerobes).

Sapico et al. reviewed their experience with diabetic bacteremia in association with infected feet over 2½ years.[35] Eleven cases were found, all of which were monomicrobial. *B. fragilis* was isolated 4 times; *S. aureus* 3 times; and *Bacteroides* spp. (nonfragilis), *E. coli*, group B streptococcus, and viridans groups streptococcus were each isolated once. It is worth noting that, even though severe foot infections in the diabetic patient are generally polymicrobial, the bacteremia associated with it is usually monomicrobial. The clinical significance of this observation is uncertain.

The role of bacteria in the nonhealing diabetic foot ulcer without associated gangrene, tissue necrosis, or cellulitis is unclear. Physical factors, such as chronic pressure over a bony prominence from ill-fitting footwear superimposed on an insensate foot, may be the most crucial factor leading to chronicity. Poor vascularity may also aggravate the situation. The microbiology of these ulcers may differ from that of an ulcer with concomitant tissue necrosis and frank gangrene.[36,37] The lesions are much more frequently monomicrobial, often involving gram-positive aerobic cocci such as *S. aureus*, coagulase-negative staphylococci, and enterococci. Anaerobes appear to be less commonly isolated in these settings.

MANAGEMENT OF DIABETIC PATIENTS WITH INFECTED FEET

General Principles

The management of diabetic patients with infected feet has to be individualized. Factors that have to be considered include manifestations of sepsis, the extent of tissue necrosis and gangrene, the adequacy of the vascularity to the involved limb, the extent and severity of the soft tissue infection, the presence and extent of bone involvement, the severity of the peripheral neuropathy, the presence and severity of foot deformity, and the metabolic control of the diabetic state. The metabolic control of the diabetic state should be prompt and aggressive. If the patient is not in adequate diabetic control, insulin therapy should be initiated. With the availability of capillary blood glucose monitoring at the bedside, rapid correction of hyperglycemia can be achieved. Oral agent therapy should be continued only if the control is satisfactory.

Surgical intervention is of paramount importance in most of these infections. Debridement of infected tissue and/or amputation at the appropriate level may be indicated. Early incision and drainage will decrease the inoculum size of the infecting organisms and may enhance local healing. Prior to definitive surgical procedure, a trial of appropriate antimicrobial therapy may be indicated to maximize the control of cellulitis and the extent of the infection in the potential surgical site. Obviously, as much of the limb as is necessary for future rehabilitation and ambulation has to be preserved without compromising control of infection.

In cases of streptococcal cellulitis or erysipelas, there may not be any open wounds that need surgical debridement, and good response may be achieved with antibiotic therapy directed at group A streptococcus. Needle aspiration of the advancing edge of the cellulitis for culture may occasionally be helpful.

Some patients may benefit from vascular reconstruction, since patients with nonhealing or poorly healing ulcers secondary to vascular insufficiency may heal following vascular surgery. These decisions will have to be guided by vascular studies such as the Doppler ultrasound with waveform analysis and/or transcutaneous oximetry. The subject of vascular reconstruction is discussed in another chapter.

All necrotic tissue has to be debrided until healthy, bleeding tissue is reached. If necrotizing fasciitis is present, then the area should be "filleted" by aggressively removing all the necrotic fascia and surrounding tissue, draining all purulent material, and leaving the involved area open and irrigated frequently with sterile normal saline solution. If necessary, daily debridements in the surgical suite may be performed. In the case of nonclostridial anaerobic myonecrosis, the necrotic nonviable muscles have to be totally removed. The surgical management of osteomyelitis is discussed separately in chapters 12, 18, and 20.

Table 11-3. Simplified Classification of Currently Available Antibacterial Agents

β-Lactam antibiotics
- Penicillins
  - Natural penicillins (penicillin G, penicillin V)
  - Penicillinase-resistant semisynthetics (methicillin, nafcillin, oxacillin, cloxacillin, dicloxacillin)
  - Extended spectrum
    - Ampicillin, amoxicillin
    - Carboxy penicillins (carbenicillin, ticarcillin)
    - Ureidopenicillins (pipericillin, mezlocillin, azlocillin)
    - Combination with β-lactamase inhibitors (amoxacillin-clavulanate, ticarcillin-clavulanate, ampicillin-sulbactam)
- Cephalosporins
  - First generation (cephalothin, cefazolin cephapirin, cephalexin, cefaclor, cephradine, cefadroxil
  - Second generation (cefamandole, ceforanide, cefonicid, cefuroxime, cefoxitin, cefotetan, cefmetazole)
  - Third generation (cefotaxime, moxalactam, cefoperazone, ceftizoxime, ceftriaxone, ceftazidime)
- Carbapenems (imipenem-cilastatin)
- Monobactams (aztreonam)

Aminoglycides (streptomycin, kanamycin, gentamicin, tobramycin, netilmicin, amikacin)

Lincosamides (lincomycin, clindamycin)

Macrolides (erythromycin)

Tetracycline (tetracycline, minocycline, doxycycline)

Chloramphenicol

Polypeptides (colistin, polymyxin B)

Nitroimidazoles (metronidazole)

Glycopeptides (vancomycin)

Quinolones (norfloxacin, ciprofloxacin)

Antimicrobial Agents

The recent availability of a multitude of newer antimicrobial agents has been a substantial boon to clinicians in general. However, the introduction of so many new agents in such a short space of time has also generated a significant amount of confusion. To help resolve some of this confusion, we will briefly discuss the salient points associated with these antimicrobial agents. Table 11-3 shows a simplified classification of the available antibacterial agents.

β-Lactam Antibiotics

Penicillins

Penicillins encompass a broad range of agents from penicillin G and ampicillin to the newer extended-spectrum penicillins such as piperacillin and mezlocillin. Ticarcillin and carbenicillin also belong to this group and have basically extended the gram-negative spectrum of activity of the older penicillins such as penicillin G or ampicillin. For example, ticarcillin and carbenicillin show activity against some *Enterobacter* spp. and *Pseudomonas aeruginosa* that ampicillin does not possess. However, both antibiotics are uniformly inactive against *Klebsiella* spp. and activity against *Enterococcus* spp. is limited. The newer extended-spectrum penicillins, such as mezlocillin and piperacillin, have improved gram-negative activity, including *Klebsiella* spp.,

Serratia spp., and *Providencia* spp., and also possess good activity against *Enterococcus* spp. and *B. fragilis*. Some gram-negative bacillii, including *P. aeruginosa*, may show resistance to carbenicillin or ticarcillin but may be sensitive to piperacillin or mezlocillin. One should keep in mind that these extended-spectrum penicillins are susceptible to the β-lactamase activity of most of *S. aureus*, coagulase-negative staphylococci, and the β-lactamase–producing strains of *Haemophilus influenzae* and are therefore not indicated for infections caused by these organisms. Nafcillin or oxacillin are distinctly more active against *S. aureus* compared to the newer penicillins, with the exception of methicillin-resistant *S. aureus* or *S. epidermidis* (MRSA or MRSE). Piperacillin and mezlocillin are also less likely to produce platelet aggregation dysfunction as compared to carbenicillin and ticarcillin, which possess the incriminated carboxyl side chain. Piperacillin is slightly more active against *P. aeruginosa* as compared to mezlocillin, but the clinical significance of this is unclear. Azlocillin has inferior activity against gram-negative bacilli with the exception of *P. aeruginosa* and therefore has limited clinical utility.

The addition of a β-lactamase inhibitor (i.e., amoxicillin-clavulanate, ticarcillin-clavulanate) has extended the spectrum of the penicillin drugs significantly. These combinations are extremely active against *B. fragilis* and methicillin-susceptible *S. aureus* (MSSA). Ticarcillin-clavulanate has more gram-negative activity while ampicillin-sulbactam has more gram-positive activity, including activity against enterococcus. Of the three, only amoxacillin-clavulanate is orally administered.

Cephalosporins

The second and third generation cephalosporins have extended the gram-negative spectrum of activity as compared to the first generation cephalosporins, which include cephalothin, cefazolin, and cephapirin. Whereas the first generation cephalosporins are characteristically inactive against *Enterobacter* spp., the newer cephalosporins may possess activity against this particular microorganisms. A subgroup of the second generation cephalosporins, the cephamycins, includes cefoxitin and the longer acting cefotetan. The cephamycins have basically been promoted as good antianaerobic agents. Cefotetan and cefmetazole, in general, have better activity against aerobic gram-negative bacilli but are inferior in activity against some of the *B. fragilis* group of microorganisms (such as *B. thetaciotaomicron* and *B. distasonis*), as compared to cefoxitin. Both also have the potential for causing bleeding complications from prolongation of the prothrombin time due to the presence of the *N*-methyl thiotetrazol (NMTT) side chain in their structure (this compound is also possessed by cefamandole, cefoperazone, and moxalactam). The NMTT side chain also confers the potential for inducing the disulfiram reaction on ingestion of alcohol. The utility of the cephamycins against anaerobic infections is, however, limited by the increasing resistance of the *B. fragilis* group of organisms to these antibiotics.

The third generation cephalosporins, as a class, are the first group of cephalosporins that have demonstrated some activity against *P. aeruginosa*. Of these antibiotics, only ceftazidime and cefoperazone have demonstrated utility against *P. aeruginosa* infections. Ceftazidime demonstrates better in vitro activity against this organism than cefoperazone.

In vitro studies have shown that the 7-desacetyl metabolite of cefotaxime, a third generation cephalosporin, synergizes with the parent compound and may make this antibiotic more active against certain gram-negative organisms, as well as *B. fragilis*, in vivo. The clinical significance of these observations are, however, still unclear. Ceftizoxime, another third generation cephalosporin, has shown conflicting activity against *B. fragilis*, depending on the antimicrobial susceptibility testing technique used. This problem should be resolved by clinical studies.

Ceftriaxone has an antibacterial spectrum comparable to cefotaxime and ceftizoxime. Its advantage over the others is the longer half-life, allowing ceftriaxone to be administered parenterally once daily. It has the disadvantage, however, of being somewhat less active against gram-positive cocci.

The inordinate number of bleeding complications observed with moxalactam have been attributed to the presence of both the NMTT and carboxyl side chains, resulting in both prolongation of prothrombin time as well as platelet dysfunction.

These complications have relegated moxalactam to the status of a historical curiosity.

All the currently available cephalosporins are inactive against enterococci, MRSA, and MRSE.

Carbapenems

Currently, imipenem is the only representative of the carbapenems that is clinically available. The spectrum of activity of imipenem is unprecedented— it has the widest spectrum of activity of all the antimicrobials we have in our armamentarium to this point in time. Imipenem comes combined in a fixed ratio with an analogue, cilastatin. This analogue has negligible antimicrobial activity but protects imipenem from hydrolysis by an enzyme found in the human proximal renal tubule, dehydropeptidase. Cilastatin, therefore, increases the level of imipenem found in the urine, may increase the serum levels to some extent, and, most importantly, protects the patient from nephrotoxicity associated with the metabolites. In spite of the broad spectrum of imipenem, it is consistently inactive against *E. faecium* and *P. maltophilia* and may be inactive against *P. capacia* and MRSA. Imipenem exhibits relatively higher MICs against *P. aeruginosa,* and emergence of resistance associated with the production of an outer membrane protein specifically impermeable to imipenem has been described.

Because of its propensity to induce seizures, its use for patients with seizure tendency and/or significant renal dysfunction should be limited. Careful dose adjustment should be done when the drug is used in renal insufficiency. Patients allergic to penicillins may sometimes also be allergic to imipenem.

Monobactams

Aztreonam is presently the sole representative of the monobactams, a unique class of β-lactams. Unlike the newer extended-spectrum β-lactams, this antibiotic is remarkably narrow in spectrum. It is active against most gram-negative bacilli (including *P. aeruginosa*) but is almost totally inactive against gram-positive organisms and against anaerobes. Patients allergic to other β-lactams appear to tolerate this antimicrobial quite well.

Aminoglycosides

Tobramycin is slightly more active against susceptible *P. aeruginosa* as compared to gentamicin, but the clinical significance of this difference is unclear. Amikacin frequently is active against microorganisms that have developed resistance to the other aminoglycosides. However, amikacin has an increased tendency to cause auditory, as compared to vestibular, toxicity. Nephrotoxicity among these agents may be comparable.

Lincosamides

Clindamycin is much superior to lincomycin in terms of antibacterial activity and absorption when given orally. Classicially, clindamycin has been active against gram-positive cocci as well as anaerobes (including *B. fragilis*). It is frequently inactive against MRSA, and increasing *B. fragilis* resistance has been reported in several institutions.

Macrolides, Tetracyclines, Chloramphenicol, Polypeptides

The macrolides and tetracyclines are now seldom used because of the development of widespread resistance in a vast range of microorganisms. The potential bone marrow toxicity of chloramphenicol has drastically limited it usefulness.

Nitroimidazoles

Metronidazole is one of the most active and bactericidal drugs against gram-negative anaerobic bacilli such as *B. fragilis*. Some gram-positive anaerobes and microaerophiles may, however, be resistant, and aerobes are also uniformly resistant to this drug.

Glycopeptides

Vancomycin is still quite active against most gram-positive cocci and bacilli and is the drug of choice for MRSA infections. Adverse reactions include the red man syndrome (histamine release phenomenon associated with rapid IV infusion) and some potential for nephro- and ototoxicity (less than that of aminoglycosides). Disturbing reports of the emergence of resistance in enterococci and coagulase-negative staphylococci have recently appeared in the literature.

Quinolones

Unlike norfloxacin, which has very limited absorption after oral intake, ciprofloxacin can be administered orally for the treatment of systemic infections. Ciprofloxacin shows impressive activity against *S. aureus* (including some MRSA) as well as against gram-negative aerobic bacilli (including *P. aeruginosa*). Its activity against streptococci and anaerobes, however, is quite limited. Care must be exercised when ciprofloxacin is given together with xanthines, such as theophyllines or caffeine, since elevated levels of the latter may result in side effects such as central nervous system stimulation and seizures.

Combinations of a variety of antimicrobial agents may result in indifference, synergism, additive effects, or antagonism. It is generally believed that a combination of bacteriostatic drugs (i.e., tetracycline or chloramphenicol) with bactericidal drugs (such as β-lactams) may result in clinical antagonism. Combinations of β-lactam agents are usually additive, but occasionally can be antagonistic. A β-lactam drug that is a good inducer of β-lactamase production (i.e., imipenem, cefoxitin) may "derepress" β-lactamase production in certain gram-negative bacilli, such as *P. aeruginosa, E. cloacae, S. marcescens,* and *Citrobacter* spp. This "derepression" may then result in hyperproduction of β-lactamase by these bacteria, resulting in accelerated hydrolysis of a non-β-lactamase stable antibiotic (i.e., penicillin G, ticarcillin, ampicillin) that is simultaneously administered with the inducer drug. These β-lactamase hyperproducers may elaborate enough of the enzyme to bind the antibiotics that diffuse into the periplasmic space of the bacteria, thereby preventing their binding to the target proteins and effectively neutralizing their antimicrobial activity.

Antibiotic Therapy

In most instances, the initial choice of antimicrobial agent(s) is made prior to knowledge of microbiologic cultures results. This decision will, therefore, have to be based on the most likely probabilities, in turn based on what previous studies have yielded in the past, and on the prevailing microbial flora seen in one's particular institution. The severity of the illness may also play a role in the choice of antimicrobial therapy, and combination therapy is most commonly utilized in the presence of systemic manifestations of sepsis and of severe local infections. The antimicrobials may be changed later, depending on the clinical response and the culture and sensitivity results. One should make sure that reliable cultures were taken and that appropriate anaerobic transport media and anaerobic culture techniques were implemented.

If the infection is relatively mild (as in the case of minimal cellulitis, mild purulence in a pre-existent ulcer, or an infected blister) and there are no clinical manifestations of sepsis, monoantibiotic therapy may be instituted while awaiting culture and sensitivity results. In the absence of necrotic tissue, foul-smelling discharge, and frank gangrene, it is more common to isolate single microorganisms, and anaerobes are relatively uncommon.[36] In this setting, the gram-positive aerobic cocci are usually the dominant organisms. Included among these are *S. aureus* as well as coagulase-negative staphylococci. Non-group D streptococci (including group B streptococci), as well as enterococci, may also be isolated. First generation cephalosporins will cover the first two microorganisms but will be inactive against the third. Ticarcillin-clavulanate and imipenem will be adequate for most coagulase-positive and -negative staphylococci, but the former may not be active against several strains of enterococci and the latter is predictably inactive against *E. faecium.* Ampicillin-sulbactam will provide more adequate coverage for the gram-positive organisms but is somewhat limited in its coverage of gram-negative bacilli. Gram-negative enteric bacilli may also be occasionally isolated in this setting. The first-generation cephalosporins are not as active against these organisms as the newer agents.

In the presence of more severe infections, especially when tissue necrosis and gangrene are present, when the infectious process is rapidly progressive, and/or when toxemia, hypotensive shock, and other signs of sepsis are present, more broad-spectrum empiric antimicrobial therapy is indicated while awaiting culture and sensitivity results. In addition to staphylococci and enterococci, anaerobes such as *B. fragilis* and gram-negative enteric aerobic bacilli, including *P. aeruginosa*, are frequently isolated. The rational approach to the empiric choice of antimicrobial agents in these polymicrobial infections includes a good knowledge of the general susceptibility patterns of the organisms most likely to be isolated in such settings. It is also important to be familiar with the antibiotic susceptibility patterns in one's individual institution. As an example, the *B. fragilis* group of microorganisms is generally resistant to penicillin G and ampicillin, but its susceptibility to anti-anaerobic drugs such as clindamycin may be different, in general, to its susceptibility 10 years ago, and the clindamycin susceptibility may vary from one institution or locality to another.[38] When we examined the antimicrobial susceptibility of anaerobic isolates (including *B. fragilis*) isolated 7 to 8 years ago from infected diabetic foot lesions in our institution, all our isolates belonging to the *B. fragilis* group were susceptible to clindamycin and 11 out of 13 were susceptible to cefoxitin.[39] Recently, however, we have observed that resistance to clindamycin has increased to at least 10 percent and resistance to cefoxitin to about 20 percent (unpublished observations). Metronidazole is excellent against the gram-negative anaerobic bacilli but has limited activity against gram-positive anaerobic and microaerophilic cocci. Imipenem, ticarcillin-clavulanate, and ampicillin-sulbactam all have excellent activity against almost all anaerobic bacteria.[38,40]

There is a reluctance to use aminoglycosides in the diabetic patient with evidence of diabetic nephropathy since there is existing evidence that patients with pre-existent impairment in renal function are more likely to develop nephrotoxicity with aminoglycoside use.[41] The choice of an anti-pseudomonal antimicrobial agent will likely be the anti-pseudomonal β-lactams or the quinolones. The anti-pseudomonal β-lactams include the older agents (carbenicillin and ticarcillin), the newer ones (piperacillin, mezlocillin, azlocillin), the third generation cephalosporins (ceftazidime and cefoperazone), and the novel class of monobactams (aztreonam). At the time of this writing, the quinolones have been available only as oral drugs (ciprofloxacin) and are more appropriate in the setting as long-term outpatient therapy, particularly when bone infection is present.

With severe infections and/or in the presence of sepsis and toxemia, it may be prudent to use a combination of at least two antimicrobial agents as preliminary empiric therapy pending knowledge of deep tissue culture and sensitivity. These combinations should be effective against the most commonly isolated microorganisms in this setting. Thus, the regimen should include coverage for *S. aureus*, anaerobic bacteria including *B. fragilis*, gram-negative enteric bacilli, and aerobic streptococci, including enterococci. A reasonable combination, for example, is that of ampicillin-sulbactam plus aztreonam or ceftazidime (or an aminoglycoside, if renal function is unimpaired). This regimen will cover almost all of the microorganisms most likely to be encountered in this setting.

Other possible useful combinations for severe polymicrobial infections include the time-proven regimen of clindamycin, ampicillin, and gentamicin. Aztreonam can be substituted for gentamicin. Cefoperazone, cefotaxime, ceftizoxime, or ceftriaxone can be combined with ampicillin and possibly clindamycin, vancomycin, nafcillin, or oxacillin to provide adequate anti-staphylococcal coverage, especially when either ceftazidime or cefoperazone is used. The latter two antibiotics, however, are considerably more active against *P. aeruginosa* than the other cephalosporins. Care must be exercised to adjust β-lactam dosages in the presence of renal insufficiency, since combinations of multiple β-lactam agents can potentially predispose to seizures. The combination of ampicillin, metronidazole, and gentamicin (or aztreonam) can provide reasonably wide coverage. Mezlocillin or piperacillin in combination with a drug with good antistaphylococcal coverage such as nafcillin or clindamycin is another reasonable option. Ceftazidime or cefoperazone plus metronidazole may be suboptimal for staphylococcal as well as enterococcal coverage. We feel that single-antibiotic therapy with either cefoxitin or cefotetan for severe infections may leave too many important microorganisms inadequately covered. These second generation cephalosporins may not provide optimal coverage for *S. aureus*, *Enterococcus* spp. and other aerobic streptococci, *P. aeruginosa* and possibly other enteric aerobic gram-negative bacilli, as well as some *Bacteroides* spp. belonging to the *B. fragilis* group. Again, it is of utmost importance to be familiar with the antimicrobial susceptibility patterns of certain microorganisms in one's particular institution. This is of particular concern with microorganisms such as *B. fragilis*, *S. aureus*, *P. aeruginosa*, as well as other gram-negative aerobic bacilli. In less severe infections, however, when one can afford to wait for culture and sensitivity results, single drug therapy with ticarcillin-clavulanate, ampicillin-sulbactam, or imipenem may be adequate.

In a polymicrobial infection, it has not been totally clarified whether one needs antibiotic coverage for all the microorganisms present in the infected tissue. These infections have been felt to be "synergistic," in that the microorganisms involved seem to support each other. In a model of subcutaneous abscess in a genetically diabetic mouse, we had previously shown that a combination of certain microorganisms enhances each other's ability to produce and sustain subcutaneous abscesses in the genetically diabetic mouse, more so than in its nondiabetic littermate.[22] In the presence of severe infection, we have been inclined not to ignore certain microorganisms in favor of others.

The duration of antimicrobial therapy has to be individualized according to the severity of infection, the presence or absence of septic complications, and the presence or absence of bone involvement. Mild cellulitis in the absence of gangrene, necrotic tissue, and bone involvement may respond to a 7- to 10-day course of antibiotics (with debridement, as necessary). More extensive tissue involvement may require longer therapy, depending on the extent of infection. If there is an attempt to salvage infected bone, prolonged antibiotic therapy may be necessary. Bamberger et al.[42] reported on good results using either a 4-week course of intravenous antimicrobials or a combination of shorter course intravenous therapy (i.e., 2 weeks) followed by prolonged oral therapy amounting to a total course of about 3 months. Our oral therapy armamentarium has been enhanced by the availability of new drugs such as amoxicillin-clavulanate and ciprofloxacin. The former is particularly active against staphylococci (with the exception of methicillin-resistant ones), enterococci, and streptococci, and some gram-negative aerobic bacilli. It has excellent activity against *B. fragilis*. It has no activity, however, against *P. aeruginosa*. Ciprofloxacin has good activity against gram-negative aerobic bacilli, including *P. aeruginosa*, and has reasonably good activity against *S. aureus*. It has very limited activity, however, against streptococci and is virtually inactive against *B. fragilis*.

Table 11-4 shows the antimicrobial activity, dosage, and administration of some of the more clinically useful antimicrobial agents that are particularly useful in the management of diabetic foot infections.

Table 11-4. Some of the More Commonly Employed Antimicrobial Agents for Diabetic Foot Infections

Classification	*Agent*	*Spectrum of Activity*	*Usual Adult Dosage and Administration*	*Comments*
Parenteral				
Penicillins	Ampicillin	Gram-positive cocci including enterococci, but not MRSA + MRSE most *S. aureus* and coagulase-negative staphylococci; limited activity vs. gram-negative bacilli; inactive vs. *P. aeruginosa*, *B. fragilis* groups	2 g IV q4–6h	Susceptible to β-lactamase
	Oxacillin	Gram-positive cocci except for enterococci, MRSA, MRSE; inactive vs. *B. fragilis*	2 g IV q4–6h	Should not be used for penicillin-allergic patients

(Continued)

Table 11-4. *(continued)*

Classification	*Agent*	*Spectrum of Activity*	*Usual Adult Dosage and Administration*	*Comments*
	Piperacillin or mezlocillin	Gram-positive cocci including enterococci but not MRSA or MRSE; active vs. most gram-negative bacilli including *Pseudomonas*; active vs. some *B. fragilis*	3 g IV q4–6h	Susceptible to β-lactamase
Cephalosporins	Cephalothin (or cephapirin)	Gram-positive cocci except for enterococci, MRSA, MRSE; some gram-negative bacilli but not *Pseudomonas*, indole-positive proteins, *Enterobacter*, *Acinetobacter*, or *Serratia*; inactive vs. *B. fragilis*	2 g IV q4–6h	5–10% of patients allergic to penicillin may not tolerate cephalosporins
	Cefazolin	Same as above	0.5–1.0 g q6–8h	Same as above; more susceptible to β-lactamase activity
	Cefotaxime	Gram-positive cocci but not enterococci, MRSA, MRSE; gram-negative bacilli but not *Pseudomonas, Acinetobacter*; variable vs. *B. fragilis*	2 g q6–8h	Third generation cephalosporin
	Ceftizoxime	Same as above	2–4 g q8h	Same as above
	Ceftazidime	Same as above, but active vs. *P. aeruginosa* and some other *Pseudomonas* spp.	1–2 g q8h	Same as above
Penicillin–β-lactamase inhibitor combination	Ampicillin-sulbactam	Gram-positive cocci including enterococci, but not MRSA or MRSE; gram-negative bacilli, but not *Pseudomonas, E. cloacae*; excellent activity vs. *B. fragilis*	Same dose as ampicillin	
	Ticarcillin-clavulanate	Same as above but less active vs. enterococci; more active vs. gram-negative bacilli	3.0 g of ticarcillin Iv of 4–6h	
Carbapenem	Imipenem-cilastatin	Active against most gram-positive or -negative organisms but not *E. faecium*, *P. maltophilia*, some *P. cepacia* and corynebacteria; excellent activity vs. *B. fragilis*	0.5–1.0 g IV q6–8h	Possible cross allergenicity with penicillins; seizures have occurred in some patients

Table 11-4. *(continued)*

Classification	*Agent*	*Spectrum of Activity*	*Usual Adult Dosage and Administration*	*Comments*
Monobactam	Aztreonam	Active vs. gram-negative bacilli including *P. aeruginosa* but not *P. maltophilia, P. cepacia, Acinetobacter*; inactive vs. gram-positive, cocci and anaerobes	1–2 g IV q6–8h	Can be used in patients with known allergy to penicillins and cephalosporins
Aminoglycosides	Gentamicin or tobramycin	Limited activity vs. gram-positive cocci such as *S. aureus*; active vs. gram-negative bacilli including *Pseudomonas* (some have developed resistance)	3–5 mg/kg/day in 3 equally divided doses depending on renal function, serum levels	May be nephrotoxic and ototoxic (special concern in diabetics with nephropathy)
	Amikacin	Same as above; may be active vs. gram-negative bacilli resistant to gentamicin or tobramycin	15 mg/kg/day divided q8 or 12h (adjust with renal function, serum levels)	Same as above
Lincosamides	Clindamycin	Active vs. gram-positive cocci except enterococci, some MRSA or MRSE; active vs. most *B. fragilis*, but variable activity vs. *Clostridia*	300–900 mg IV q8h	Resistance in *B. fragilis* isolates may vary according to institution or geograhic location
Glycopeptides	Vancomycin	Active vs. gram-positive cocci including MRSA, MRSE, and enterococci; inactive vs. most gram-negative bacilli and gram-negative anaerobes	500 mg IV q8h to 1 g IV q12h	Should not be infused IV faster than 1 hour (may cause red man syndrome)
Nitroimidazoles	Metronidazole	Active vs. anaerobes; no acitivity against aerobes	500 mg q6h	Concurrent ingestation of alcohol can produce a disulfiram-like reaction
Oral				
Penicillins	Ampicillin	Same as parenteral ampicillin	250–500 mg PO q6h	Should not be administered with food
	Amoxicillin	Same as above	250–500 mg PO q8h	May be given with food
Penicillin-β-lactamase inhibitors	Amoxicillin-clavulanate	Similar spectrum as parenteral ampicillin/sulbactam	250–500 mg of amoxicillin (each with 125 mg clavulanate PO q8h	May cause diarrhea
Cephalosporins	Cephalexin or cephradine	Same as parenteral cephalothin	250–500 mg PO q6h	May be absorbed better without food

(Continued)

Table 11-4. *(continued)*

Classification	*Agent*	*Spectrum of Activity*	*Usual Adult Dosage and Administration*	*Comments*
	Cefixime	Same activity vs. gram-positive cocci but not enterococci, MRSA, MRSE; active vs. many gram-negative bacilli but not *Enterobacter*, and *Pseudomonas*; inactive vs. *Bacteroides* spp.	200 mg PO q12h or 400 mg PO daily	New oral third generation cephalosporin
Lincosamides	Clindamycin	Same as parenteral form	150–300 mg PO q6h	Same as parenteral form
Quinolones	Ciprofloxacin	Active vs. *S. aureus* (including most MRSA and MRSE); limited activity against some other gram-positive cocci; active vs. gram-negative bacilli including *P. aeruginosa*; inactive vs. *B. fragilis*	500–750 mg PO q12h	Should not be given to children or pregnant women
Nitroimidazoles	Metronidazole	Same as parenteral form	500–750 mg PO q8h	Same as parenteral form

Abbreviations: MRSA, methicillin-resistant *S. aureus*; MRSE, methicillin-resistant *S. epidermidis.*

REFERENCES

1. Wheat LJ: Infection and diabetes. Diabetes Care 3:187, 1980
2. Doroghazi RM, Nad 1 JB, Hyslop NE et al: Invasive external otitis: report of 21 cases and review of literature. Am J Med 71:603, 1981
3. Abramson E, Wilson D, Arky RA: Rhinocerebral phycomycosis in association with diabetic ketoacidosis. Ann Intern Med 66:735, 1967
4. Pillsbury HC, Fischer ND: Rhinocerebral mucormycosis. Arch Otolaryngol 103:600, 1977
5. Mentzer RM, Jr, Golden GT, Chandler JG, Horsley JS III: A comparative appraisal of emphysematous cholecystitis. Am J Surg 129:10, 1975
6. Albengowe CW, McManamon PJM: Acute emphysematous cholecystitis. Can Med Assoc J 111:1112, 1974
7. Michaeli J, Mozle P, Perlberg S et al: Emphysematous pyelonephritis. J Urol 131:203, 1984
8. Thorley JD, Jones SR, Sanford JP: Perinephric abscess. Medicine 53:441, 1974
9. Gibbons GW, Eliopoulos GM: Infection of the diabetic feet. p. 97. In Kozak GP, Hoar CS, Jr, Rowbotham JL et al (eds): Management of Diabetic Foot Problems. WB Saunders, Philadelphia, 1984
10. Bagdade JD, Root RK, Bulger RJ: Impaired leukocyte function in patients with poorly controlled diabetes. Diabetes 23:9, 1974
11. Molinar DM, Palumbo PH, Wilson WR, Ritts RE: Leukocyte chemotaxis in diabetic patients and their first degree relatives. Diabetes suppl. 2, 25:880, 1976
12. Repine JE, Clawson CC, Goetz FE: Batericidal function of neutrophils from patients with acute bacterial infections and from diabetes. J Infect Dis 142:869, 1980
13. Katz S, Klein B, Elian I et al: Phagocyte activity of monocytes from diabetic patients. Diabetes Care 6:479, 1983
14. Tan JS, Anderson JL, Watanakunakorn C, Phair JP: Neutrophil dysfunction in diabetes mellitus. J Lab Clin Med 85:26, 1975
15. Mahmoud AAF, Rodman HN, Mandel MG, Warren KS: Induced and spontaneous diabetes mellitus and suppression of cell-mediated immunologic responses: granuloma formation, delayed dermal reactivity, and allograft rejection. J Clin Invest 57:362, 1976

16. Salvapandian AJ: Infections of the foot. p. 401. In Jahss MH (ed): Disorders of the Foot. WB Saunders, Philadelphia, 1982
17. Siebart WT, Dewan S, Williams TW Jr: Pseudomonas puncture wound osteomyelitis in adults. Am J Med Sci 283:83, 1982
18. Greene NE, Bruno J III: Pseudomonas infections of the foot after puncture wounds. So Med J 73:146, 1980
19. Johnson PH: Psuedomonas infections of the foot following puncture wounds. JAMA 204:170, 1968
20. George WL: Other infections of skin, soft tissue, and muscle. p. 485. In Finegold SM, George WL (eds): Anaerobic Infections in Humans. Academic Press, San Diego, 1989
21. Leslie CA, Sapico FL, Bessman AN: Infections in the diabetic host. Comp Ther 15:23, 1989
22. Bessman AN, Sapico FL, Tabatabai MF, Montgomerie JZ: Persistence of polymicrobial abscesses in the poorly controlled diabetic host. Diabetes 36:448, 1986
23. Zierold AA: Gangrene of the extremity in the diabetic. Ann Surg 110:723, 1937
24. Weiss L: The pathogenicity of *Bacteroides melaninogenicus* and its importance in surgical infections. Surgery 13:683, 1943
25. Ziment I, Davis A, Finegold SM: Joint infection by anaerobic bacteria. Arthritis Rheum 12:627, 1969
26. Louie TJ, Bartlett JG, Tally FP, Gorbach SL: Aerobic and anaerobic bacteria in diabetic foot ulcers. Ann Intern Med 85:461, 1976
27. Sharp CS, Bessman AN, Wagner FW, Jr, Garland D: Microbiology of deep tissue in diabetic gangrene. Diabetes Care 1:289, 1978
28. Sharp CS, Bessman AN, Wagner FW, Jr et al: Microbiology of superficial and deep tissues in infected diabetic gangrene. Surg Gynecol Obstet 149:217, 1979
29. Mackowiak PA, Jones SR, Smith JW: Diagnostic value of sinus-tract cultures n chronic osteomyelitis. JAMA 239:2772, 1978
30. Fierer J, Daniel D, Davis C: The fetid foot: lower extremity infections in patients with diabetes mellitus. Rev Infect Dis 1:210, 1979
31. Sapico FL, Canawati HN, Witte JL et al: Quantitative aerobic and anaerobic bacteriology of infected diabetic feet. J Clin Microbiol 12:413, 1980
32. Sapico FL, Witte JL, Canawati HN et al: The infected foot of the diabetic patient: quantitative microbiology and analysis of clinical features. Rev Infect Dis suppl. 1, 6:171, 1984
33. Wheat JL, Allen SD, Henry M et al: Diabetic foot infections: bacteriologic analysis. Arch Intern Med 146:1935, 1986
34. Scher KS, Steele FJ: The septic foot in patients with diabetes. Surgery 104:661, 1988
35. Sapico FL, Bessman AN, Canawati HN: Bacteremia in diabetic patients with infected lower extremities. Diabetes Care 5:101, 1982
36. Leslie CA, Sapico FL, Ginunas VJ, Adkins RH: Randomized clinical trial of topical hyperbaric oxygen for treatment of diabetic foot ulcers. Diabetes Care 11:111, 1988
37. Lipsky BA, Pecoraso RE, Larson S: Microbiology and treatment of acute lower extremity infections in diabetic outpatients. Abstracts of the Intensive Conference on Antimicrobial Agents and Chemotherapy, 1:287, 1987
38. Cuchural GJ Jr, Tally FP, Jacobus NV et al: Susceptibility of the *Bacteroides fragilis* group in the United States: analysis by site of isolation. Antimicrob Ag Chemother 32:717, 1988
39. Ginunas VJ, Canawati HN, Sapico FL: Anaerobic bacteria isolated from foot infections in diabetic patients: in vitro susceptibility to nine antibiotics. Clin Ther 6:457, 1984
40. Rolfe RD, Finegold SM: Comparative in vitro activity of new beta-lactam antibiotics against anaerobic bacteria. Antimicrob Ag Chemother 20:600, 1981
41. Moore RD, Smith CR, Lipsky JJ et al: Risk factors for nephrotoxicity in patients treated with aminoglycosides. Ann Intern Med 100:352, 1984
42. Bamberger DM, Dans GP, Gerding DN: Osteomyelitis in the feet of diabetic patients: long-term results, prognostic factors, and the role of antimicrobial and surgical therapy. Am J Med 83:658, 1987

12

Osteomyelitis of the Diabetic Foot

Jason H. Calhoun, M.D., M.Eng.
Jon T. Mader, M.D.

Osteomyelitis is a common problem in the diabetic foot. In one series of more than 1,000 diabetic foot infections, osteomyelitis was the most common initial presentation.[1,2] The compromised blood supply and decreased sensation in the diabetic foot make diagnosis and treatment of osteomyelitis difficult. Poor blood glucose control, poor patient compliance with treatment regimens, progressive vascular changes of diabetes mellitus, as well as smoking, drinking, obesity, and other systemic problems hinder the healing process. Complete cure of osteomyelitis is the ideal aim of treatment. In these compromised hosts, however, suppression of the infection or, if necessary, eradication of the disease by amputation of the extremity, is often the best possible treatment. We support a team approach to the management of osteomyelitis in the diabetic patient, including staging of the osteomyelitis and use of multiple specialists to deal successfully with the anatomic, neurovascular, and bacterial difficulties encountered in osteomyelitis of the diabetic foot.[3-6]

DIABETIC FOOT INFECTIONS

Diabetic foot infections can be classified by the depth of soft tissue and bone involvement. The widely used Wagner classification separates diabetic foot infections into ulcers, osteomyelitis, or gangrene.[7-10] Within the category of osteomyelitis several different systems for subclassification have been proposed. We have found that classifying osteomyelitis by the anatomy of the infection and the quality of the host is helpful in understanding, diagnosing, and treating diabetic osteomyelitis. We will briefly review Wagner's system of diabetic foot infection and then discuss staging of osteomyelitis in the diabetic foot.

Wagner's system is valuable for evaluating, planning treatment, documenting, and comparing treatment of all diabetic foot infections (Fig. 12-1 and Table 12-1).[7,8] Wagner's grade 0 infection is cellulitis in a diabetic patient's foot. This foot is at risk for developing ulcers, osteomyelitis, or gangrene (Fig. 12-2). Therapy of Wagner's grade 0 infection is directed toward outpatient control of the infection. Broad spectrum oral antibiotics active against gram-positive organisms are used empirically. If rapid improvement is not seen by 48 hours, additional antimicrobial agents directed against enterococcus or gram-negative organisms may be needed. After the infection has cleared, patient education and preventive therapy decrease the risk of future problems. The "at risk" foot may benefit from revascularization procedures if ischemia exists (ischemic index < 0.45 or transcutaneous $O_2 < 20$ mm).[7,8,11-15] Diabetic foot care school or surgical correction of hallux valgus, toenail prob-

Table 12-1. Therapy for Wagner Stages of Diabetic Foot Infections[a]

Grade	*Therapy*
0	Antibiotics, prophylactic surgery
1	Antibiotics, ST&B evaluation, LWC, debridement
2	Same, aggressive debridement
3	Same, debridement-resection-amputation
4	Same, amputation
5	Same, higher amputation

Abbreviations: ST&B, soft tissue and bone; LWC, local wound care.

[a] Outline of recommended therapy for diabetic foot infections.

lems, hammer toes, metatarsal prominence, other weight-bearing abnormalities, or Charcot joints may also be helpful.[7,8,16]

Wagner grade 1 and 2 lesions are superficial and deep ulcers. The diagnostic challenge for ulcers is proving that osteomyelitis is not present. Once this is done, the cellulitis and purulence can be controlled with short courses of culture-directed antibiotics, local wound care with dressings, total con-

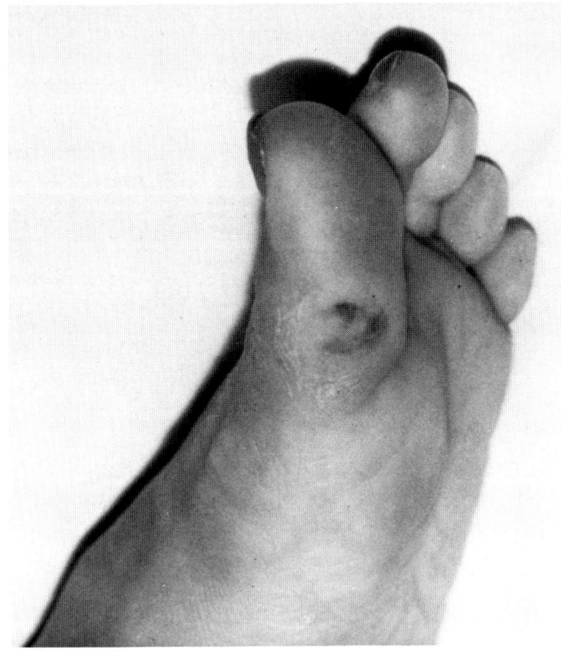

Fig. 12-2. Grade 0. Foot at risk. A 38-year-old white woman with diabetes controlled with oral hypoglycemics. Hyperkeratotic skin was treated with sanding for 3 years.

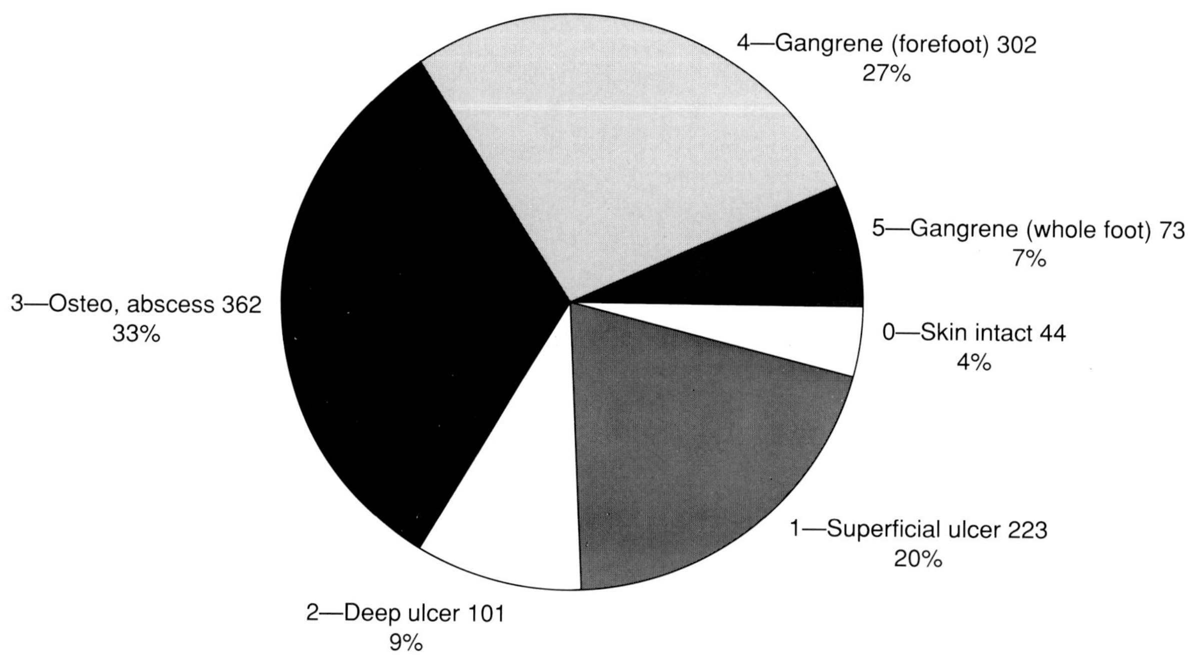

Fig. 12-1. Experience at University of Texas Medical Branch from 1968 to 1988 with 1,105 diabetic foot infections.

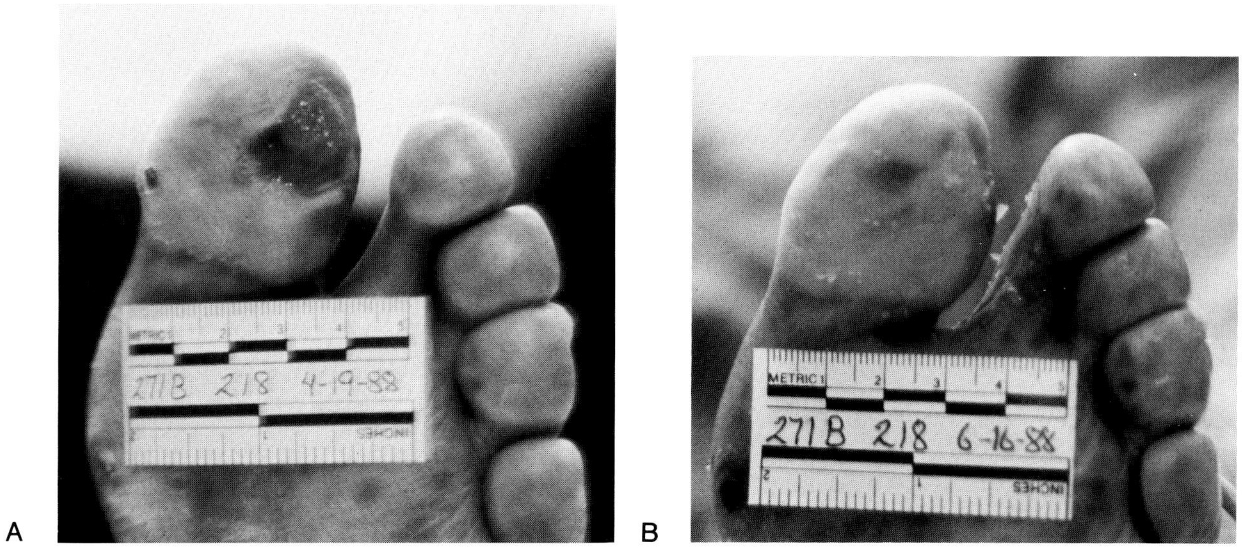

Fig. 12-3. (**A**) Grade 1. Diabetic ulcer in a 48-year-old Latin American man with insulin-dependent diabetes mellitus. The patient was treated with oral antibiotics for 2 weeks, with minimal debridement and wet-to-dry dressings. (**B**) The ulcer healed in 2 months. It recurred once and responded to the same therapy.

tact casts,[17,18] and minimal debridements. Ulcers generally heal in compliant patients if the surrounding soft tissue has a good blood supply (Fig. 12-3). Therapy is directed toward ulcer healing and preventing progression to osteomyelitis or gangrene. As in Wagner grade 0 infections, surgical procedures to revascularize ischemic areas or correct deformities may be indicated after the infection has been controlled.

Grade 3 lesions in the Wagner classification of diabetic foot infections are osteomyelitis or deep abscesses. At our institution, osteomyelitis is more common than deep abscesses by about 20:1 and osteomyelitis is the most common diabetic foot in-

Table 12-2. Microbiology of Diabetes Mellitus Osteomyelitis over a 20-Year Period at UTMB

	% Cultured[a]			
Organism	*1969–1973*	*1974–1978*	*1979–1983*	*1984–1988*
Staphylococcus aureus	66	28	43	51
(% MRSA)			(14)	(16)
Streptococcus sp.	33	61	62	24
Enterococcus		22	39	23
Staphylococcus epidermidis			36	27
(% MRSE)			(17)	(2)
Diphtheroids	33	17	19	23
Proteus mirabilis	33	17	37	20
Pseudomonas aeruginosa		6	22	14
M. morganii	33	22	6	7
Escherichia coli			16	9
Anaerobes			34	35
Polymicrobial	33	83	87	76

Abbreviations: MRSA, methicillin-resistant *S. aureus;* MRSE, methicillin-resistant *S. epidermidis.*

[a] Represents the percentage of the patients who cultured a specific bacteria for Wagner grade 3 (osteomyelitis) diabetic foot infections.

fection seen (Fig. 12-1). Although osteomyelitis can develop in the diabetic foot with intact, sensate, or well-vascularized soft tissue, it is uncommon. Infections usually start with minor trauma, infected nail beds, followed by cellulitis and ulcers. As the soft tissue breaks down, multiple bacteria colonize the ulcer (Table 12-2). Although treatment by debridement and long-term culture-directed antibiotics or amputation has the best chance of curing the infection,[1,19] it may be best to simply suppress the infection and maintain the functional integrity of the limb.[20] Even after successfully arresting or suppressing the infection, recurrence or new bone infection occurs in many patients. Resection of the involved bone or amputation of the limb may become necessary.[7,8]

Wagner's grade 4 lesions are partial foot gangrene and grade 5 lesions are full foot gangrene (Fig. 12-4). Diagnosis is usually straightforward and the treatment is amputation. The important treatment decision is when and how much to amputate. Decision making is aided by transcutaneous oxygen levels, ischemic indices, and arterial pressure waveforms. Clinical assessment of tissue viability with preoperative palpation of skin temperature differences and blanching followed by intraoperative observation of tissue bleeding is extremely important. Antibiotics are used to resolve cellulitis and prevent gas gangrene or necrotizing fasciitis. Some patients with only one or two small toes involved and no pain may be treated with observation, allowing the gangrenous toes to demarcate and autoamputate.[21] Although this is not usually successful, some patients prefer this. We prefer debridement of the necrotic tissue to prevent the possibility of gas gangrene or necrotizing fasciitis followed by close observation and amputation at a level with a good enough blood supply to allow healing.

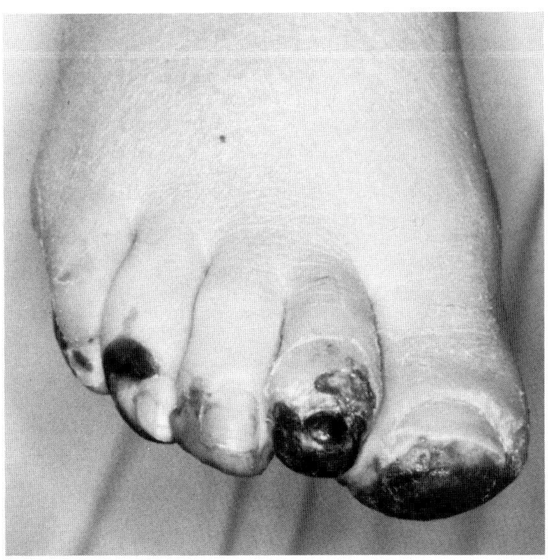

Fig. 12-4. Grade 4. Gangrene of the foot. A 45-year-old white man with insulin-dependent diabetes mellitus. All toes were amputated.

STAGING DIABETIC OSTEOMYELITIS

Osteomyelitis is difficult to treat even in nondiabetic patients. Numerous authors have offered classification systems to aid in the understanding, diagnosis, and treatment of osteomyelitis. Kelly's system is based on the multiple etiologies of osteomyelitis.[22] Waldvogel et al. classified adult osteomyelitis as resulting from contiguous spread, hematogenous seeding, or peripheral vascular disease.[23] Mays et al. used the size of defect to classify osteomyelitis.[24] Cierny and Mader, of the University of Texas Medical Branch (UTMB), staged adult long bone osteomyelitis by the anatomy of the bone infection and by host factors.[25] In over 1,500 cases of osteomyelitis treated at UTMB since 1980 (one-third of these being diabetic patients), we have found that the Cierny-Mader system is the most universally applicable and helps define treatment algorithms most accurately.

The Cierny-Mader system stages osteomyelitis according to the depth of the bone involvement and the quality of the overlying tissue. Each infection is assigned both a number stage for the anatomy of the infection and a letter stage for the host's capabilities. The number describes the area of the bone that is infected, and the letter describes the quality of the host defenses. This system can be modified to include joint and soft tissue infection (Tables 12-3 and 12-4). By staging the infection, treatment-based algorithms can be developed (Fig. 12-5).

A stage I infection is a simple infection with no

Table 12-3. The UTMB Staging System for Musculoskeletal Infections

Anatomic Type	*Bone Osteomyelitis*	*Septic Arthritis*	*Soft Tissue Cellulitis*
I Simple	Medullary OM	Simple SA (Acute)	Cellulitis
II Superficial	Superficial OM	SA with chondrolysis	Ulcer
III Localized	Local OM	SA with localized OM	Abscess
IV Diffuse	Diffuse OM	Unstable joint	Permeative[a]

Physiologic Class

A Host	Good immune system and delivery
B Host	Compromised locally (Bl) or systemically (Bs)
C Host	Requires suppressive or no treatment; minimal disability; treatment worse than disease; not a surgical candidate

Clinical Stage
Type + class = clinical stage
Example: Stage IV (Bs) osteomyelitis = a diffuse lesion in a systemically compromised host[b]

Abbreviations: OM, osteomyelitis; SA, septic arthritis.
[a] Permeative soft tissue infection includes gangrene, necrotizing fasciitis, etc.
[b] Compromising factors, see Table 12-4.

permanent anatomic damage. This is medullary osteomyelitis in a bone, acute septic arthritis in a joint, or cellulitis of soft tissue. Stage II is either superficial periosteal or cortical osteomyelitis, chondrolysis, subacute septic arthritis, or ulcerated soft tissue. In stage III, the infection is deeper but remains localized. It involves both the cortex and the medullary canal for osteomyelitis, bone about the joint for septic arthritis, or an abscess in soft tissue. A stage IV infection is a diffuse infection, diffuse osteomyelitis (nonunion), end stage septic arthritis (unstable joint), or a permeating necrotizing infection (gas gangrene, necrotizing fasciitis).

An A host is a physiologically normal host. The B host has systemic or local tissue factors that compromise healing. These range from systemic problems (malnutrition, immune deficiency, diabetes mellitus) to local factors (open wounds, scarring, vessel disease). Every diabetic patient is, at best, a B host because of systemic compromise; locally compromising factors may be present as well (usually ischemia and/or neuropathy). The last host classification is the C host: this patient is not a surgical candidate because surgery would be worse than the disease, either because of minimal disability, significant anaesthetic risk, or patient choice.

Table 12-4. Systemic or Local Factors That Affect Immune Surveillance, Metabolism, and Local Vascularity

Systemic (s)	*Local (l)*
Malnutrition	Chronic lymphedema
Renal, liver failure	Venous stasis
Alcohol abuse	Vessel compromise
Immune deficiency	Arteritis
Chronic hypoxia	Extensive scarring
Malignancy	Radiation fibrosis
Diabetes mellitus	Loss of sensation
Extremes of age	
Immunosuppression	
Steroid therapy	
Tobacco abuse (> 1½ packs per day)	
IV drug abuse	

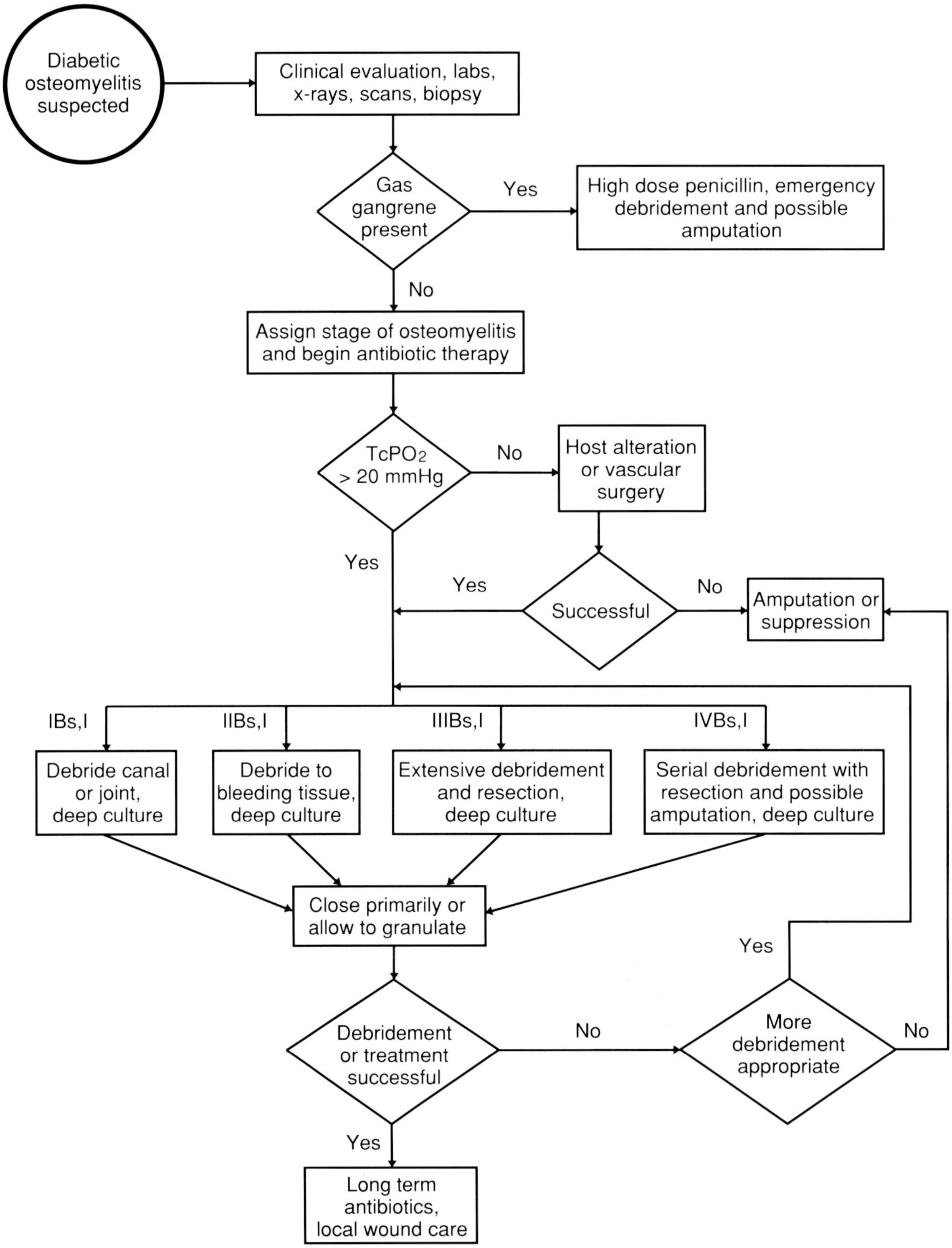

Fig. 12-5. Treatment algorithm for diabetic osteomyelitis.

DIAGNOSIS OF OSTEOMYELITIS

Presentation

Infections in the diabetic patient can be difficult to diagnose. Even in the absence of infection, diabetic dermatitis or hyperpigmentation can make the extremities look erythematous.[6] Neurotrophic arthropathy and autonomic dysfunction can cause the extremity to be swollen.[16,26] Poor diet and insulin therapy or progression of diabetes can cause elevated glucose levels. These changes, however, can also be indications of infection.

Patients can present with cellulitis around an ulcer or swollen area. They may give a history of an ingrown toenail, a hyperkeratotic area that fissured, minor trauma, or they may have no awareness of the cause. Usually these patients do not have systemic sepsis. Early osteomyelitis, abscesses, gas gangrene, and "flare-ups" of chronic osteomyelitis, however, may cause bacteremia and systemic signs of sepsis such as fever, uncontrolled glycosemia, and even diabetic coma. Foot infection is a very common cause for hospital admission in the diabetic patient.

Pain is usually absent because the tissue has no sensation. Many diabetic patients with chronic ulcers and osteomyelitis do not complain about foot problems, so health care personnel and family members can help with routine foot examinations. Many of our patients are referred by other health professionals who have either found the foot problem as an incidental part of a clinical examination or who have been following the patient and observed an increase in the infection.

The etiology of diabetic foot osteomyelitis is usually contiguous spread of bacteria and necrosis from pressure ulcers and, occasionally, ingrown toenails or trauma such as puncture wounds or lacerations (Fig. 12-6).

The most common site of presentation is in the forefoot (Fig. 12-7). This is because loss of protective sensation and blood supply starts distally in the toes and progresses proximally. The distal phalanges are most commonly involved, followed by the metatarsal heads (see Figs. 12-9 to 12-11 and 12-13). With midfoot deterioration due to Charcot joint, the tarsal bones may become prominent, cause ulcers, and become infected (see Fig. 12-12). The next most commonly involved bone is the calcaneus because of its weight-bearing status and limited soft tissue. The joints are often involved

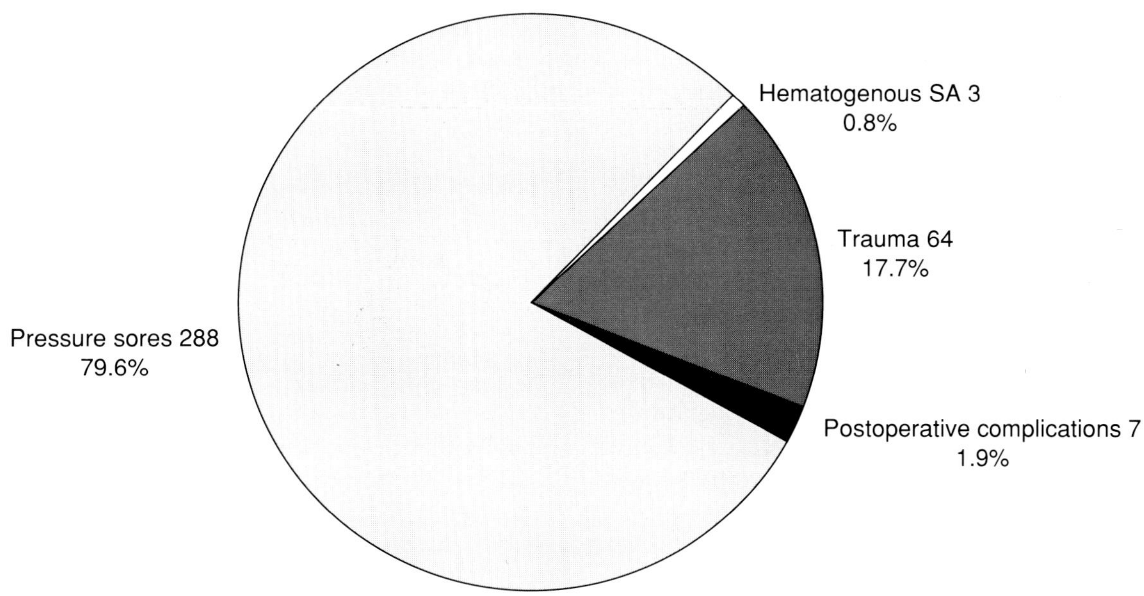

Fig. 12-6. Etiology of diabetic osteomyelitis seen at University of Texas Medical Branch from 1968 to 1988 (362 cases).

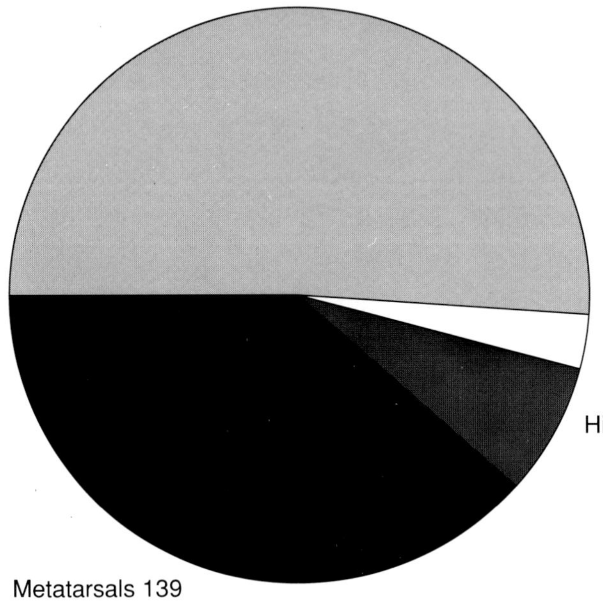

Fig. 12-7. Sites of infection in diabetic osteomyelitis (362 cases).

about these bones. Occasionally the ankle joint is infected by hematogenous seeding or from ulcers on the medial or lateral malleolus (see Fig. 12-15).

History and Physical

The duration and severity of a patient's diabetes is variable. If the diabetes has been poorly controlled because it was undiagnosed, was brittle, received ineffective treatment, or was present in a noncompliant patient, the neuropathy and depth of infection are usually worse. Other medical problems (hypertension, heart, kidney, liver, or vessel disease) and a medication history are important factors in staging and treating diabetic patients (Tables 12-4 and 12-5). Family, social, and employment history should be known so support and rehabilitation can be planned.

The physical examination gives information about other medical problems (eyes, heart, lungs, liver, kidney, gastrointestinal tract, and urinary) as well as the blood and nerve supply to the extremities. Palor, shiny skin, hair loss, diabetic hyperpigmentation, gangrene, muscle atrophy, and gait abnormalities may be observed. Decreased temperature, pulselessness, poor capillary refill, and exact level of compromised sensation are important. Capillary refill can be estimated with blanch tests at different levels; normal refill after

Table 12-5. Chronic Diseases in 380 Diabetic Patients Admitted for Foot Infections

Disease	*Patients (%)*
Hypertension	44.8
Congenital heart disease	14.6
Chronic renal failure	10.4
Coronary artery disease	9.8
Cerebrovascular disease	5.8
Hypothyroidism	3.5
Alcoholism	2.7
COPD	2.3
Tuberculosis	2.1
Peptic ulcer	1.9
Asthma	1.5
Total	99.4

Abbreviation: COPD, chronic obstructive pulmonary disease.

blanch is 2 seconds. The feet can be elevated above the heart with the patient supine and then on standing normal venous refill occurs in less than 15 seconds; moderate ischemia is present if refill takes 15 to 25 seconds, severe ischemia if it takes 25 to 40 seconds, and very severe ischemia if it takes greater than 40 seconds.[6] Subcutaneous air from gas gangrene can be palpated.

A complete neurologic and joint examination is important. Active and passive range of motion and muscle strength all decrease with muscle atrophy of the intrinsic and extrinsic muscles. Inability to sense pain allows repetitive stress loading and minimal trauma that causes ulcers. A pin wheel is a fast and easy way to measure pain and light touch.

Radiographs

The most important study to obtain for the evaluation of these infections is radiographs.[27] Gas gangrene can be seen as subcutaneous defects in the soft tissue (Fig. 12-8). The radiographs for osteomyelitis may initially show osteoporosis and soft tissue swelling. Early bone changes in osteomyelitis are thinning of cortical bone and loss of trabecullae in cancellous bone (Fig. 12-9A). These are followed by cystic changes as the infection grows. Progressive bone and joint destruction is followed by complete bone and joint loss (Fig. 12-9B). Cortical scalloping indicates periosteal ischemia and not necessarily infection (Fig. 12-10).[28] It is important to differentiate bone destruction due to stress fractures or Charcot joint and infection (Fig. 12-11A & B and 12-12B).[29-31] Xeroradiographs, magnification, or "hot lights" aid the sensitivity of the radiographs.[32]

Cultures

The second most important study after radiographs in diagnosing osteomyelitis is wound culture.[33-35] Swab cultures of ulcers or draining sinuses are not very accurate but are a helpful first step.[36,37] Swab cultures typically identify only about 66 percent of the pathogenic bacteria. *Enterococcus* and gram-negative bacteria are inadequately identified with swab cultures. Blood cultures or tissue injection cultures may be helpful for bacteremia sepsis or cellulitis that does not respond to first choice antimicrobials.[38] Chronic osteomyelitis is, however, an infection in ischemic tissue and is effectively "walled off" from the rest of the tissues so bacteria are not usually seen in the blood or local tissues. Bone cultures are necessary for accurate diagnosis and treatment.

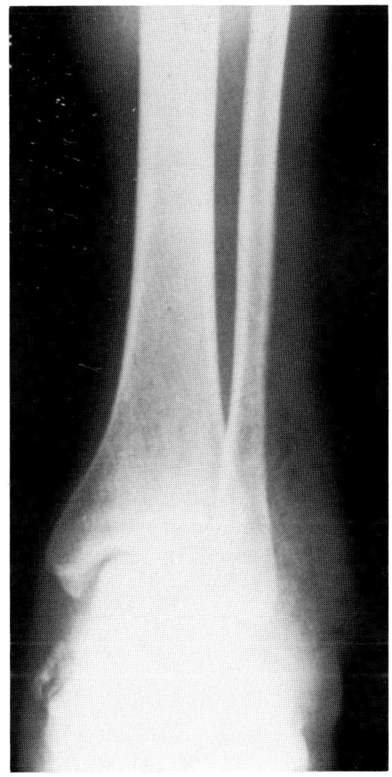

Fig. 12-8. Gas gangrene of the foot. A 44-year-old white woman with insulin-dependent diabetes mellitus had an ulcer on the heel that became necrotic. The ulcer went untreated until she developed life- and limb-threatening gas gangrene. She was treated with debridement, penicillin, and hyperbaric oxygen. Gram stain and cultures were positive for *Clostridium difficile*. The entire foot is now healed and has no ulcer.

Diabetic foot osteomyelitis is usually polymicrobial.[39,40] *Staphylococcus aureus* is the most common bacteria, followed by nonenterococcal *Streptococcus*, *S. epidermidis*, and *Enterococcus* sp. *Proteus mirabilis* and *Pseudomonas aeruginosa* are seen frequently. Anaerobes are cultured in about one-third of the patients (Table 12-2).[35,41,42]

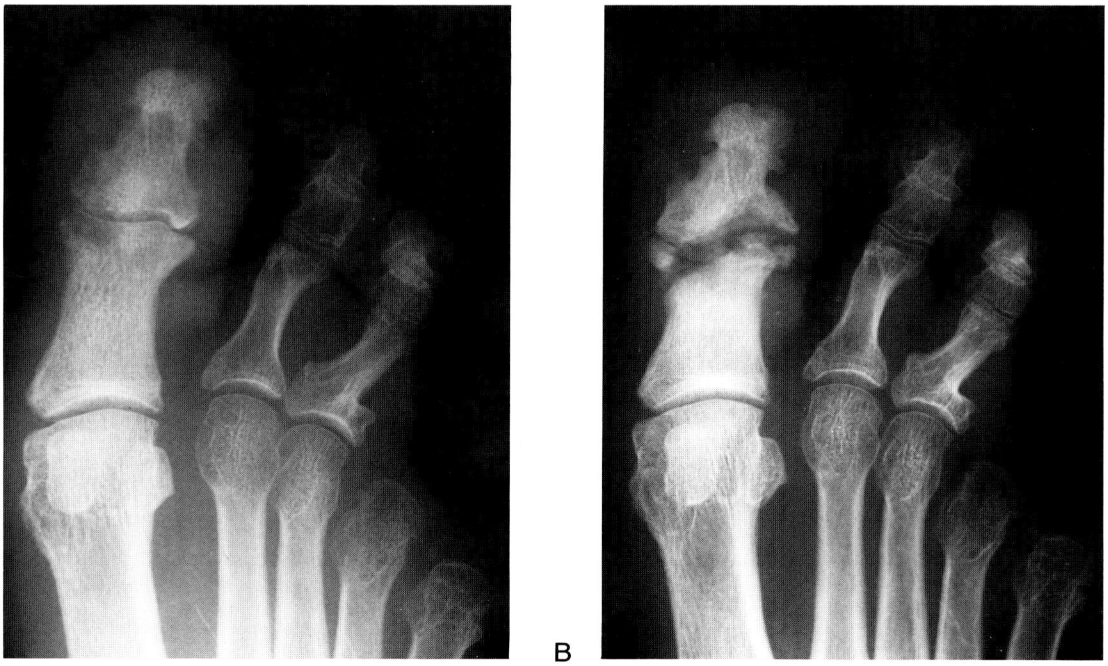

A B

Fig. 12-9. (A) Early bone changes. A 45-year-old white man with insulin-dependent diabetes mellitus shows early cortical bone lysis about the medial aspect of the interphalangeal joint of the great toe. (B) Same patient 3 months later with progressive radiograph changes.

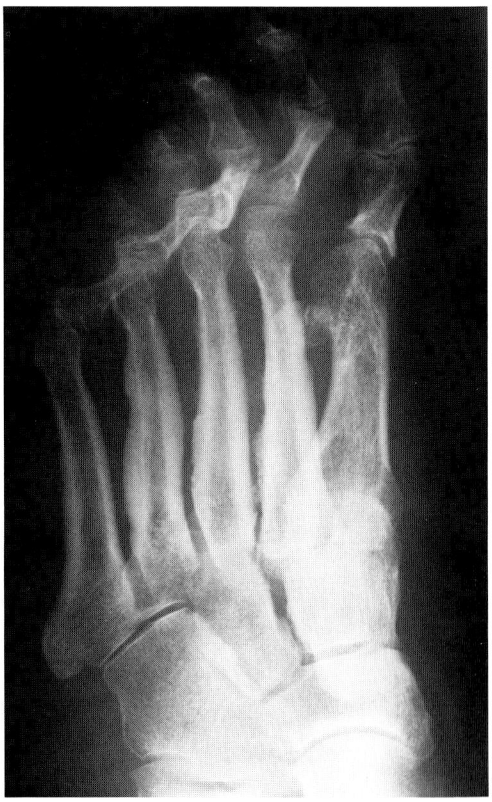

Fig. 12-10. Periosteal ischemia. A 60-year-old white woman with insulin-dependent diabetes mellitus shows scalloping on metatarsals due to ischemia. She had very little loss of sensation.

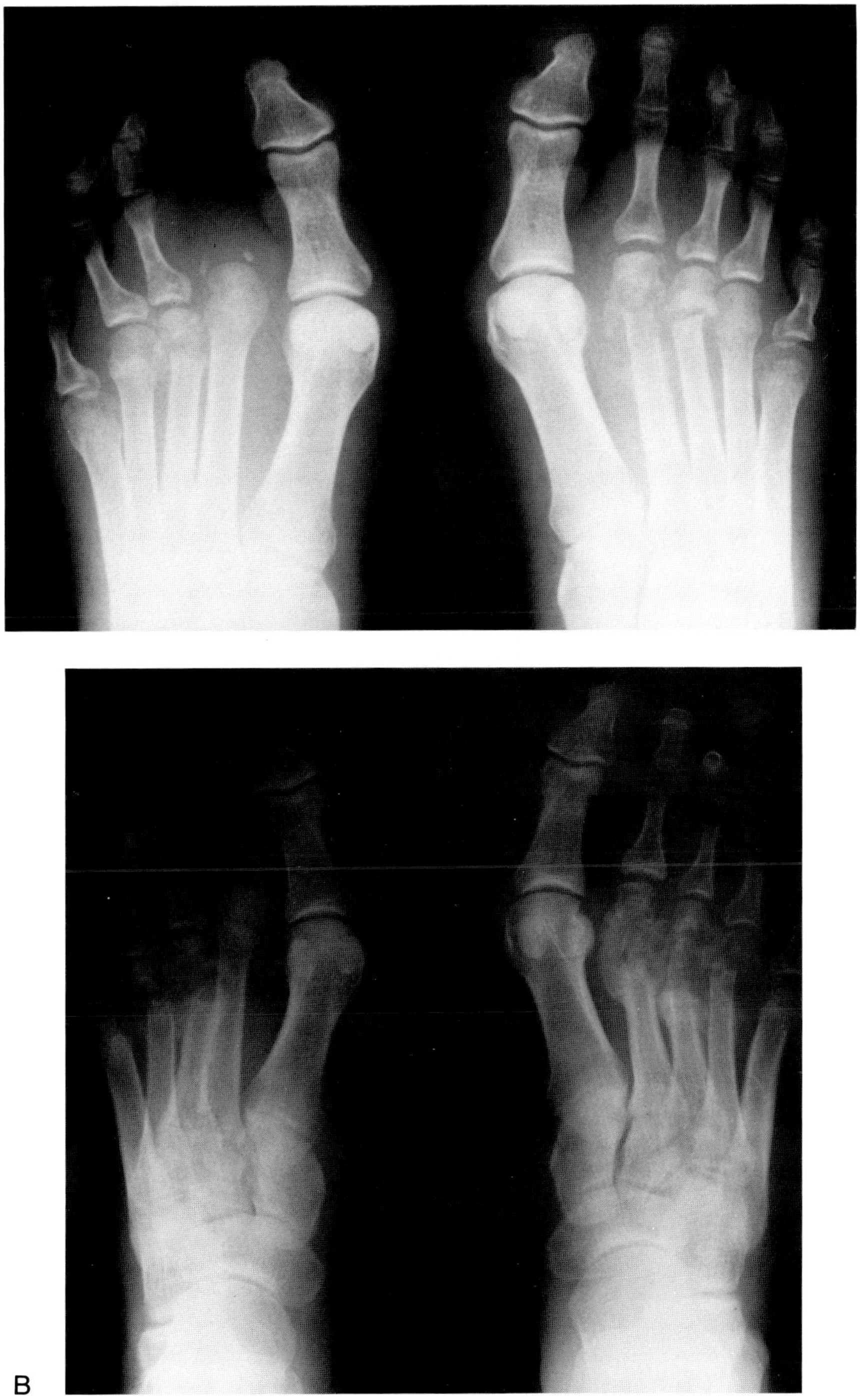

A

B

Fig. 12-11. (**A**) Noninfected Charcot changes in a 43-year-old white man with insulin-dependent diabetes mellitus. There is diabetic neuropathy to the midthigh, stress fractures of left third and fourth metatarsal shafts and right second, third, and fourth metatarsal shafts, and involvement of the metatarsophalangeal joints. (**B**) Exuberant callus formation at 10 weeks. *(Figure continues.)*

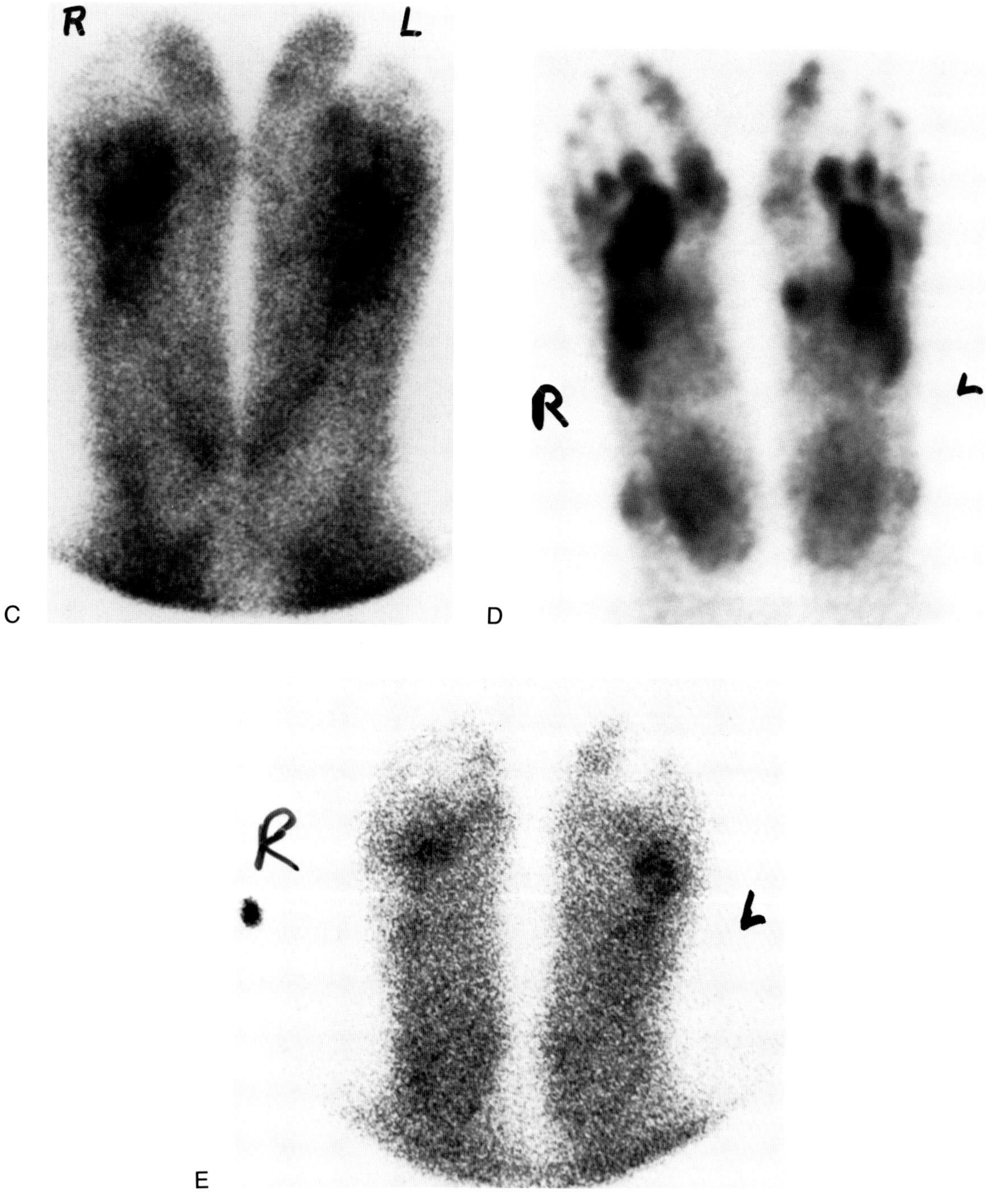

Fig. 12-11 *(Continued)*. (**C**) Technetium scan of the same patient. A blood pool scan shows increased soft tissue uptake due to vascular changes; this is seen after fractures or infections. (**D**) Technetium bone image shows metatarsal fractures and bone turnover at phalanges and midfoot due to Charcot joints. Multiple planes of nuclear medicine scans are helpful in diagnosing osteomyelitis. (**E**) Gallium white blood cell scan shows increased uptake, but it does not correlate with technetium scans. Therefore, no infection is diagnosed with scans.

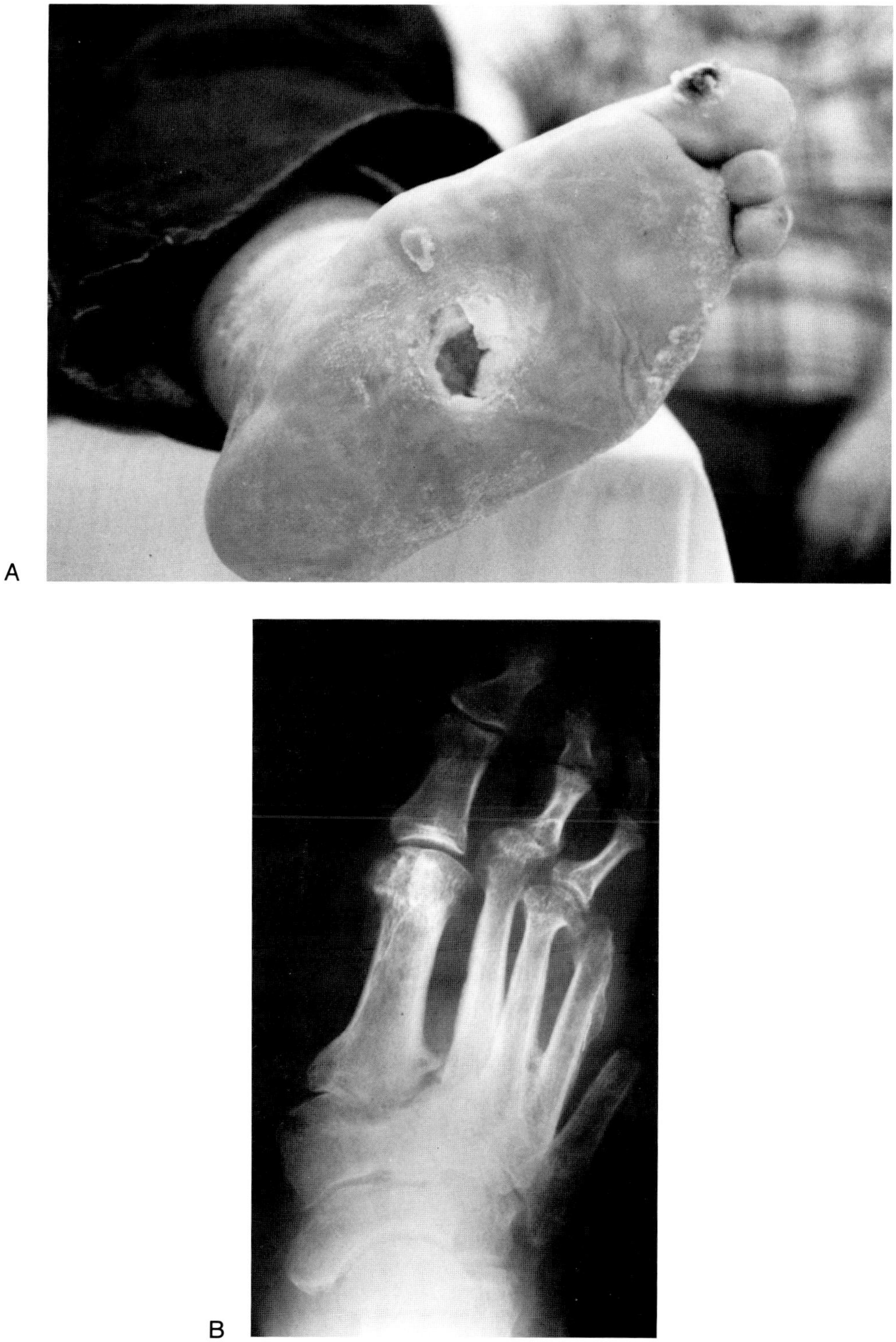

Fig. 12-12. (A) Infected Charcot foot in a 54-year-old white man with insulin-dependent diabetes mellitus. The patient had a 3-year history of drainage through an ulcer caused by midfoot collapse. (B) Radiograph of same patient showing midfoot Charcot joint with collapse. *(Figure continues.)*

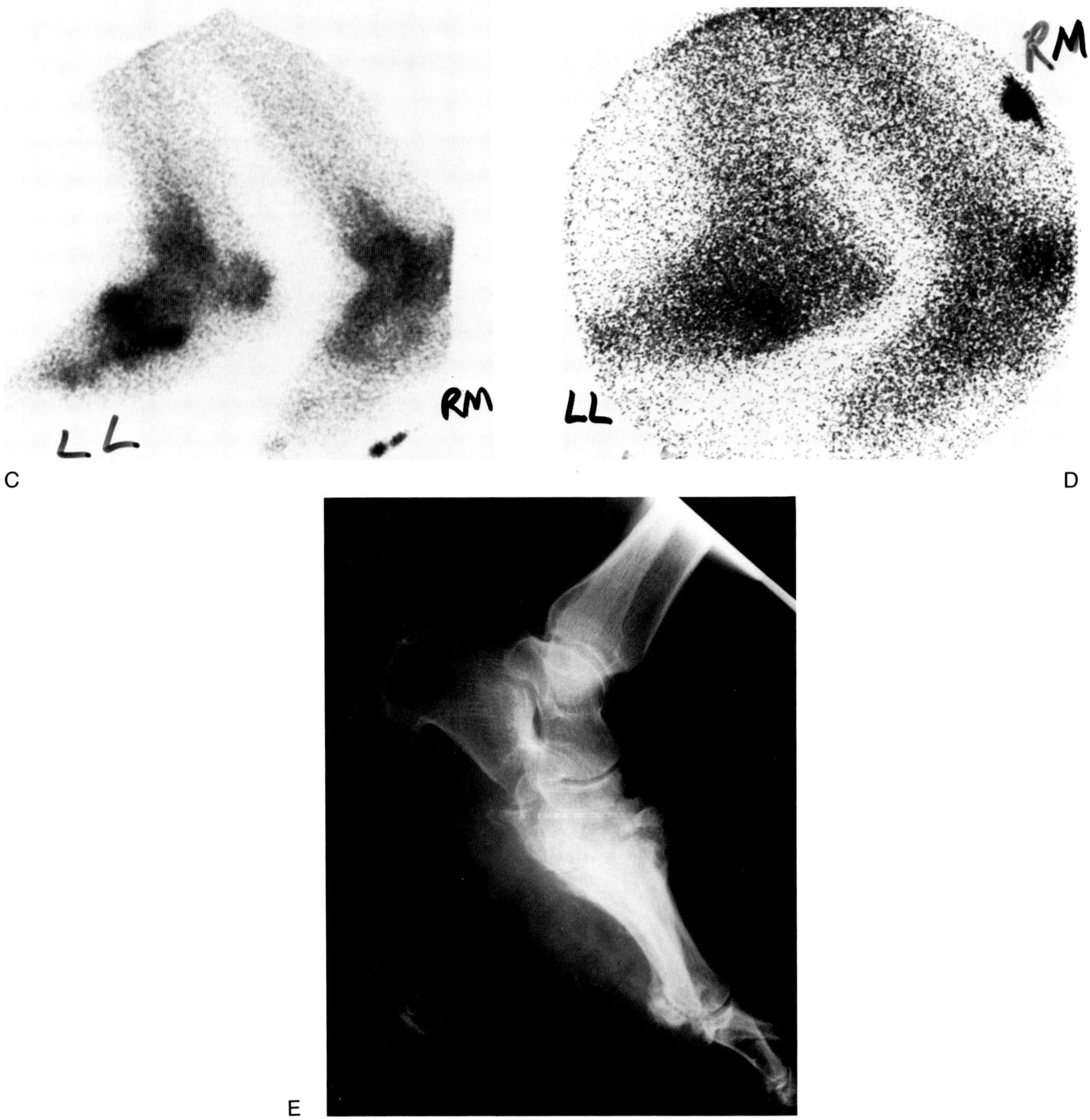

Fig. 12-12 *(Continued)*. **(C)** A technetium bone scan shows an increased uptake to midfoot. LL, left lateral view; RM, right medial view. **(D)** An indium chloride abscess scan shows infection that correlates with the bone scan; therefore, osteomyelitis is present. **(E)** The same patient is shown treated with debridement, wedge excision of cuboid and ulcer, closed primarily, antibiotics, and wound care. The wound dehisced postoperatively due to noncompliance and is now treated with local wound care. No osteomyelitis is present and the wound is closing. There was limited success with downstaging the infection from a Wagner grade 3 (osteomyelitis) to grade 2 (deep ulcer).

Positive bone biopsy cultures are definitive proof that osteomyelitis is present.[33,34] Tissue is usually obtained prior to starting antimicrobial therapy, or after the patient has been off antibiotics for 48 hours so that residual antibiotics will not retard bacterial growth. It is not necessary, however, to discontinue antibiotics if severe cellulitis, fasciitis, or gangrene (dry, wet, or gas) is present. In these cases, antibiotics usually cannot penetrate to the bone infection, or if they can, the local pH and low oxygen tension will not allow them to function, so antibiotic inhibition of bacterial growth on cultured material is not a problem.[43] A bone biopsy can be taken in the clinic or emergency room with or without local anesthesia (usually the foot is insensate) or in the operating room if extensive debridement is necessary. Aerobic and anaerobic cultures are taken, and a bone sample is sent to pathology for histiologic confirmation of diagnosis. Confirmation of the diagnosis of osteomyelitis by a radiologist or pathologist may be requested by third party payers.

Laboratory Studies

Laboratory values are not directly diagnostic of osteomyelitis but do help in determining the presence of bacteremia and the quality of the host's defenses. The white blood cell count, sedimentation rate, and glycosylated hemoglobin are usually elevated in systemic sepsis, but normal in chronic osteomyelitis. A complete blood count, clotting factor levels, basic electrolytes, liver enzymes, iron, and serum protein are obtained to define the nutritional status and healing capabilities of the patient.

Scans

Technetium and white blood cell scans obtained in patients with osteomyelitis show increased radiotracer uptake in the involved bone. Severe ischemia and gangrene prevent radiotracer imaging. White blood cell scans with gallium and indium can delineate infection, but it may be difficult to differentiate osteomyelitis from cellulitis or Charcot joint (Figs. 12-11C–E, 12-12, and 12-13). A few days of antibiotic therapy prior to scanning to decrease cellulitis improves the accuracy of abscess scans. Soft tissue infections appear diffuse on such scans, whereas bone infections demonstrate specific bone anatomy. Scans, however, do not always differentiate between infected and noninfected Charcot joints. Scans are helpful in showing the extent of osteomyelitis but may not be diagnostic for osteomyelitis in the diabetic.[28,44–50]

Presentation Summary

When a patient presents to our clinic with the signs and symptoms of osteomyelitis, the first tests obtained are radiographs and blood for routine laboratory studies. If an ulcer is present, wound swab cultures are taken (aerobic, anaerobic, and Gram stain). The lesion is debrided of all infected or necrotic tissue. A 2-minute sterile scrub with hexachlorophene or tincture of iodine is followed by use of a curette or metatarsal rongeur to obtain a sample of infected bone (Fig. 12-14). A #17 surgical blade is useful for excising hyperkeratotic skin that harbors bacteria and impedes ulcer healing. Deep soft tissue and bone cultures (aerobic, anaerobic, and Gram stain) are sent for study. If an abscess or joint infection is present, a sterile aspiration for culture is done. The patient is scheduled for bone and indium white blood cell scans. All of the results are then compiled for the diagnosis and staging of osteomyelitis.

The different Cierny-Mader stages of diabetic osteomyelitis present quite differently. All diabetic patients are systemically compromised hosts ("Bs"). Other systemic compromises can also be present: uncontrolled glycosemia, malnutrition, alcoholism, autoimmune deficiencies, renal or liver failure, steroid or immune suppression medication, and cigarette smoking. These factors need to be documented and corrected before surgical therapy. The most common local host compromising factors are vessel disease, neuropathy, and soft tissue defects (ulcers). These must be addressed as part of the surgical and postoperative therapy. Furthermore, septic arthritis should be rapidly diagnosed and aggressively treated, otherwise

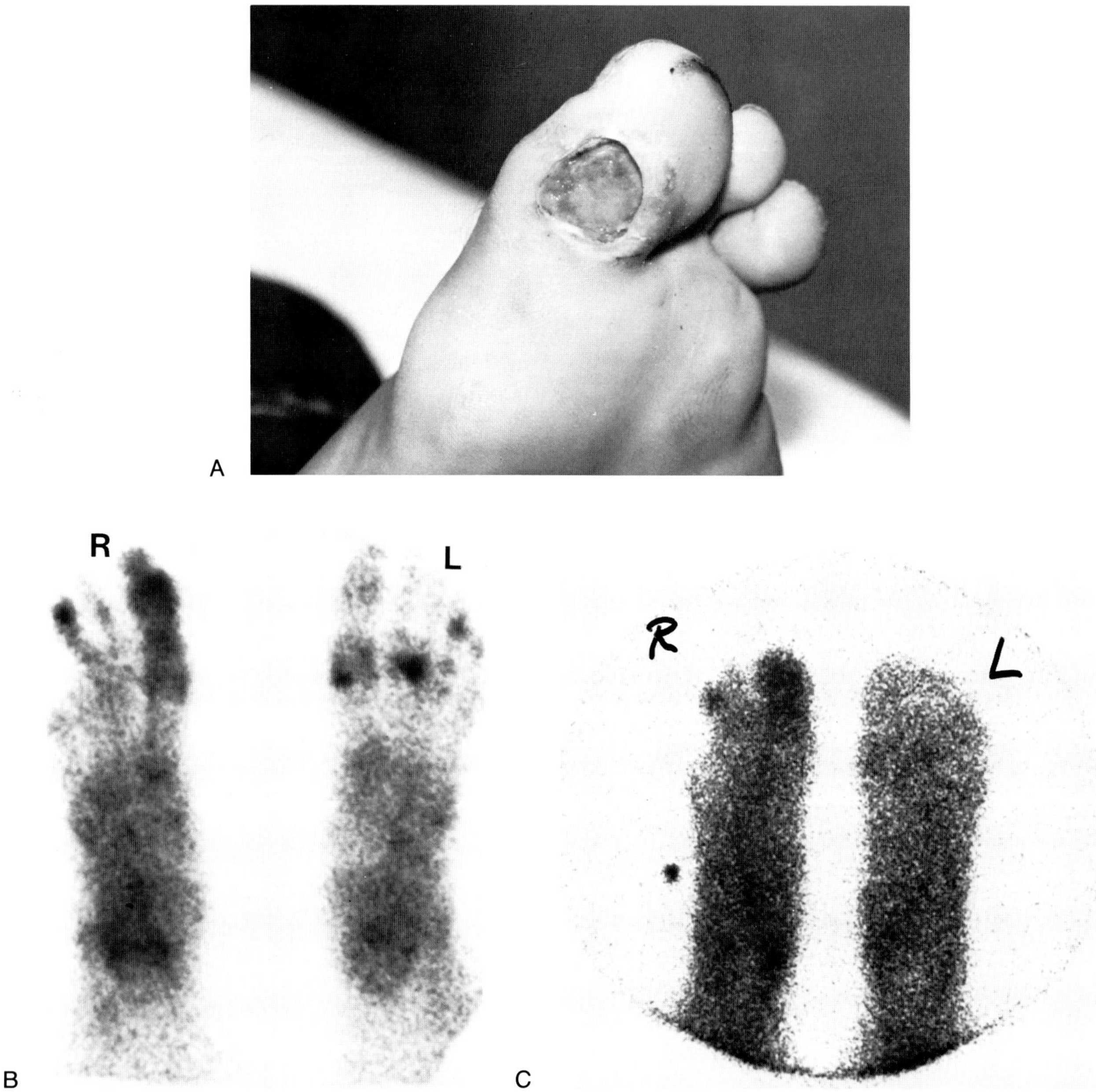

Fig. 12-13. (**A**) A 47-year-old white man with insulin-dependent mellitus shows chronic osteomyelitis of the right great toe. The clinical photograph shows deep ulcer. Radiographs of this patient are shown in Figure 12-9. (**B**) Plantar view of same patient. Technetium scan shows uptake in right great toe at interphalangeal joint. (**C**) Indium chloride scan also shows increased uptake in great toe confirming diagnosis of osteomyelitis.

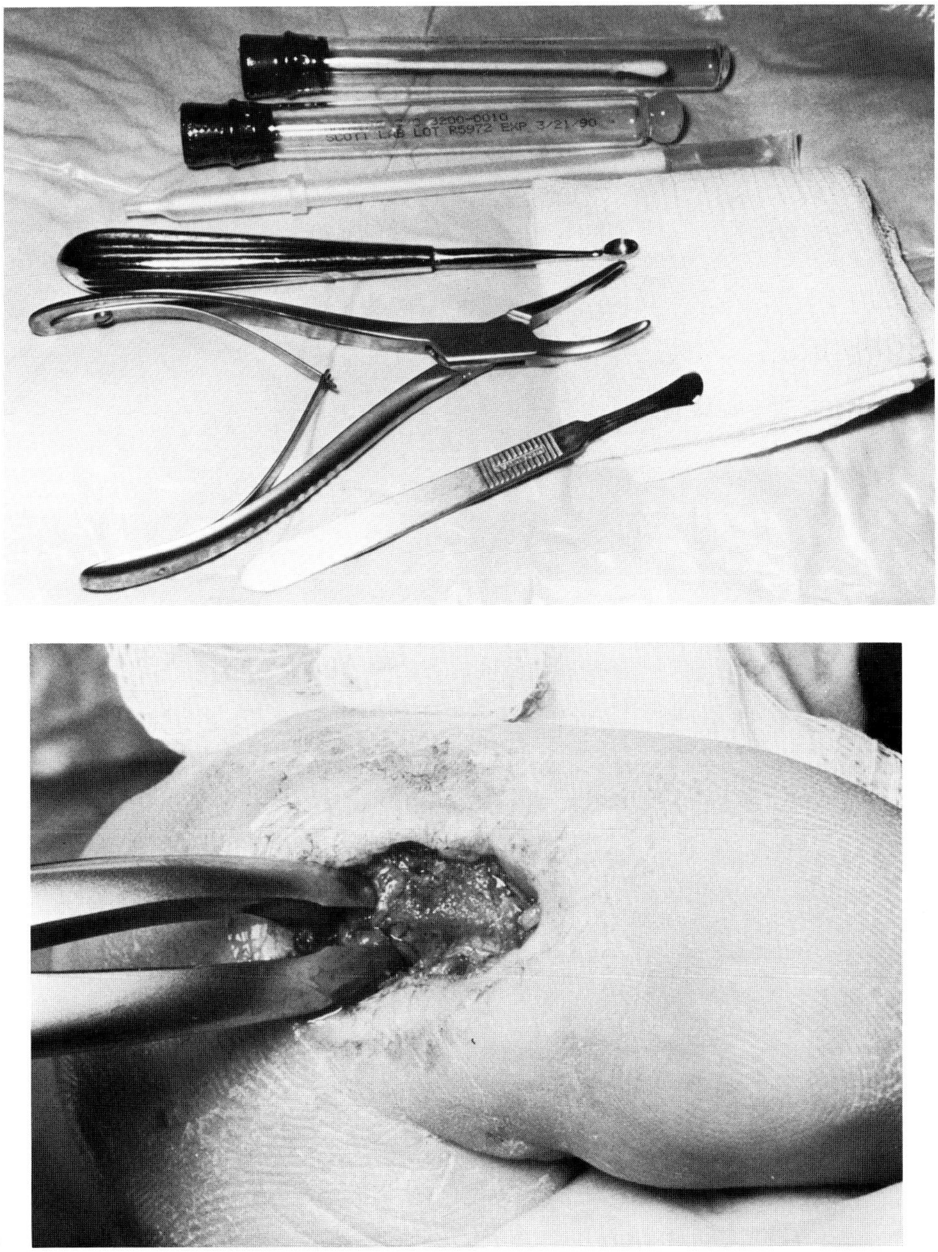

A

B

Fig. 12-14. **(A)** Instruments needed for debriding and culturing diabetic osteomyelitis. A #17 Bard-Parker scalpel, rongeur, currette, and aerobic and anaerobic cultures. **(B)** A 59-year-old white male insulin-dependent diabetic patient with proximal phalangeal osteomyelitis. Culture biopsy taken with rongeur.

chondrolysis and osteomyelitis produce severe deformities.

Stage I osteomyelitis (medullary) usually presents without an ulcer. It is caused by hematogenous seeding. Erythema and edema are present if the blood supply is adequate. Pain is present if deep sensation remains. The sedimentation rate and glycosylated hemoglobin may be elevated. Radiographs may show medullary lysis of trabecullae and endosteal scalloping. Bone or abscess scans may be the only way to diagnose medullary osteomyelitis (Fig. 12-15).

Stage I septic arthritis is a simple joint infection. Swelling and edema may be present. Radiographs may show soft tissue swelling. Scans show joint involvement (Fig. 12-16).

Stage II osteomyelitis is a superficial cortical infection with no medullary involvement. It usually presents with an ulcer over a bony prominence. Cellulitis, erythema, edema, and drainage may be present. Sedimentation rate and glycosylated hemoglobin may also be elevated. Radiographs show

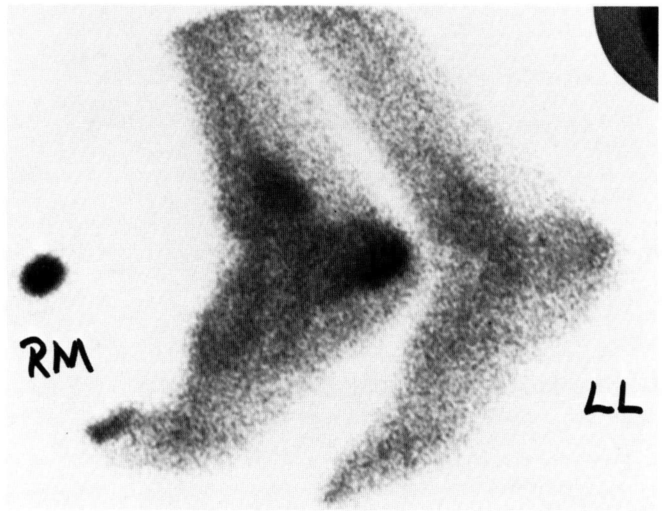

A

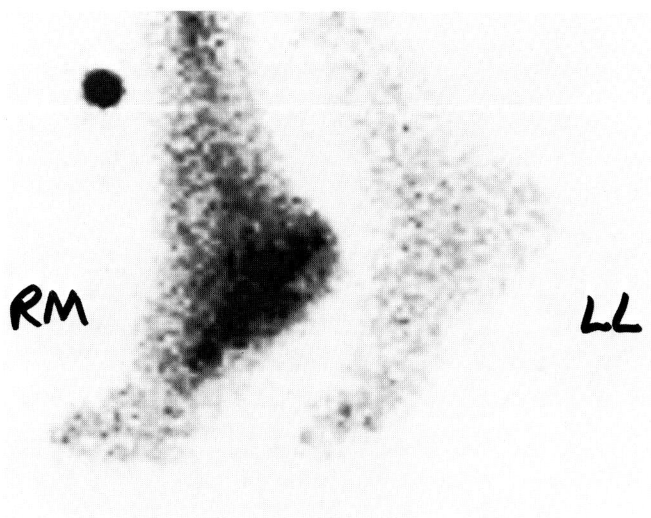

B

Fig. 12-15. **(A & B)** A 69-year-old non-insulin-dependent diabetic black woman with calcaneal osteomyelitis. There was no skin lesion or history of injury. Radiographs appeared normal. Technetium and indium chloride scans are positive for medullary osteomyelitis. The patient was treated with debridement and closure, and 6 weeks of intravenous antibiotics. Two years later she was still healed. **RM**, right medial view; **LL**, left lateral view.

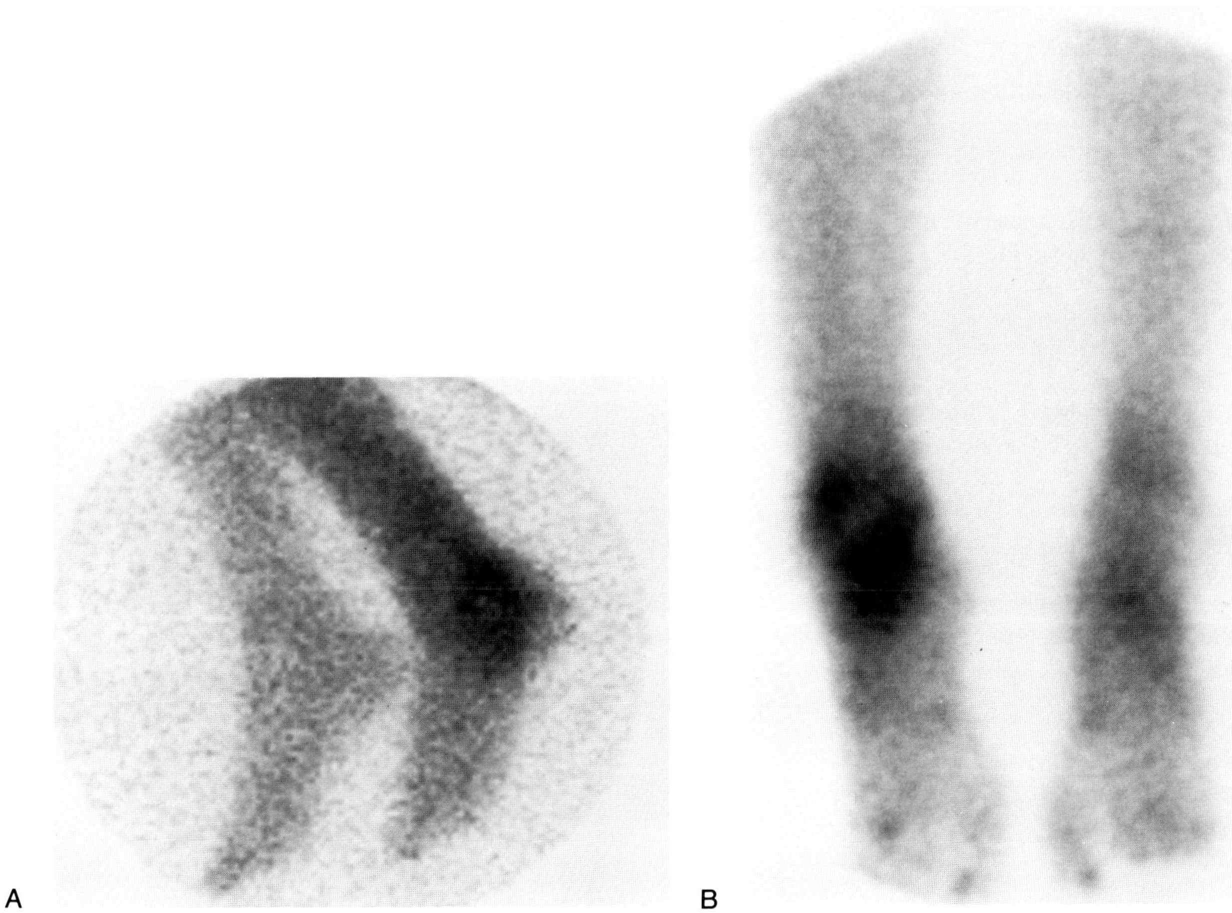

Fig. 12-16. (**A & B**) This 32-year-old insulin-dependent diabetic white woman with severe diabetic neuropathy and septic right ankle due to ulcer on the lateral malleolus that seeded the joint was treated with debridement of the ankle, IV antibiotics, and casting. She had been treated for this problem three times in 12 months due to noncompliance. Amputation was required.

minimal changes, but scans show slightly increased uptake in the area. It may be difficult to differentiate stage II osteomyelitis from cellulitis on the basis of radiographs and scans. Inspection or palpation of the ulcer reveals that it is in direct continuity with bone (Fig. 12-9).

Stage II septic arthritis is a simple joint infection that has progressed to chondrolysis. Superficial osteomyelitis may also be present. This is usually a result of the infection being present long enough to start destroying cartilage (subacute, i.e., 1 to 2 weeks). Radiographs show loss of joint space.

Stage III osteomyelitis is a localized cortical infection with medullary involvement. This is a combination of stage I and II, so it presents very similar to a "deep" stage II. Radiographs and scans show more bone involvement.

Stage III septic arthritis is a joint infection that has progressed to localized osteomyelitis. This is stage III osteomyelitis that involves a joint or chronic (i.e., > 2 weeks) stage II septic arthritis that has progressed to osteomyelitis (Fig. 12-9).

Stage IV osteomyelitis is a diffuse infection of the cortex and cancellous bone and may involve the joints (stage IV septic arthritis). These infections usually have an ulcer unless a hematogenously infected joint is the problem (Fig. 12-12).

TREATMENT

Osteomyelitis is difficult to cure, even in normal bone, because of bone's limited blood flow. An infection in bone results when bacteria are able to colonize ischemic or injured areas where the blood supply is not adequate to combat the infection with its normal defenses. As bacteria grow in this ischemic bone, they cause further bone death by vessel injury from decreases in pH, oxygen, and nutrients and increases in pressure and metabolites. When bone's blood supply is further limited by diabetic vasculitis and then by osteomyelitis, cure is more difficult.[51,52]

Normal oxygen tension in bone is 40 to 50 mmHg and arterial blood is 60 to 70 mmHg.[53] Osteomyelitic bone in animals has a 50 to 75 percent reduction in oxygen tension.[53,54] Oxygen tension level in the skin of diabetic patients is frequently reduced to levels that prevent healing of surgical wounds or ulcers.[11,12] Therefore, the oxygen tension of infected bone in the diabetic patient is about one-quarter that of the overlying soft tissue, which may also be very low. This ischemia is accompanied by metabolic and pH changes that decrease or prevent normal immunologic defenses and antibiotic penetrance and efficacy, and increase bacterial growth. Furthermore, the diabetic individual has decreased phagocytosis by polymorphonuclear leukocytes and decreased T-cell function. These factors make diabetic osteomyelitis a challenge to treat.

Treatment Stages

Stage I Infection

Algorithm directed treatment is possible when the osteomyelitis is classified (Fig. 12-5). For stage I osteomyelitis (medullary), stage progression to stage III or IV is by erosion through the cortex and skin or into joints. Similarly, stage I septic arthritis progresses to stage II by destruction of cartilage. Prevention of stage progression or arrest of the infection is the treatment goal. With a good blood supply and sensation, treatment may be as simple as arrest with culture-directed antibiotics. If the infection is not responsive to antibiotics, arrest is achieved by debridement and reculturing, with intravenous antibiotics for 6 weeks. Debridement of osteomyelitis is accomplished by medullary reaming with a bone scalpel (Midas Rex) for large bones (midfoot, hindfoot, distal tibia, or fibula) or curettes for the small bones. Care is taken not to damage the cortical blood supply with overly aggressive reaming or soft tissue dissection. Septic arthritis requires aspiration and culture-directed antibiotics. If the infection does not respond, arthrotomy with irrigation, debridement, and reculturing is needed, followed by intravenous antibiotics for 3 to 4 weeks.

With ischemia, a successful arrest is difficult because antibiotics may not penetrate or a surgical incision may not heal. Adjunctive therapy is helpful to stimulate healing. Hyperbaric oxygen, revascularization procedures, nasal oxygen, and hemorrheologic agents (Trental) have all been tried with limited success.[55–60] With a good blood supply but insensate tissue, arrest is possible. Postoperative foot care is of paramount importance so ulcers and reinfection do not occur.[61] With both ischemia and insensate tissue, arrest is difficult, stage progression is common, and suppression or amputation may be the best that can be achieved (reclassified to a IC).

Stage II Infection

Stage II osteomyelitis is a superficial cortical infection caused by an ulcer. Progression to stage III or IV occurs by erosion through the remaining cortex and skin. If a good blood supply and sensation are both present, treatment for early infections is with antibiotics and local wound care, minimal debridements, wet-to-dry dressings, or total contact casts that allow the ulcer to granulate closed. For more chronic infections, arrest is obtained with debridement or partial ray resection and closure by primary or secondary intention. Long-term antibiotics are needed. Stage II septic arthritis usually requires aspiration, debridement of joint loculations, adhesions, and necrotic cartilage, followed by long-term antibiotics.

With ischemia or neuropathy, successful arrest of a stage II infection is difficult because not only is there poor antibiotic penetration and poor surgical wound healing, but there is often a soft tissue defect as well. Adjunctive therapy is more often needed. With both ischemia and insensate tissue, arrest is very difficult, so suppression, stage progression, and amputation are seen more often than in stage I.

Stage III Infection
Stage III osteomyelitis is a localized cortical infection with medullary involvement with an ulcer usually present. Stage III septic arthritis is an infection that has been present long enough for bone to become involved. Progression to stage IV occurs by erosion through the opposite cortex and skin. With a good blood supply and sensation, successful treatment of stage III osteomyelitis can be obtained with antibiotics and local wound care, aggressive debridements, wet-to-dry dressings, or total contact casts that allow the ulcer to granulate closed. For more chronic infections, arrest is usually obtained with multiple, aggressive debridements or partial ray resection and closure by primary or secondary intention. Long-term antibiotics are also needed.

Similarly, with stage III septic arthritis, treatment is directed toward debriding the chronic joint loculations and adhesions and the bone cysts and sequestrations. Simple aspiration is less successful and multiple debridements may be necessary. Culture-directed antibiotics are given for 4 to 6 weeks. "Dead space" management of the void left from ischemic tissue removal or joint involvement may be needed in the form of antibiotic beads, muscle flaps, or tissue advancements.[25,62]

Ischemia and neuropathy make a successful arrest of a stage III infection very difficult because of the extensive bone involvement. Adjunctive therapy becomes even more important and reclassification to stage IIIC is common, so suppression, amputation, or stage progression are seen.

Stage IV Infection
Stage IV osteomyelitis is diffuse infection of the cortex and cancellous bone and may involve the joints (stage IV septic arthritis). These infections are the most challenging to arrest because extensive necrotic tissue is infected. These infections usually have an ulcer or sinus unless a hematogenously infected joint is seen and has not self-drained. Even with a good blood supply and sensation, successful arrest is seldom obtained with antibiotics, local wound care, or aspirations. Arrest may be obtained with multiple, aggressive debridements, partial ray resections, total ray resections, joint resections, resection arthroplasties, or amputations. Closure is by either primary or secondary intention. Long-term antibiotics are needed unless an amputation is done through non-infected tissue. If an amputation is done through infected tissue, the wound is not closed immediately. Antibiotics are administered and the wound is closed after the soft tissue infection has resolved.

Ischemia and neuropathy increase the difficulty in obtaining an arrest, so adjunctive therapy and reclassification to stage IVC is common and suppression and amputation are often seen.

Treatment Goals

There are three possible treatment goals for diabetic osteomyelitis: arrest, amputation, and suppression. Which option is selected is determined by the stage of the osteomyelitis and the patients' goals.

Arrest
The term *arrest* is used instead of *cure* for osteomyelitis because once a bone is chronically infected, bacteria are "locked" into haversian canals that died from the infection or from normal bone turnover. These quiescent bacteria may be distant from the active infection and cannot be removed with debridement or antibiotics. They remain quiescent until the local environment changes so they can colonize. The only way to remove them is to remove the entire bone (amputate, enucleate, or ray resection). "Arresting" osteomyelitis means to debride the infection to the subthreshold level of bacteria so local tissue and antibiotics can heal the wound. Unfortunately, this is difficult for diabetic patients because of rapidly progressing ischemia from accelerated atherosclerosis.

Arresting a bone infection in the diabetic patient is difficult because of ischemia in the bone. Some bone can be surgically debrided if the soft tissue is viable for coverage. Debridement includes removal of all dead and infected tissue. Ideally, debridement is carried just to viable tissue with good bleeding. The *paprika sign*, or punctate bleeding, of cortical bone is used in long bone osteomyelitis surgery to identify healthy bone. Although bleeding of diabetic bone is limited by the ischemia, bone is debrided so minimal infection remains and punctate bleeding is observed in the bone and soft tissue. Therefore, even in the diabetic patient the paprika sign is helpful. This facilitates good antibiotic penetrance, improved oxygen supply, minimal continued necrosis, and the best chances for healing.

Clinical judgment and experience in the operating room is very important.[7,8] Preoperative evaluation of blood supply and protective nerve function is combined with intraoperative observation of bleeding to obtain the best chance for healing. Gangrene or transcutaneous oxygen tension ($tcPO_2$) levels less than 10 mmHg prevent local ulcer healing.[13] Surgery is done without the tourniquet inflated so soft tissue and bone bleeding can be evaluated and tissue and vessels are not damaged. Punctate tissue bleeding is needed to heal skin edges. Debridement of soft tissue is done with sharp disposable blades because dull blades damage tissue. Debridement of large bones (metatarsal heads, tarsal, and hindfoot) can be done with a bone scalpel (Midas Rex) that allows easy visualization of punctate bone bleeding. Debridement of small bones (phalanges and metatarsal shafts) is best done with a sharp metatarsal rongeur and small curettes. Skin and tissue edges are closed with no tension and nonabsorbable sutures. If the skin edges do not close easily, more bone is resected or the bone is allowed to granulate closed. This is done because skin grafting to granulated bone is not very effective. It may be necessary to return to the operating room for further debridement if the wound does not close primarily, or necrosis or infection progresses.

Cultures of the "advancing edge" of the bone infection are most accurate in establishing the appropriate antibiotics.[36,37] Deep wound or bone cultures are taken at the patient's initial presentation. Empiric antibiotics are given preoperatively to decrease cellulitis and edema. Initially, broad spectrum gram-positive and gram-negative antimicrobials are used. These antibiotics are modified with intraoperative cultures for long-term intravenous therapy (initial presentation deep wound and bone cultures plus intraoperative cultures; swab cultures are discounted). Long-term intravenous therapy is possible with indwelling Silastic catheters.[62] Compliance and bone penetration is improved with this approach. Six weeks of postoperative intravenous antibiotics is recommended.

Patient compliance is important to arrest the infection. Foot care, protective dressing changes, home IV therapy, and follow-up visits are all under their control. It is a mutual decision by the patient and physician to proceed with any treatment option, and a successful arrest of the infection can only be obtained through hard work by the patient, the family, and the entire health care team.

Amputation

Amputation is a second treatment option.[7,8,63] Osteomyelitis with gangrene or severe ischemia is best treated with ablation. Osteomyelitis of the toe can be resolved with enucleation of the phalanx from the toe or amputation of the toe. Osteomyelitis of the metatarsals can be treated with the total ray resection if there is viable soft tissue. Midfoot osteomyelitis can be treated with enucleation of the bone or a midfoot amputation. Calcaneal, talar, or distal tibial osteomyelitis can be treated with enucleation or a Syme's or below the knee amputation. Amputation levels are largely determined by soft tissue viability that is gauged by the ischemic index, transcutaneous oxygen, or clinical judgment. Wagner has much experience in the former. Wyss et al. and Christensen et al. found that tissue with a $tcPO_2$ level of 40 mmHg gives a high amputation healing rate and tissue with a $tcPO_2$ of 20 mmHg a low healing rate.[11,12] We use $tcPO_2$ values, preoperative physical examinations, and intraoperative observations of bleeding.

Suppression

Suppression is the third treatment option. Because surgical wounds heal poorly in the diabetic individual, many patients are candidates for suppression therapy. With our staging system for musculoskeletal infections, if the patient and physician decide that the treatment to arrest the infection is worse than the disease, that the disability is minimal, or that the patient is not a good surgical candidate, then the stage is reset to a C and suppression, amputation, or no treatment is selected.

Suppressive therapy requires the highest

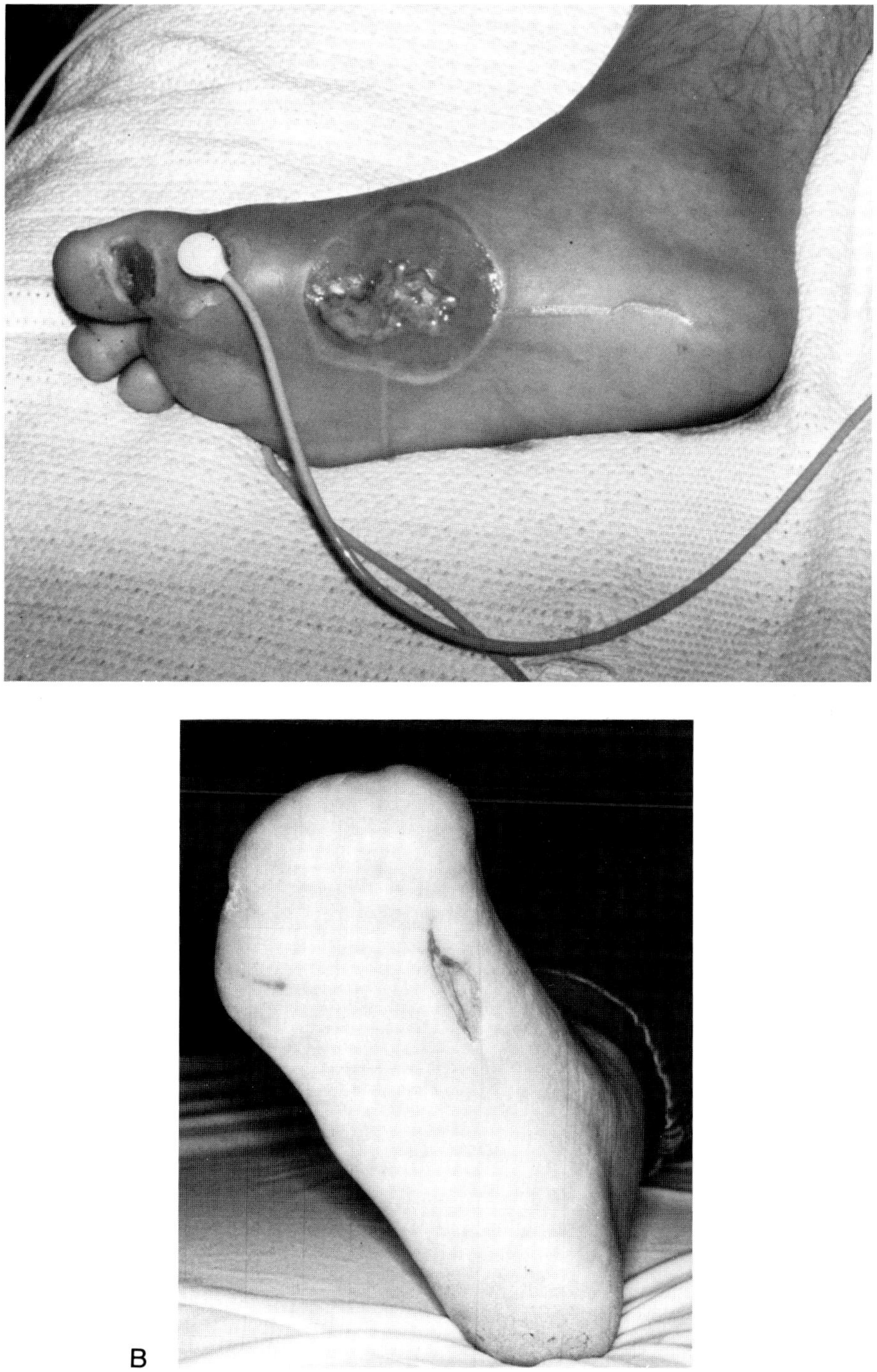

A

B

Fig. 12-17. (**A**) Clinical photograph of a 47-year-old white man with insulin-dependent diabetes mellitus. The patient was treated starting in February 1987 with local care (for radiograph from this time, see Fig. 12-9**A**). He was not compliant, the superficial ulcer on the great toe worsened and he developed a plantar abscess. (**B**) The patient's toes were amputated and his plantar wound debrided. He had IV antibiotics and skin grafting to the plantar wound, and has been healed for 12 months.

amount of patient compliance and physician clinical time. If the infection is not progressive or causing systemic sepsis, then out-patient therapy is reasonable. An open wound is debrided in the clinic. Local wound care is done at home, and suppressive antibiotics are used to control cellulitis or progression of infection. Suppressive antibiotics are guided by clinical response and cultures. Antibiotics are used sparingly for short courses (1 to 2 weeks). Local wound care depends on the patient's infection and capabilities. Usually patients are able to keep the hyperkeratotic ulcer edge soft with daily callus care of sanding, cleaning, and lotion. Hyperkeratotic skin edges and necrotic tissue are sharply excised in the clinic. Debridement is as previously described to punctate bleeding of the skin edge, deep tissue, and bone. It is important to remove necrotic deep tissue such as fascia and tendons (Fig. 12-14B).

The wound is dressed with dry gauze until hemostasis is obtained and then dressed wet-to-dry until the infection is under control. Wet-to-dry dressings are continued if the wound and the patient respond to them. We prefer saline dressings since saline is not cytotoxic, but others use acetic acid, Dakin's solution, or Betadine. The dressings simply keep the wound soft and clean to allow granulation. Total contact casts, Una boots, zinc oxide gauze, dry dressings, or foam boots may be used but generally work better in foot infections that do not involve the bone.[18]

The success of suppressive care depends greatly on the patient. Some patients are not able to return to clinic for follow-ups, are not able to control their serum glucose levels, are not able to afford dressings, antibiotics, and therapy, or are not able to do simple foot care (Fig. 12-17). These patients are usually treated with amputation; otherwise their infection progresses.

Other patients fight a long battle of two steps forward and one step back. Their wounds heal, and as they decrease their foot care, the infection flares up and therapy is resumed all over again. Very few patients resolve their osteomyelitis with this approach. The wound usually remains open but occasionally closes. The osteomyelitis remains quiescent, so bipedal gait is maintained and hospital admission or surgery is avoided.

Suppressive therapy is usually most successful with a good blood supply, a compliant patient, and bone that is not directly weight bearing. The toes, metatarsal shafts, and midfoot bones respond best, but once an ulcer develops under the metatarsal heads or calcaneus, it is difficult to get this area to heal until all of the bone in contact with the weight-bearing surface is removed. These patients may respond better to more aggressive surgical therapy.

Many patients choose suppression therapy even when no success is possible. Infected Charcot joints (Fig. 12-12A) or severe soft tissue loss that may only be cured with multiple debridements or amputation can be prevented from progressing with suppressive therapy. At UTMB, as we learn more about diabetic osteomyelitis and the difficulties with treatment, we treat an increasing number of patients with suppression.[44]

DIFFICULTIES

The main difficulties with treating osteomyelitis in the diabetic foot are poor quality soft tissue, poor patient compliance, and confused physician management. Ischemia is a major cause of soft tissue breakdown and development of diabetic osteomyelitis. Soft tissue ischemia may respond to arterial bypass surgery. Soft tissue loss may occasionally be treated with muscle flaps or skin grafts, if the proximal arterial supply is adequate. Neuropathy may be a difficult problem, separate from ischemia (Fig. 12-10).[26] Management of neuropathy requires meticulous foot care and special shoes. With patient compliance, osteomyelitis with severe neuropathy in the absence of ischemia can be managed successfully.

Most diabetic patients with osteomyelitis of the foot have a combination of ischemia and neuropathy. Management is to initially decrease the infection (cellulitis) with local care and antibiotics, and then to correct the ischemia (bypass), to protect the neuropathic foot, and, finally, to arrest or suppress the osteomyelitis. If the ischemia is severe and cannot be corrected, then suppression or amputation may be used.

Patient compliance and physician management are improved with a team management approach of all the specialists. Patients may become frustrated and depressed and require psychiatrists and psychologists. Difficult insulin therapy requires endocrinologists. Kidney problems require nephrologists. The multiple medical problems require family physicians and internal medicine specialists to coordinate care. Infectious disease experts can help with antimicrobial therapy. Foot, vessel, and extremity care require podiatrists, vascular surgeons, orthopaedists, and general surgeons. Postoperative care requires physical therapists, occupational therapists, and rehabilitation experts. Family and financial concerns are aided by social service workers and counselors.

CONCLUSION

Osteomyelitis in the diabetic patient is a frequent and difficult problem. Diagnosis is usually straightforward but can be difficult. Treatment depends on the stage of the osteomyelitis and on the patients' and physicians' goals. Therapy ranges from arrest to suppression to amputation. Understanding the pathophysiology of diabetic osteomyelitis and working through this challenging problem is rewarding for both the patient and the physician.

ACKNOWLEDGMENT

We wish to acknowledge Billy R. Ledbetter, Jr., for his assistance in the preparation of this manuscript.

REFERENCES

1. Calhoun JH, Cantrell J, Lacy J et al: Treatment of diabetic foot infections: Wagner classification, therapy and outcome. Foot Ankle 9(3):101, 1988
2. Calhoun JH, Valdez R, Mader JT et al: Microbiology of diabetic foot infections: Wagner classification and trends. American Academy of Orthopaedic Surgeons, 56th Annual Meeting, Las Vegas, February 9, 1989
3. Donovan DL, File TM: Team approach in the management of diabetic foot infections. J Foot Surg 26(1):S12, 1987
4. Edmonds ME, Blundell MP, Morris ME et al: Improved survival of the diabetic foot: the role of a specialized foot clinic. Q J Med 60(232):763, 1986
5. LeFrock JL, Joseph WS: A team approach to infections of the lower extremity in the diabetic patient. J Foot Surg, suppl. 1, 26:S1, 1987
6. Levin ME: The diabetic foot: pathophysiology, evaluation, and treatment. Ch. 1. In Levin ME, O'Neal LW (eds): The Diabetic Foot. 4th Ed. CV Mosby, St. Louis, 1988
7. Wagner FW, Jr: The diabetic foot and amputation of the foot. p. 421. In Mann RA (ed): Surgery of the Foot. 5th Ed. CV Mosby, St. Louis, 1986
8. Wagner FW, Jr: A classification and treatment program for diabetic, neuropathic, and dysvascular foot problems. A.A.O.S. Instruct Course Lect 27:143, 1979
9. Apelqvist J, Castenfors J, Larsson J et al: Wound classification is more important than site of ulceration in the outcome of diabetic foot ulcers. Diabetic Med 6(6):526, 1989
10. Kahn O, Wagner W, Bessman AN: The pathogenesis of diabetic foot infections—immunopathy, angiopathy and neuropathy. J Foot Surg, suppl. 1, 26:S7, 1987
11. Wyss CR, Harrington RM, Burgess EM, Matsen FA: Transcutaneous oxygen tension as a predictor of success after an amputation. J Bone Joint Surg 70A(2):203, 1988
12. Christensen KS, Falstie JN, Christensen ES, Brochner MJ: Results of amputation for gangrene in diabetic and non-diabetic patients. J Bone Joint Surg 70A(10):1514, 1988
13. Karanfilian RG, Lynch TG, Zirul VT et al: The value of laser Doppler velocimetry and transcutaneous oxygen tension determination in predicting healing of ischemic forefoot ulcerations and amputations in diabetic and non-diabetic patients. J Vasc Surg 4(5):511, 1986
14. Oishi CS, Fronek A, and Golbranson FL: The role of non-invasive vascular studies in determining levels of amputation. J Bone Joint Surg 70A(10):1520, 1988
15. Matsen FA, Wyss CR, Pedegana LR et al: Transcutaneous oxygen measurement in peripheral vascular disease. Surg Gynecol Obstet 150:525, 1980
16. Jacobs RL, Karmondy AM: Charcot foot. p. 1248. In

Jahss MH (ed): Disorders of the Foot. WB Saunders, Philadelphia, 1982
17. Sinacore DR: Total-contact casting in the treatment of diabetic neuropathic ulcers. Ch. 15. In Levin ME, O'Neal LW (eds): The Diabetic Foot. 4th Ed. CV Mosby, St. Louis, 1988
18. Mueller MJ, Diamond JE, Sinacore DR et al: Total contact casting in treatment of diabetic plantar ulcers: controlled clinical trial. Diabetes Care 12(6):384, 1989
19. Bamberger DM, Daus GP, Gerding DN: Osteomyelitis in the feet of diabetic patients: long term results, prognostic factors, and the role of antimicrobial and surgical therapy. Am J Med 83(4):653, 1987
20. Robson MC, Edstrom LE: Conservative management of the ulcerated diabetic foot. Plast Reconstr Surg 59:551, 1977
21. Collens WS, Vlahos E, Dobkin GB et al: Conservative management of gangrene in the diabetic patient. JAMA 181(8):692, 1962
22. Kelly JP, Wilkowske CJ, Washington JA: Chronic osteomyelitis in the adult. p. 120. In Current Practice in Orthopaedic Surgery. CV Mosby, St. Louis, 1975
23. Waldvogel FA, Medoff G, Swartz MN: Osteomyelitis: a review of clinical features, therapeutic considerations, and unusual aspects. N Engl J Med 282:198, 260, 316, 1970
24. May JW, Jr, Jupiter JB, Weiland AJ, Byrd HS: Current concepts review: clinical classification of posttraumatic tibial osteomyelitis. J Bone Joint Surg 71A(9):1422, 1989
25. Cierny G, III, Mader JT, Penninck JJ: A clinical staging system for adult osteomyelitis. Contemp Orthop 10:17, 1985
26. Greene DA: Neuropathy in the diabetic foot: new concepts in etiology and treatment. p. 76. In Levin ME, O'Neal LW (eds): The Diabetic Foot. 4th Ed. CV Mosby, St. Louis, 1988
27. Griffiths HJ: Diabetic osteopathy. Orthopedics 8(3):398, 401, 1985
28. Hardy DC, Staple TW, Picus D, Gilula LA: Imaging of the diabetic foot. Ch. 9. In Levin ME, O'Neal LW (eds): The Diabetic Foot. 4th Ed. CV Mosby, St. Louis, 1988
29. Hart TJ, Healey K: Diabetic osteoarthropathy versus diabetic osteomyelitis. J Foot Surg 25(6):464, 1986
30. Kristiansen B: Ankle and foot fractures in diabetics provoking neuropathic joint changes. Acta Orthop Scand 51:975, 1980
31. Frykberg RG: Osteoarthropathy. Clin Pod Med Surg 4(2):351, 1987
32. Lee SM, Lee RG, Wilinsky J et al. Magnification radiography in osteomyelitis. Skel Radiol 15(8):625, 1986
33. Little JR, Kobayshi GS: Infections of the diabetic foot. Ch. 7. In Levin ME, O'Neal LW (eds): The Diabetic Foot. 4th Ed. CV Mosby, St. Louis, 1988
34. Wheat LJ: Diagnostic strategies in osteomyelitis. Am J Med 78(6B):218, 1985
35. Wheat LJ, Allen SD, Henry M et al: Diabetic foot infections. Bacteriologic analysis. Arch Intern Med 146(10):1935, 1986
36. Calhoun JH, Lacy J, Cobos J et al: Diagnostic Value of Wound Cultures in Diabetic Osteomyelitis. American Orthopaedic Foot and Ankle Society, Summer Meeting. St. Paul, MN, August 5, 1988
37. Mackowiak PA, Jones SR, Smith JW: Diagnostic value of sinus tract cultures in chronic osteomyelitis. JAMA 239:2772, 1978
38. Sapico FL, Bessman AN, Canawati HN: Bacteremia in diabetic patients with infected lower extremities. Diabetes Care 5(2):101, 1982
39. Axler DA: Microbiology of diabetic foot infections. J Foot Surg, suppl. 1, 26:S3, 1987
40. Sapico FL, Witte JL, Canawati HM et al: The infected foot of the diabetic patient: quantitative microbiology and analysis of clinical features. Rev Infect Dis, suppl. 1, 6:171, 1984
41. Ginunas VJ, Canawati, HN, Sapico FL: Anaerobic bacteria isolated from foot infections in diabetic patients: in-vitro susceptibility to nine antibiotics. Clin Ther 6(4):457, 1984
42. Louie TJ, Bartlett JG, Tally FP, Gorbach SL: Aerobic and anaerobic bacteria in diabetic foot ulcers. Ann Intern Med 85(4):461, 1976
43. Mader JT, Brown GH, Guckian JC et al: A mechanism for the amelioration by hyperbaric oxygen of experimental staphylococcal osteomyelitis in the rabbits. J Infect Dis 142:915, 1980
44. Sayle B, Fawcett H, Mader JT, Calhoun JH: Indium^{111} chloride imaging in the diabetic foot. J Nucl Med 29(2):279, 1988
45. Simon WH, Joseph WS: Clinical imaging with indium 111 oxine-labelled leukocyte scan: review and case report. Clin Podiatr Med Surg 5(2):329, 1988
46. Yuh WT, Corson JD, Baraniewski HM et al: Osteomyelitis of the foot in diabetic patients: evaluation with plain film, 99mTc-MDP bone scintigraphy, and MR imaging. Am J Roentgenol 152(4):795, 1989
47. Seldin DW, Heiken JP, Feldman F, Alderson PO: Effect of soft-tissue pathology on detection of pedal osteomyelitis in diabetics. J Nucl Med 26(9):988, 1985
48. Shafer RB, Edeburn GF: Can the three-phase bone

scan differentiate osteomyelitis from metabolic or metastatic bone disease? Clin Nucl Med 9(7):373, 1984
49. Visser HJ, Jacobs AM, Oloff L, Drago JJ: The use of differential scintigraphy in the clinical diagnosis of osseus and soft tissue changes affecting the diabetic foot. J Foot Surg 23(1):74, 1984
50. Shih WJ, Magoun S, Purcell M, Domstad P: Malunion of a femoral fracture mimicking osteomyelitis in three phase bone imaging. Clin Nucl Med 13(1):38, 1988
51. Colwell JA, Lopes-Virella MF, Winocour PD, Halushka PV: New concepts about the pathogenesis of atherosclerosis in diabetes mellitus. Ch. 2. In Levin ME, O'Neal LW (eds): The Diabetic Foot. 4th Ed. CV Mosby, St. Louis, 1988
52. Brookes M: The Blood Supply of Bone: An Approach to Bone Biology. Butterworth (Publishers), London, 1971
53. Mader JT, Calhoun JH: Long bone osteomyelitis: an overview. J Am Podiatr Med Assoc 79(10):476, 1989
54. Esterhai JL, Pisarello J, Brighton CT et al: Treatment of chronic refractory osteomyelitis with adjunctive hyperbaric oxygen. Orthop Rev 17:809, 1988
55. Baroni G, Porro T, Faglia E et al: Hyperbaric oxygen in diabetic gangrene treatment. Diabetes Care 10(1):81, 1987
56. Sargent WQ: Hemorheology. Ch. 3. In Levin ME, O'Neal LW (eds): The Diabetic Foot. 4th Ed. CV Mosby, St. Louis, 1988
57. Sicard GA, Walker WB, Anderson CB: Vascular surgery. Ch. 10. In Levin ME, O'Neal LW (eds): The Diabetic Foot. 4th Ed. CV Mosby, St. Louis, 1988
58. Mader JT, Hicks CA, Calhoun JH: Bacterial osteomyelitis: Adjunctive hyperbaric oxygen therapy. Orthop Rev 18(5):581, 1989
59. Leslie CA, Sapico FL, Ginunas VJ, Adkins RH: Randomized controlled trial of topical hyperbaric oxygen for treatment of diabetic foot ulcers. Diabetes Care 11(2):111, 1988
60. Knighton DR, Fiegel VD, Halverson T et al: Oxygen as an antibiotic. Arch Surg 125:97, 1990
61. Boulton AJ, Kubrusly DB, Bowker JH et al: Impaired vibratory perception and diabetic foot ulceration. Diabetic Med 3(4):335, 1986
62. Couch L, Cierney G, Mader J: Inpatient and outpatient use of the Hickman catheter for adults with osteomyelitis. Clin Orthop 219:226, 1987
63. Fisherman SA: Diabetic osteomyelitis: long term attempts at salvage with eventual mortality. J Foot Surg 27(4):310, 1988
64. Wilson KH, Kauffman CA: Oral antibiotic therapy for osteomyelitis of the foot in diabetic patients. South Med J 78(2):223, 1985

13

Noninvasive Evaluation of the Lower Extremity Arterial System

Anton N. Sidawy, M.D., F.A.C.S.
Kathleen M. Curry, P.A.-C., R.V.T.

In the last two decades the noninvasive vascular laboratory has emerged as a major advance in the screening, diagnosis, management, and follow-up of patients with peripheral vascular disease. The noninvasive vascular laboratory has not only improved the quality of care we can offer our patients, but it has also given us a better understanding of the natural evolution of the atherosclerotic disease process. Hemodynamic measurements of the peripheral circulation can now be carried out with essentially no risk whatsoever to the patient. Sound waves and magnetic fields can also be used to answer clinical questions that only a few years ago could not be resolved without an angiogram. That is not to say that the angiogram is obsolete. On the contrary, the angiogram remains the standard against which all other tests are judged. The development of noninvasive vascular testing fundamentally represents an effort to supplant the angiogram, along with its attendant risks to the patient. This is a goal worthy of the undertaking, but it has not yet been achieved. The noninvasive vascular laboratory has been particularly useful for the screening and follow-up of diabetic patients, who are generally at high risk for developing peripheral vascular disease.[1]

While technologic advances have brought sophisticated testing equipment to the bedside of the vascular patient, the paramount importance of a thorough history and physical examination must be continually kept in mind. The history and the presenting symptoms usually bear heavily on decisions regarding the patient's optimal management, and they often determine whether or not aggressive intervention will be required. A careful examination to determine both the presence and quality of lower extremity pulses frequently allows accurate prediction of the location and severity of vascular disease. In fact, palpation of pulses was the first noninvasive vascular test. An absent pulse typically indicates an occlusion proximal to the artery examined. The quality of the pulse should also be noted, since a reduction in its strength is likely to mean a hemodynamically significant stenosis above that level.

In this chapter we will discuss the noninvasive studies that complement the clinical evaluation of the patient with vascular disease. In general, non-

Table 13-1. Noninvasive Diagnosis of Peripheral Vascular Disease

Indirect Methods
Doppler ultrasound and Doppler pressure
Doppler signal waveform
Ankle doppler pressure and ankle-brachial index
Doppler segmental pressures
Photoplethysmography
Toe pressure measurement
Skin perfusion pressure
Pulse volume recording
Contour
Amplitude
Transcutaneous oxygen tension
Laser doppler flux
Isotope clearance
Direct Methods
Duplex scanning
Magnetic resonance imaging

invasive vascular studies are used to confirm the presence of peripheral vascular disease and to detect its severity and location. They enhance our diagnostic accuracy and help us to predict whether ulcerations and amputation sites will heal. As outlined in Table 13-1, these tests can be divided into indirect and direct studies. Until recently most tests were of the indirect category. These tests give information about physiologic parameters such as flow and pressure but do not provide an image of the vessel under study. Recent technologic advances such as duplex scanning and magnetic resonance imaging now offer noninvasive methods for direct visualization of the arterial system.

DOPPLER ULTRASOUND AND DOPPLER PRESSURES

Doppler ultrasound is the most widely used device in the evaluation of lower extremity arterial flow. There are many instruments now available, ranging from a pocket-size device to the large stationary Doppler. The examiner evaluates the audible signal using headphones or a loudspeaker. A tracing of the waveform, which becomes a part of the patient's record, can be made by the addition of a strip chart recorder.

The Doppler Signal Waveform

The normal arterial Doppler waveform is triphasic. A systolic upward deflection is followed by a diastolic downward deflection. There is then a smaller upward and downward deflection indicating diastolic forward flow (Fig. 13-1A). This triphasic wave can be directly visualized on a strip recording and also can be audibly appreciated by the experienced examiner. The waveform configuration changes with arterial disease (Fig. 13-1B). It is difficult for the novice to differentiate an acoustically normal from an abnormal Doppler signal. While an arterial Doppler signal denotes the presence of blood flow in the underlying artery, it does not directly indicate the adequacy of flow. This is tested with other Doppler studies, such as the ankle Doppler pressure, the ankle brachial index, and the segmental pressures.

The Ankle Doppler Pressure

While segmental Doppler pressure examination of the lower extremity at different levels provides important information regarding the level of arterial occlusion, the ankle-brachial index (ABI) is probably the test used most often for evaluating the severity of lower extremity ischemia. If an appropriately sized cuff is used, the values correlate well with intra-arterial pressures.[2,3] The cuff is applied snugly around the ankle, and the Doppler probe is used to detect flow in the dorsalis pedis and the posterior tibial arteries. The higher pressure of the two is considered the ankle pressure. Obviously only the systolic pressure is measured with this technique. This ankle systolic pressure is normally slightly higher than the brachial pressure measured the same way using the same Doppler technique.[4] If the ankle pressure is considerably higher than the brachial pressure, then the examiner should be suspicious of highly calcified vessels causing artificially increased ankle pressures. These elevations should not be solely attributed to stiffness of the arteries due to age but diabetic disease should be suspected as a reason.[3-6] Incompressible vessels leading to falsely high systolic pressure were found in the lower extremities of more than one-third of diabetic patients exam-

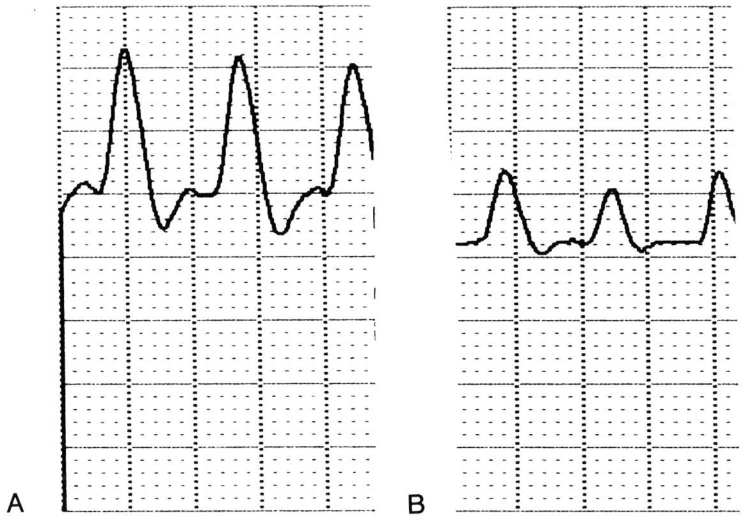

Fig. 13-1. (**A**) Normal arterial Doppler waveform. The wave is triphasic with a systolic upward deflection, a diastolic downward deflection followed by diastolic upward and downward deflection. (**B**) Abnormal arterial Doppler waveform. Decreased amplitude and loss of the diastolic forward flow due to peripheral vascular occlusive disease.

ined.[7] Vessel stiffness is not limited to diabetic patients since almost one-fifth of patients with this condition are nondiabetic individuals.[8] Ouriel and Zarins found that the absolute ankle pressure was the best predictor of limb viability.[9] A pressure higher than 60 mmHg identified 86 percent of the viable lower extremities, and a pressure lower than 60 mmHg correctly identified 77 percent of the nonviable extremities. In viable limbs, however, the ABI was a good indicator of the severity of ischemia.[9]

The Ankle-Brachial Index

Since the systemic blood pressure is variable in the same individual over a relatively short period of time, the absolute ankle pressure can deviate without reflecting a significant change in vascular occlusive disease. It is common practice to use the ABI as a means of standardizing measurements of ankle pressure. The normal ABI is 1.0 or slightly higher since the normal ankle Doppler pressure is slightly higher than the brachial pressure. The ABI correlates well with the severity of ischemia. Patients with intermittent claudication usually have an ABI between 0.5 and 0.8. Patients with more severe ischemia as evidenced by rest pain or tissue loss have an ABI of less than 0.5.[4,10,11] In addition the ABI is also helpful in the follow-up of peripheral arterial disease. A decline in the ABI from one examination to the next suggests worsening of the degree of vascular occlusion. It is felt that the ABI must change by 0.15 or more before it is considered significant.[12]

Segmental Pressures

While the ABI gives an overall assessment of the blood flow to the distal lower extremity, it does not give information regarding the location of the vascular obstruction. When the ABI signals the presence of arterial occlusion, segmental pressures may be helpful in localizing it. Pneumatic cuffs are placed at high thigh, low thigh, below knee, and ankle level. The brachial pressure in both arms is also obtained using the same Doppler pressure technique. The presence of a gradient between measurements obtained from two consecutive cuffs in the same extremity indicates a significant stenosis or a complete occlusion in the arterial segment between the two cuffs. The thigh pressure is usually about 30 mmHg higher than the brachial pressure in normal subjects. A thigh pressure that is significantly less than expected is indicative of an aortoiliac stenosis or occlusion. Unfortunately, the upper thigh cuff cannot be used to localize the occlusion very accurately. The cuff cannot be placed in such a way that it occludes the common femoral artery to measure the pressure in only that segment. A low pressure detected from the inflation of the upper thigh cuff may indicate an aortoiliac or common, superficial, or deep femoral occlusion. One attempt to overcome this deficiency is a square cuff designed to compress the common femoral artery in the groin. Our approach is to correlate the pressure gradient with the quality of the femoral pulses. If the high thigh pressure is low and the ipsilateral femoral pulse is absent, then the occlusion is in the aortoiliac segment. If the high thigh pressure is low and femoral pulse is of good quality, then the stenosis or occlusion is in the femoral arteries below the pulse.

The patient's level of activity can affect blood flow to the lower extremities. Patients with intermittent claudication are asymptomatic at rest and become symptomatic when walking. Their lower extremity pressures and ABI change with activity. At rest the blood supply to the extremity is adequate for the metabolic needs. With exercise, the oxygen requirement of the muscles increases. The increased demand is usually met in a normal subject by vasodilation of the muscular arterioles, which leads to increased cardiac output and an increase in the blood flow to the extremity. In the presence of a hemodynamically significant stenosis, however, the limb beyond the arterial occlusion is supplied by the collateral circulation, which is a high resistance system. Dilation of muscular arterioles in response to exercises, in the presence of an arterial stenosis causes a drop in the Doppler pressures distal to the obstruction. The use of exercise testing unmasks a stenosis that is not hemodynamically significant at rest.[13] The same effect can be obtained using the reactive hyperemia technique. It is performed by occluding the arterial blood flow to an extremity using cuff inflation for 5 minutes. When the cuff is deflated, Doppler pressures distal to the stenosis will fall because the blood is shunted to supply the ischemic muscles.[14] When Laing and Greenhalgh attempted to develop a standard exercise test, they found that the pressure decline occurs after only 1 minute of exercise at 4 km/h on a 10 percent slope. This test was safe and sensitive enough to diagnose asymptomatic mild peripheral vascular disease.[15] Exercise testing and reactive hyperemia are valuable techniques that can be used to differentiate claudication due to ischemic pain from that due to spinal compression or other nonvascular etiologies in patients with relatively normal Doppler pressures and ABI.[16]

PHOTOPLETHYSMOGRAPHY

Photoplethysmography (PPG) uses a diode that emits infrared light into the tissue. This light is reflected back from the blood in the cutaneous microcirculation. The intensity of the reflected light depends on the amount of blood in the microcirculation, which in turn is indicative of the degree of ischemia.[17,18] PPG is used to estimate the cutaneous blood flow when the Doppler pressure cannot be adequately measured. This is particularly important in the case of highly calcified vessels, where an artificially high ankle Doppler pressure is obtained.[8] In addition PPG is used to measure toe blood pressure. A Doppler pressure cannot be obtained because there is not enough room on the toe to place both the cuff, to occlude the digital artery, and the Doppler probe, to listen to it. In this situation the photocell is placed at the tip of the toe and the occluding cuff at its base (Fig. 13-2) and skin flow can be measured and recorded (Fig. 13-3). Many factors play a role in the accuracy of toe pressures, including the presence of hypertension, the temperature of the examination room, and the size of the cuff used.[19] Toe pressure is of special value in the evaluation of Buerger's disease and Raynaud's phenomenon where the arterial disease is usually distributed distal to the ankle vessels, making the value of ankle pressures limited.[20] The toe pressure considered to be the lower limit of normal was found to be 50 mmHg.[21]

Skin Perfusion Pressure

PPG can also be used to obtain skin perfusion pressure to predict healing of ulcers[22] and of amputation sites. A skin perfusion pressure of 21 mmHg or above was found to correlate with

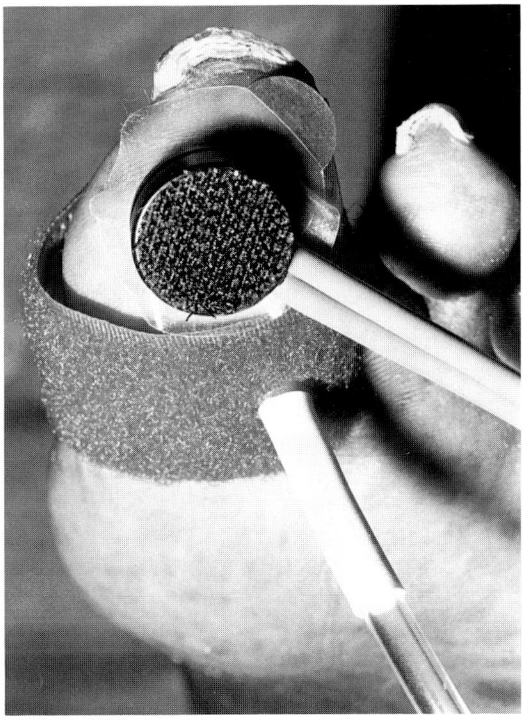

Fig. 13-2. Photoplethysmography. The figure shows the placement of the digital occluding cuff at the base of the toe with the photocell placed at its tip to record skin blood flow during inflation and gradual deflation of the cuff.

healing and decreased complication rate of the amputation site. For this measurement the PPG probe is placed under the cuff to detect the pressure that allows blood perfusion of the skin directly under the cuff to begin.[23] The skin perfusion pressures are usually lower than Doppler pressures, and they are also influenced by the presence of hypertension.[24]

PULSE VOLUME RECORDING

The pulse volume recorder (PVR) employs a segmental plethysmograph to measure and record the changes in extremity or digit volume that take place in response to arterial pulsation.[25–27] Pressure cuffs are placed around an extremity or a digit and inflated with a known amount of air until a certain pressure is obtained. In order for the PVR results to be reproducible, the size and the location of the cuffs should be standardized. The size of the thigh cuff is 18 cm and the calf and ankle cuff 12 cm.[27] The changes in the volume of the limb or the digit are then recorded. In addition, the systolic pressures can be recorded by using a proximal cuff inflation to occlude the arterial flow (occluding cuff) and another distal cuff to measure the pres-

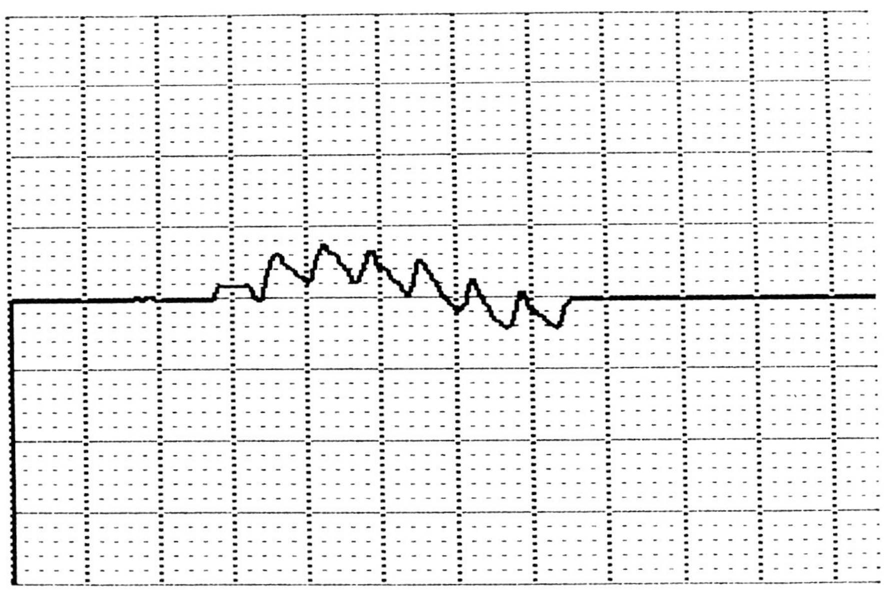

Fig. 13-3. Photoplethysmography recording. A recorded strip showing skin blood flow waves. These waves disappear with inflation of the cuff and complete interruption of blood flow.

sure (measuring cuff). The pressure measured will then be that of the level of the occluding cuff. The contour and amplitude of the recorded pulse volume changes are then studied. These measurements are reproducible if the cuff location, pressure, and volume remain constant.

PVR Contour

The contour of a normal PVR wave is peaked, with brisk anacrotic and dicrotic deflections and a dicrotic notch (Fig. 13-4A). The abnormal PVR waveform due to arterial occlusion is characterized by a flattened wave, the absence of the dicrotic notch, and a decrease in the anacrotic and dicrotic components of the wave. The absence of the dicrotic notch is a characteristic sign of vascular occlusion (Fig. 12-4B).[27]

PVR Amplitude

The amplitude of the PVR waveform reflects the volume of blood flow into the examined area. Factors that affect blood flow in general play an important role in the amplitude of the PVR waveform, especially cardiac output and blood pressure. In arterial occlusive disease, however, there is a marked decrease in the amplitude of the waveform, which is usually reproducible from one study to another.[25]

Clinical Applications of PVR in the Diabetic Foot

Noncompressible vessels in diabetic patients often cause the ankle pressure to be falsely elevated.[8] In this situation the PVR can play an important role in the evaluation of diabetic foot problems such as rest pain and foot ulcers. As reported by Raines et al., foot pain is probably due to ischemia if the amplitude of the waveform at the ankle is less than 15 mm, and foot ulcers are unlikely to heal if the amplitude is less than 5 mm. These criteria were the same in diabetic and nondiabetic individuals. In contrast the cutoff for ankle pressure needed to be 25 mm higher in diabetic patients for the same conclusions to be true.[28] Gibbons and his group used forefoot PVR measurement to predict healing of forefoot amputations in diabetic patients and compared the results with ankle systolic pressure. They found that neither the ankle systolic

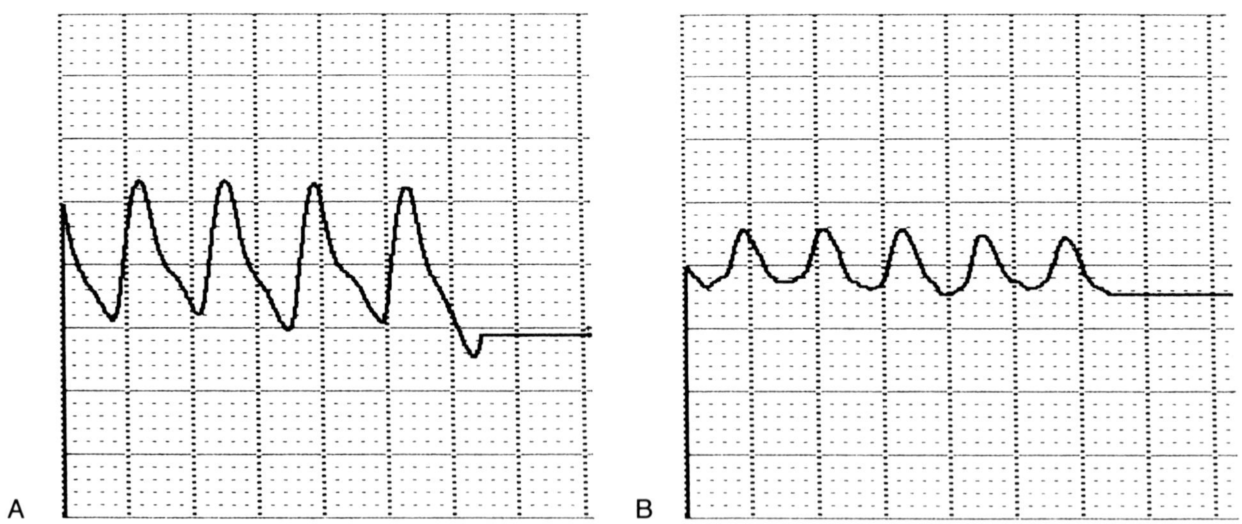

Fig. 13-4. (A) Normal pulse volume recording waveform (PVR). Anacrotic and dicrotic deflections with a dicrotic notch. (B) Abnormal PVR waveform. Decrease in the anacrotic and dicrotic components of the wave with loss of the dicrotic notch.

pressure nor the PVR were very accurate in predicting healing.[29] However, if one examines the pulses and then considers the PVR and pressure measurements, it is frequently possible to arrive at a valid evaluation of the diabetic foot, to predict healing, and to localize the level of vascular occlusion.

TRANSCUTANEOUS OXYGEN TENSION

The transcutaneous oxygen tension ($tcPO_2$) employs a modified Clark electrode[30] to measure the partial pressure of oxygen that diffuses through heated skin. This electrode uses a thermistor-controlled heating coil to keep the skin at a certain temperature in order to maintain cutaneous vasodilation.[31,32] The usual electrode temperature is 45°C, which elevates the skin temperature to 43°C.[33] The advantage of $tcPO_2$ in evaluating peripheral vascular disease is that it measures the amount of oxygen available at the skin level. This measurement is highly useful in patients with arterial calcification where ankle pressures are not accurate. This method can also detect localized areas of decreased perfusion that were found to cause delayed healing of skin lesions in spite of good blood supply to the extremity following successful revascularization. Patients with these types of foot lesions were found to have markedly depressed $tcPO_2$ in the area of the nonhealing lesion itself.[34] Many factors affect the level of $tcPO_2$ in normal subjects. They include age,[35] arterial oxygen tension, room temperature, and the amount of blood flow to the area examined.[36,37] The $tcPO_2$ level was found to correlate with the severity of peripheral vascular disease when patients with ischemic symptoms were compared to controls.[38] Diabetic patients with no evidence of peripheral vascular disease were found to have significantly lower $tcPO_2$ in the foot. The same was also found in the arm of diabetics after induction of hyperemia by cuff occlusion. The authors postulated that these results may reflect an abnormality in capillary flow in diabetic patients.[39] In diabetic patients, $tcPO_2$ correlated much better with symptoms and arteriographic findings of peripheral vascular disease than did other noninvasive studies.[35,40–42] Transcutaneous oxygen tension was found to be an accurate predictor of tissue healing in diabetic and nondiabetic patients alike.[35] Many investigators examined the relationship between the level of $tcPO_2$ and the propensity for healing. It was found that healing is likely if $tcPO_2$ is above 35 to 40 mmHg and unlikely below 20 to 26 mmHg.[43–45] If arterial oxygen tension changes for some reason, the absolute $tcPO_2$ measurement may change in the same subject from one examination to another without a change in the severity of peripheral vascular disease. In order to account for the effect of the variation of arterial oxygen tension on $tcPO_2$, the use of the $tcPO_2$ regional index is favored. The $tcPO_2$ regional index is obtained by dividing each $tcPO_2$ measurement obtained from the lower extremity by the $tcPO_2$ measurement obtained from a reference point, which is usually located on the chest. For example, the generally lower $tcPO_2$ measurements found in older patients remain stable with age when normalized by measurements on the chest.[35] It was found that wounds with a $tcPO_2$ regional index below 0.4 are unlikely to heal, and wounds with $tcPO_2$ level above 0.6 are likely to heal.[46,47] In our experience the $tcPO_2$ regional index is very helpful in evaluating the severity of ischemia in the diabetic foot and is useful for predicting the ability of a diabetic foot lesion to heal.

LASER DOPPLER FLUX

Laser Doppler flux (LDF), or velocimetry, provides a direct and continuous measurement of superficial skin capillary blood flow velocity. A helium-neon laser beam is directed at the dermal capillary network. When it is reflected by the moving red blood cells in the capillaries, the light beam is scattered and shifted to different wavelengths. The wavelength depends on the velocity and angle of red blood cell flow in relation to the laser Doppler probe in a surface area of 1 to 1.5 mm^2 with a 1 to 1.5 mm depth of the examined tissue. The velocities of the reflected light are recorded, and the mean velocity measurement is displayed as a digital readout in millivolts.[48–50] Many factors affect the measurement of LDF, including room temperature,[51] blood hemoglobin content, epidermal thickness, and skin pigmentation.[52] Karanfilian and colleagues reported on the correlation between healing and the laser Doppler pulse wave amplitude (LD-PWA) and laser Doppler skin blood flow velocity (LD-SBFV). They compared these results to the use of $tcPO_2$. Using LD-PWA values greater than 4 mV and LD-SBFV values greater than 40 mV as criteria for healing in diabetic and nondiabetic patients, they found that the sensitivity of LDF was markedly lower than that of $tcPO_2$ (79 percent versus 100 percent, respectively).[50] The LDF probe, however, is not heated, which may account for the decreased accuracy when compared with the $tcPO_2$ heated probe, a point made by Matsen et al.[53]

ISOTOPE CLEARANCE

^{133}Xe is a gas isotope that, when injected into tissue, is removed by crossing the capillary cell membrane via diffusion down a concentration gradient. Lassen and colleagues were able to demonstrate that muscular blood flow can be measured by monitoring the rate of removal of ^{133}Xe injected in skeletal muscle.[54,55] The presence of infection or cellulitis may give inconsistent results when healing is correlated with blood flow measured by isotope clearance.[56] Chimoskey suggested the use of this technique in the measurement of skin blood flow.[57] Healing correlated more with blood flow measurements than with angiographic patterns. This may be due to the extensive collateral circulation network that supplies enough blood to an extremity to allow healing in spite of major arterial occlusion.[58]

Skin Blood Flow Measurement

Regional differences in skin blood flow were documented, in healthy volunteers, by Tsuchida. Using ^{133}Xe clearance, he found that skin blood flow has the tendency to decrease gradually from the face down to the dorsum of the feet.[59] Moore correlated the skin blood flow measurement with the healing of amputation sites. He injected ^{133}Xe intradermally in the midline area at the level of the amputation incision. A scintillation probe was used and connected to a rate meter. The skin blood flow rate was calculated as described by Moore. All amputation sites with flow rates above 2.6 ml/100 g of tissue per minute healed primarily.[60] These results were confirmed by using the gamma camera technique and were not affected by the presence of diabetes.[56]

Skin Perfusion Pressure

Skin perfusion pressure can be measured using ^{133}Xe clearance. In order to determine the amputation level, Holstein injected ^{133}Xe intradermally at the area of the amputation skin incision. Then he placed a blood pressure cuff over the injection site. The rate of ^{133}Xe removal was monitored by a scintillation counter. The cuff was inflated until the ^{133}Xe clearance curve became flat, and the cuff pressure measured. That point corresponded to the skin perfusion pressure. Holstein found that when the skin perfusion pressure was above 40 mmHg, all amputations healed. A skin perfusion pressure below 20 mmHg was consistent with nonhealing.[61] These results were later repeated using ^{133}I-antipyrine. Again a perfusion pressure of less than 20 mmHg was inconsistent with healing of amputation sites, whereas incisions in an area with a perfusion pressure above 40 mmHg healed.[55] Faris and Duncan modified Holstein's technique and used an intradermal ^{99m}Tc-pertechnetate injection of the dorsum of the foot. In diabetic patients, they found that a skin perfusion pressure above 40 mmHg allowed the healing of ulcers and surgical incisions performed for the operative treatment of gangrene of the foot.[62]

DUPLEX SCANNING

Duplex scanning employs a combination of a real-time B-mode sonography and a pulse Doppler. This design allows two-dimensional visualization of the blood vessel in question and different planes surrounding it. In addition, it detects the blood flow velocities in the vessel scanned and gives an analyzed spectrum of these velocities. The generated data from the B-mode and the spectrum analyzer can be stored on a video tape for later study. The degree of the angle the sound beam makes with the axis of the vessel is displayed on the screen, and it should remain constant, usually at about 60°, to standardize the results of the study.[63] The space inside the artery where flow velocities are being sampled is marked on the screen along the sound beam line, and it is called the sample volume (Fig. 13-5). The vessel is localized by the B-mode real-time sonography and studied in longitudinal and cross-sectional projections. Then the sample volume is positioned in the center of the bloodstream, and the study is continued using Doppler signal analysis. Both the B-mode sonogram and the signal analysis provide important information as to the presence, absence, and degree of severity of arterial occlusive disease.

B-Mode Ultrasound Imaging

B-mode gives a real-time image of the part of the body scanned, including the vessel in question. It helps to identify the artery being examined, positions the sample volume in the center of the bloodstream (a location consistent with adequate sampling) or any other location desired to detect disturbances in blood flow, and gives an anatomic description of the arterial wall, including detection of calcified plaques, ulcers, thrombi, and aneurysmal dilations. This mode is not accurate in estimating the degree of stenosis, especially in areas of soft plaques and thrombi. The length of each artery is scanned by moving the scan head along its axis. In order to confirm the patency of the artery and to detect the presence of atherosclerotic lesions, the areas in question are examined in both longitudinal and cross-sectional projections, keeping the sample volume in the center of the bloodstream while sampling the flow velocities. To measure the diam-

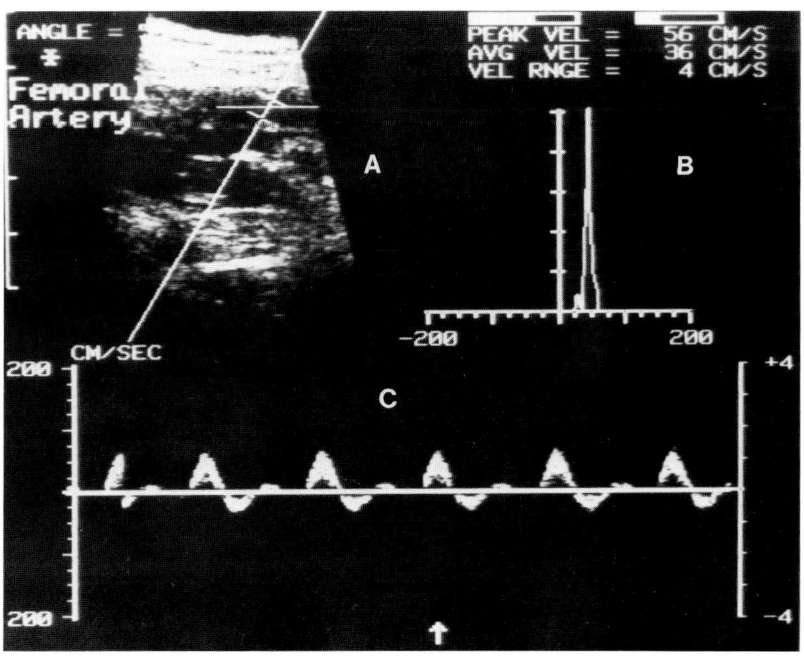

Fig. 13-5. Duplex scan of a normal femoral artery. **(A)** B-mode sonogram showing the sample volume positioned in the center of bloodstream making a 59° angle with the direction of the sound beam. **(B)** Measured peak systolic velocity at 56 cm/s. **(C)** Spectrum waveform showing clear window with forward flow at the end of the diastole.

eter of an artery, the B-mode is used and the walls of the artery are visualized. A marker is then placed on each of the opposing walls, and the distance between the two is measured by the scanner's software. If a narrowing is visualized, then more time is spent studying it in multiple projections, with measurement of multiple flow velocities.

Doppler Signal Analysis

A spectral analysis of Doppler signals is provided by dedicated software (fast Fourier transform [FFT]) of the duplex scanner. It is displayed on the screen as individual velocities, with time on the horizontal axis and velocity (cm/s) on the vertical axis. The collection of all the individual velocities constructs the spectral waveform. The waveform consists of brisk systolic forward flow directed toward the probe, followed by a diastolic reverse flow directed away from the probe, and then by another small forward flow at the end of diastole. The window is the space bordered by the wave and the horizontal axis. The window is usually clear in normal study (Fig. 13-5). The waveform should be studied for its contour, window, and spectral width. Peak systolic and end-diastolic velocities and frequencies are also measured. Changes in these characteristics indicate the degree of the arterial stenosis as reported by Jager and his colleagues.[64] The patterns are as follows:

1. Less than 20 percent narrowing: Broadening of the spectrum with the peak systolic velocity and the contour of the waveform remaining normal.
2. Twenty to 49 percent narrowing: Increase in the peak systolic velocity with broadening of the spectrum. The contour of the waveform remains unchanged.
3. Fifty to 99 percent narrowing: Marked increase in the peak systolic velocity and spectral broadening with loss of the reverse flow.
4. Complete arterial occlusion: No flow is detected in the artery.

The results of duplex scanning of the lower extremity were compared to conventional arteriography. In detecting greater than 50 percent diameter stenosis, this noninvasive technique had a sensitivity of 82 percent, specificity of 92 percent, positive predictive value of 80 percent, and negative predictive value of 93 percent.[65]

The duplex scanner is an operator-dependent instrument. It requires a substantial amount of experience. It is also a time-consuming study. When these difficulties are overcome, however, this instrumentation becomes very useful in the diagnosis of peripheral vascular disease. With the new color flow duplex imager, the technician can accurately and rapidly identify the vessels. The imager displays the flow in the vessels in different colors depending on the direction of the flow either toward or away from the examining probe. This is especially important in small or highly stenotic vessels with markedly decreased flow. The accuracy of this method ranges from 77 to 97 percent, depending on the artery studied.[66] Lower extremity bypasses can also be examined periodically in the course of the postoperative follow-up to determine the presence and progression of various lesions that can influence patency.[67]

The use of the duplex scanner in lower extremity vascular diagnosis is becoming more common. It is not only enhancing our ability to diagnose peripheral vascular disease in a direct noninvasive fashion, but it is also increasing our knowledge of the natural history of the development and progress of atherosclerotic disease.

MAGNETIC RESONANCE IMAGING

The newest development in the direct noninvasive diagnosis of peripheral vascular disease is magnetic resonance imaging (MRI). In healthy subjects, cross-sectional and sagittal views of the aorta and pelvic arteries have revealed a uniformly thin wall around the circumference of the vessels with no wall irregularities or intimal thickening. In contrast, views of atherosclerotic arteries revealed markedly thickened walls with lesions protruding into the lumen of the artery, lumen narrowing, and calcified plaques.

Overall MRI findings correlated with those demonstrated arteriographically in 91 percent of the cases. The MRI revealed the angiographic lesions in 100 percent of patients with atherosclerotic and vascular graft occlusion, 75 percent of those with

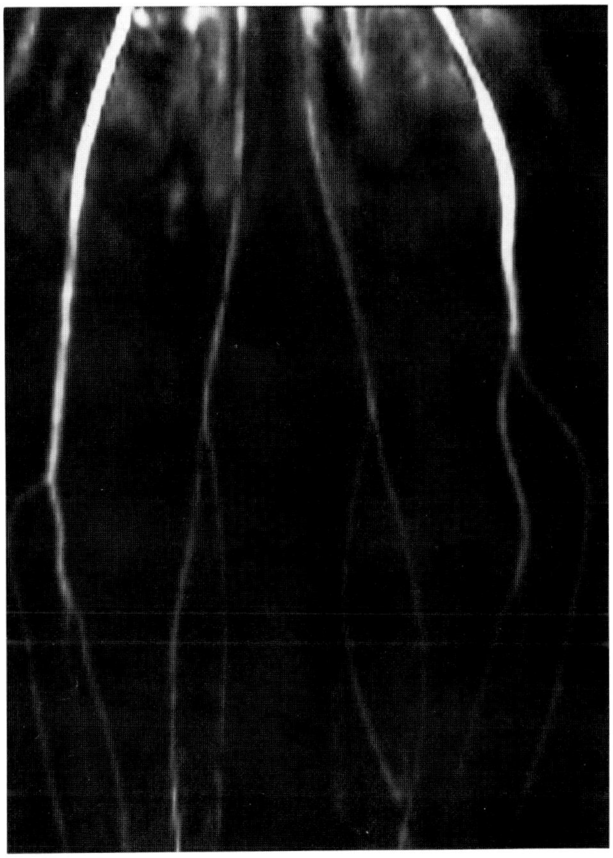

Fig. 13-6. Phase contrast magnetic resonance angiography. showing the superficial femoral, popliteal, tibial, and peroneal arteries. Note the high takeoff of the anterior tibial artery especially on the left. (Courtesy Fred L. Steinberg, M.D., Division of Vascular Radiology, Massachusetts General Hospital, Boston, MA.)

arteriographically significant stenoses, and 92 percent of those with atherosclerotic plaques protruding into the arterial lumen.[68,69] MRI is also capable of measuring and displaying intra-arterial blood flow velocity[70,71] and three-dimensional reconstruction of blood vessels using special techniques.[72,73] The sectional morphology, however, is not an optimal way to study the blood vessels since they are present in different planes. Using MRI-gated subtraction of a systolic from a diastolic image leaves only the signal from the pulsatile arteries, deleting the static background.[74] This allows the creation of flow-dependent contrast and the representation of arteries in a two-dimensional image, resembling conventional arteriography.[75] Using different strategies to enhance phase contrast magnetic resonance angiography, Steinberg and his colleagues were able to image lower extremity vasculature including the popliteal, tibial and peroneal arteries[76] (Fig. 13-6). This evolving technology is an exciting development and may someday replace angiography in the evaluation of certain patients with vascular disease.

The noninvasive vascular laboratory offers important tools to help the clinician identify, early on, foot lesions caused by ischemic disease so attention would be directed to improve the blood supply to the extremity to promote healing and avoid major amputations.

REFERENCES

1. Marinelli MR, Beach KW, Glass MJ et al: Non-invasive testing vs. clinical evaluation of arterial disease: a prospective study. JAMA 241:2031, 1979
2. Stegall HF, Kardon MB, Kemmerer WT: Indirect measurement of arterial blood pressure by Doppler ultrasonic sphygmomanometry. J Appl Physiol 25:793, 1968
3. Bollinger A, Barras JP, Mahler F: Measurement of foot artery blood pressure by micromanometry in normal subjects and in patients with arterial occlusive disease. Circulation 53:506, 1976
4. Carter SA: Clinical measurements of systolic pressures in limbs with arterial occlusive disease. JAMA 207:1869, 1969
5. Carter SA: The effect of age, cardiovascular disease, and vasomotor changes on transmission of arterial pressure waves through the lower extremities. Angiology 29:601, 1978
6. Christensen T, Neubauer B: Increased arterial wall stiffness and thickness in medium-sized arteries in patients with insulin-dependent diabetes mellitus. Acta Radiol 29:299, 1988
7. Gibbons GW, Wheelock FC: Problems in the non-invasive evaluation of the peripheral circulation in the diabetic. Pract Card 8:115, 1982
8. Vincent DG, Salles-Cunha SX, Bernhard VM, Towne JB: Non-invasive assessment of toe systolic pressures with special reference to diabetes mellitus. J Cardiovasc Surg 24:22, 1983
9. Ouriel K, Zarins CK: Doppler ankle pressure. Arch Surg 117:1297, 1982

10. Yao JST, Hobbs JT, Irvine WT: Ankle systolic pressure measurements in arterial diseases affecting the lower extremities. Br J Surg 56:676, 1969
11. Jager KA, Langlois Y, Roederer GO, Strandness DE: Non-invasive assessment of lower extremity ischemia. p. 97. In Bergan JJ, Yao JST (eds): Evaluation and Treatment of Upper and Lower Extremity Circulatory Disorders. Grune & Stratton, Orlando, FL, 1984
12. Baker JD, Dix D: Variability of Doppler ankle pressures with arterial occlusive disease: an evaluation of ankle index and brachial-ankle pressure gradient. Surgery 89:134, 1981
13. Sumner DS, Strandness DE: The effect of exercise on resistance to blood flow in limbs with an occluded superficial femoral artery. Vasc Surg 4:229, 1970
14. Fronek A, Johansen KH, Dilley RB et al: Ultrasonically monitored post occlusive reactive hyperemia in the diagnosis of peripheral arterial occlusive disease. Circulation 48:149, 1973
15. Laing SP, Greenhalgh RM: Standard exercise test to assess peripheral arterial disease. Br Med J 280:13, 1980
16. Carter SA: Response of ankle systolic pressure to leg exercise in mild or questionable arterial disease. N Engl J Med 287:578, 1972
17. Gunderson J: Segmental measurements of systolic blood pressure in the extremities including the thumb and great toe. Acta Chir Scand, suppl. 426:15, 1974
18. Hurley JJ, Hershey FB, Auer AI, Binnington HB: Non-invasive evaluation of peripheral arterial status: the physiologic approach. p. 119. In Levin ME, O'Neal LW (eds): The Diabetic Foot. CV Mosby, St. Louis, 1988
19. Carter SA, Lezak JD: Digital systolic pressures in the lower limb in arterial disease. Circulation 43:905, 1971
20. Hirai M, Shionoya S: Intermittent claudication of the foot and Beurger's disease. Br J Surg 65:210, 1978
21. Carter SA: Role of pressure measurements in vascular disease. p. 317. In Bernstein EF (ed): Non-invasive Diagnostic Techniques in Vascular Disease. CV Mosby, St. Louis, 1985
22. Lee BY, Trainer FS, Kavner D et al: Assessment of the healing potentials of ulcers of the skin by photoplethysmography. Surg Gynecol Obstet 148:232, 1979
23. Van den Broek TAA, Dwars BJ, Rawerda JA, Bakker FC: Photoplethysmographic selection of amputation level in peripheral vascular disease. J Vasc Surg 8:10, 1988
24. Nielsen PE, Poulsen HL, Gytelberg F: Skin blood pressure measured by a photoelectric probe and external counter pressure. Scand J Clin Lab Invest 31:137, 1973
25. Darling RC, Raines JK, Brener BJ, Austen WG: Quantitative segmental pulse volume recorder: a clinical tool. Surgery 72:873, 1972
26. Raines JK, Jaffrin MY, Rao S: A non-invasive pressure pulse recorder: development and rationale. Med Instrum 7:245, 1973
27. Raines KR: The pulse volume recorder in peripheral arterial disease. p. 563. In Bernstein EF (ed): Non-invasive Diagnostic Techniques in Vascular Disease. CV Mosby, St. Louis, 1985
28. Raines JK, Darling RC, Buth J et al: Vascular laboratory criteria for the management of peripheral Vascular disease of the lower extremities. Surgery 79:21, 1976
29. Gibbons GW, Wheelock FC, Hoar CS et al: Predicting success of forefoot amputations in diabetics by non-invasive testing. Arch Surg 114:1034, 1979
30. Clark LC: Monitor and control of blood and tissue oxygen tensions. Trans Am Soc Artif Intern Organs 2:41, 1956
31. Huch R, Lubbers DW, Huch A: Quantitative measurement of partial oxygen pressure on the skin of adults and new-born babies. Pflugers Arch 337:185, 1972
32. Huch A, Huch R, Arner B, Rooth G: Continuous transcutaneous oxygen tension measured with a heated electrode. Scand J Clin Lab Invest 31:269, 1973
33. Huch A, Huch R: Technical, physiological and clinical aspects of transcutaneous PO_2 measurements. In Taylor D, Whamond J (eds): Non-invasive Clinical Measurements. University Park Press, Baltimore-London-Tokyo, 1977
34. Rhodes GR, Cogan F: "Islands of ischemia": transcutaneous $TCpO_2$ documentation of pedal malperfusion following lower limb revascularization. Am Surg 51:407, 1985
35. Cina C, Katsamoutis A, Megerman J et al: Utility of transcutaneous oxygen tension measurements in peripheral arterial occlusive disease. J Vasc Surg 1:362, 1984
36. Spence VA, Walker WF: Tissue oxygen tension in normal and ischemic human skin. Cardiovasc Res 18:140, 1984
37. Takagi-Smith M, Byrne P, Ameli FM et al: The measurement of transcutaneous oxygen tension ($TCpO_2$) and its application in the vascular laboratory. Bruit 8:213, 1984
38. Clyne CAC, Ryan J, Webster JHH, Chant ADB: Ox-

ygen tension on the skin of ischemic legs. Am J Surg 143:315, 1982

39. Railton R, Newman P, Hislop J, Harrower ADB: Reduced transcutaneous oxygen tension and impaired vascular response in type I (insulin-dependent) diabetes. Diabetologia 25:340, 1983
40. Hauser CJ, Klein SR, Mehringer CM et al: Assessment of perfusion in the diabetic foot by regional transcutaneous oximetry. Diabetes 33:527, 1984
41. Hauser CJ, Klein SR, Mehringer CM et al: Superiority of transcutaneous oximetry in non-invasive vascular diagnosis in patients with diabetes. Arch Surg 119:690, 1984
42. Lalka SG, Malone JM, Anderson GG et al: Bernhard VM: Transcutaneous oxygen and carbon dioxide pressure monitoring to determine severity of limb ischemia and to predict surgical outcome. J Vasc Surg 7:507, 1988
43. White RA, Nolan L, Harley D et al: Non-invasive evaluation of peripheral vascular disease using transcutaneous oxygen tension. Am J Surg 144:68, 1982
44. Katsamouris A, Brewster DC, Megerman J et al: Transcutaneous oxygen level in the selection of amputation level. Am J Surg 147:510, 1984
45. Burgess EM, Matsen FA, Wyss CR et al: Segmental transcutaneous measurements of Po_2 in patients requiring below-the-knee amputation for peripheral vascular insufficiency. J Bone Surg 64:378, 1982
46. Hauser CJ, Shoemaker WC: Use of a transcutaneous Po_2 regional perfusion index to quantify tissue perfusion in peripheral vascular disease. Ann Surg 197:337, 1983
47. Hauser CJ: Tissue salvage by mapping of skin surface transcutaneous oxygen tension index. Arch Surg 122:1128, 1987
48. Nilsson GE, Tenland T, Oberg PA: Evaluation of a laser doppler flowmeter for measurement of tissue blood flow. IEEE Trans Biomed Eng 27:597, 1980
49. Karanfilian RG, Lynch TG, Lee BC et al: The assessment of skin blood flow in peripheral vascular disease by laser doppler velocimetry. Am Surg 50:641, 1984
50. Karanfilian RG, Lynch TG, Zirul VT et al: The value of laser Doppler velocimetry and transcutaneous oxygen tension determination in predicting healing of ischemic forefoot ulcerations and amputations in diabetic and nondiabetic patients. J Vasc Surg 4:511, 1986
51. Van Den Brande P, Welch W: Diagnosis of arterial occlusive disease of the lower extremities by laser doppler flowmetry. Inter Angio 7:224, 1988
52. Oberg PA, Tenland T, Nilsson GE: Laser Doppler flowmetry: a non-invasive and microvascular and continuous method for blood flow evaluation in microvascular studies. Acta Med Scand, suppl. 687:17, 1983
53. Matsen FA, Wyss CR, Robertson CL et al: The relationship of transcutaneous PO_2 and laser Doppler measurements in a human model of local arterial insufficiency. Surg Gynecol Obstet 159:418, 1984
54. Lassen MA, Lindjurg J, Munck O: Measurement of blood flow through skeletal muscle by intramuscular injection of Xenon-133. Lancet 1:686, 1964
55. Lassen MA, Holstein P: Use of radioisotopes in assessment of distal blood flow and distal blood pressure in arterial insufficiency. Surg Clin North Am 54:39, 1974
56. Malone JM, Leal M, Moore WS et al: The "gold standard" for amputation level selection: xenon-133 clearance. J Surg Res 30:449, 1981
57. Chimoskey JE: Skin blood flow by ^{133}Xe disappearance validated by venous occlusion plethysmograph. J Appl Physiol 32:432, 1972
58. Moore WS, Malone JM: Amputation level determination using isotope clearance techniques. p. 602. In Bernstein EF (ed): Non-invasive Diagnostic Techniques in Vascular Disease. CV Mosby, St. Louis, 1985
59. Tsuchida Y: Regional differences in the skin blood flow at various sites of the body by xenon 133. Plast Reconstr Surg 80:705, 1987
60. Moore WS: Determination of amputation level: measurement of skin blood flow with ^{133}Xe. Arch Surg 107:798, 1974
61. Holstein P: Distal blood pressure as guidance in choice of amputation level. Scand J Clin Lab Invest, suppl. 128, 31:245, 1973
62. Faris I, Duncan H: Skin perfusion pressure in the prediction of healing in diabetic patients with ulcers or gangrene of the foot. J Vasc Surg 2:536, 1985
63. Jager KA, Ricketts HJ, Strandness DE: Duplex scanning for the evaluation of lower limb arterial disease. p. 619. In Bernstein EF (ed): Non-invasive Diagnostic Techniques in Vascular Disease. CV Mosby, St. Louis, 1985
64. Jager, KA, Phillips DJ, Martin RL et al: Non-invasive mapping of lower limb arterial lesions. Ultrasound Med Biol 11:515, 1985
65. Kohler TR, Nance DR, Cramer MM et al: Duplex scanning for diagnosis of aortoiliac and femoropopliteal disease: a prospective study. Circulation 76;1074, 1987
66. Cossman DV, Ellison JE, Wagner WH et al: Comparison of contrast arteriography to arterial mapping

with color-flow duplex imaging in the lower extremities. J Vasc Surg 10:522, 1989
67. Bartlett ST, Killewich LA, Fisher C, Ward RE: Duplex imaging of in situ saphenous vein bypass grafts and late failure reduction. Am J Surg 156:484, 1988
68. Herfkens RJ, Higgins CB, Hricak H et al: Nuclear magnetic resonance imaging of atherosclerotic disease. Radiology 148:161, 1983
69. Wesbey GE, Higgins CB, Amparo EG et al: Peripheral vascular disease: correlation of MR imaging and angiography. Radiology 156:733, 1985
70. Von Schulthess GK, Higgins CB: Blood flow imaging with MR: spin-phase phenomena. Radiology 157:687, 1985
71. Stahlberg F, Henriksen O, Thomsen C et al: Determination of flow velocities from magnetic resonance multiple spin-echo images: a phantom study. Acta Radiol 28:643, 1987
72. Hale JD, Valk PE, Watts JC et al: MR imaging of blood vessels using three-dimensional reconstruction: methodology. Radiology 157:727, 1985
73. Cline HE, Lorenson WE, Herfkens RJ, Johnson GA, Glover GH: Vascular morphology by three-dimensional magnetic resonance imaging. Magnetic Resonance Imaging 7:45, 1989
74. Wedeen VJ, Meuli RA, Edelman RR, Geller SC, Frank LR, Brady TJ, Rosen BR: Projective MRI angiography of pulsatile flow with magnetic resonance. Science 230:946, 1985
75. Meuli RA, Wedeen VJ, Geller SC, Edelman RR, Frank LR, Brady TJ, Rosen BR: MR gated substraction angiography: Evaluation of lower extremities. Radiology 159:411, 1986
76. Steinberg FL, Ycel EK, Dumoulin CL, Souza SP: Peripheral vascular and abdominal applications of MR flow imaging techniques. Magn Reson Med 14:315, 1990

14

Lower Extremity Arteriography in the Diabetic Patient

Kenneth R. Stokes, M.D.
Frank B. Pomposelli, M.D.
H. Esterbrook Longmaid III, M.D.

Atherosclerosis in the diabetic patient is the leading cause of morbidity and mortality, accounting for 75 percent of diabetic deaths.[1] Overall, 16 percent of diabetics have peripheral vascular disease, 20 times more common than nondiabetic patients, and up to 20 percent of these patients have gangrene. The degree of atherosclerotic occlusive disease is related to the duration of diabetes, with 15 percent involvement at 10 years and 45 percent at 20 years after initial diagnosis.[2] The severity of diabetes correlates with the severity of tibial-peroneal atherosclerotic disease but not large vessel disease.[3] Other risk factors such as smoking, hypertension, and obesity further increase the severity of the atherosclerotic disease.[4] The incidence in the female is nearly equal to that of the male and affects both pre- and postmenopausal females. Individuals are also affected at a younger age.[3]

It is important to realize that peripheral vascular disease in the diabetic patient is often diffuse with involvement of both the large arteries including the aorta, and involvement of the arteries of the calf and foot.[5] The tibial and peroneal arteries, however, can be severely affected without involvement of more proximal vessels, a distribution rarely seen in the nondiabetic individual. Atherosclerosis in the arteries of the foot is present in 40 percent of diabetic patients. Vascular disease is also more prevalent in the profunda femoris artery and geniculate arteries, and the ability to develop collateral circulation is reduced.[6] For this reason, stenoses or occlusions produce more serious symptoms in the diabetic than in the nondiabetic patient. A solitary severe stenosis or multiple relatively mild stenoses in the iliac, femoral, popliteal, or calf arteries can lead to frank gangrene.

In the diabetic patient, atherosclerotic plaques show an increased propensity for ulceration and cracking; otherwise they are indistinguishable from those in the nondiabetic individual. The arteries are characterized by extensive calcification occurring in up to 25 percent of cases of adult onset diabetes.[7] This medial calcinosis involves the intima and media and results in the typical radiographic "pipestem" or "trolley track" appearance (Fig. 14-1). This calcification is not associated with arterial occlusion, however. Its distribution is important to evaluate since dense calcification may make an arterial bypass anastomosis impossible to perform.

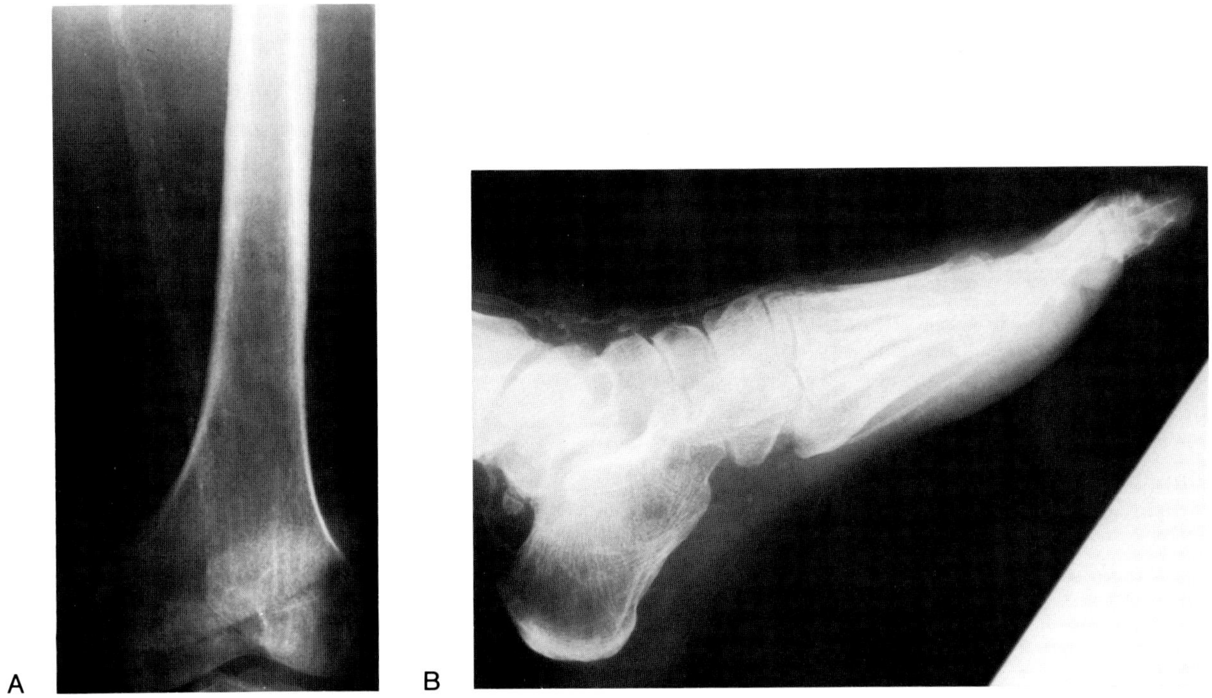

Fig. 14-1. (**A**) "Pipestem" or "trolley track" calcification of medial calcinosis in the popliteal artery. (**B**) Medial calcinosis involving pedal arteries typical of diabetes mellitus.

INDICATIONS

Indications for arteriography of the lower extremity in the diabetic patient are disabling claudication, ischemic rest pain, ischemic ulceration, and gangrene. Since atherosclerotic occlusive disease is so diffuse with multiple levels of arterial involvement, pedal arteries may be patent even though the pedal pulses are nonpalpable, and noninvasive examination shows no evidence of flow. Also, the presence of palpable foot pulses does not exclude significant proximal vascular disease.[8] Arteriography should therefore be performed if ischemic symptoms are present regardless of the status of the peripheral pulses. Certainly no patient should have an amputation without previous arteriographic evaluation.

TECHNIQUE

Preangiographic orders are similar to those for nondiabetic patients.[9] Because of the increased incidence of renal impairment in the diabetic patient, renal status should be carefully evaluated. All patients should be well hydrated before, during, and after the angiogram (e.g., 5 percent dextrose and 50 percent normal saline at 75 to 100 cc/h) preferably starting the night before the procedure. The degree of hydration should be followed closely since many of these patients have coronary artery disease. Any oral diabetic medication is withheld while those patients taking insulin receive half of the morning dose. Those patients scheduled for the afternoon receive a liquid breakfast. Following the procedure, patients are allowed to eat immediately. Blood sugar levels are followed closely at all times and adjusted by sliding-scale insulin administration if necessary.

Arteriography is preferably performed through the common femoral artery or, if necessary, the axillary or proximal brachial artery. Whether the common femoral artery is punctured ipsilateral or contralateral to the more severely diseased lower extremity is a matter of preference. With the use of no. 4 or 5 French catheters, the incidence of hematoma formation or arterial injury following catheterization of the ipsilateral femoral artery is small and, if present, does not significantly hinder peripheral bypass.

If the contralateral approach is used, iliac angioplasty can be readily performed by crossing over the aortic bifurcation with either a cobra or Simmons catheter. In addition a superficial femoral angioplasty or even a popliteal angioplasty can be performed with this approach without performing a second antegrade puncture in the ipsilateral femoral artery.

If the femoral arteries cannot be catheterized or if a femoral bypass graft is present, our preferred access is through the proximal left brachial artery or, if necessary, the right brachial artery. This vessel is catheterized using the standard Seldinger technique at the junction of its proximal one-third and distal two-thirds. Because of its relative small size, a no. 4 French pigtail catheter is preferred. Placement of the catheter into the abdominal aorta is easily performed even in the presence of a tortuous thoracic aorta. By placing the pigtail tip in the direction of the descending aorta, a guidewire can then be advanced into the distal aorta without difficulty. All patients receive 1,000 units of intravenous heparin after catheterization to help prevent pericatheter thrombosis. If catheterization is difficult or the artery is thought to be small, a vasodilator such as nifedipine (10 mg sublingual) is given to prevent spasm. Because of the possibility of subclavian artery disease, any dampening of the left brachial pulse or decrease in the left arm blood pressure represents a contraindication to catheterization.

Translumbar arteriography is reserved for the

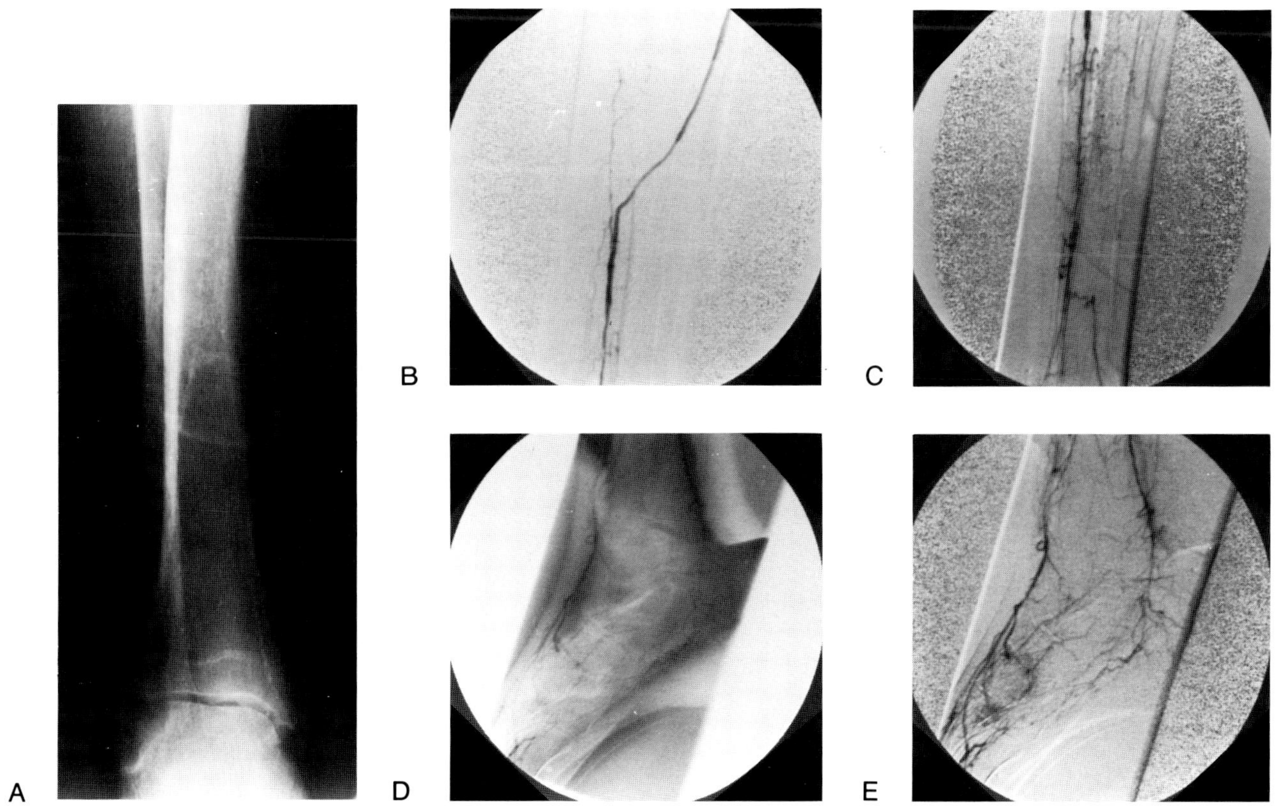

Fig. 14-2. Use of selective digital arteriogram to visualize pedal arteries not evident on routine arteriogram. (**A**) Routine aortic injection in a patient with occluded superficial femoral artery and popliteal-to-peroneal artery bypass graft fails to opacify the distal vasculature. (**B**) Selective digital arteriogram reveals vein graft entering the peroneal artery, which is severely diseased distally. (**C**) Posterior tibial artery is reconstituted above the ankle. (**D**) Lateral scout view and (**E**) lateral digital arteriogram of the foot reveal reconstitution of the dorsal pedal artery at the ankle and a severely diseased posterior tibial artery.

patient in whom transbrachial or transfemoral catheterization is not possible. This technique, especially the low (L2) puncture, is otherwise avoided because of the dense calcification and extensive distal aortic atherosclerotic disease frequently present. Selective iliac injection and angioplasty are also more difficult or not possible from this approach.

If aortoiliac disease is suspected clinically or by noninvasive examinations, the aorta and iliac arteries are best evaluated by routine arteriography. However, if not suspected or in the renally compromised patient, digital subtraction arteriography (DSA) may be performed with less than half the contrast load of routine arteriography. Typically, 30 ml of Conray-30 (Mallinckrodt Medical Inc., St. Louis, MO) is injected for the digital aortogram compared with 40 ml of Conray-60 or the equivalent for routine aortography.

Peripheral arteriography may be unilateral or bilateral depending upon the clinical symptoms and renal status. Routine bilateral iliofemoral arteriography allows the best visualization of the iliac and femoral arteries. If the atherosclerotic disease is limited, this aortic injection may visualize both lower extremities. However, because of the diffuse nature of the atherosclerosis and poor collateral flow, visualization of the tibial and pedal arteries is often suboptimal, requiring selective catheterization and additional injections of contrast medium. For these reasons, instead of aortic injection, we routinely use digital subtraction arteriography by selective external iliac injection to evaluate the lower extremities (Fig. 14-2).

Anteroposterior and lateral views of the foot are routinely obtained to evaluate the patency of the dorsalis pedis and posterior tibial artery below the ankle since bypass to these vessels is possible when more proximal vessels are occluded[10,11] (Figs. 14-3 and 14-4). It is important to evaluate the arterial anatomy in the foot as the long-term patency of distal bypass grafts is dependent on patency of the pedal arch.[12–14]

With multiple levels of arterial occlusion, patent distal arteries, especially the pedal arteries, may not be visualized even with selective injection and DSA. Moreover, because of poor inflow, pedal arteries that appear small on arteriography may only be constricted and at surgery may be quite large (Fig. 14-5). To better visualize these vessels, intra-arterial nitroglycerine (200 to 400 μg) can be injected to produce arterial dilatation and improve opacification. Papaverine (30 mg) or tolazoline (Priscoline, 25 to 40 mg) can also be used.[15–18] Because of the extensive medial calcinosis often present and the poor flow to the distal calf, effects of these drugs may be somewhat limited. The use of a thigh tourniquet to cause reactive hyperemia has been described.[19,20] This has proven unreliable and in the diabetic patient appears to be not as effective as intra-arterial vasodilators.

It should be remembered that limitations of flow in the arterial tree distal to multiple levels of occlusion may make vessels appear smaller on the arteriogram than their true size and that patent pedal arteries may not be visualized even when using all of the above techniques. In circumstances of limb-threatening ischemia or possible limb amputation, the final determinant of the suitability of a pedal vessel for bypass should be surgical exploration; we have successfully performed bypasses in 6 of 12 patients in whom a weak Doppler signal was present over the dorsalis pedis artery, although this vessel was not visualized on arteriography.[14]

Digital Subtraction Arteriography

In DSA, televised fluoroscopic images of the arteriogram are first digitalized for computer processing. A noncontrast "mask image" is then electronically subtracted from postinjection images. Resultant images contain only contrast-filled structures free of background detail. This is then computer enhanced and displayed on a video monitor for evaluation.[21–27]

Although DSA has been much maligned because of suboptimal or even unusable early equipment, the image quality of DSA now approaches that of routine arteriography. Because of the advantages in patients with severe atherosclerotic disease, it has largely supplanted routine arteriography in our institution.[28–31] The advantages of DSA over routine arteriography are as follows:

1. High contrast resolution. Such resolution results in a reduction in the volume of injected contrast and improved visualization of periph-

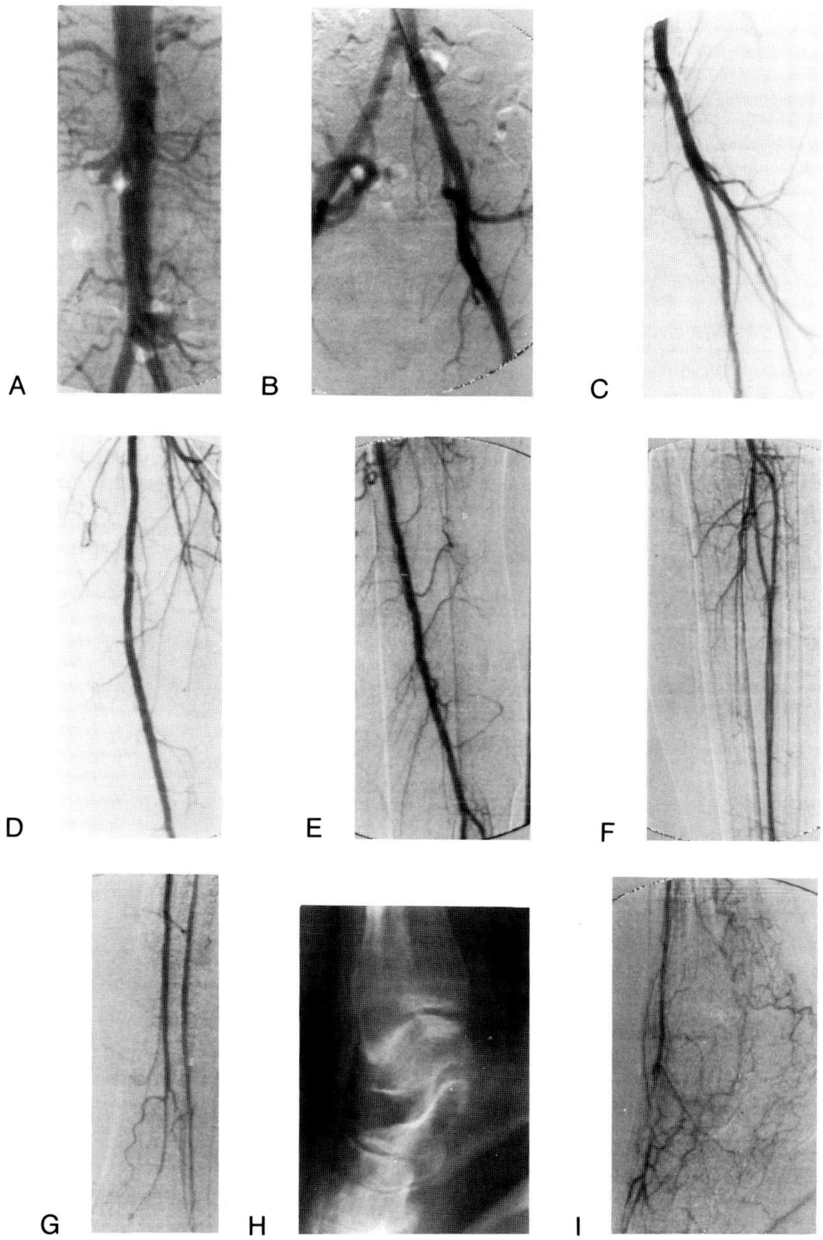

Fig. 14-3. Use of DSA to evaluate distal vasculature for bypass surgery. Digital abdominal aortogram and left leg arteriogram in a 50-year-old diabetic man with gangrenous forefoot. Except for severe renal vascular disease, (**A**) aorta and (**B**) left iliac arteries are unremarkable. (**C, D**) The superficial femoral artery and (**E**) the popliteal artery are irregular but patent. (**F**) The anterior tibial and peroneal arteries are patent while the posterior tibial artery is occluded at midcalf. (**G**) AP view of ankle reveals the distal anterior tibial and peroneal arteries. (**H**) Lateral scout view of the foot and (**I**) lateral digital arteriogram reveal short occlusion of the dorsalis pedis artery which is then reconstituted distally. The plantar arch does not fill. Bypass graft was placed distal to dorsalis pedis occlusion.

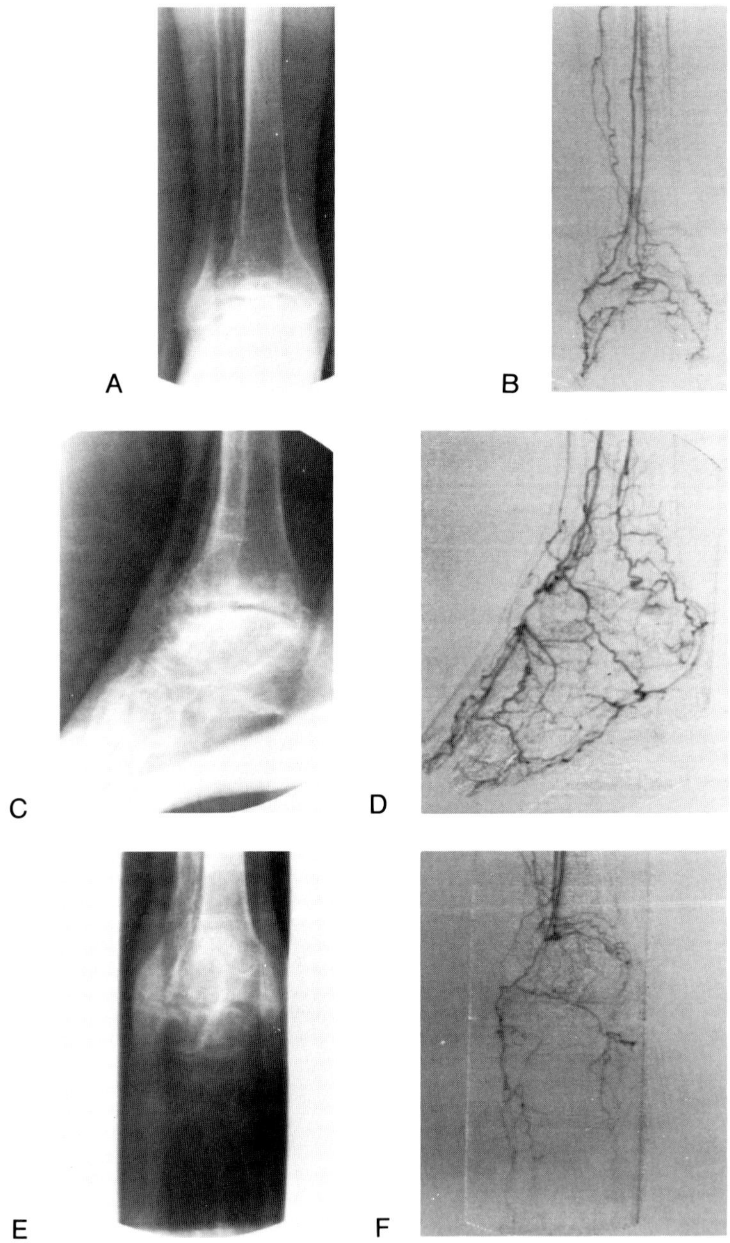

Fig. 14-4. Evaluation of pedal vasculature for bypass surgery. (**A**) Anterioposterior (**AP**) ankle scout film and (**B**) digital subtraction arteriography (**DSA**) reveal patent anterior tibial and peroneal arteries to the ankle. (**C**) Lateral foot scout film and (**D**) DSA reveal occlusion of the distal anterior tibial artery with questionable dorsalis pedis artery reconstitution at the tarsal level. (**E**) AP foot scout view and (**F**) DSA reveal occlusion of the dorsalis pedis and posterior tibial arteries with the questionable distal dorsalis pedis artery actually representing a collateral vessel (confirmed at surgery). Patient eventually required amputation.

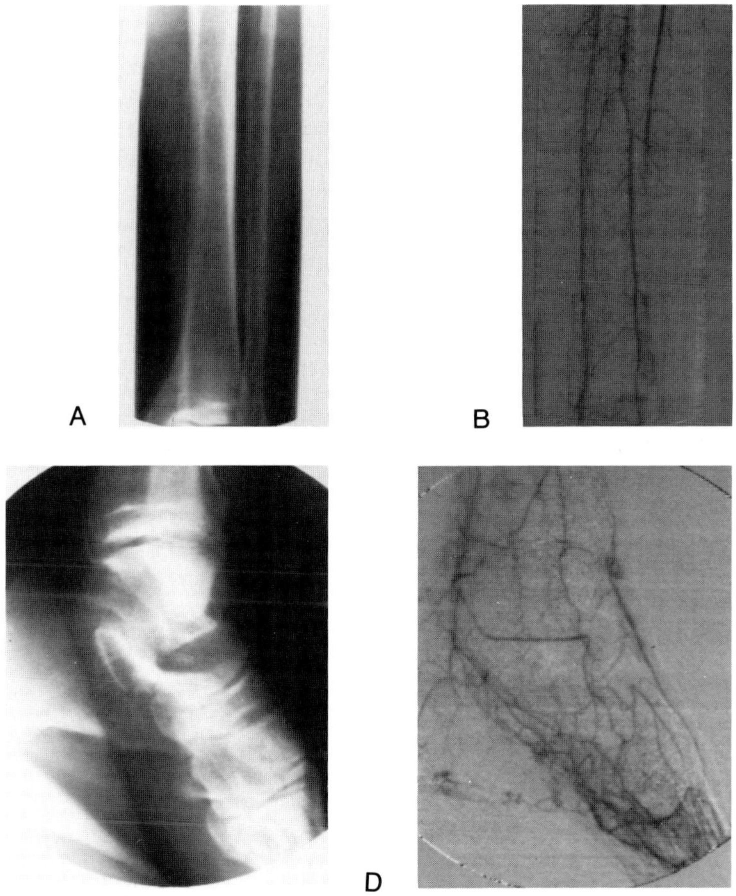

Fig. 14-5. Evaluation of pedal vasculature. (**A**) Anteroposterior nonsubtracted view and (**B**) digital subtraction arteriogram (DSA) of the calf reveal anterior tibial artery occlusion with patent but severely diseased posterior tibial and peroneal arteries. (**C**) Lateral scout view of the foot and (**D**) DSA reveal posterior tibial occlusion at the ankle. Collateral vessels reconstitute the dorsalis pedis artery, which appears small, at the ankle. At surgery, this artery was found to be larger and of better quality than its radiographic appearance suggests and in situ vein graft was placed.

eral arteries. This allows visualization of minimally opacified pedal arteries that would not be evident on routine arteriography. Improved arterial visualization also allows less selective arterial catheterization. In addition, large field image intensifiers (14–16 inches) now used in DSA allow examination of a larger area of the limb resulting in fewer contrast injections.

2. Less contrast-related discomfort. The less concentrated ionic contrast used in lower volumes results in less discomfort without the necessity of using less painful but expensive nonionic contrast agents.
3. Reduced cost of examination. In addition to saving the cost of nonionic contrast, there is a significant savings in the quantity of radiographic film used with DSA. Film processing and storage costs are also reduced.

The disadvantage of DSA is decreased spacial resolution. Spacial resolution of digital arteriography is 2 to 3 line pairs per millimeter as opposed to 5 to 6 line pairs per millimeter of routine arteriography. Although arteries less than 1 mm can be visualized, they are not adequately seen for diagnostic evaluation. Decreased spacial resolution also results in a loss of edge sharpness in larger vessels. There is also a loss of fine detail in larger arteries, most evident in the aorta. This is partially due to decreased resolution and partially due to image subtraction and can result in an underestimation of the degree of atherosclerosis within the aorta and iliac arteries. Consequently, we routinely obtain intra-arterial pressures to evaluate the significance of any questionable aortoiliac atherosclerotic disease.

COMPLICATIONS

Arteriographic complications are related to arterial catheterization, contrast reaction, and contrast-induced renal failure. Hessel et al. reported a complication rate of 1.73 percent for femoral catheterization comprising hematoma (0.26 percent), occlusion or thrombosis (0.14 percent), false aneurysm (0.05 percent), and arteriovenous fistula (0.01 percent).[32] Distal embolization is extremely rare. The overall complication rate for axillary artery catheterization was 3.29 percent and translumbar catheterization was 2.89 percent. Fatal complications occur in 0.03 to 0.06 percent of patients.[33]

In our experience, hematoma formation and thrombosis are slightly more common with the high brachial or axillary approach than with the femoral approach. In a series of 600 brachial catheterizations, we experienced 6 immediate brachial arterial occlusions, all of which responded to full heparinization. None of these patients received an initial 1000-unit intravenous heparin bolus that we now employ. Since initiating this heparin bolus following brachial arterial catheterization, no thrombosis has occurred. Over the entire series, five patients required evacuation of a large hematoma causing brachial nerve compression. A single patient with arteritis experienced distal embolization to the hand. No vertebral neurovascular complications have occurred.

True contrast reactions occur in 0.14 percent of patients and involve urticaria, bronchospasm, laryngospasm, laryngeal edema, and cardiopulmonary arrest. Fatal reaction occurs in 0.02 percent of arteriograms.[34–36] If a history of previous reaction is present, we premedicate the patient with prednisone (50 mg PO every 6 hours for 24 hours), diphenylhydramine (Benadryl, 50 mg IM or IV), and cimetidine (300 mg PO or IV).[37,38] We also use nonionic contrast, which appears to have a lower incidence of contrast reaction.[39,40]

Patients with diabetic nephropathy have an increased incidence of contrast-induced renal failure, varying from 9 to 22 percent.[41,42] Defining contrast-induced renal failure as an increase of 25 percent in the serum creatinine level, Parfrey et al. found 11.8 percent incidence in the well-hydrated diabetic patient with pre-existing renal failure (baseline creatinine of 1.7 to 5 mg/dl).[41] Few patients required dialysis. Diabetic patients without pre-existing renal failure had a 2 percent incidence of mild contrast-induced renal failure, a rate comparable to nondiabetic individuals with normal renal function. In patients with baseline creatinine levels greater than 5 mg/dl, acute renal failure occurs in nearly all patients and is often irreversible.[43,44] Other factors that increase the incidence of contrast-related renal failure include congestive heart failure, hyperurcemia, proteinuria, advanced age (60 years), dehydration, myeloma, and concomitant administration of nephrotoxic medication.[35,45–47]

In order to limit nephrotoxicity, the quantity of contrast injection should be kept to a minimum. In high risk patients (creatinine level > 2.0 to 2.5), aortoiliac arteriography can be omitted in the presence of strong femoral pulses and normal noninvasive exams. Selective injection of the involved limb instead of bilateral leg arteriography and the use of DSA can greatly reduce the quantity of contrast injected.

All patients should be well hydrated with overnight intravenous fluids depending upon cardiac status. The patient should be further hydrated following the examination. Although controversial, patients with serum creatinine levels greater than 2 to 2.5 mg/dl receive 25 percent mannitol infused at a rate of 20 cc/h starting 1 hour before the arteriogram and continuing for 6 hours afterward. In addition, 100 mg of furosemide is injected for each mg/dl of creatinine level above 2.0. The patient is well hydrated before the procedure and urinary output is replaced with 5 percent dextrose in 0.45 percent saline with 30 mEq of potassium chloride per liter.[48] At this time, nonionic contrast has not been shown to reduce the incidence of contrast-induced renal failure.[39,40,49]

PERCUTANEOUS TRANSLUMINAL ANGIOPLASTY

Since the first arterial dilatation by Dotter in 1963 and the development of the modern double lumen angioplasty balloon by Gruntzig in 1974, percutaneous transluminal angioplasty has firmly established its role as either primary or adjunctive treatment of lower extremity atherosclerotic occlusive disease.[50,51] The mechanism of dilatation has been understood only recently.[52-54] Dilatation fractures the endothelial plaque, causes intima and media dehiscence, and stretches the media and adventia, resulting in a dilated lumen. This plaque separation and underlying dissection result in an intimal flap visualized on 70 percent of postdilatation arteriograms.[56] In a period of days, the dissection is remodeled by thrombus deposition and organization. By one month, this remodeling results in a smooth luminal surface within the dilated segment.

The decision as to whether or not a patient is a candidate for angioplasty or any interventional procedure designed to improve lower extremity circulation, including surgery, is based on the history, physical examination, noninvasive examination, and arteriogram. In general, a clinical assessment is made of either the degree of disability due to intermittent claudication or the threat to further limb viability from the presence of ischemic rest pain, ulceration, and/or gangrene. Although controversial, angioplasty can be used with claudication that is severe enough to affect the individual's life-style, but not severe enough for surgical revascularization. These patients are ideal in that usually the stenoses are short, easily crossed, and easily dilated. However, both the patient and other physicians involved should understand that, although unusual, complications do occur. Although long-term patency rates are much reduced, angioplasty should also be considered in those patients with diffuse or multisegmental disease who are too ill for surgical revascularization.

We have found that performing diagnostic arteriography and, if needed, angioplasty at the same time is efficient and spares the patient the potential risks of subsequent contrast studies—an especially important consideration in the diabetic patient with underlying renal insufficiency. An open line of communication in the spirit of cooperation between the arteriographer and vascular surgeon can greatly facilitate the arteriographer's task of making treatment decisions while the patient is in the process of being studied. When the greater expense and morbidity of surgery are weighed against the generally lower patency rates of angioplasty, the choice of which procedure to perform is usually straightforward. In more difficult situations, however, this cooperative relationship is essential to tailoring the best treatment to the individual's clinical situation.

The basic techniques for angioplasty are the same in the diabetic patient as in the nondiabetic patient and are well described.[58-61] Once the lesion has been crossed with the angiographic guidewire, the balloon catheter can easily be exchanged for the existing diagnostic catheter and then angioplasty performed (Fig. 14-6). At our institution, patients routinely receive 3,000 units of intravenous heparin at the time of the angioplasty and are maintained on aspirin (80 mg/day) following the procedure. Infrapopliteal arteries are fully heparinized for 24 hours following the procedure.

The type of balloon catheter used is a matter of personal preference. For 10- and 12-mm iliac arteries, we prefer the Olbert angioplasty catheter (Medox Surgimed, Inc., Oakland, NJ). Its design eliminates the large "wings" found on other deflated balloons and we feel this results in a smaller, less irregular arterial puncture site after removal. For small arteries, we presently use any of the "thin-wall" no. 5 French catheter high pressure balloons now available (Advanced Cardiovascular Systems, Inc., Mountain View, CA: CR Bard, Inc., Billerica, MA). These balloon catheters will tolerate inflation pressures up to 10 atmospheres, which is often necessary with densely calcified atherosclerotic plaques. These high pressure balloons are also less likely to be damaged by calcified lesions than previous no. 5 French catheter balloons and the thin balloon wall and small catheter size result in a smaller and less traumatized puncture site on

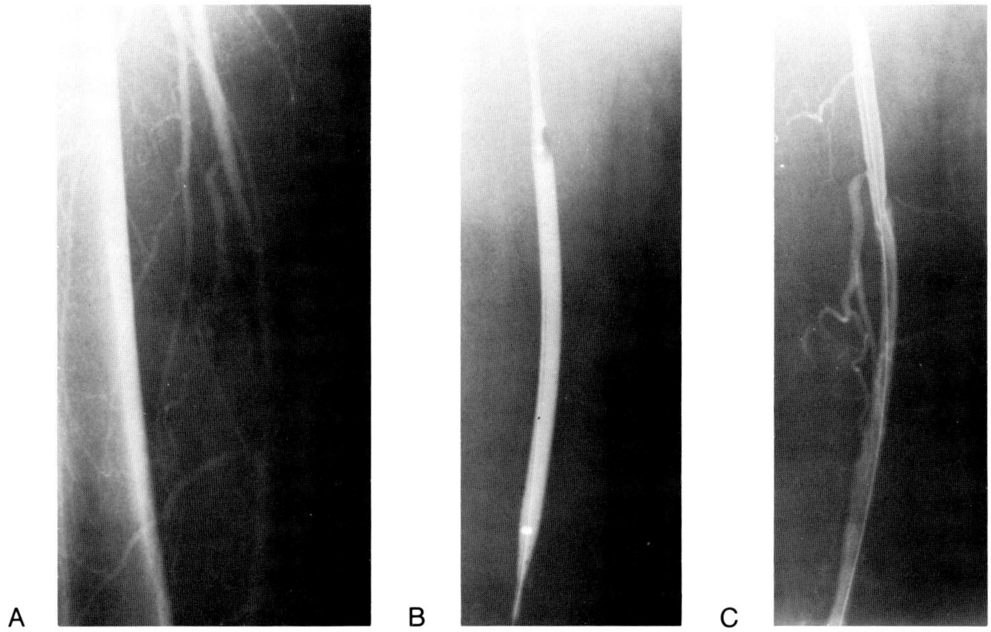

Fig. 14-6. Superficial femoral angioplasty. (**A**) Severe stenosis of the mid superficial femoral artery. (**B**) Expanded 5-mm-diameter angioplasty balloon. (**C**) Postangioplasty injection revealing luminal irregularity typical of arterial dissection.

removal. For arteries less than 3 mm in size, coronary angioplasty catheters are used.

Complication rates vary, although they are generally decreasing with improved techniques and catheter designs.[61] A review of 1,968 procedures resulted in an overall complication rate of 5.1 percent with 0.6 percent requiring surgical repair. The rate of individual complications are as follows (with the rate of surgical intervention given in parenthesis): hematoma, 2.5 percent (0.12 percent); thrombosis, 1.3 percent (0.2 percent); distal embolization, 0.8 percent (0.15 percent); false aneurysm, 0.25 percent (0.15 percent); and perforation, 0.25 percent (0.05 percent).[62]

Generally, the larger the artery and the shorter the stenosis, the better the long-term patency rates, the short iliac artery stenosis being an ideal lesion. Long stenoses or multiple stenoses greater than 8 cm have a lower long-term patency.[57] Generally, chronic occlusions have a lower patency rate than stenoses, although short occlusions have similar results to stenoses of similar length.[57,58] Acute occlusions, either embolic or thrombotic, or occlusions of unknown age should not be treated solely by angioplasty since distal embolization of recently formed thrombus can result. If the patient's limb can tolerate continuing ischemia and there are no contraindications, a trial of lytic therapy can be used to eliminate any fresh thrombus and the underlying stenosis can then be angioplastied.

Little information is available on long-term angioplasty results in the diabetic patient. Our review of 122 angioplasties evaluated by life table analysis revealed results comparable to nondiabetic patients with similar severity of vascular disease, findings supported by others.[57,58,63,64] Significantly better results were obtained in both iliac and femoral angioplasties in those patients with patent, although diseased, two- or three-vessel runoff ("good runoff") than with more severe diffuse disease with no runoff or one-vessel runoff ("poor runoff"). Of these patients, 76 percent were insulin-dependent and 71 percent had rest pain, ulceration, or gangrene.

Of 66 successful iliac angioplasties, the overall patency rate was 85 percent at 1 year, 67 percent at 3 and 4 years, and 34 percent at 5 years (Fig. 14-7).

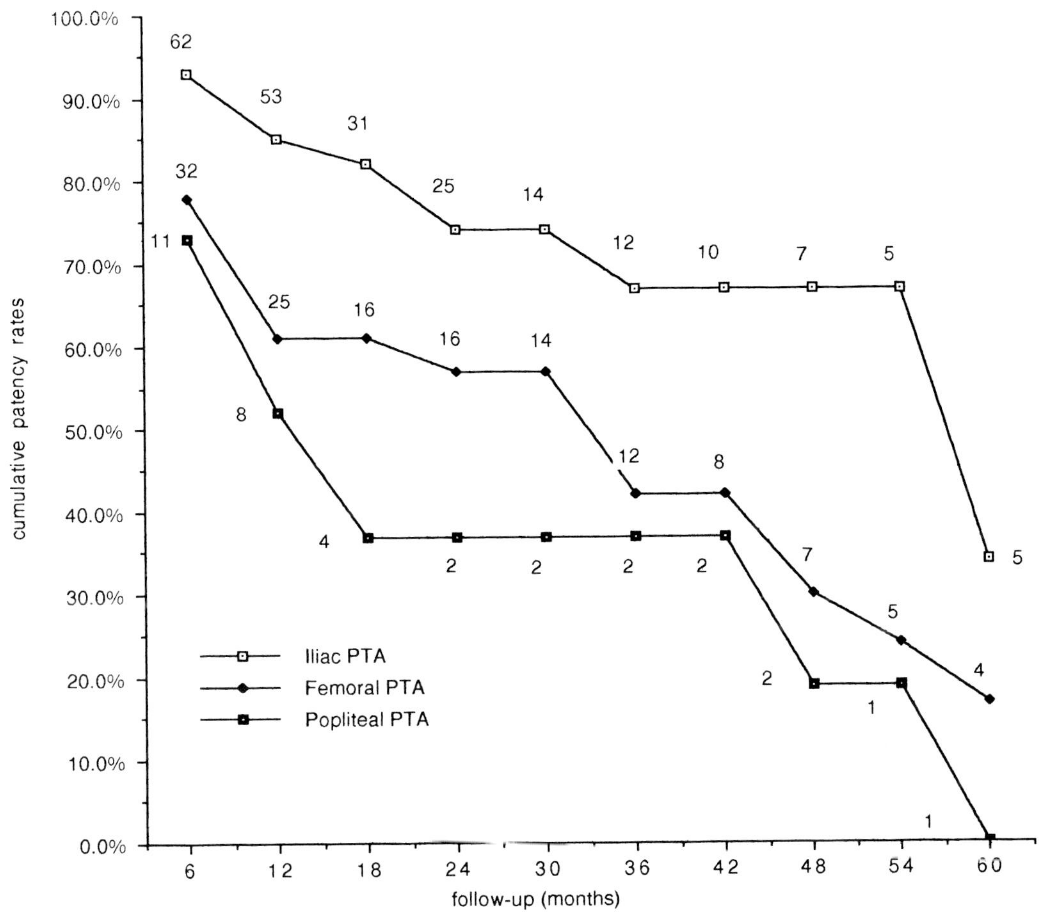

Fig. 14-7. Life table analysis of patency rates for successful iliac, femoral, and popliteal angioplasties. PTA, percutaneous transluminal angioplasty.

Of these patients, 49 percent presented with good runoff, while 51 percent presented with poor runoff. The 3- and 5-year patency rates of iliac angioplasties with good runoff were 76 percent, as opposed to 60 percent 3-year and 20 percent 5-year patency rates with poor runoff (Fig. 14-8).

Review of 40 superficial femoral angioplasties revealed overall patency rates of 61 percent at 1 year, 42 percent at 3 years, and 17 percent at 5 years. Patients with good runoff had patency rates of 82 percent at 1 year, 46 percent at 3 years, and 46 percent at 5 years, while patients with poor runoff had 48 percent 1-year, 40 percent 3-year and 8 percent 5-year patency rates (Fig. 14-9).

Sixteen popliteal angioplasties were performed for limb salvage, all with poor runoff (Fig. 14-7). Patency rates were 52 percent at 1 year and 37 percent at 3 years. None were patent at 5 years.

Not infrequently, a diabetic patient with limb-threatening ischemia will have multiple segments of atheroslerotic disease involving the aortoiliac segment, superficial femoral artery, and proximal infrapopliteal vessels (so-called inflow/outflow disease). When ischemic tissue loss or gangrene is present in the foot, bypass of the aortoiliac segment (inflow disease) without bypassing of the more distal occlusions (outflow disease) may not allow healing. In these circumstances the vascular surgeon is faced with two unappealing options: either to perform a lengthy combined procedure involving the simultaneous correction of both inflow and outflow disease or to sequentially perform the inflow procedure first followed by the outflow procedure several days later. This exposes the patient to the morbidity and mortality associated with two separate surgical procedures. When iliac angioplasty is

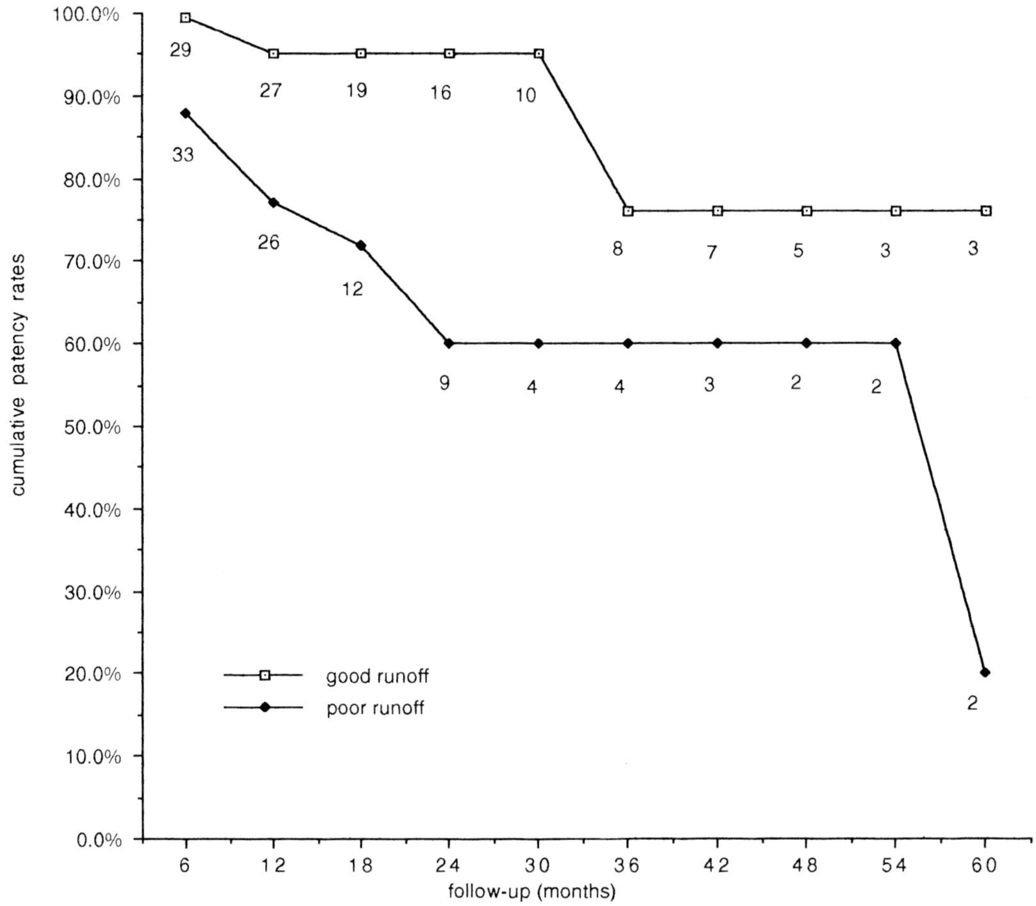

Fig. 14-8. Patency of iliac angioplasty with respect to runoff.

possible, the potential morbidity to the patient can be significantly reduced by alleviating the need for the inflow surgical procedure.

Percutaneous transluminal angioplasty has also had an impact on atherosclerotic lesions occurring below the inguinal ligament. Occasionally a patient may require distal tibial reconstruction but will not have an adequate length of venous conduit for bypass. When angioplasty of the superficial femoral artery is possible, the length of vein necessary for bypass can be reduced by performing the proximal anastomosis with the popliteal artery at the knee instead of with the usual common femoral artery at the groin. Although the durability of percutaneous transluminal angioplasty below the inguinal ligament is significantly lower than seen with surgical procedures, it still may be the appropriate primary procedure in patients with isolated superficial femoral artery stenoses with disabling claudication when the risks of surgery are great or when venous conduit is not available.

INTRA-ARTERIAL THROMBOLYSIS

Although thrombolytic agents have been used to treat arterial thrombosis since 1955,[65,66] only recently has this technique in the form of regional intra-arterial thrombolysis been used extensively.[67–70] Early studies involved the use of streptokinase administered in relative low doses directly into the thrombosed artery. We presently use urokinase, which has been found to be more effective and safer with fewer systemic thrombolytic side

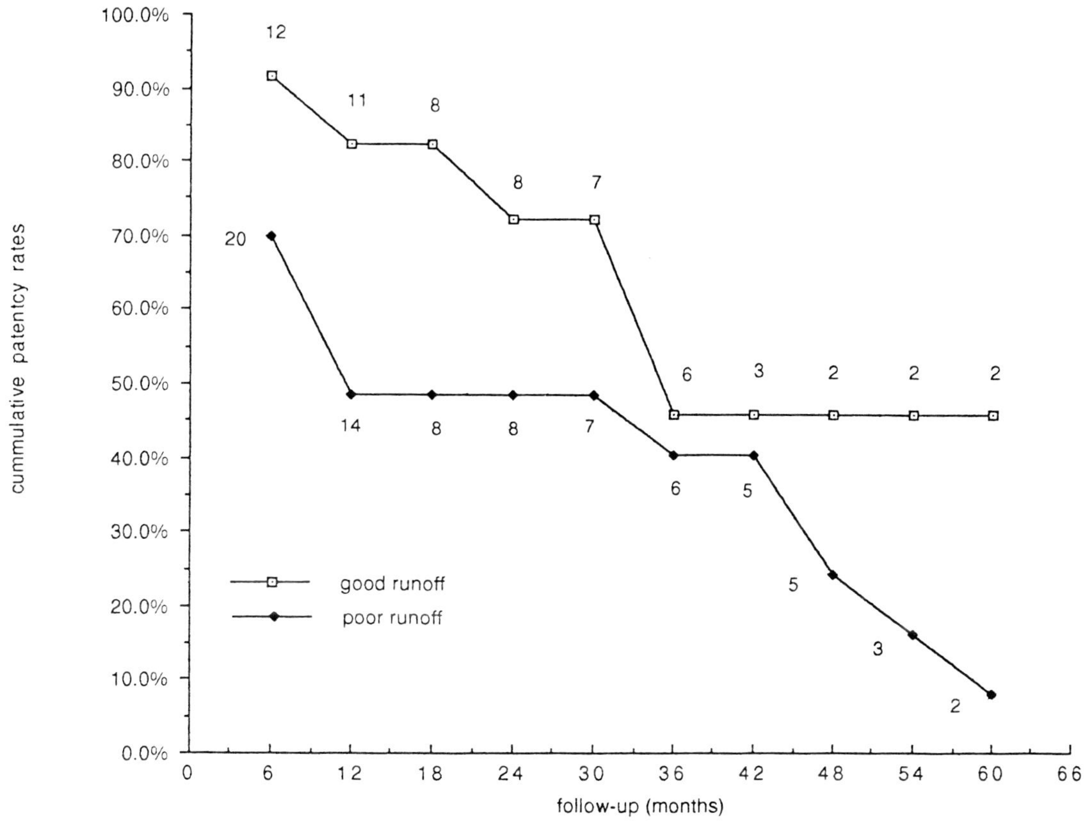

Fig. 14-9. Patency of femoral angioplasty with respect to runoff.

effects than streptokinase, although urokinase is more expensive.[71-73]

Urokinase (UK) is a nonantigenic thrombolytic agent derived from human fetal renal cell cultures. It lyses thrombus by directly activating plasminogen. Its half-life is approximately 20 minutes; however, its anticoagulant effects persist for hours due to depletion of clotting factors and fibrinogen. At this time an additional thrombolytic agent, tissue plasminogen activator (TPA) is under investigation. It is an endogenous agent that activates plasminogen only in the present of fibrin. Although experience is limited, initial results suggest TPA is as effective as UK but is less expensive and may require shorter infusion times.[74,75]

The basic technique of local intra-arterial thrombolysis involves the placement of an arteriographic infusion catheter selectively into the thrombosed artery and, if possible, into the thrombus itself. This allows the direct infusion of relatively low doses of urokinase into the thrombus, resulting in improved thrombolysis but without the bleeding complications associated with high-dose systemic therapy. Dosage regimens for UK vary with the most popular being a constant infusion of 40,000 to 80,000 units/h, or the initial infusion of 240,000 units/h for 2 hours followed by 60,000 units/h.[71,76,77]

During infusion, patients are monitored closely in an intensive care unit. Repeat angiography is performed periodically both to evaluate the extent of lysis and to reposition the catheter into the residual thrombus if necessary. The infusion is continued until there is no further lysis for a period of 12 to 24 hours or if complications such as hemorrhage necessitate termination of the infusion. Generally the longer the length of infusion, the more likely that systemic bleeding complications will occur. When infusion is complete, the underlying cause of the thrombosis, such as atherosclerotic narrowing, should be treated immediately either by surgery or angioplasty. Since lytic therapy may be prolonged, it should be performed only when the limb is in no immediate danger of loss.

Intra-arterial thrombolytic therapy can be successfully used for occluded native arteries and occluded bypass grafts. It is also useful in the treatment of postarteriographic or postangioplasty arterial thrombosis. The more acute the thrombosis, the more likely thrombolytic therapy will be successful, with lysis of acute thromboses in up to 90 percent of cases. In general, thrombolytic therapy is successful in approximately 80 percent of all cases.[71,76–79]

The most frequent complication is that of hemorrhage. For that reason, contraindications to thrombolytic therapy involve those conditions in which bleeding is likely to occur, such as recent surgery or trauma, pregnancy, recent stroke, central nervous system tumor or other pathology, or active internal bleeding. In the diabetic, the possibility of retinal hemorrhage should be considered. Other complications include pericatheter thrombosis and distal embolization. These conditions generally can be treated with continued thrombolytic therapy.

NEW INTERVENTIONAL DEVICES

Percutaneous Atherectomy Devices

The recent development of atherectomy devices has resulted in an additional potential modality for the percutaneous treatment of atherosclerotic disease. As opposed to angioplasty, which disrupts the plaque and stretches the arterial wall, atherectomy devices mechanically remove atheromatous material. At this time only three devices have been approved for vascular use: the Simpson Atherectomy Catheter (Atherocath, Devices for Vascular Intervention, Redwood City, CA); the Transluminal Endarterectomy Catheter (TEC, Interventional Technologies Inc., San Diego, CA); and the Kinsey Dynamic Angioplasty Catheter (KDAC, Therateck International, Miami, FL).[80–82]

The Simpson catheter is the only device designed to remove the bulk of the plaque, restoring patency without angioplasty. It is useful in relatively short stenoses or occlusions only and not applicable to diffuse disease. Hypothetically, removal of atheromatous material results in a smoother surface with less turbulence and a lower incidence of dissection, improving long-term patency rates compared with angioplasty. Using this device, Althous et al. reported a 1-year patency rate of 92.5 percent, which compares favorably to most angioplasty series.[83]

The remaining two devices "bore" a small hole through the occluded artery to allow passage of an angiographic guidewire. Both require adjunctive angioplasty to completely open the artery. Neither of these devices has been studied in the diabetic patient and no long-term results are yet available in the nondiabetic patient. Wholey et al. reported a 14 percent recurrence with stenoses and a 24 percent recurrence with occlusions treated with the TEC catheter.[84]

Too little experience exists with the Kinsey catheter for evaluation. Snyder et al. successfully recanalized 14 of 23 superficial femoral arteries using open surgical techniques; however, only 4 of these were totally occluded arteries.[85] Wholey et al. recanalized 7 of 8 totally occluded femoral arteries percutaneously; however, 4 reoccluded early and 1 suffered distal embolization with only three arteries patent at 17 to 18 months.[86]

Laser Angioplasty

After initial enthusiasm for the use of lasers in recanalizing femoral and popliteal arteries, the technique has been found to have limited usefulness. Limited data on long-term patency are available in the nondiabetic patient and none specifically in the diabetic patient. In the hands of an experienced angiographer, most severe stenoses and short occlusions can easily be crossed with standard catheter and guidewire techniques. The laser can be successfully used, however, to cross femoral and popliteal occlusions not otherwise possible. Like some atherectomy devices, the laser, whether argon or Nd:YAG and whether a hot tip, sapphire tip, or direct fiber design, only forms a 2-3-mm path through the occlusion to permit passage of a guidewire for subsequent angioplasty. In this respect, it has been a successful technique with up to 90 percent of total occlusions being recanalized.[87,88] The long-term patency rates, however, have not been shown to be appreciably better than angioplasty alone.

Because of the expense of the laser unit, exceeding $100,000 in some cases in addition to the cost of installation and operation, it is difficult to recommend it over mechanical atherectomy catheters that have similar success. Additional laser systems are being investigated, the most notable of which are the excimer laser and the directed laser (MCM Smart Laser, MCM Laboratories, Mountain View, CA).[89-91] Their efficacy is not yet determined.

Also under investigation is a radiofrequency thermal angioplasty system.[92,93] A radiofrequency generator heats a hot-tip probe that is then used in the same fashion as the hot-tip laser. The uses and shortcomings are the same as the laser, although this system will be appreciably less expensive. At this time little clinical data are available.

REFERENCES

1. Gibbons GW, Freeman D: Vascular evaluation and treatment of the diabetic. Clin Pod Med Surg 4:377, 1986
2. Melton LJ, Macken KM, Palumbo RJ, Elveback LR: Incidence and prevalence of clinical peripheral vascular disease in a population-based cohort of diabteic patients. Diabetes Care 3:650, 1980
3. Janka HV, Standl F, Mehnert H: Peripheral vascular disease in diabetes mellitus and its relation to cardiovascular role factors: screening with the Doppler ultrasonic technique. Diabetes Care 3:207, 1980
4. McGil HC, Jr: Diabetes and vascular lesions. In Moskowitz J (ed): Diabetes and Atherosclerosis Connection. Juvenile Diabetes Foundation Medical Series, New York, 1981
5. Sternby NH: Atheroslcerosis and diabetes mellitus. Acta Pathol Microbiol Scand, suppl., 194:152, 1968
6. King TA, Depalma RG, Rhodes RS: Diabetes mellitus and atherosclerotic involvement of the profunda femoris artery. Surg Gynecol Obstet 159:553, 1984
7. University Group Diabetes Program: A study of the effects of hypoglycemic agents on vascular complications in patients with adult-onset diabetes. Design, methods and baseline results. Diabetes, suppl. 2, 19:747, 1970
8. Andros G, Harris RW, Dulauna LB et al: The need for arteriography in diabetic patients with gangrene and palpable foot pulses. Arch Surg 119:1260, 1984
9. Kadir S: Preangiographic evaulation. p. 78. In: Diagnostic Angiography. WB Saunders, Philadelphia, 1986
10. Kozak BE, Bedell JE, Rosch J: Small vessel leg angiography for distal vessel bypass grafts. J Vasc Surg; 8:711, 1988
11. Dardik H, Ibrahim IM, Sussman B et al: Morphologic structure of the pedal arch and its relationship to patency of crural vascular reconstruction. Surg Gynecol Obstet 152:645, 1981
12. Imparato AM, Kim GE, Mandayag M, Haveson S: Angiographic criteria for successful tibial arterial reconstruction. Surgery 74:830, 1973
13. O'Mara CS, Flinn WR, Neiman HL et al: Correlation of foot arterial anatomy with early tibial bypass patency. Surgery 89:743, 1981
14. Pomposelli FB, Jepsen SJ, Gibbons GW et al: Efficacy of the dorsal pedal bypass for limb salvage in diabetic patients: short term observations. J Vasc Surg 11:745, 1990
15. Neubauer B: Intra-arterial tolazoline in angiography of the foot. Acta Radiol Diag 19:793, 1978
16. Abramson DI: Drugs used in peripheral vascular diseases. Am J Cardiol 12:203, 1963
17. Kahn PC, Callow AD: Selective vasodilation as an aid to angiography. Am J. Radiogr 94:213, 1965
18. Murphy RA Jr, McClure JN, Jr, Cooper FW et al: The effect of priscoline, papaverine and nicotinic acid on blood flow in the lower extremity of man. A comparative study. Surgery 27:655, 1950
19. Hishida Y: Peripheral arteriography using reactive hyperemia. Jpn Circ J 27:349, 1963
20. Kahn PC, Boyer DN, Moran JM et al: Reactive hypermia in lower extremity arteriography: an evaluation. Radiology; 90:975, 1968
21. Kruger RA: Image data acquisition, processing, storage and display. Cardiovasc Intervent Radiol 6:183, 1983
22. Kruger RA, Riederer SJ: Basic Concepts of Digital Subtraction Angiography. GK Hall Medical Publishers, Boston, 1984
23. Mistretta CA, Ort MG, Cameron JR et al: A multiple image subtraction technique for enhancing low contrast, periodic objects. Invest Radiol 8:43, 1973
24. Ovitt TW, Capp MP, Christenson P et al: Development of a digital video subtraction system for intravenous angiography. Proc Spie 206:73, 1979
25. Vizy KN: Electronic imaging fundamentals: basic theory. Cardiovasc Intervent Radiol; 6:183, 1983
26. Harrington DP, Boxt LM, Murray PD: Digital sub-

traction angiography overview of technical principles. Am J. Radiol 139:781, 1982
27. Ovitt T, Newell JD II: Digital subtraction angiography: technology, equipment, and techniques. Radio Clin North Am 23:177, 1985
28. Turski PA: Digital subtraction angiography: current status and use in intraarterial injection. Radiology 145:303, 1982
29. Kaufman SL, Chang R, Kadir S: Intraarterial digital subtraction angiography in diagnostic arteriography. Radiology 151:323, 1984
30. Katzen BT: Peripheral abdominal, and interventional applications of DSA. Radiol Clin North Am 23:227, 1984
31. Foley WD, Milde MW: Intraarterial digital subtraction angiography. Radiol Clin North Am 23:293, 1985
32. Hessel SJ, Adams DF, Abrams HL: Complications of angiography. Radiology 138:273, 1981
33. Lang FK: A survey of the complications of percutaneous retrograde arteriography. Radiology 81:257, 1963
34. Shehadi WH, Toniolo G: Adverse reactions to contrast media. A report from the Committee on Safety of Contrast Media of the Interventional Society of Radiology. Radiology 137:299, 1980
35. Moore RD, Steinberg EP, Powe NR: Frequency and determinants of adverse reactions induced by high-osmolarity contrast media. Radiology 170:727, 1989
36. Sheladi WH: Contrast media adverse reactions: occurrences, recurrences, and distribution patterns. Radiology 143:11, 1982
37. Greenhuger P, Patterson R, Kelly M et al: Administration of radiographic contrast media in high risk patients. Invest Radiol, suppl., 15:540, 1980
38. Myers G, Bloom FL: Cimetidine (Tagamet) combined with steroids and H_1 antihistamines for the prevention of serious radiographic contrast material reactions. Cath Cardiovasc Diagn 7:65, 1981
39. Wolf GL, Arenson RL, Cross AP, A prospective trial of ionic vs nonionic contrast agents in routine clinical proactice and comparison of adverse effects. Am J Radiol 152:939, 1989
40. Kinnison ML, Powe NR, Steinberg EP: Results of randomized controlled trials of low- versus high-osmolarity contrast media. Radiology 170:381, 1989
41. Parfrey PS, Griffiths SM, Barrett BJ et al: Contrast material-induced renal failure in patients with diabetes mellitus, renal insufficiency, or both. N Engl J Med 320:143, 1989
42. D'Elia JA, Gleason RE, Alday M et al: Nephrotoxicity from angiographic contrast material: a prospective study. Am J Med 72:719, 1982
43. Harkonen S, Kjellstrand CM: Exacerbation of diabetic renal failure following intravenous pyelography. Am J Med 63:939, 1977
44. Weinrauch LA, Healy RW, Leland OS et al: Coronary angiography and acute renal failure in diabetic azotemic nephropathy. Ann Intern Med 86:56, 1977
45. McGill HC, Jr: Diabetes and vascular lesions. In Moskowitz J (ed): Diabetes and Atherosclerosis Connection. Juvenile Diabetes Foundation Medical Series, New York, 1981
46. Cochran ST, Wong WS, Roe DJ: Predicting angiography induced acute renal function impairment: clinical risk model. Am J. Radiol 141:1027, 1983
47. Byrd L, Sherman RL: Radiocontrast-induced acute renal failure: a clinical and pathophysiologic review. Medicine 58:270, 1979
48. Berkseth RO, Kjellstrand CM: Radiologic contrast-induced nephropathy. Clin North Am 68:351, 1984
49. Schwab SJ, Hjatky MA, Pieper KS et al: Contrast nephrotoxicity: a random controlled trial of a nonionic and ionic radiographic contrast agent. N Engl J Med 320:149, 1989
50. Dotter CT, Judkins MP: Transluminal treatment of arteriosclerotic obstruction: description of a new technique and a preliminary report of its application. Circulation 30:654, 1964
51. Gruntzig A, Hopff H: Perkutane recakanalisation chronischer arterieller vershlusse mit newen. Dilatation skatheter. Dtsch Med Wochenschr 99:2502, 1974
52. Castenenda-Zuniga WR, Formanek A, Tadavarthy M et al: The mechanism of balloon angioplasty. Radiology 135:565, 1980
53. Lyon RT, Zarins CK, Lu C-T et al: Vessel, plaque and lumen morpology after transluminal balloon angioplasty: quantitative study in distended human arteries. Arteriosclerosis 3:306, 1987
54. Zarins CK, Lu C-T, Gewertz BL et al: Arterial disruption and remodeling following balloon dilatation. Surgery 92:1086, 1982
55. Dondelinger RF, Rossi P, Kurdziel JC: Interventional Radiology. Thieme, New York, 1990
56. Zarins, CK, Lu CT: Grewertz BL et al: Arterial disruption and remodeling following balloon dilatation. Surgery 92:1086, 1982
57. Hewes RC, White RI, Murray RR et al: Long-term results of superficial artery angioplasty. Am J Radiol 146:1025, 1986
58. Johnston KW, Rae M, Hogg-Johnston SA et al: Five-

year results of a prospective study of percutaneous transluminal angiography. Ann Surg 206:403, 1987
59. Katzen B, Van Breda A: Transluminal angioplasty of the iliac arteries. Sem Intervent Radiol, suppl., 2(2):196, 1985
60. Van Breda A, Katzen B: Femoral angioplasty. Sem Intervent Radiol, suppl., 1(4):251, 1984
61. Gardiner GA, Meyerovitz MF, Stokes KR et al.: Complications of transluminal angioplasty. Radiology 159:201, 1986
62. Walden R, Siegel Y, Rubinstein ZJ et al: Percutaneous transluminal angioplasty. J Vasc Surg 3:583, 1986
63. Stokes KR, Strunk HM, Campbell DR et al: Five-year results of iliac and femoropopliteal angioplasty in diabetic patients. Radiology 174:977, 1990
64. Lally ME, Johnston KW, Andrews D: Percutaneous transluminal dilatation of peripheral arteries: an analysis of factors predicting early success. J Vasc Surg 1:704, 1984
65. Tillet WS, Johnson AJ, McCarthy WF: The intravenous infusion of the streptococcal fibrinolytic principle (streptokinase) into patients. J Clin Invest 34:169, 1955
66. Dotter CT, Rosch J, Seaman AJ. Selective clot lysis with low-dose streptokinase. Radiology 1111:31, 1974
67. Katzen BT, van Breda A: Low dose streptokinase in the treatment of arterial occlusions. Am J Radiol 136:1171, 1981
68. Totty WG, Gilula LA, McClellan BL et al: Low-dose intravascular fibrinolytic therapy. Radiology; 143:59, 1982
69. Becker CJ, Rabe FE, Richmond BD et al: Low-dose fibrinolytic therapy: results and new concepts. Radiology 148:663, 1983
70. Mori KW, Bookstein JJ, Heeney DJ et al. Selective streptokinase infusion: clinical and laboratory correlates. Radiology 148:677, 1983
71. McNamara TO, Fischer R: Thrombolysis of peripheral arterial and graft occlusions: improved results using high dose urokinase. Am J Radiol 144:769, 1985
72. Gardiner GA, Koltum W, Kandarpa L et al: Thrombolysis of occluded femoropopliteal grafts. Am J Radiol 147:621, 1986
73. Belkin M, Belkin B, Bucknam CA et al: Intraarterial fibrinolytic therapy, efficacy of streptokinase versus urokinase. Arch Surg 121:769, 1986
74. Meyerovitz MF, Goldhaber SZ, Reagan K et al: Tissue plasminogen activator versus urokinase: randomized controlled trial in peripheral arterial occlusion. Presented at annual meeting of the RSNA, Chicago, December 1988
75. Graor RA, Risius B, Yound JR et al: Peripheral artery and bypass graft thrombolysis with recombinant human tissue type plasminogen activator. Circulation 72(4):III-XV(58), 1985
76. Van Breda A, Katzen BT, Picus D, Steinberg DL: Intra-arterial urokinase infusion for treatment of acute and chronic arterial occlusions. Radiology 1161:104, 1986
77. Van Breda A, Waltman AC: Low dose thrombolysis for arterial disease of the lower extremities. Int Angiol 12:75, 1983
78. Van Breda A, Robinson JC, Feldman L: Local thrombolysis in the treatment of graft occlusions. J Vasc Surg 1:103, 1984
79. Lammer J, Pilger E, Neumayer K, Schreyer H: Intra-arterial fibrinolysis: long-term results. Radiology 161:159, 1986
80. Simpson JB, Johnson DE, Thapliyal HV et al: Transluminal atherectomy: a new approach to the treatment of atherosclerotic vascular disease. Circulation, suppl., 72:111, 1985
81. Kensey KR, Nash JE, Abrahams C et al: Recanalization of obstructed arteries with a flexible, rotating tip catheter. Radiology 165:387, 1987
82. Maynar M, Reyes R, Cabreara V et al: Percutaneous atherectomy with Simpson atherectomy device in the management of arterial stenosis. Sem Intervent Radiol 5:247, 1988
83. Althaus SJ, Minneapolis MN, Maynar M et al: Clinical-pathologic-angiographic correlation following transluminal atherectomy. Presented at the annual RSNA meeting, Chicago, 1989
84. Wholey MH, Jarmolowski CR, Rein D et al: Multicenter trial with the transluminal endarterectomy catheter in 200 patients with peripheral vascular occlusive disease. Presented at the annual RSNA meeting, Chicago, 1989
85. Snyder SO, Wheeler JR, Gregory RT et al: Kensey catheter-early results with a transluminal atherectomy tool. J Vasc Surg 8:541, 1988
86. Wholey MH, Smith JAM, Godlewski P: Recanalization of total arterial occlusions with the Kensey dynamic angioplasty catheter. Radiology 172:95, 1989
87. Sanborn TA, Cumberland DC, Greenfield AS et al: Percutaneous laser thermal angioplasty: initial results and one-year follow up in 129 femoropopliteal lesions. Radiology 168:121, 1988
88. Nordstrom LA, Young EG: Direct laser recanalization of occluded superficial femoral and iliac ar-

teries: primary success and low complication rates. Sem Intervent Radiol 5:277, 1988
89. Murphy-Chutorian D: The concept of a directed laser. p. 442. In Moore WS, Ahn SS (eds): Endovascular Surgery. WB Saunders, Philadelphia, 1989
90. Mok WY: Construction of the MCM smart laser. p. 453. In Moore WS, Ahn SS (eds): Endovascular Surgery. WB Saunders, Philadelphia, 1989
91. Litvack F, Grundfect WS, Adler L et al: Percutaneous excimer-laser and excimer-laser-angioplasty of the lower extremities: results of initial clinical trial. Radiology 172:331, 1989
92. Litvack F, Grundfect WS, Adler L et al.: Percutaneous "hot tip" angioplasty in man by a radiofrequency catheter systems, abstracted. J Am Coll Cardiol 11:103A, 1988
93. Grundfest WS, Litvack F, Hickey A et al: Radiofrequency thermal angioplasty for the treatment of peripheral vascular occlusive disease: Preliminary results of a clinical trial. J Am Coll Cardiol (in press)

15

Vascular Surgery of the Lower Extremity

Gary W. Gibbons, M.D.

Prior to the discovery of insulin, coma and infection were the most common causes of death in the diabetic. Vascular disease now accounts for 75 percent of deaths of diabetic patients. While the severity of diabetes is not crucial to the development of atherosclerosis, the relationship between the two exceeds the commonly recognized risk factors for atherosclerosis.[1] These include hypertension, hyperlipidema, obesity, cigarette smoking, hypercoagulability, and genetics.

Peripheral vascular disease is 20 times more common in diabetic than in nondiabetic patients. While diabetic patients have a 17-fold increased risk of developing gangrene over nondiabetic individuals, it is not assumed that this is totally the result of atherosclerosis.[2] It is the triopathy of neuropathy, vascular insufficiency, and an inability to handle infection normally that either singularly or, more commonly, in combination make the diabetic patient uniquely susceptible to the development of foot problems. While this chapter discusses vascular surgery, it must be remembered that effective treatment must be directed at these three primary pathologic situations.

The economic impact of lower extremity ischemia in the diabetic patient is important. The incidence of type 2 diabetes is increasing, with 564,868 newly diagnosed cases reported in 1987. A study that assesses the direct and indirect cost of diabetes and its complications at $20.4 billion in the United States for 1987 is startling.[3] Twenty-five percent of diabetic persons will seek the advice of a health care professional for a foot- or leg-related problem at some point during the course of their diabetes. Diabetic foot problems account for 20 percent of all hospital admissions for diabetic patients, and more in-hospital days are spent treating diabetic foot problems than all other complications of diabetes. The majority of major amputations in this country are performed on diabetic patients, which is not surprising.[4,5] Unfortunately, many of these are performed needlessly because of misconceptions that still persist regarding the appropriate treatment of diabetic foot or leg problems.[6] This chapter discusses the misconceptions relating to effective management of ischemia in the diabetic lower extremity.

Ischemia again is only one component of diabetic foot problems, and effective treatment begins with prevention. Patient and physician education and understanding correlate directly with the development of foot problems.[7] Many diabetic patients remain free of foot problems yet have diminished or even absent pulses at the femoral, popliteal, pedal, or at all levels. The role of proper foot care, therefore, cannot be overemphasized. While good control of diabetes will not prevent foot problems or ischemia, it could possibly delay them. Controlling the other risk factors is also essential. Smoking increases the prevalence and progression of arterial occlusive disease in the diabetic patient, and it is associated with a higher mortality. Daily foot inspection, proper hygiene, and appropriate shoeing are essential. Periodic vascular evaluation is a prerequisite for successful management. Most important is the need to report any change or new foot lesion immediately. The diabetic patients' greatest fears are gangrene and amputation, and oftentimes these fears overwhelm their need to report a problem early.

OPTIMAL MANAGEMENT

Optimal management of the diabetic patient with lower extremity ischemia requires an understanding of four essential components: (1) nonexistence of an occlusive microvascular disease of the diabetic foot, (2) specific pattern of atherosclerotic vascular disease, especially involvement of the tibial-peroneal vessels, (3) specific techniques or arteriography, and (4) modern approaches to arterial reconstruction.[8]

There is a continued misconception that diabetic patients have arterial or occlusive disease involving the foot that impairs perfusion and causes ulceration. It was thought that this "small vessel disease" occurred even in patients with palpable pedal pulses and therefore "all diabetics have poor circulation." This has led to a hopeless attitude held by many health care professionals treating diabetic foot problems, and certainly it is responsible for the inappropriate care extended to many. Logerfo and Coffman's careful review of vascular and microvascular disease of the foot in the diabetic patient puts to rest the notion of an arteriolar microvascular lesion in the diabetic foot.[9] Put simply, tissue perfusion in the ischemic diabetic foot can be restored by appropriate vascular reconstructions.

While the pathology of atherosclerosis is similar in both diabetic and nondiabetic patients, several major distinguishing factors characterize the diabetic person. In the diabetic individual there is a predilection for macrovascular occlusive disease involving the more distal tibial-peroneal vessels between the knee and the foot.[10] This is evidenced by the fact that 40 percent of diabetic patients who present with gangrene or ulceration have a palpable popliteal pulse. As stated before, the foot vessels are usually spared. Involvement of the distal profunda femoris artery and infrageniculate is more prevalent, and the ability to develop collateral circulation when major vessel occlusion occurs is markedly diminished.[11] It is for this reason that a femoral artery occlusion in the diabetic patient may produce more serious symptoms and complications in the distal leg and foot than the same occlusion would produce in the nondiabetic person. It is also why multiple areas of occlusions or stenosis involving the aortoiliac and leg vessels have more serious consequences for the diabetic and not because of any involvement of the foot arteries.

Diabetic arteries frequently contain extensive calcification involving the intimal plaque and also the media, which is known as medial calcinosis or Monckeberg's sclerosis. Medial calcinosis frequently results in a rigid, noncompressible artery, but usually does not occlude the lumen. It is responsible for erroneous noninvasive segmental systolic pressure results and makes surgical or laser manipulation more difficult.

Up-to-date arteriography is essential for successful vascular reconstruction. Arteriography is detailed in another chapter, but several points need to be emphasized for the vascular surgeon. First, the increased incidence of renal failure associated with arteriography in the diabetic requires not only careful preparation, but the avoidance of major revascularization procedures immediately following arteriography (except in urgent or emergency situations).[12] Precise arteriography is mandatory for successful vascular reconstruction and the vascular surgeon should accept nothing less. This includes visualization of the foot arteries whenever possible. It is important for the vascular surgeon to understand that the clinical pathology and severity of the involved vessels at the time of operation is usually worse than shown on the arteriogram. This is especially true for the arterial digital subtraction technique, which tells the surgeon that there is a patent vessel but does not quantitate nor qualitate its atherosclerotic involvement.

The diagnosis of diabetic peripheral vascular disease is generally more difficult to make when compared to the nondiabetic individual for all the reasons previously mentioned. While assessment of peripheral vascular disease is detailed elsewhere, key points deserve emphasis. Clinical evaluation, judgment, and experience are still essential for assessing vascular insufficiency in the diabetic lower extremity and are only complemented by noninvasive testing.[13] We have found no noninvasive tests that uniformly predict healing with or without surgery.[14] An excellent rule of thumb is to proceed with arteriography when there is a question of ischemia associated with an unresolving diabetic foot problem.

CLINICAL PRESENTATION AND INDICATIONS FOR SURGICAL INTERVENTION

The clinical presentation of patients with major artery occlusion and/or hemodynamically significant stenosis varies depending on activity level and adequacy of collateral pathways. Some patients (diabetic persons included) with major vessel disease are asymptomatic. Clinical presentation is detailed in the inflow and outflow disease sections to follow.

Conservative management of peripheral vascular disease is always the first line of treatment. Good control of the diabetes, the cessation of smoking, reduction in or maintenance of an ideal weight, control of hypertension, and a tailored exercise program are essential in this endeavor. One cannot say enough about the need for proper foot care and hygiene to avoid the complications of ischemic neuropathy. Periodic review of medications and the discontinuance of β blockers are often necessary, especially in patients whose claudication worsens. While the use of Trental (pentoxifylline) is somewhat controversial, I believe that it should be tried since it may improve the walking distance in a number of diabetic patients with claudication.

More invasive intervention is indicated when conservative medical care has failed or would be inappropriate. The main indications for intervention continue to be (1) progressive claudication (walking distance usually less than one-half block) that interferes with the patient's life-style or work, (2) rest or night pain, and (3) the development of ischemic ulcerations or necrotic (gangrene) lesions of the foot. It should be remembered that intermittent claudication is not a precursor of limb loss, especially in its early stages. Conservatism is justified since only 10 to 15 percent of patients worsen and progress to more limb-threatening symptoms.[15] There is evidence that in the diabetic patient, claudication is more progressive, especially in those patients who continue to smoke.[16] Rest pain and ischemic ulceration are considered limb-salvaging indications. These extremities are imminently threatened. Obviously more aggressive intervention is dependent on the patient's associated risk factors and well-being.

AORTOILIAC (INFLOW) OCCLUSIVE DISEASE

The nature of the muscle groups involved with claudication helps to distinguish aortoiliac occlusive disease from femoral-popliteal occlusive disease. The initial manifestation of occlusive disease in the distal aorta and/or iliac arteries is intermittent claudication involving the muscles of the thigh, hip, and buttock as well as the calf. Claudication is almost always relieved by rest and the severity is determined by the distance that the patient can walk, usually measured in blocks. Claudication in the diabetic patient with neuropathy may not necessarily take the form of pain and may be described by some patients as a "numbness" or "dead feeling" in the leg or foot when walking a given distance. Oftentimes this is worse when one is going up an incline or hurrying. It is always relieved by rest and never occurs when standing or sitting. Claudication must also be distinguished from symptoms or nerve-root irritation caused by spinal stenosis, intervertebral disc herniation, or even diabetic neuropathy itself.

Male patients with aortoiliac occlusive disease may also complain of erectile dysfunction because of associated internal iliac or pudendal artery occlusion. Symptoms may progress to those of the classic Leriche syndrome.[17] Aortoiliac occlusive disease uncommonly causes ischemic rest pain or ischemic tissue loss, except in cases of embolization. This is not necessarily the case for the diabetic patient, since the collateral circulation that usually develops around aortoiliac occlusive disease may be limited and because of associated femoral, popliteal, or tibial-peroneal occlusive disease. So the diabetic patient with severe diffuse vessel occlusive disease may remain asymptomatic for claudication or early rest pain masked by neuropathy until some minor trauma results in ischemic ulceration. In the diabetic patient, impotence is also associated with diabetic autonomic neuropathy, sometimes confusing the diagnosis.

Microembolization of arteriosclerotic debris to the terminal vessels of the foot (blue toe syndrome) is another symptom of significant arteriosclerotic aortoiliac occlusive disease. This occurs less commonly in diabetic patients, again because of associated distal occlusive disease. The sudden appearance of dusky blue toes with pregangrenous skin changes may be more indicative of rapidly progressing distal disease rather than embolization in the diabetic patient.

PREOPERATIVE ASSESSMENT AND PREPARATION

Once the need for vascular reconstruction is determined by arteriography, preoperative assessment and preparation are similar for inflow and outflow procedures and will be discussed here. With atherosclerotic occlusive disease being more generalized in the diabetic patient, careful preoperative assessment is mandatory prior to any surgical procedure. Coronary artery disease and left ventricular dysfunction are the leading causes of morbidity and mortality in all of our major vascular reconstructions. Sensory neuropathy obscures cardiac symptoms (especially in patients with functional limitations), allowing significant coronary artery disease and left ventricular dysfunction to go unrecognized in a number of diabetic patients. An electrocardiogram is obtained, and if any significant abnormalities exist, or if the patient has a history of significant coronary artery disease or left ventricular dysfunction, further workup is indicated. The single most important factor in preoperative assessment and risk is the presence of a previous myocardial infarction.[18] The next most important factor is the time interval from the initial infarction to the time of the perioperative period.[19] Goldman and co-workers have demonstrated the association of left ventricular function and perioperative mortality.[20]

Further cardiac workup includes echocardiography and possible thallium persantine stress testing. A recent study at our institution demonstrated that thallium persantine stress testing was not as quantitative as it was hoped to be, since as many as 70 percent of diabetic patients undergoing major vascular reconstruction had positive tests.[21] Areas of significant redistribution by thallium persantine stress testing may lead to cardiac catheterization and even balloon dilation or coronary bypass prior to elective major vascular surgery.

Noninvasive carotid artery evaluation is routinely performed in those patients who have a carotid bruit or a history of transient ischemic attacks or carotid disease. Renal function is assessed by obtaining blood-urea-nitrogen (BUN) and creatinine levels pre- and postangiogram and during administration of any nephrotoxic agents.

Pulmonary function is important to assess, especially in patients with a smoking history. Like the presence of coronary artery disease, compromised pulmonary function may influence the type of revascularization procedure proposed and certainly influences the anesthesia recommended. Arterial blood gases at rest, forced expiratory volume at 1 second (FEV_1 = approximately 1 L) and forced vital capacity (FVC = approximately 1,500 ml) may indicate the need for more extensive preoperative pulmonary testing and treatment as needed. Preoperative incentive spirometry and pulmonary toilet are beneficial, but routine bronchodilator therapy is not recommended.

WOUND CARE AND ANTIBIOTICS

Since the majority of vascular reconstructions in diabetics are performed because of limb-threatening conditions, control of infected ulcers is essential prior to any revascularization procedure. Diabetic patients do not tolerate infection, yet systemic signs and symptoms occur late or are even absent. Because of neuropathy, deep limb-threatening infection may be masked by overriding callus or what is thought to be a superficial ulceration. These areas must be carefully probed, and all necrotic tissue and pus debrided and dependently drained prior to any thought of revascularization.[22]

Polymicrobial infections are the rule for limb-threatening ulcers (average isolates, three per ulcer) with anaerobes present in over 40 percent of our cases.[23] Gram staining and deep cultures are obtained for aerobic and anaerobic bacteria. Broad spectrum intravenous antibiotics are initiated to cover suspected organisms and are changed based on sensitivity and the response of the wound. It must be remembered that local ischemia inhibits a proper host defense, promotes anaerobic or facultative growth, limits antibiotic delivery or penetration, and delays wound healing. This justifies initial treatment with broad spectrum intravenously administered antibiotics, especially in patients manifesting systemic toxicity or gastroparesis. Potentially nephrotoxic antibiotics are monitored very carefully and we try to limit their use prior to angiography.

As important as the antibiotics are, however, as mentioned previously, early aggressive surgical debridement and dependent drainage are equally important, especially to sterilize lymphatic pathways adjacent to potential vascular reconstruction vessels and incisions. Antibiotics are continued throughout the intraoperative and postoperative period, with monitoring of changes in any newly revascularized, previously infected wound.

PERIOPERATIVE MANAGEMENT

Perioperative management of lower extremity vascular surgery is similar for any major vascular reconstruction in the diabetic patient and is considered here.

Anesthesia and Monitoring

Because of the diffuse and generalized nature of atherosclerosis in the diabetic patient, every effort should be made to optimize the patient's cardiac, renal, and cerebral vascular status preoperatively, intraoperatively, and postoperatively. Once the preoperative risk and the procedure needed are determined, the choice of anesthesia is really an individual decision. To date there are no randomized series supporting one type of anesthesia as safer for the diabetic patient. General endotrachial, spinal, or epidural anesthesia are all effective and used in our hospital.[24]

In the operating room an arterial line is placed whenever feasible, as is a Foley catheter. Swan-Ganz monitoring is routine, since many of these patients have silent coronary artery disease and/or are on a variety of medications, including diuretics and cardiac drugs. Aggressive but judicious fluid management can be individually tailored to best optimize cardiac, renal, and cerebral vascular perfusion. Selecting and monitoring the newer and more sophisticated pharmacologic agents is much easier and safer. In the last 10 years routine Swan-Ganz monitoring is probably most responsible for reducing the intra- and immediate postoperative complication rate (mainly cardiac) in all our series of bypasses. Arterial blood gas, serial blood sugar, potassium, and hematocrit levels are monitored intra- and postoperatively, since fluctuations do occur frequently and require appropriate treatment.

The only advantage of epidural anesthesia may be less nausea and vomiting postoperatively, and it can provide effective postoperative pain management for several days in a monitored setting. Invasive postoperative monitoring is continued until the patient's overall condition is stable, which may be 24 hours or up to 1 week. It is wise to continue to monitor patients until it is proven that they are able to mobilize and eliminate third-space fluid; this generally starts on postoperative day 2 or 3. One should never be lulled into thinking that because the first 24 hours postoperatively are uneventful, the diabetic patient is out of danger. Daily monitoring of weight, serial blood electrolytes, BUN, creatinine, blood sugar, and hematocrit levels are important, as is a carefully maintained intake and output record.

Ambulation

Ambulation is delayed until invasive monitoring is terminated. Weight bearing is obviously prohibited in patients with open dependent ulcers or healing local procedures, including amputations or revisions. In these patients bed exercises and chest physiotherapy are appropriately ordered. In patients without foot restrictions, ambulation may be delayed 1 or 2 days to let the incision stabilize. It is not deferred for 1 week, which was thought in the past to be necessary for diabetic patients. Because of neuropathy, ambulation should also progress slowly in patients who have been non-weight-bearing because of a local problem. An acute Charcot foot, disruption of a local procedure, or worsening of an ulcer are all complications of too rapidly progressed ambulation. Carefully molded healing sandals are also appropriate for individual feet.

TREATMENT (AORTOILIAC OCCLUSIVE DISEASE)

Endarterectomy

Endarterectomy consists of removal of the atheromatous disease in the artery with the intima and sizable portion of the media. This can be performed by opening the artery longitudinally or opening it above and below the diseased area and removing the above-mentioned area with a loop dissector. A cuff is usually left in the distal section, which must be carefully secured with tacking sutures to prevent dissection when flow is reestablished. One of the earliest treatment modalities used, endarterectomy can be performed alone or in conjunction with bypass grafting. Excellent results have been achieved with aortoiliac endarterectomy confined to patients who have principally aortic disease with little involvement of the iliac arteries.[25] With the advances in durable synthetic graft materials, aortoiliac endarterectomy has been largely replaced by aortoiliac or aortobifemoral bypass grafting. Iliac artery endarterectomy has been generally replaced by transluminal angioplasty or bypass grafting. Endarterectomy today is most commonly used in conjunction with bypass grafting, especially in preparing the proximal aortic cuff for graft insertion. For diabetic patients, it has been our belief that endarterectomy of the distal graft insertion site or beyond should be avoided, thereby leaving the distal intima as undisturbed as possible. Because of the more diffusely calcified and extensive nature of the atherosclerotic plaque in diabetic arteries, it is better to do a patch angioplasty with vein or graft material rather than relying on endarterectomy to open the outflow tract (see "Profundaplasty").

Bypass Grafting

As stated previously, the advent of suitable (Dacron, Gortex) graft materials and refinement in cardiovascular sutures and their needles make aortoiliac or aortofemoral bypass grafting the preferred method of treatment for symptomatic aortoiliac occlusive disease. While a knitted Dacron prosthesis may provide a more stable pseudo-intima than a woven prosthesis, the choice of graft material in high flow areas such as the aortoiliac or aortofemoral segment is most influenced by the particular preferences of the surgeon.

Controversy continues as to how the proximal anastomosis of an aortic bifurcation graft should be performed[26,27] (Figs. 15-1 to 15-3). Most vascular

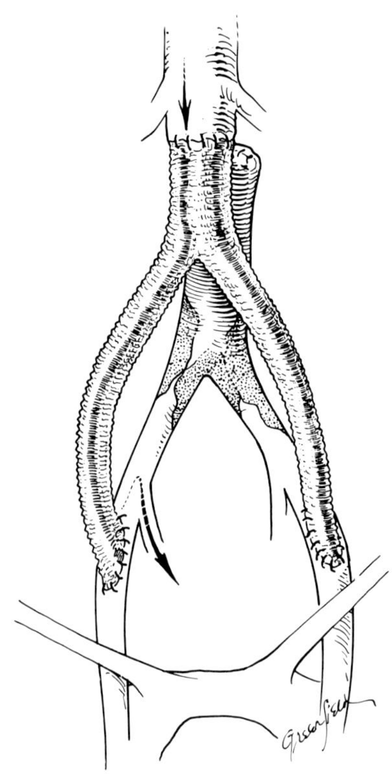

Fig. 15-1. Aortoiliac bypass graft with end-to-end anastomosis to aorta. (From Hoar and Campbell,[64] with permission.)

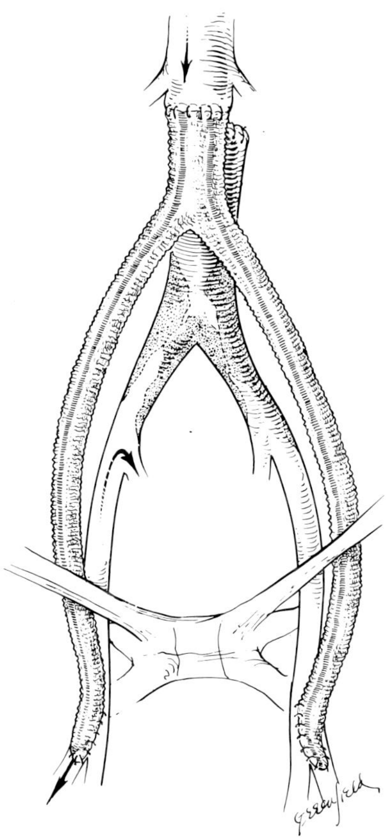

Fig. 15-2. Aortofemoral bypass graft with end-to-end anastomosis to aorta. (From Hoar and Campbell,[64] with permission.)

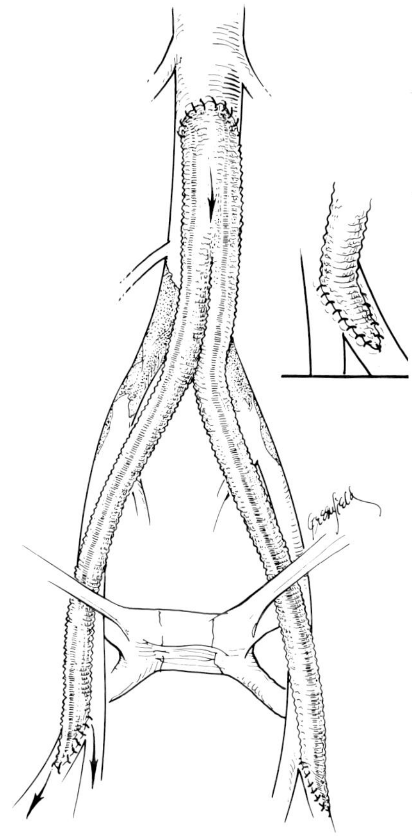

Fig. 15-3. Aortofemoral bypass graft with end-to-side anastomosis to aorta. (From Hoar and Campbell,[64] with permission.)

surgeons prefer the end-to-end technique of proximal anastomosis with transection of the aorta between clamps, about 1 to 3 cm below the renal arteries, and oversewing the distal end. This allows endarterectomy or thrombectomy of the proximal aortic stump under direct vision as needed in constructing the proximal anastomosis, a point sometimes applicable to the diabetic patient with a heavily calcified area that prohibits suture placement. The main advantage, however, is that it does not project anteriorly as does the end-to-side anastomosis, thereby allowing better closure of the retroperitoneum and protecting the graft from overlying bowel more readily. It also does not require reestablishment of flow in the more distal diabetic aorta where extensive calcified plaque and thrombus may be loosened by application of the distal clamp, increasing susceptibility to embolization distally as flow is restored. Whether the end-to-end technique results in less competitive flow, thereby increasing graft patency, is speculative. Available controlled studies do not support one graft technique as being superior to the other. Configuration of the stenosis or obstruction, or both, in the aortoiliac segment may best determine which type of proximal anastomosis to perform. The end-to-end technique is probably most appropriate when there will be no hemodynamic disadvantage from the interruption of forward flow to the distal abdominal aorta. Patients with complete distal aortic occlusion are examples where the technique is desirable. The end-to-side technique may be best reserved for those patients who would lose the perfusion of an important hypogastric or inferior mesenteric artery if the forward flow in the aorta were sacrificed at the time of surgery. It is important to try to preserve the inferior mesenteric artery whenever possible, and at least one hypogastric artery.

In males it is essential to limit the dissection in the terminal aorta and proximal left common iliac artery in order to preserve as much of the autonomic nerve plexus that sweeps over this area as possible. Awareness of sexual dysfunction secondary to inadequate hypogastric artery perfusion is important, and such dysfunction should be considered in the decision process as to which bypass to perform. One should not just assume that sexual dysfunction is secondary to diabetic autonomic neuropathy. These considerations should be discussed with the patient preoperatively.

Diabetic medial calcinosis may have a profound effect on the type of bypass performed. On three occasions I have abandoned an aortic bifurcation graft because the entire abdominal aorta was totally calcified, negating any type of cross clamping. Even when a soft area of infrarenal aorta permits cross clamping, the diabetic patient tends to have more associated calcium involving the intima and media, making handling and suturing more difficult. Vascular clamps must be applied carefully. The newer refined vascular cutting needles on 2-0 or 3-0 monofilament suture material has been advantageous. Systemic heparinization is preferred prior to any cross clamping, and flushing the anastomosis to remove any loose debris and mural thrombus is necessary before the clamps are removed. The grafts are tunneled retroperitoneally along anatomic pathways whenever possible. Generally the ureters should lie above the graft prostheses.

The use of the aortobifemoral graft as opposed to an aortoiliac bypass tends to negate the effect of unsuspected or progressive atherosclerosis in the remaining iliac vessel. The recipient vessel chosen should be the most widely patent vessel from which there is good runoff to support continued patency of the graft. Running the distal anastomosis down to or even through the origin of the profunda femoris will ensure an adequate outflow tract. This is especially important in diabetic patients with tandem superficial femoral artery or distal tibial occlusions and also in patients with disease that originates in the profunda femoris artery. Extended profundaplasty is best closed with autogenous tissue patches of either saphenous vein or endarterectomized superficial femoral artery rather than extension of the graft over the area or relying on endarterectomy as discussed previously. Other factors that contribute to long-term patency are matching graft size with the vessel into which it is implanted and avoiding any graft limb redundancy. The femoral exposure should be such that there is no damage to the proximal saphenous vein, since this vein may be needed later for distal bypass grafting. Transected inguinal nodes or lymphatics must be carefully interrupted to prevent lymphatic leakage. The distal anastomosis is usually carried out under 2½ power magnification and using appropriately sized monofilament cardiovascular suture and fine cardiac cutting needles when needed.

Careful closure of the femoral wound is essential to prevent lymphatic leaks and infections. Administration of pre- and perioperative antibiotics has reduced the incidence of groin infection. Careful consideration must be given to the diabetic with an open infected foot ulcer (see the section "Wound Care and Antibiotics"). Simultaneous femoral-popliteal or femorodistal reconstruction must be carefully considered in diabetics with extensive tissue loss of the forefoot or heel where restoration of pulsatile flow may be necessary to achieve healing. The combined procedure increases the operating time, surgical trauma, and morbidity, especially in patients with associated risk factors such as coronary artery disease. Careful selection of patients, modern anesthetic technique, and careful perioperative monitoring have allowed successful combined reconstruction in selected cases.

Results

Initial patency rates for aortobifemoral grafts approach 100 percent, with many centers reporting a 5-year cumulative patency rate of over 80 percent and a 10-year patency rate approaching 75 percent.[25,27,28] Previous reports noted poor graft patency, poor limb salvage, and poor survival in diabetic patients undergoing aortic reconstruction for occlusive disease.[29,30] This was probably the result of the more diffuse nature of atherosclerosis in diabetic patients, especially in the outflow vessels of the lower extremities.[30] Because these series had a relatively low number of diabetic patients and dif-

Table 15-1. Patient Profile: 100 Consecutive Patients Undergoing Aortic Reconstruction for Occlusive Disease

	Diabetics (N = 57)	*Nondiabetics (N = 43)*
Age, years	60.4 mean (range, 37–79)	58.6 mean (range, 33–37)
Sex, no. (%)	35 M (61) 22 F (39)	17 M (40) 26 F (60)
Smoking,[a] no. (%)	52 (91)	39 (90)
Hypertension,[b] no. (%)	28 (49)	20 (47)
Cardiac,[c] no. (%)	22 (39)	13 (30)
CVA/TIA, no. (%)	6 (11)	4 (9)
Chronic renal failure,[d] no. (%)	7 (12)	3 (7)

Abbreviations: M, male; F, female; CVA, cardiovascular accident; TIA, transient ischemic attack.
[a] Greater than 20 pack-years.
[b] Receiving drug therapy.
[c] Angina, myocardial infarction, congestive heart failure, arrhythmia, and/or ischemic electrocardiogram.
[d] Serum creatinine concentration greater than 2.0 mg/dl (180 μmol/l).
(From Bartlett et al.,[31] with permission.)

fered from our experience, we reviewed our experience with a largely diabetic population in 1986.[31] We reported on 100 consecutive patients receiving aortic bifurcation grafts strictly for occlusive disease between 1969 and 1982. The study group consisted of 57 diabetic patients and 43 nondiabetic patients, and surprisingly, patient profiles were similar (Table 15-1). Indications for aortic reconstruction differed, with 68 percent of operations in diabetic patients performed for limb salvage compared with 47 percent in the nondiabetic group (Table 15-2). All 100 patients survived the operation and left the hospital with open grafts. There was a cumulative graft patency of 94 percent at 5 years for each group. While the rate of subsequent distal reconstruction and limb loss was somewhat higher in the diabetic group, this suggested more progressive distal arterial disease in the diabetic group and not an unsuccessful outflow procedure. Significant was the fact that 33 percent of the diabetic patients were dead at 4 years, a survival rate one-half that of nondiabetics.

Table 15-2. Indications for Aortic Reconstruction

	Disabling Claudication, No. (%)	*Threatened Limb Loss*	
		Rest Pain	*Ulcer/Gangrene, No. (%)*
Diabetics (N = 57)	18 (32)	13	26 (68) (51 limbs/39 patients)
Nondiabetics (N = 43)	23 (53)	13	7 (47) (25 limbs/20 patients)

(From Bartlett et al.,[31] with permission.)

Table 15-3. 30-Day Complications after Aortic Reconstruction

	Diabetics (N = 57)	*Nondiabetics (N = 43)*
Cardiac	11 (4 Mi)	8 (1 Mi)
CVA/TIA	2	0
Pulmonary	2 Atelectasis 1 Embolus	4 Atelectasis 1 Pneumonia
Phlebitis	0	1
Groin[a]	4	0
ATN	1	2
Urinary tract infection	1	4

Abbreviations: MI, myocardial infarction; CVA, cardiovascular accident; TIA, transient ischemic attack; ATN, acute tubular necrosis.
[a] Fat necrosis, hematoma, superficial infection.

Peri- and postoperative complications (Table 15-3) were primarily cardiac in origin, demonstrating the diffuse nature of diabetic vascular occlusive disease, and this finding intensified our efforts to identify particularly high risk patients. Certainly careful preoperative assessment, increased perioperative monitoring with routine Swan-Ganz catheters, judicious fluid management, modern pharmacologic management, and blood pressure control as discussed in the section "Perioperative Management," were important reasons why we had such an acceptable complication rate and no mortality.

One interesting aspect of our results was comparing complications associated with aortoiliac versus aortofemoral grafts. In the diabetic group, 23 patients had aortoiliac, 28 had aortofemoral, and 6 had aortoiliac-femoral bypasses. There were 9 femoral-popliteal concomitant procedures. It was our feeling prior to the study that aortoiliac grafting was safer for the diabetic patient because of a concern for groin complications in the diabetic person with an impaired resistance to infection. This theoretical advantage of aortoiliac grafting in diabetic patients was not substantiated by this study, and we concluded that aortofemoral bypass grafting was safe for the diabetic patient with symptomatic aortoiliac occlusive disease.

Profundaplasty

Endarterectomy of the origin and or proximal portion of the deep femoral artery is beneficial, especially when combined with some form of inflow operation mentioned previously. Profundaplasty as an isolated procedure will rarely heal an ischemic foot ulcer.[32] It may improve rest pain in poor risk patients who cannot undergo distal bypass grafting, or it may allow the patient to live in symbiosis with a foot ulcer. Proximal profundaplasty is also beneficial when performed in conjunction with a distal bypass graft to maintain patency and to maximize all available outflow. In general it is better to perform a vein patch angioplasty than to get involved with extensive endarterectomy of the common and profunda artery segment in the diabetic patient (see the previous section on endarterectomy).

ALTERNATIVES FOR INFLOW PROCEDURE

While aortoiliac and aortofemoral bypass grafting can be performed successfully with low morbidity and mortality in many patients, less extensive or extra-anatomical procedures may be preferable or necessary in certain instances. The extent and location of the occlusive disease are important determinants, as is the patient's risk for surgery and general anesthesia. With the routine use of Swan-Ganz monitoring and aggressive intraoperative and perioperative management, patients previously considered as exceptionally high risk for major surgery are now able to better tolerate the major vascular reconstructions described previously.

If the occlusive disease is limited to one common or external iliac artery, a unilateral aortic or iliac to femoral artery bypass may suffice (Fig. 15-4B). This can be done through a retroperitoneal flank incision and provides a graft that follows the anatomic plane. It requires less dissection than the aortobifemoral approach and has better long-term patency than axillofemoral bypass grafting, if that is the only alternative. Another alternative, especially in the high risk patient, would be to perform a contralateral iliac or femoral to femoral bypass graft (Figs. 15-4A and 15-5).

For the patient with bilateral iliac artery disease, where the aorta or a proximal segment of one of the common iliac arteries is not involved, consideration for an ileofemoral combined with femoral bypass graft must be weighed against the standard aortofemoral bypass graft, especially in high risk cardiac or pulmonary patients (Fig. 15-4C). Another alternative in the patient with bilateral proximal disease, where there is only a short stenotic segment of one iliac system, is to perform transluminal balloon angioplasty followed by a femorofemoral bypass graft several days later. Long-term results with all these grafts are reasonably good, and the type of bypass to be performed must be weighed and carefully considered for each patient.[33–36] For the particular patient with an infected groin, the obturator bypass as described by Shaw and Baue may provide the best solution.

The final alternative to aortoiliac or femoral re-

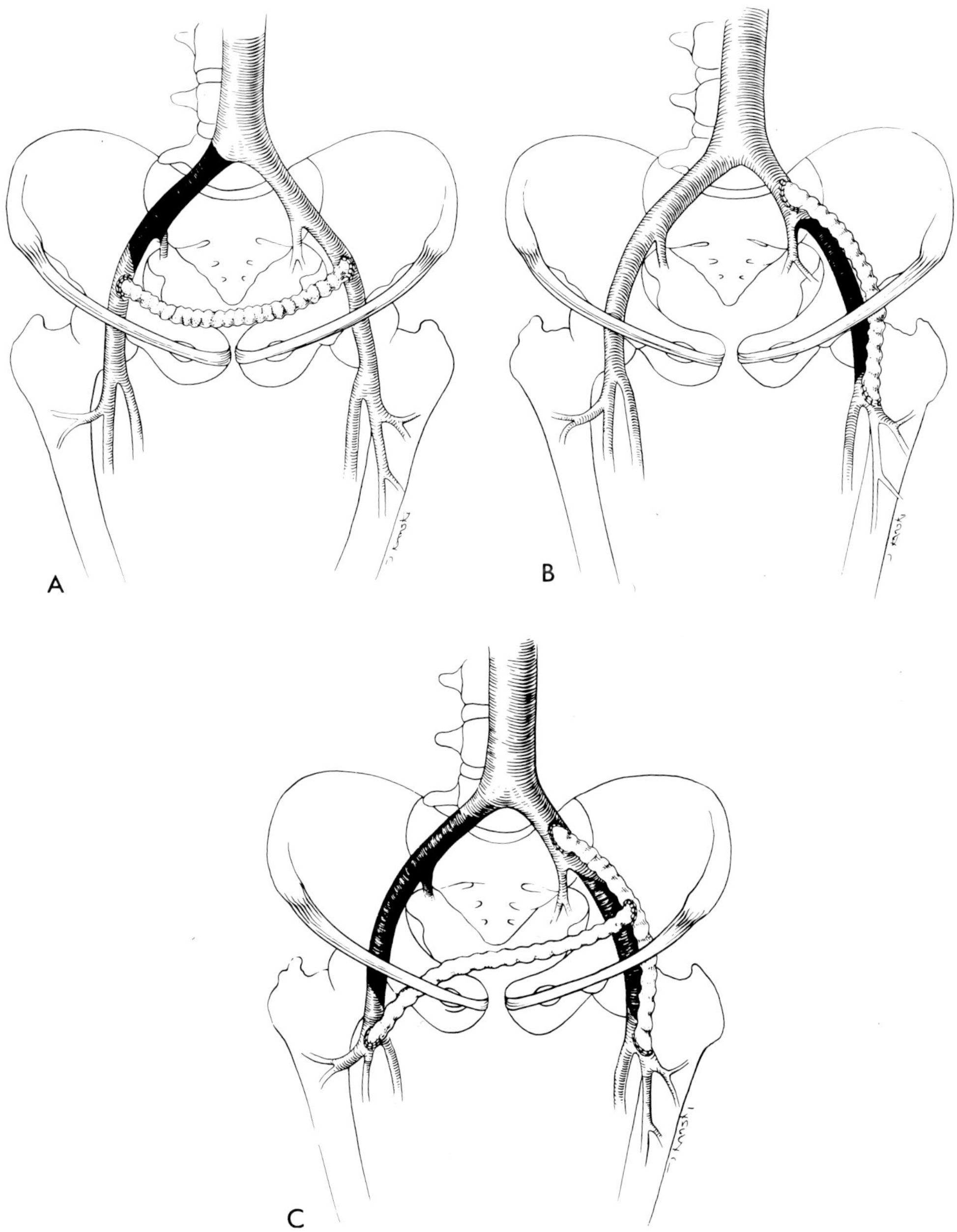

Fig. 15-4. A patent common or external iliac artery may be used as a donor vessel for (A) ilioiliac, (B) iliofemoral, or (C) iliobifemoral bypasses in appropriate patients who would otherwise require axillofemoral reconstruction. (From Mannick et al.,[66] with permission.)

construction is the axillofemoral or axillobifemoral bypass graft.[37] In the past this operation has been limited to the very elderly and high risk patient who otherwise would be subjected to primary amputation. The axillobifemoral graft is preferred to a unilateral axillofemoral graft because of better 5-year cumulative patency.[38] This graft is pictured in Figure 15-6. It is extra-anatomic in nature and can be performed under light general anesthesia and/or even local anesthesia, except for the tunneling

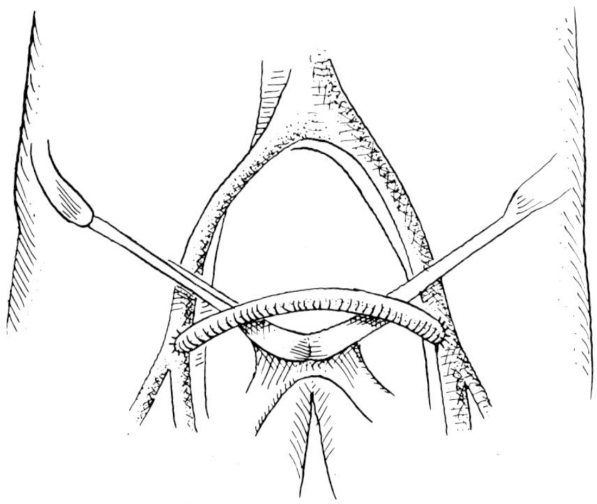

Fig. 15-5. The femorofemoral bypass graft is illustrated with the preferred C configuration of the subcutaneous tunnel constructed well above the pubis. (From Mannick et al.,[66] with permission.)

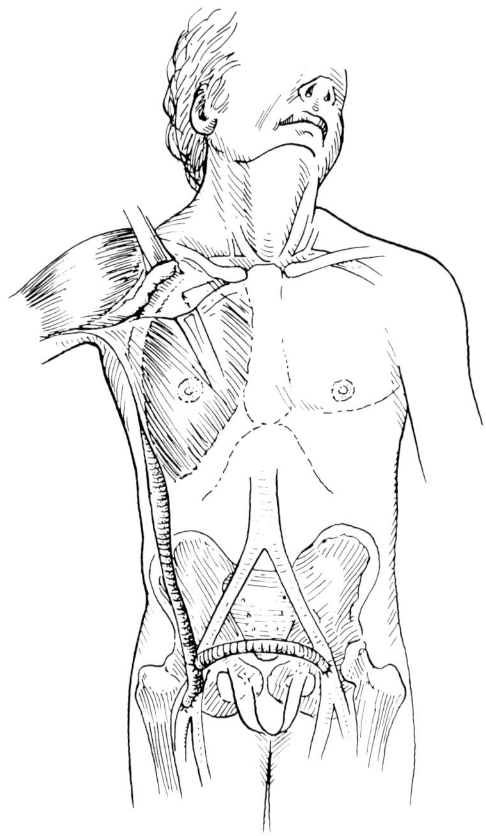

Fig. 15-6. Subcutaneous axillobifemoral bypass graft completed with proximal anastomosis to the right axillary artery, right distal anastomosis to the common and deep femoral arteries, and extension of the prosthesis with side limb to left common femoral artery. (From Mannick et al.,[66] with permission.)

part. Synthetic grafts are used, the most common of which is PTFE. The 5-year cumulative patency in this group of patients averages 70 percent in most series. When these grafts do fail, they frequently can be salvaged by thrombectomy under local anesthesia in about 25 percent of patients. While these results are certainly inferior to standard aortoiliac or bifemoral bypass grafting, they still offer hope to the high risk patient who otherwise faces major amputation.

Lumbar Sympathectomy

Mention must be given to lumbar sympathectomy, which has little if any place in the treatment of diabetic peripheral vascular disease. Most long-term diabetic patients have already undergone autosympathectomy, and our experience with this procedure was most disappointing.

ANGIOPLASTY AND LASER THERAPY

While Dotter and Judkins first introduced percutaneous catheter dilation of stenotic areas of arteries in 1963, the technique really was popularized by Gruntzig, who in 1974 devised and developed a double-lumen balloon catheter for percutaneous transluminal angioplasty (PTA).[39,40] Advances in technology and plastics have allowed for the development of smaller, stronger, and safer catheters. Balloon angioplasty is a controlled form of arterial injury whereby the radial force of the balloon causes a splitting of the intima along one edge of the plaque, thus partially shearing the plaque from the outer wall. An axial or rotary shift of the plaque occurs as the lumen and the outer layers are further stretched, and this entire process accounts for 90 percent of the changes to the lumen.[41] When the balloon is deflated, the force of the flowing arterial blood stabilizes the area until the injury heals (usually 4 to 6 weeks).

Indications and Patient Selection

Optimal lesions suitable for balloon dilation are short (less than 2 cm) hemodynamically significant stenoses in arteries that are otherwise disease free. The iliac arteries lend themselves to the best initial and long-term results, with overall initial and long-term success rates greater than 90 and 80 percent, respectively, for short stenotic lesions.[42] Longer stenoses (greater than 5 cm), multiple stenoses, and total occlusions lend themselves less well to balloon dilation. Appropriate patient selection is a necessity for initial and long-term success of PTA. PTA should not compete with bypass surgery and comparison of results is inappropriate since case selection for each treatment modality is quite different. The morphology and location of the particular atherosclerotic lesion and associated disease, patient risk, and longevity must be considered. PTA is the treatment of choice for symptomatic short (less than or equal to 5 cm), discrete iliac stenosis. Longer segments, multiple lesions, and extensive diffuse occlusive disease are better treated with bypass, providing the patient is an acceptable risk. Patients with occlusive distal disease and a favorable iliac stenosis may be best served with an initial PTA of the iliac segment followed by a distal bypass 2 to 3 days later. Poor-risk patients with bilateral iliac disease, where one side lends itself to dilation, may then have a femoral-to-femoral or ileofemoral crossover graft in 2 to 3 days under regional anesthesia. PTA has proven cost effective. It rarely jeopardizes a later or future surgical approach, and the two specialties should complement one another for the best results. Cooperation and communication are a necessity for appropriate patient selection, planning, and timing of combined procedures, and for immediate management of complications. This is especially true for the diabetic whose atherosclerotic disease tends to be diffuse with more distal extensive occlusive lesions and frequent medial calcinosis.

Complications

There is a learning curve in successful performance of balloon dilation, and complications correlate with experience, skill, and judgment. PTA carries all the complications associated with angiography, and dye load must be kept in mind when treating diabetics. Groin hematoma is the most frequent complication and is of concern in less than 5 percent of patients. Retroperitoneal dissection, false passage, intimal flaps, thrombosis, and embolization occur less commonly. PTA of complete iliac occlusions carries a high embolization rate (greater than 10 percent), precluding its usefulness in this setting at most centers. Technical failure and hemodynamic failure have many causes, but combined account for less than 5 percent of failures of iliac arteries. This increased to 20 percent for femoropopliteal PTAs in Rutherford's series. Rutherford believes the overall complication rate of iliac PTA can and should be held to just under 10 percent.[43] Half of these complications should not affect the outcome, while the other half results in technical or hemodynamic failure, requiring surgery in about 1 percent. Hemodynamic deterioration occurs most frequently during the first 12 months following PTA, and it is associated most frequently with myointimal hyperplasia. After 12 months, progression of atherosclerotic disease is the primary cause of deterioration or failure.

Laser Technology

Developments in laser technology raised hope that laser recanalization of totally occluded peripheral arteries under controlled circumstances and with minimal morbidity would provide an ideal cost-effective treatment. Without doubt, it has become the most media-hyped treatment modality currently sought for occlusive vascular disease, but without long-term patency and limb salvage rates truly known. In fact current laser delivery systems only create small channels (less than 2 mm) through occluded arteries and require balloon angioplasty to provide lumen size sufficient to allow adequate blood flow. As previously noted, PTA success is limited to short localized lesions with decreasing initial and long-term success the more distal one goes. Seeger, et al. note that current laser systems are most appropriate for the treatment of isolated lesions less than 15 cm in length involving the middle or distal superficial femoral artery, above knee popliteal, or isolated common iliac artery occlusions.[44] One-half of their patients evaluated for possible laser recanalization were initially excluded because of inappropriate disease location. Only one occlusion below the knee was successfully treated, and no patients with severe tibial artery occlusion that precluded surgical reconstruction were successfully treated. No patient with disease involving more than one level (iliac, femoral-popliteal, tibial) in the treated extremity had successful laser recanalization.

Overall, clinically successful laser recanalization can be accomplished approximately 50 percent of the time.[45,46] Three factors (lesion location, lesion length, and localized versus diffuse arterial disease) when considered together most influence successful laser recanalization. Again, localized lesions of the common iliac, middle, and distal superficial femoral artery and above the knee popliteal artery fared the best in Seeger et al.'s review, but only 10 to 15 percent of patients with peripheral vascular disease appear to have this pattern. In our experience it would apply to an even smaller diabetic population because of the pattern of their atherosclerotic occlusive disease and the high frequency of intimal plaque and medial calcification that makes laser recanalization even more difficult. Since the diabetic patient rarely has only one of the favorable factors influencing outcome, success may be less than 12 percent. Compared to the initial and long-term favorable results of tibial and pedal bypass grafting, at the present time current laser recanalization techniques have an extremely limited application to the diabetic patient with critical lower-extremity ischemia.

Angioscopy

One new and exciting technology partly developed in our institution under the direction of Dr. Arnold Miller has been routine angioscopy—the endoscopic examination of the interior of blood vessels and bypass grafts. The development of ultrathin flexible fiberoptic endoscopes and a pressurized irrigation system have allowed angioscopy to be routinely performed during vascular reconstructions. Our initial experience with intraoperative angioscopy shows it to be feasible, safe, and clinically useful in distal bypass grafting.[47] Following completion of the distal anastomosis, the angioscope and irrigation catheter can be placed through a side branch into the vein graft, and the vein can be inspected along its entire course, as can proximal and distal anastomoses and native arteries. The adequacy of valve lysis in in situ or nonreversed grafts can be determined, and now valve lysis is routinely performed under angioscopic control. This technique has reduced our need for intraoperative angiography and has reduced the incidence of early graft occlusion (30 days) from 10 to 4 percent.[48] Angioscopy has also been of great use in inspecting the adequacy of thrombectomy or of lysis of clot by urokinase in patients operated on for graft occlusions. It is hoped that in the future, angioscopy will be able to provide direct visualization of percutaneous laser recanalization or balloon dilation of peripheral as well as coronary arteries.

FEMORAL-POPLITEAL-TIBIAL OUTFLOW REVASCULARIZATION

This section discusses restoration of circulation below the inguinal ligament (outflow procedures) when significant symptoms are manifested by stenosis or occlusions of the common femoral, superficial femoral, profunda femoral, popliteal, and/or tibial-peroneal arteries. Like disease of the aortoiliac segment, hemodynamically significant stenosis or occlusions can exist in the infrainguinal arterial tree and yet the patient may exhibit minimal or no symptoms. The adequacy of collateral pathways and the patient's activity level again are important in how these occlusions manifest themselves clinically. The criteria for infrainguinal vascular reconstruction is the same as that for aortoiliac occlusive disease. Claudication, however, usually begins below the knee level, but again in the diabetic patient may not always take the form of pain. Because of associated neuropathy, the patient may not be able to describe classical claudication or describe it as a numbness or dead feeling in the leg or foot when walking a given distance, which is relieved by rest. The differential diagnosis of claudication at this level is the same as described previously and may be quite challenging in the diabetic patient. While rest pain may be mimicked by severe neuropathy, it has enough of the distinguishing clinical features of severe ischemia that accompany it to make its diagnosis less problematic. Ischemic ulceration and/or gangrene is obvious to the experienced observer.

In all of our reported series of infrainguinal bypasses in diabetic patients, the major indication for revascularization was limb salvage either because of rest pain or ischemic tissue loss. This is in contrast to series reporting large numbers of nondiabetic patients, and again is secondary to the more diffuse pattern of atherosclerosis in the diabetic lower extremity and its predilection for the more distal arteries. Forty percent of diabetic patients who present with ischemic tissue loss or gangrene will have a palpable popliteal pulse, in sharp contrast to the nondiabetic population.

The clinical examination and vascular laboratory tests are detailed in other chapters, and this chapter will discuss treatment options. It really was not until the early 1950s when dos Santos introduced the concept of arteriography that arterial reconstruction of the lower extremity was realized.[49] The dos Santos endarterectomy or resection of an occluded arterial segment with replacement by sterilized homographs from cadavers were the early procedures of choice. The French devised the end-to-side anastomosis above and below the occluded segment, allowing the patient's artery to remain open and intact, and thus preserving any functioning artery remaining. Kunlin was the first to popularize the long venous bypass graft, and in this country Robert Linton's success with the reversed saphenous vein bypass established this method as the procedure of choice for reconstruction below the inguinal ligament.[50] Despite the advances in arterial bypass techniques and in graft material, the saphenous vein continues to be the conduit of choice to provide satisfactory long-term patency. When this vein is limited because of size and length, then lesser saphenous vein or arm vein is the next conduit of choice. Synthetic grafts such as reinforced expanded polytetrafluoroethylene (PTFE) have limited indications except in above knee segments of occlusion or as a patch if vein is unavailable.

One of the most important advances allowing successful revascularization of the diabetic lower extremity was the development of digital arterial subtraction angiography. This method made visualization of distal tibial-peroneal or pedal vessels possible where routine angiography had failed. Advances in suture material with newer cardiac cutting needles have been of great benefit for sewing the frequently encountered calcified diabetic artery. The advances in instrumentation have also proven beneficial for occluding diabetic arteries. Since the development and successful use of the Fogerty balloon catheter and occlusion clamps, newer devices such as Silastic vessel loops and intraluminal coronary vessel occluders are now standard for distal bypass grafting in diabetic patients. Advances in magnification make the use of magnification of approximately $2\frac{1}{2}$ times routine in performing successful bypasses.

Criteria for Revascularization

Once it has been determined that a bypass is needed to restore circulation to a clearly threatened limb, there are several clear-cut requirements to assure patency and success. Obviously patients who have severe dementia or mental deterioration who do not ambulate are certainly not candidates for a bypass. Patients with extensive tissue destruction, where even if circulation was restored there would be questionable limb salvage, must be carefully evaluated as to whether a primary below the knee amputation may better suit their needs. Bedridden patients with longstanding flexion contractions are also not candidates for reconstruction. Preoperative assessment of risk has already been discussed (aortoiliac section) and identifies patients able to withstand lower extremity revascularization. Preoperative preparation, anesthesia, and perioperative management have likewise been considered.

The ideal situation for a lower extremity bypass would be an occlusion of the superficial femoral artery with an open popliteal artery below and good runoff via the three distal vessels onto the foot (Fig. 15-7). This is seldom the situation for the diabetic patient. Specifically, the type of bypass performed will most often depend on the outflow vessels visualized during arteriography and the reason for which the bypass is being performed. One would prefer a femoral to popliteal artery bypass graft in patients whose only symptom is disabling claudication or early rest pain. I would not recommend a femoral to distal tibial, peroneal, or pedal bypass for patients with claudication. These grafts should really be limited to those patients with limb-threatening ischemia. Diabetic patients who have extensive tissue loss or gangrene of the foot probably need pulsatile flow to the foot whenever possible. Because of limited collateral vessels, very distal tibial or pedal bypasses may not eliminate claudication in the calf. Limited collateralization may also partially explain why amputation is still necessary in some patients despite a functioning tibial-peroneal graft.

Revascularization of the diabetic lower extremity has a proud and rich history at the New England Deaconess Hospital and the Joslin Clinic. The growth and modernization of vascular surgery principles and techniques as applied to the diabetic are best understood by reviewing this experience. In 1969 Dr. Frank Wheelock reported the first large experience of 104 consecutive reversed saphenous vein bypasses in diabetic patients at the New England Deaconess Hospital and Joslin Clinic.[51] Eighty-six percent of these grafts were performed for critical limb ischemia. There was an initial success of 98 percent, with one death and one early graft failure, an incredible tribute to this pioneer, the institutions, and a team approach. Of interest was the fact that in 69 of the 103 successful bypasses, only one pedal pulse could be felt postoperatively, "the pedal pulses being absent because of blocks in the tibial arteries of the calf," according to Dr. Wheelock in his discussion. The Doppler was yet to be invented. Sixty percent of the patients had gangrene and postbypass 4 toe amputations and 23 transmetatarsal amputations were performed to achieve limb salvage. Only one of these procedures failed, and it was in a limb with a functioning bypass graft. At 2 years patency was 91 percent, and 72 percent of the grafts were still patent at 5 years. One-third of the patients, however, were dead at 5 years, in contrast to most series reporting on nondiabetic patients.

In the discussion following this landmark paper presented before the International Cardiovascular Society in 1969, Wheelock noted that only about 20 percent of diabetic patients with advanced ischemia were bypass candidates. Of the diabetic patients in trouble already, 40 percent had palpable popliteal bypasses that he did not think he could improve upon. At that time artery grafts were about equal in number per year to major amputations at our institution, and routine distal bypass grafting in the diabetic patient was yet to come.

It became obvious that infrapopliteal bypass grafting was possible for the diabetic, even when the tibial-peroneal arteries were calcified or a pedal arch was not seen on standard arteriography.[52,53] Our initial results of 41 infrapopliteal reconstructions in 39 patients was quite encouraging. Ninety percent of these patients were diabetic and all procedures were performed for tissue necrosis or gangrene. There was no perioperative mortality and an acceptable morbidity. Initial limb salvage and graft patency was 90 percent, and at 2 years was 80 percent.

The advances noted earlier (routine magnification, finer vascular suture material with cardiac cutting needles, refinements in instrumentation, and better arteriography) were all responsible for our enthusiasm toward more distal bypass grafting. The reintroduction of the in situ saphenous vein bypass technique together with a modified valvulotome by Leather and associates in the 1970s added to our enthusiasm, since it seemed particularly suited to the diabetic patient with proximal tibial disease and limb-threatening ischemia.[54,55] The in situ technique leaves the saphenous vein in its anatomical bed except proximally and distally at the anastomoses (Fig. 15-8). The valves are cut and side branches ligated. Its greatest advantage is probably related to the fact that the larger end of the vein is anastomosed to the larger artery and the smaller end to the smaller tibial artery, creating less size mismatch as seen with the reversed vein technique. Since its adoption in 1983, the ability to salvage limbs previously thought to be unreconstructable changed dramatically. In 1985 a retrospective review of our vascular division's experience was carried out.

Patients undergoing vascular reconstruction in the last year (July 1982 to June 1983) of the pre–in situ era (group 1) were compared to those (group 2) operated on from July 1984 to June 1985 when we had mastered the technique of in situ bypass grafting. When the groups were separated into the 2 years of the study, there was no significant difference noted in the incidence of age, sex, diabetes, smoking, or other risk factors.

Certain differences, however, did become ap-

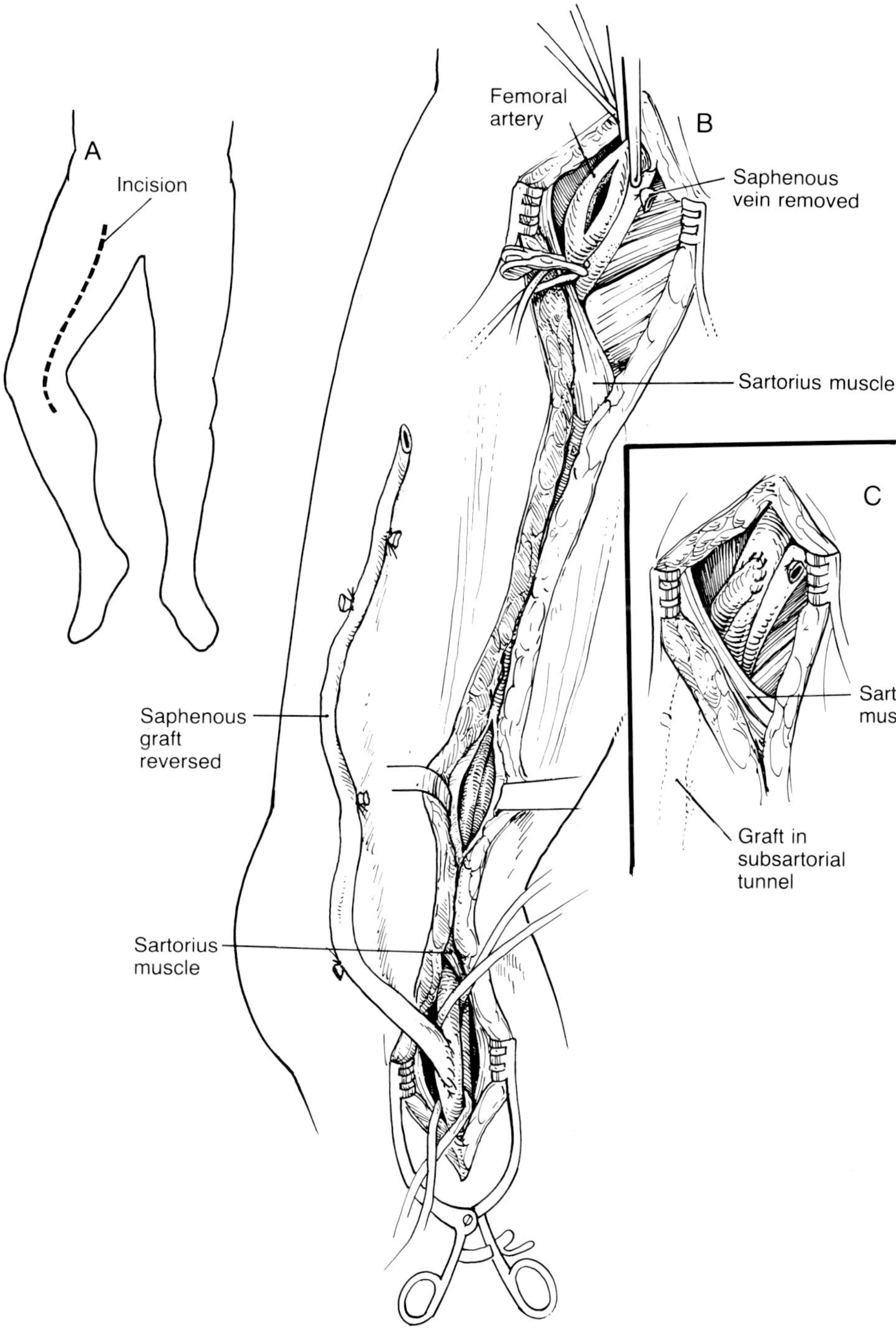

Fig. 15-7. Standard femoral-to-popliteal artery reversed saphenous vein bypass. **(A)** Continuous incision along the course of the greater saphenous vein. **(B)** Distal anastomosis is completed and the graft is ready for tunneling through the subsartorial plane to the common femoral artery. **(C)** Completed femoral anastomosis. (From Wheelock and Gibbons,[65] with permission.)

parent. In group 1, 122 limbs were at risk and 39 (27.8 percent) underwent primary major amputation. Of these, 5 were above the knee amputations and 34 were below the knee amputations. Of these amputations, 28 (72 percent) were on limbs considered to be unreconstructable after arteriography. The rest were carried out because of lack of conduit (4), cardiac disease (1), and uncontrolled sepsis (4). In 5 cases distal disease necessitated amputation despite a functioning graft. In group 2, 129 limbs were at risk and 13 (9.3 percent) underwent primary amputation. Two of these were above the knee amputations and 11 were below the knee amputations. Six of these extremities were considered to be unreconstructable after arteriography and 5 were amputated because of uncontrolled sepsis. Seven patients required an amputation despite a functioning graft.

The perioperative mortality was 9.8 percent in group 1 and decreased to 0.8 percent in group 2. All perioperative deaths were secondary to myocardial infarction. Immediate graft failure resulted in secondary amputations in 6.8 percent of patients in group 1 and 4.2 percent in group 2. Vein utilization was greatly improved in group 2, with only 4.2 percent of veins being inadequate as opposed to 15.6 percent in group 1. Also significant was the fact that only 40 percent of bypasses were to the tibial vessels in group 1, while 64 percent were to the tibial vessels in group 2.

The 6-month graft patency for group 1 was 81 percent versus 92 percent for group 2. For tibial vessels, the patency rate was 77 percent for group 1 versus 92 percent for group 2. The type of conduit certainly affected outcome for both groups, with the 6-month patency for vein grafts being 90 percent; for composite vein and synthetic grafts, 63 percent; and synthetic grafts alone, 79 percent. None of the synthetic grafts went to the tibial vessel. In group 2, the in situ saphenous vein technique was used for 66 percent of the grafts with a 6-month patency of 96 percent.

Our own as well as others' experience noted better patency rates for tibial grafts than popliteal grafts when using the in situ technique[56] (Fig. 15-8). We felt that this may be secondary to the acute angulation of the vein graft when the in situ vein was anastomosed directly to the popliteal artery. This procedure was abandoned in favor of the standard reversed saphenous vein bypass graft or a nonreversed vein graft (depending on vein artery size match), where in both cases the graft was tunneled along the anatomic course of the artery (Fig. 15-7).

While other reports note comparable patency rates for reversed saphenous vein grafts to distal tibial vessels, the in situ technique has remained our procedure of choice.[57] The increase in our vein utilization is unquestionable, as was the better size match of artery and vein at each anastomotic site. Also of interest is the fact that the reduction in perioperative mortality was the result of increased awareness of associated cardiac risk factors and the routine use of Swan-Ganz monitoring as described in the section on preoperative assessment and intraoperative monitoring. The most significant finding, however, was a reduction in the primary major amputation rate from 28 to 9.3 percent for diabetic patients presenting with critical limb-threatening ischemia.

During this time it became apparent that there were limitations to standard arteriography and to determining which patients had sufficient runoff to sustain a distal bypass. Our increasing experience demonstrated that while runoff into a patent foot arch was not a prerequisite for successful distal bypass grafting, it may be a prerequisite to limb salvage in cases where there is extensive gangrene or tissue loss where pulsatile flow to the forefoot is needed. Our previous occasional disappointing

Fig. 15-8. In situ saphenous vein bypass. (**A**) Continuous incision similar to one for reversed saphenous vein. (**B**) Transection of saphenous vein at common femoral vein junction and preparation for anastomosis to common femoral artery. Saphenous vein is kept in its anatomical position. (**C**) Common femoral anastomosis completed and blood flows into graft to point of first competent valve. Valvulotome is inserted via branches along course of vein and valves are incised. (**D**) Completed graft with the major portion of the saphenous vein lying in anatomical position. The needle is inserted via the proximal branch and completion arteriogram is performed after all vein branches are ligated. (From Wheelock and Gibbons,[65] with permission.)

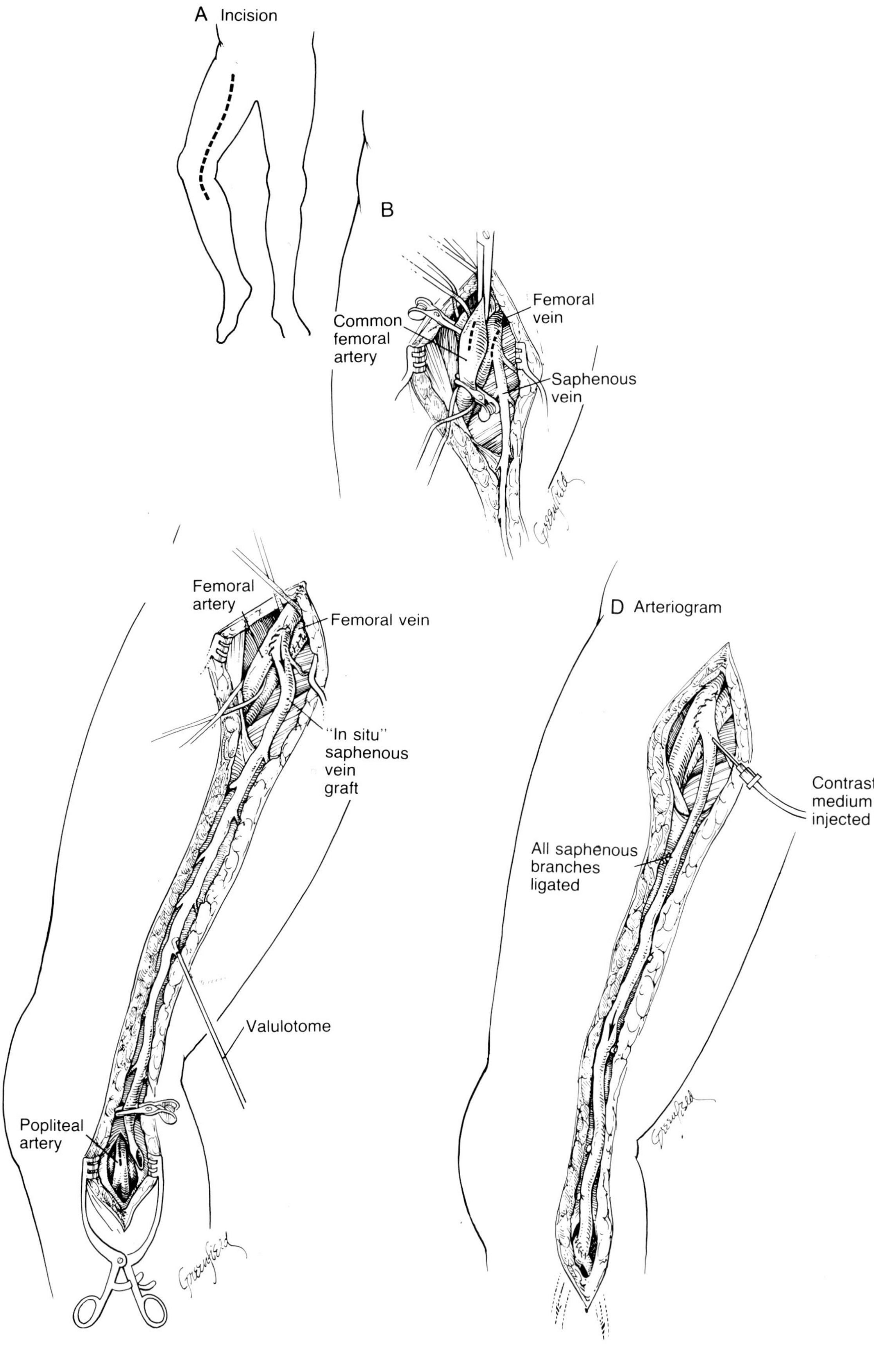

A Incision
B
Common femoral artery
Femoral vein
Saphenous vein
Femoral artery
Femoral vein
"In situ" saphenous vein graft
Valulotome
Popliteal artery
D Arteriogram
Contrast medium injected
All saphenous branches ligated

need for major amputation despite a functioning graft (7 patients in group 2) supported a more aggressive approach to visualizing the complete distal arterial circulation involving the foot. Arterial digital subtraction arteriography was a great advance in this endeavor. While not quantifying or qualifying the degree of atherosclerotic involvement, this new angiographic technique provides excellent distal visualization with a minimum of contrast and discomfort to the patient. Patency of the pedal and distal posterior tibial arteries and their branches in the foot (disproving any notion of small vessel disease) challenged our skills to bypass to these vessels when the tibial vessels were extensively diseased or obstructed. Encouraged by the reports of others and our own early experience, we felt these procedures had far more potential than just a desperate attempt at limb salvage.[58]

PEDAL ARTERY BYPASS

We recently reviewed our combined experience of pedal artery bypass at the New England Deaconess Hospital between August 1986 and May 1989, wherein 104 bypasses were attempted in 96 patients.[59] The patient profile is presented in Table 15-4; 94 percent of these patients had diabetes, with 34 percent having associated cardiac disease. Twenty-seven percent of patients had previous peripheral vascular reconstruction. All procedures were performed for limb salvage, with 42 percent of patients having associated infection of the extremity requiring initial debridement and administration of intravenous antibiotics prior to revascularization. The mean preoperative ankle brachial index was 0.64, and all patients had less than 5 boxes on pulse volume recording forefoot tracings.

Table 15-4. Profile of 104 Patients Undergoing Dorsalis Pedis Bypass

Prior Condition	*Patients, No., %*
Diabetes	90 (94)
Angina/MI	33 (34)
Previous vascular surgery	28 (27)
Previous amputation	41 (42)
Ipsilateral TMA	6 (6)

Abbreviations: MI, myocardial infarction; TMA, transmetatarsal amputation.

Table 15-5. Dorsalis Pedis Bypass

	No. of Bypasses (N = 97)
Inflow Source	
Femoral	48
Popliteal	45
Tibial	2
Femoral-tibial graft	2
Nature of Conduit	
In situ	48
Reversed vein	21
Nonreversed vein	16
Arm vein	6
Composite	6

All patients underwent arterial digital subtraction arteriography. The usual pattern of disease demonstrated occlusion of all three tibial vessels, either proximally or distally, and no demonstrable continuity with a reconstituted pedal or posterior tibial artery below the ankle. Angiography successfully visualized the dorsalis pedis artery in 92 patients, and in 12 the artery was not visualized despite an audible Doppler signal.

In the 92 cases where the dorsalis pedis artery was visualized, 91 bypasses were successfully performed. In the 12 cases where the pedal artery was explored because of an audible signal, but visualization by angiogram failed, 6 successful bypasses were performed (5 of the other 6 patients underwent below the knee amputation). Therefore 97 cases were available for analysis.

All bypasses were performed with vein, with the type of bypass varying with the adequacy of the inflow source and the size and adequacy of the vein (Table 15-5). Our technique of the pedal bypass is detailed in our review and will not be discussed here (Fig. 15-9). Routine intraoperative angioscopy became an important adjunct to intraoperative angiography during this time to ascertain vein size, quality, and adequacy of valve lysis, and to evaluate the anastomoses.

Two patients died within 30 days of surgery (1.92 percent) and 6 bypasses failed within this period (16.1 percent). Further postbypass reconstructive foot surgery was required by 33 patients, and all patients who were discharged with patent

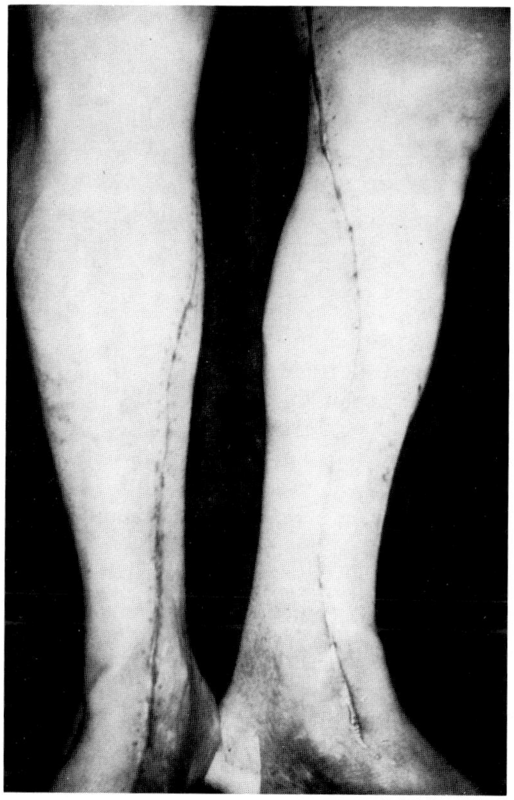

Fig. 15-9. Dorsalis pedis bypass and angiogram.

grafts had their feet saved. Actuarial life table analysis of graft patency, limb salvage, and patient survival rate was 82, 87, and 80 percent, respectively, at 18 months.

Diabetic patients presenting with extensive tissue loss or gangrene of an ischemic forefoot or heel probably need the restoration of pulsatile flow to the foot to achieve healing. This may be the reason why some blind popliteal segment or tibial reconstructions without vessel continuity to the foot remain patent but fail to achieve limb salvage. The dorsalis pedis artery is the recipient vessel of choice for bypass grafting under those circumstances. Additionally, bypass to a distal peroneal artery where there is continuity via collateral flow with the dorsalis pedis artery on the forefoot has been preferentially replaced by the dorsalis pedis graft, since the pedal graft is a technically less demanding procedure. Should the bypass fail, there may be fewer consequences to healing a below the knee amputation. Sometimes healing a below the knee amputation is more difficult when it has been preceded by a deep dissection of the lower leg.[60] The 50 percent success rate achieved with blind exploration of the pedal artery when an audible Doppler signal is present but visualization by arteriography fails supports an attempt at exploration before proceeding with a major amputation. This is especially important in patients who have already had a major amputation of the other extremity and are facing certain limb loss if circulation is not restored. The same can be said for a distal posterior tibial artery, especially when the primary foot problem is located in the heel or proximal plantar foot. It is apparent that there has been a further reduction of the 9.3 percent primary major amputation rate as a result of pedal or distal posterior tibial bypass grafting, and our post-bypass local forefoot amputation requirements have changed dramatically since the Wheelock era. In our efforts to preserve as much of the foot as possible to achieve maximum function, the number of transmetatarsal amputations performed post pedal bypass has dramatically declined in favor of more localized procedures. The return of pulsatile forefoot flow makes this possible. Arterial reconstruction in the diabetic patient is not recommended for the occasional vascular surgeon. Diabetic arteries are frequently extensively calcified and tibial and pedal arteries not infrequently take only a 1 mm probe. Diabetic patients generally have greater associated risk factors and certainly a team approach utilizing all health care disciplines is needed to achieve success.

COST VERSUS BENEFIT ANALYSIS

Diagnostically related groups (DRGs) and health care cost constraints certainly have placed additional burden on caring for diabetic patients with ischemic lower extremity problems. There is no question that limb salvage surgery is expensive, but really no more so than the alternative of major amputation.[61,62] It should be remembered that 30 to 50 percent of diabetic patients will have a limb-threatening contralateral extremity problem in the next few years.[63] While life expectancy for the diabetic with critical limb ischemia is reduced, the subjective factors such as quality of life and the ability to live and function independently are foremost in their minds. The diabetic's greatest fear is amputation, and we believe the benefits of an aggressive revascularization program outweigh the risks and costs even if this requires an initial lengthy period of hospitalization.

REFERENCES

1. Ganda OP: Pathogenesis of macrovascular disease in the human diabetic. Diabetes 29:931, 1980
2. Warren S: Le Compte PM, Legg MA: The Pathology of Diabetes Mellitus. 4th Ed. Lea & Febiger, Philadelphia, 1966
3. Jacobs J: The economic impact of diabetes. American Diabetes Association 48th annual meeting, New Orleans, June 11–14, 1988
4. Haimovici H: Amputation of the lower extremity. p. 893. In Haimovici H (ed): Vascular Surgery Principles and Techniques. McGraw-Hill, New York, 1976
5. Wheelock FC, Jr, Gibbons GW: Lower extremity amputations. p. 273. In Jarret F (ed): Vascular Surgery of the Lower Extremity. CV Mosby, St Louis, 1985
6. Gibbons GW: Diabetic foot sepsis. p. 412. In Brewster D (ed): Problems of Vascular Surgery. Yearbook Medical Publishers, Chicago, 1989
7. Kozak GP, Hoar CS, Jr, Rowbotham JL et al (eds): Management of Diabetic Foot Problems. WB Saunders, Philadelphia, 1984
8. Logerfo FW, Gibbons GW: Ischemia in the diabetic foot: modern concepts and management. Clinical Diabetes. 7:72, 1989
9. Logerfo FW, Coffman JD: Vascular and microvascular disease of the foot in diabetics: implications for foot care. N Engl J Med 311:1615, 1984
10. Strandness DE, Jr, Priest RE, Gibbons GW: Combined clinical & pathologic study of diabetic and nondiabetic peripheral arterial disease. Diabetes 13:366, 1964
11. Fing TA, DePalma RG, Rhodes RS: Diabetes mellitus and atherosclerotic involvement of the profunda femoris artery. Surg Gynecol Obstet 159:553, 1984
12. Cruz C, Hricak H, Samhouri F et al: Contrast medial for angiography: effect on renal function. Radiology 158:109, 1986
13. Gibbons GW, Wheelock FC, Jr, Hoar CS, Jr, et al: Predicting success of forefoot amputations in diabetics by non-invasive testing. Arch Surg 114:1034, 1979
14. Gibbons GW, Wheelock FC, Jr, Siembieda C, Hoar CS, Persson AB: Non-invasive prediction of amputation level in diabetic patients. Arch Surg 114:1253, 1979
15. Imparato AM, Kim GE, Davidson T, Crowley JG: Intermittent claudication: its natural course. Surgery 78:795, 1975
16. Stemmer EA: Influence of diabetes mellitus on the patterns and complication of vascular occlusive disease. p. 543. In Moore WS (ed): Vascular Surgery. Grune & Stratton, Orlando, FL, 1986
17. LeRiche R, Morel A: The syndrome of thrombotic obliteration of the aortic bifurcation. Ann Surg 127:193, 1948
18. Kosinski EJ, Pippin JJ, Kozak GP: Preoperative evaluation of the diabetic patient. p. 133. In Kozak GP, Hoar CS, Jr, Rowbotham JL et al (eds): Management of Diabetic Foot Problems. WB Saunders, Philadelphia, 1984
19. Tarhans, Moffitt EA, Taylor WF: Myocardial infarction after a general anesthesia. JAMA 220:1451, 1972
20. Goldman L, Caldera DL, Nossbaum SR et al: Multifactorial index of cardiac rush in nonvascular surgical procedures. NEJM 297:845, 1977
21. Lane SE, Lewis S, Pippin JJ et al: Predictive value of quantitative dipyridamole-thalium scintigraphy in assessing cardiovascular risk after vascular surgery in diabetes mellitus. Am J Cardiol 64:1275, 1989
22. Gibbons GW: The diabetic foot: amputation and drainage of infection. J Vasc Surg 5:791, 1987
23. Gibbons GW, Eliopoulas G: Infection of the diabetic foot. p. 91. In Kozak GP, Hoar CS, Jr, Rowbotham JL et al (eds): Management of Diabetic Foot Problems. WB Saunders, Philadelphia, 1984
24. Pierce Ellison C, Kupeli IA: Anesthesia in the diabetic patient. p. 150. In Kozak GP, Hoar CS, Jr, Rowbotham JL et al (eds): Management of Diabetic Foot Problems. WB Saunders, Philadelphia, 1984
25. Brewster DC, Darling RC: Optimal methods of aortoiliac reconstruction. Surgery 84:739, 1978
26. Pierce GE, Turrentine M, Stringfield et al: Evaluation of end to side vs. end to end proximal anastomosis in aortobifemoral bypass. Am J Surg 117:1580, 1982
27. Mannick JA, Whittemore AD, Couch NP: Aortoiliac occlusive disease. p. 489. In Moore WS (ed): Vascular Surgery. 2nd Ed. Grune & Stratton, Orlando, FL, 1986

28. Crawford ES, Bomberg RA, Glaser DH et al: Aortoiliac occlusive disease: factors influencing survival and function following reconstructive operation over a 25-year period. Surgery 90:1055, 1981
29. Moore WS, Malone JM: Vascular reconstruction in the diabetic patient. Angiology 29:741, 1978
30. Malone JM, Moore WS, Goldstone J: The natural history of bilateral aortofemoral bypass grafts for ischemia of the lower extremities. Arch Surg 110:1300, 1975
31. Bartlett FF, Gibbons GW, Wheelock FC, Jr: Aortic reconstruction for occlusive disease: comparable results in diabetics. Arch Surg 121:1150, 1986
32. Towne JB: Combined superficial femoral artery disease and profunda disease: profundaplasty versus distal bypass. p. 260. In Brewster DC (ed): Common Problems in Vascular Surgery. Year Book Medical Publishers, Chicago, 1989
33. Whittemore AD, Mannich JA: The ischemic leg. p. 293. In McLean LD (ed): Advances in Surgery. Year Book Medical Publishers, Chicago, 1981
34. Brief DK, Brener FJ, Alpert J, Parsonnet V: Crossover, femoro-femoral grafts followed up five years or more. Arch Surg 110:1294, 1975
35. Plecha FR, Pones WJ: Extra anatomic bypasses for aorto-iliac disease in high risk patients. Surgery 80:480, 1976
36. Velto RM: The treatment of unilateral iliac artery obstruction with a transabdominal, subcutaneous; femorofemoral graft. Surgery 52:342, 1962
37. Blaisdell FW, Hall AD, Lim RC, Jr, et al: Aorto-iliac substitution utilizing subcutaneous grafts. Arch Surg 172:775, 1970
38. Logerfo FW, Johnson WC, Carson JD et al: A comparison of the late patency rates of axillo-bilateral femoral and axillounilateral femoral grafts. Surgery 81:33, 1977
39. Dotter CT, Judkins MD: Transluminal treatment of arteriosclerotic obstruction: description of a technique and a preliminary report of its application. Circulation 30:654, 1964
40. Gruntzig A: Perkutane transliminel rekanalization chronischer Arterienverschlusse mit einer neuen. p. 43. Dilations-Technike, Derlag Gerjardt Wizstock Baden-Baden, Germany, 1977
41. Castaneda-Zuniga WR, Farmanek A, Todavarthy M et al: The mechanism of balloon angioplasty. Radiology 135:565, 1980
42. Rutherford RB, Patt A, Kumpe DA: The current role of percutaneous transluminal angioplasty. In Greenhalgh R (ed): Vascular Surgery: Issues and Current Practice. Grune & Stratton, London, 1986
43. Rutherford RB, Kumpe DA: Transluminal angioplasty in aortoiliac disease. Surg Rounds 12:17, 1989
44. Seeger JM, Abela GS, Silverman SH, Jablonski SK: Initial results of laser recanalization in lower extremity arterial reconstruction. J Vasc Surg 9:10, 1989
45. Myler RR, Cumberland DA, Clark DA, et al: High & low power thermal laser angioplasty for total occlusions & restenosis in man. Circulation 76, suppl. 23: 230, 1987
46. Abela GS, Seeger JM, Khoury AI, et al: Laser recanalization of peripheral arteries of humans: Acute & long term effects. Circulation 76, suppl. IV:409, 1987
47. Miller A, Campbell DR, Gibbons GW, et al: Routine intraoperative angioscopy in lower extremity revascularization. Arch Surg 124:604, 1989
48. Miller A, Jepson SA, Gibbons GW et al: Continued experience with routine intraoperative angioscopy for monitoring infrainguinal bypass grafting. Surgery (accepted for publication)
49. Dos Santos JC, Lamas A, Calcas J: L'arteriographie des membres de l'aorte et des ses branches abdominales. Bull Mem Soc Nat Chir (Paris) 55:587, 1929
50. Linton RR: Some practical considerations in surgery of blood vessels. Surgery 38:817, 1955
51. Wheelock FC, Jr, Filtzer HS: Femoral grafts in diabetics. Arch Surg 99:776, 1969
52. Reichle FA, Rankin KP, Tyson RR et al: Long-term results of femoroinfrapopliteal bypass in diabetic patients with severe ischemia of the lower extremities. Am J Surg 137:653, 1979
53. Veith FJ, Gupta SK: Femoral-distal artery bypasses. p. 141. In Bergan JJ, Yao JST (eds): Operative Techniques in Vascular Surgery. Grune & Stratton, Orlando, FL, 1980
54. Maini BS, Mannick JA: Affect of arterial reconstruction on limb salvage: a ten year appraisal. Arch Surg 113:1297, 1978
55. Leather RP, Shah DM, Buchbinder D et al: Further experience with the saphenous vein used in situ for arterial bypass. Am J Surg 142:506, 1981
56. Leather RP, Karmody AM: In situ saphenous vein arterial bypass for the treatment of limb ischemia. p. 175. In Mannick JA et al (eds): Advances In Surgery. Year Book Medical Publishers, Chicago, 1986
57. Taylor LM, Jr, Edwards JM, Phinney ES, Parter JM: Reversed vein bypass to infrapopliteal arteries: modern results are superior to or are equivalent to in situ bypass for patency and for vein utilization. Arch Surg 205:90, 1987
58. Buchbinder D, Pasch AR, Rollins DL et al: Results of

arterial reconstruction of the foot. Arch Surg 121:673, 1986
59. Pomposelli FB, Jepsen SJ, Gibbons GW et al: Efficacy of the dorsalis pedis bypass for limb salvage in diabetic patients. J Vasc Surg 11:745, 1990
60. Reinhold RB, Gibbons GW, Wheelock FC, Jr, Hoar CS, Jr: Femoral-popliteal bypass in elderly diabetic patients. Am J Surg 137:549, 1979
61. Mackey WC, McCullough JL, Conlon TP et al: The costs of surgery for limb-threatening ischemia. Surgery 99:26, 1986
62. Veith FJ, Ascer E, Gupta SK, Sprayregen S: Femoral-popliteal-tibeal occlusive disease. p. 513. In Moore WS (ed): Vascular Surgery. 2nd Ed. Grune & Stratton, Orlando, FL, 1986
63. Goldner MG: The fate of the second leg in a diabetic amputee. Diabetes 9:100, 1960
64. Hoar CS, Jr, Campbell DR: Aortoiliac reconstruction. p. 159. In Kozak GP, Hoar CS, Jr, Rowbotham JL et al (eds): Management of Diabetic Foot Problems. WB Saunders, Philadelphia, 1984
65. Wheelock FC, Jr, Gibbons GN: Arterial reconstruction: femoral-popliteal-tibial. p. 173. In Kozak GP, Hoar CS, Jr, Rowbotham JL et al (eds): Management of Diabetic Foot Problems. WB Saunders, Philadelphia, 1984
66. Mannick JA, Whittemore AD, Couch NP: Aortoiliac occlusive disease. p. 489. In Moore WS (ed): Vascular Surgery. 2nd Ed. Grune & Stratton, Orlando, Fl, 1986

16

Diabetic Neuropathic Osteoarthropathy: The Charcot Foot

Lee J. Sanders, D.P.M.
Robert G. Frykberg, D.P.M., F.A.C.F.S.

> How often have not I seen persons, not yet familiar with this arthropathy, misunderstand its real nature, and wholly preoccupied with the local affection, even absolutely forget that behind the disease of the joint there was a disease far more important in character, and which in reality dominated the situation . . . J.M. Charcot[1]

Charcot's intuitive statement referred to sclerosis of the posterior columns of the spinal cord, which he believed to be responsible for the development of neuropathic joints in patients with tabes dorsalis.[1–4] His meticulous observations of patients with locomotor ataxia and his astute statements about the importance of neuropathy, more than 120 years ago, apply equally well to diabetes mellitus with its neuropathic influence and ravaging effects on the bones and joints of the foot and ankle.

Multiple factors contribute to the development of bone and joint destruction in diabetic patients. Peripheral neuropathy with loss of protective sensation, autonomic neuropathy with increased blood flow to bone, and trauma have emerged as the most important determinants. Diabetic neuropathic osteoarthropathy (DNOAP) may also be due to metabolic factors that tend to weaken bone, renal disease, renal transplantation, steroid-induced osteoporosis, and decreased cartilage growth activity. Notwithstanding, the mechanism for development of neuropathic bone and joint lesions is not completely understood. This enigma was shared by Virchow, who had expressed his opposition to Charcot's *French theory* for the etiology of the arthropathy of ataxic patients, by saying "the trophic influence of the nerves is still a dark chapter."[5]

HISTORICAL PERSPECTIVE

J. K. Mitchell, in 1831, while an attending physician at the Pennsylvania Hospital, was the first to suggest a relationship between a spinal cord lesion, "caries of the spine," and the sudden attack of acute rheumatism of the lower extremities.[6] He observed a patient with "one ankle, and the knee of the opposite leg tumified, red, hot and painful . . . (where) the usual treatment by leeches, purgatives and cooling diaphoretics, with evaporating lotions, had the effect of transferring the symptoms to the other ankle and knee, and finally to the hip." Mitchell's disappointment with the results of this treatment caused him to suspect that the cause of the irritation might lie in the affected spine. In an attempt to examine experimentally the spinal origin of rheumatism, Mitchell described his successful treatment of a 56-year-old man of "vigorous constitution and active habits" who was confined to bed with severe pain in his right heel and ankle, immediately followed by redness, heat, and tumefaction with rapid spread to the opposite limb. He noted that local blood-letting with "the application of seventeen cups to the lumbar region" was effective in relieving pain and enabling movement of the legs. Mitchell concluded that his treatment was ". . . most potent when applied to that part of the spine, which supplies with nerves the parts in a state of active inflammation."

It is interesting to note that Mitchell made a distinction between the treatment of rheumatism and neuralgia. His success was greatest in the treatment of acute rheumatism and diminished as the process passed through a chronic phase. *Neuralgia,* however, was seldom cured, "neuralgia, a disease which spontaneously disappears; but is scarcely ever, in this city, cured by merely *medical* means. The art of the surgeon occasionally subdues it, and the physician often allays, but seldom removes it."

It was not until 1868, however, that J.M. Charcot brought attention to the spinal arthropathies associated with tabes dorsalis. Charcot's meticulous clinical studies of patients at the Salpêtrière, the "grand asylum of human misery" in Paris, enabled him to describe for the first time a distinct pathologic entity, the arthropathy of ataxia. He believed that lesions of the spinal cord, particularly of the gray matter, were responsible for disorders of the skin, the muscles, and the bones and joints commonly associated with the tabetic arthropathies.[1–4] "The irritative lesions of the spinal cord . . . react sometimes on the periphery, and determine various *nutritive* disorders . . . . The bones and articulations do not appear to escape this law. It follows that the arthropathies of locomotor ataxia would be . . . one of the forms of these articular affections, developed under the more or less direct influence of the spinal centre."[1] Charcot's concept of a *nutritive* trophic regulation of bones and joints, mediated by the spinal cord, became the basis of the *French theory* for the etiology of arthropathy seen in ataxic patients.[1–4,8–10]

Charcot described his observations of a *sudden* and *unexpected* arthropathy that often began without apparent cause. Fulgurant pains in the extremities often preceded the joint affection. He described a sudden onset of a generalized tumefaction of the limb with rapid changes in the articular surfaces of the joint. Crepitations in the joint would occur within a few days after the onset and would normally precede the development of the characteristic motor incoordination of tabes. He argued that these arthropathies did not result exclusively from the distension of the ligaments and capsules of the joints or from the awkward gaits of these patients. "Anatomically the enormous wear and tear shown by the heads of the bones, the extensive looseness of the ligaments of the joints, and the frequent occurrence of luxations seem to distinguish these arthropathies from the ordinary type of osteoarthritis".[1]

Volkman and later Virchow, German surgeons, were vocal in their opposition to Charcot's "nutritive" theory for the etiology of the arthropathy associated with locomotor ataxia. They believed that the joint changes in these patients were nothing more than a traumatic arthritis caused by the manner of locomotion peculiar to these patients, that is, the flinging about of their lower extremities in a disorderly manner.[1] This concept became known as the *German,* mechanical, or neurotraumatic *theory.*[7–10]

Charcot's brilliant contribution to the understanding of spinal (neuropathic) arthropathies was recognized in the *Rapport du Congrès* (Transactions of Congress) published in London in 1882, where it was written, "These bone changes constitute a distinct pathological entity. They deserve the name of *'Charcot's joint'* ".[4] Accordingly, this term has been perpetuated to describe the bone and joint changes associated with all the neuropathic arthropathies.

It was not until 1936, however, that Jordan first associated neuropathic arthropathy of the foot and ankle with diabetes mellitus.[11] In a very comprehensive paper, "Neuritic Manifestations in Diabetes Mellitus," he devoted a mere paragraph to Case 10,451, in which he described a 56-year-old woman with diabetes of 14 years' duration and peripheral neuropathy, who presented with "a rather typical, painless Charcot joint of the ankle, in addition to chronic osteomyelitis of the foot of an unusual type and without obvious etiology." The similarity of this presentation to that produced by syphilis, in the absence of positive serologic confirmation, led Jordan to consider this arthropathy as "a diabetic process of a neurologic trophic nature." When Jordan first saw this woman, he noted, "The ankle joint became swollen but not tender. Bits of bone were painlessly extruded from the toes. The lesions would heal but recur, or new ones would develop. The ankle joint became useless and instable. The process then involved the other ankle and foot." Since this early description by Jordan, the number of case reports of diabetic neuroarthropathy has steadily increased.[12-18]

DISORDERS PRODUCING CHARCOT'S JOINT

Various diseases and injuries involving the spinal cord and peripheral nerves have been reported to destroy the protective mechanisms of joints and interfere with the "nutritive" trophic regulation of bone.[1-5,7-10,19] The mechanism of destruction may be precipitated by a single injury or by repetitive moderate stress applied to the bones and joints of an insensate foot and ankle. The results are fractures, effusions, and ligamentous laxity followed by erosion of articular cartilage, fragmentation, luxation, disintegration, and collapse of the foot. The presence of peripheral neuropathy and the clinical and laboratory evidence of diabetes mellitus, tabes dorsalis, syringomyelia, spina bifida, or other cord lesions complete the picture of neuroarthropathy, or bona fide Charcot joint.

With a decline in the number of patients with tabes dorsalis, diabetes mellitus has emerged as the leading cause of neuropathic arthropathy today.[20-25] The importance of the diabetic form of neuropathic arthropathy was established in 1955, in a report by Miller and Lichtman at the Cook County Hospital and Chicago Medical School.[20] In their summary report of 17 cases they stated that "whereas tabes of syphilitic origin was formerly the usual cause of these painless deformities of the feet, with complicating soft tissue infections, ulcers and osteomyelitis, the diabetic neuropathic foot is now showing the higher incidence. Perhaps there is greater alertness in recognition".[20]

Disorders commonly cited as having the potential for producing neuroarthropathy include syringomyelia,[22,26-30] leprosy (Hansen's disease),[8,22,31,32] spina bifida,[8,28,29] meningomyelcoele,[28] congenital insensitivity to pain,[22,28] chronic alcoholism,[28,33] spinal cord injury/compression,[1-4,22,27] and peripheral nerve injuries.[27,34] Table 16-1 lists commonly cited disorders with the potential for producing neuropathic arthropathy and their sites of joint predilection. Bone and joint changes have been reported to occur in 4 to 10 percent of patients with tabes dorsalis,[26-28,35] 10 to 25 percent of patients with syringomyelia,[28,29,35] and 29 percent of patients with leprosy.[32] Spina bifida and meningomyelocele are the most common causes of neuropathic joints in children.[26,28] The key characteristic that all these disorders have in common is the absence or decrease of pain sensation in the presence of uninterrupted physical activity.

Table 16-1. Commonly Cited Disorders with Potential for Producing Neuropathic Arthropathy and Their Sites of Predilection

Disorder	*Site of Predilection*
Diabetes mellitus[a]	Foot and ankle
Tabes dorsalis[a]	Knee, shoulder, hip
Syringomyelia[a]	Shoulder, elbow
Hansen's disease	Foot, ankle, hand
Spina bifida[b]	Hip and knee
Meningomyelocele[b]	Foot and ankle
Congenital insensitivity to pain (rare)	Ankle and foot
Chronic alcoholism	Foot
Spinal-cord injury/ compression	Varies with level of involvement
Peripheral nerve injury	Ankle and knee
Severance of sciatic nerve	Ankle and knee

[a] Most common causes of neuropathic joints in adults.
[b] Most common causes of neuropathic joints in children.

INCIDENCE OF DNOAP AND PATIENT CHARACTERISTICS

The incidence of neuropathic bone and joint changes associated with diabetes mellitus has been reported to be from 0.08 to 7.5 percent.[13,14,36,37]

Pogonowska and associates reported on a clinical and radiologic survey of 242 patients in Houston, Texas.[37] They noted 6.8 percent of the cases had bone abnormalities classified as "diabetic osteopathy." Forgács, in a comprehensive literature review of data on 237 patients, estimated that DNOAP occurs in 0.3 to 0.5 percent of all diabetic patients.[14] There is the suspicion, however, that there may be many more cases that go undetected or misdiagnosed.[22–25]

Cofield and associates have reported radiographic evidence of bone and joint changes in the lower extremities of 29 percent of 333 cases of diabetics with peripheral neuropathy.[15]

The average age reported for the onset of DNOAP is approximately 57 years, with the majority of patients in their fifth and sixth decades. Of greater significance, the average duration of diabetes at the time of diagnosis of neuropathic bone changes is approximately 15 years, with 80 percent of patients being diabetic for more than 10 years, and 60 percent more than 15 years. Clohisy and associates reported on a homogeneous group of 18 adult juvenile-onset diabetic patients with an average age of 33.5 years and a 20-year history of diabetes mellitus.[16] Age therefore does not appear to be as important a factor in the development of DNOAP as the duration of diabetes mellitus.

Bilateral involvement has been reported to occur in 5.9 to 39.3 percent of the heterogeneous cases.[12,13,18,20,35] Clohisy and associates reported that 75 percent of their cases had bilateral involvement, with a very high incidence of serious fractures of the ankle and the tarsal bones[16] (Table 16-2). There does not appear to be a significant difference in sex distribution, with men and woman affected equally. In most patients, the diabetes is poorly controlled regardless of treatment with diet, oral agents, or insulin.[22]

THE NATURAL HISTORY OF DNOAP: CLASSIFICATION

Various descriptions of bone and joint changes associated with neuropathic arthropathies have appeared in the literature over the last century. Several authors have used the terms atrophic, destructive, hyperemic, and active to describe acute or early findings. The terms hypertrophic, reparative, proliferative, sclerotic, and quiescent have been used to describe chronic or late findings.[22–25,35,38,39] These descriptions are based on clinical, radiologic, and histologic observations as well as the chronicity of disease. Norman suggested that neuropathic joints be classified as *acute* or *chronic,* on the basis of the suddenness of their onset and speed of development. He believed that "since both reaction to injury and repair occur simultaneously in the joint two separate phases of development do not take place."[21] What seems to link these opposite states is the process of bony resorption and repair, as determined by the balance of osteoclastic and osteoblastic activity (Fig. 16-1).

The acute phase of neuroarthropathy is often precipitated by *minor trauma* and is characterized by swelling, local heat, erythema, laxity of ligaments, joint effusion, and bone resorption. Early findings may be indistinguishable from those of osteoarthritis and infection. Nearly all reports confirm the role of trauma in initiating the evolution of neuropathic osteoarthropathy in patients with an underlying neurologic deficit.

It has been suggested that the earliest changes in the evolution of neuropathic joints involve the soft tissues.[40] Newman has postulated that gross neuropathic changes in the ligaments were responsible for spontaneous dislocation of the foot that he observed in five cases occurring without bone destruction.[40] He believes that in those cases of neuropathic osteoarthropathy that do not begin with spontaneous fractures, ligamentous lesions may be of paramount importance, leading to spontaneous dislocation of the foot. Ligaments and joint capsule are thought to be stretched by the abnormal stresses applied to the joints, allowing them to go beyond their normal range of motion. They may be further weakened at their insertions into bone by hyperemic resorption allowing complete dislocation to take place.[27]

Charcot described *benign* and *malignant* forms of tabetic arthropathy affecting the knee, shoulder, elbow, hips, and wrists.[1] In the benign form, swelling would disappear within some weeks or months with a return to normal. In the malignant form, however, there was a serious disorder of the joint characterized by rapid disorganization and luxa-

Table 16-2. Reported Incidence of Diabetic Neuropathic Osteoarthropathy (DNOAP), 1947–1990

Reference	*No. Cases Reported*	*Incidence*	*Age (years)*	*Duration DM (years)*	*Bilateral Involvement*	*Source of Information, Important Distinctions*
Bailey and Root[36]	17	0.08% 1:1100	56 (30–69)	11.5	23.5% 4/17	George F. Baker Clinic (E.P. Joslin, medical director), New England Deaconess Hospital. All cases of neuropathic foot lesions among 20,000 consecutive cases.
Miller and Lichtman[20]	17		53		5.9% 1/17	Cook County Hospital and the Chicago Medical School. Cases seen over a 5-year period. Diabetes emerging as the #1 cause of Charcot joints.
Sinha et al.[13]	101	0.15% 1:680	2/3s 50s–60s (20–79)	83% > 10 65% > 15	23.8% 24/101	Joslin Clinic, Boston, MA. All Patients with documented radiologic features of neuroarthropathy between 1949 and 1970; 28/101 with *triopathy*.
Clouse et al.[12]	90		55 (25–78)	18 (1.5–43)	18%	Departments of Radiology and Pathology New England Deaconess Hospital and Joslin Clinic. Cases Observed between 1959 and 1972.
Forgács[14]	23	0.3 to 0.5%*	63 (48–79)	14.8		Radiological Clinic of the Semmelweis Medical University, Budapest, Hungary.* Reviewed data on 237 patients from 66 papers, plus his own 23 cases.
Cofield et al.[15]	96	29%†	56 (27–79)	81% > 10 16 (1–40)	21% 20/96	Department of Orthopedics, Mayo Medical School, Rochester, MN.† Mayo Clinic cases of diabetic patients with lower extremity peripheral neuropathy and radiographic evidence of bone/joint changes (333 patients), 1966 through 1975. Incidence represents the percentage of *neuropathic diabetics* with Charcot joint changes.
Clohisy et al.[16]	18		33.5 (25–52)	20	75% 14/18	Department of Orthopedic Surgery, University of Minn. Homogeneous group of adults with *juvenile-onset diabetes*; 15/18 *renal transplant*; 16/18 *triopathy*.
Sanders and Mrdjenovich[18]	28		79% 50s–60s 57.2 (36–70)	78% > 10 59% > 15 15.1 (1–27)	39.3% 11/28	Surgical Service, Podiatry Section VA Medical Center, Lebanon, PA. A series of 28 patients (39 extremities) with DNOAP, seen between September 1982 and December 1989. A heterogeneous group of adult diabetics.

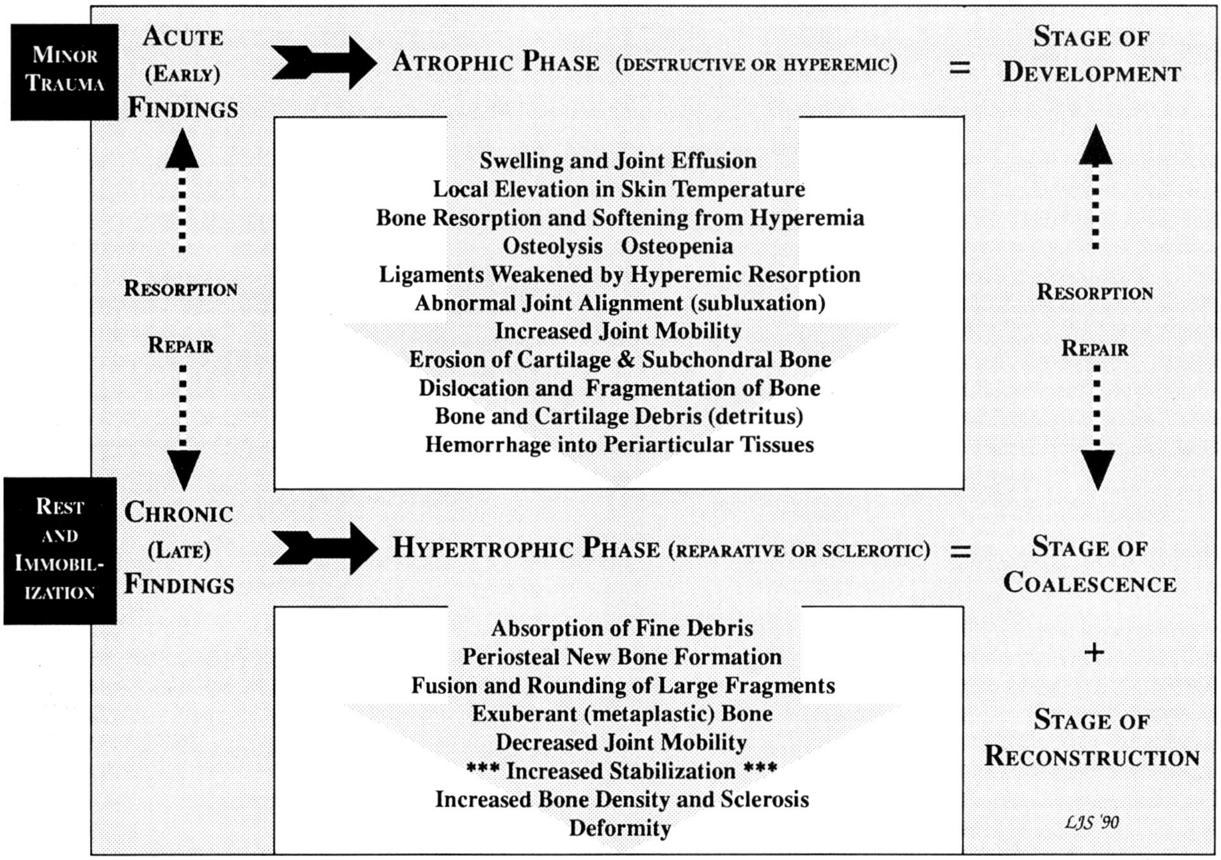

Fig. 16-1. The natural history of neuropathic osteoarthropathy in the diabetic foot and ankle.

tion, often with a cracking sound on movement of the joint. Charcot's distinction may be somewhat misleading, however, as the benign form of neuropathic arthropathy often becomes malignant or hypertrophic in the course of its development.

To qualify as an atrophic arthropathy, Schwarz and associates propose that the joint must be free of osteophytes, sclerosis, eburnation, fragmentation, and detritus.[39] In fact, these features are representative of hypertrophic, reparative, late findings.

Radiographic Findings

Radiographic findings associated with DNOAP can be broadly categorized into atrophic changes typical of the tubular bones of the forefoot and hypertrophic alterations usually found to affect the solid bones of the rearfoot.[12,22–25,39,41,42] This regional variation is not absolute, however, as atrophic lesions of the metatarsals and phalanges may heal with periosteal new bone formation, whereas the hypertrophic changes found in proximity to healing tarsal bones are preceded by areas of bony resorption during their early destructive period.[12] These changes are consistent with the natural history of the disease, wherein increased blood flow to bone results in a relative hyperemia, resorption, and softening of the bone.[8,39,42] During this hyperemic inflammatory phase the bone is soft, easily damaged, and prone to destruction,[27] especially in face of continued weight bearing on the affected extremity. Soft-tissue swelling, joint effusions, subluxations, subchondral osteopenia, and osteocartilaginous fragmentation ensue, perpetuating the destruction of the involved bones and joints.[22,42,43]

Clouse and associates, in their review of 90 cases

with 106 affected extremities, identified five types of bone reaction in diabetic osteoarthropathy.[12] Fragmentation of bone, as well as sclerosis of bone adjacent to fractures and neuropathic joints, were predominant findings in more than 70 percent of the extremities. Periosteal new bone formation was observed in 60 percent of the affected extremities and was seen to involve the metatarsals and phalanges almost exclusively. Resorption of bone, as evidenced by osteolysis of the metatarsal heads, was seen in 38 percent of the radiographs. Subchondral "osteoporosis" (osteopenia) adjacent to the articular surface of the tarsal bones or in metatarsal base at the tarsometatarsal joint was noted in 15 percent of the affected extremities. This finding most likely represents a fracture in the subchondral bone or resorption of bone secondary to a hyperemic response to injury.

Atrophic changes in skeletal tissue are characterized by the disappearance of bone, juxta-articular cortical bone defects, tapering of the metatarsal shafts, erosion of articular cartilage, joint subluxation and dislocation. Small cortical defects occur primarily in the phalangeal bases and the metatarsal heads.[37] These alterations may progress to osteolysis of the distal metatarsals with tapering of bone to produce a "sucked candy," "licked peppermint stick," or "sharpened pencil" deformity of the metatarsal heads and shafts. This leads to the appearance of "mortar and pestle" or "pencil in cup" deformities of the metatarsophalangeal joints. Atrophic changes of the phalanges are characterized by concentric resorption of the proximal phalangeal shafts resembling an "hourglass".[39,41,42]

Eichenholtz divided this disease process into three radiographically distinct stages: development, coalescence, and reconstruction.[44] The *stage of development* represents the acute, destructive period, which is distinguished by joint effusions, soft tissue edema, subluxation, formation of bone and cartilage debris (detritus), intra-articular fractures, and fragmentation of bone. This phase of bone and joint destruction is induced by minor trauma and aggravated by persistent ambulation on an insensitive foot. The consequence of trauma is a hyperemic response, which promotes additional resorption of bone and increases the susceptibility to further injury and progressive deterioration. The *stage of coalescence* is noted by a lessening of edema, absorption of fine debris, and healing of fractures. Clinical and radiographic evidence of coalescence indicates that the reparative phase of healing has begun. Rest, immobilization, and removal of weight-bearing stress are prerequisites for this stage to commence. The final phase of bone healing is the *stage of reconstruction* wherein further repair and remodeling of bone take place in an attempt to restore stability and homeostasis (Table 16-3). DNOAP can be arrested during the stage of development, if diagnosed before the disease has had a chance to mature. Early identification and treatment will ideally result in minimal joint destruction and deformity.

Hypertrophic, late bone changes associated with DNOAP are an exaggeration of those seen in osteoarthritis: cartilage fibrillation, loose body formation, subchondral sclerosis, and marginal osteophytes.[22] Neuropathic bone and joint lesions often heal with the formation of hyperplastic dense bone, especially in the midfoot. The early phase of healing is distinguished by the gradual absorption of fine debris and hematoma, with callus formation and the coalescence and reattachment of loose fragments of bone or cartilage. Proliferative changes are characteristic of this phase, with usual findings being intra and extra-articular osteophytes, exostoses, ossification of ligaments, and joint cartilage and marginal lipping at contact points.[7] Proliferation of new bone is often evidenced by exuberant overgrowth, "florid ossification" with decreased joint mobility, and increased stabilization of the foot. Fusion and rounding of large fragments are late findings.

BONE RESORPTION: NONINFECTIVE BONE DISEASE VS INFECTION

Newman described six different conditions of noninfective bone and joint pathology that he studied in 67 patients with diabetic neuropathy.[45] "Charcot osteoarthropathy" and "bone loss" were the most common conditions seen. In 12 cases the pattern of bone involvement was predominantly destructive, with severe wasting of the metatarsal shafts and phalanges. Because of the similarity of

Table 16-3. Radiographic Findings in Diabetic Neuropathic Osteoarthropathy

Stage	*Atrophic Findings*	*Hypertrophic Findings*	*Miscellaneous Findings*
1. Development	Resorption of bone: Concentric resorption of phalangeal diaphyses with an "hourglass" appearance Metatarsal osteolysis with "sucked candy" or "pencil pointing" destruction	Osteochondral fragmentation Intra-articular debris and joint mice "Rocker bottom" foot deformity	Joint effusion Subluxation Soft tissue edema Fractures Medial arterial calcification
2. Coalescence	Periosteal new bone formation	Sclerosis of bone Subchondral osteopenia Marginal osteophytes Periosteal new bone formation	Resorption of debris Decreased edema Fracture healing
3. Reconstruction		Ankylosis Trabecular remodeling Rounding of bone	Decreased sclerosis

(Modified from Frykberg and Kozak,[22] with permission.)

the radiologic findings associated with DNOAP and osteomyelitis, it is very important to differentiate these conditions.

Two mechanisms have been described for the development of bony resorption (osteolysis); one is the increased blood flow to bone and the other is through osteoclastic activity.[46] Infection may cause increased blood flow to bone through granulation tissue, as is often the case with a mal perforans ulcer. The resultant radiographic changes in bone are usually nonspecific. What initially appears to be bone destruction consistent with osteomyelitis may not be due to direct extension of infection to the bone but may instead represent osteolysis secondary to increased peripheral blood flow, inflammatory hyperemia, granulation tissue, or soft tissue infection.

Bone resorption and joint deformity, especially in the metatarsophalangeal joints, may be exaggerated by the presence of trophic ulceration and infection.[47,48] The diagnostic dilemma in these cases is which came first, the osteoarthropathy or the infection. Because the presenting symptoms of ulceration and infection often precede radiographic evaluation of the foot, it is invariably construed that any pathologic bone and joint changes must have occurred secondary to infection. This may be a grave mistake resulting in unnecessary ablative surgery. In their discussion of the role of infection in the pathogenesis of the Charcot foot and ankle, Lippman and associates determined that in four of their twelve patients, collapse preceded infection. In four other cases it seemed likely that ulceration and bacterial invasion occurred after the Charcot lesion had been established for some time.[49] Other authors have reported similar observations.[50,51] The role of infection in many of these patients should be viewed as a complication and not an etiologic factor.[37]

PATHOGENESIS OF DNOAP

The pathogenesis of diabetic neuropathic osteoarthropathy is multifactorial, with peripheral neuropathy, autonomic neuropathy, and trauma identified as dominant factors. Neuropathic and mechanical factors are obviously important, yet there are other elements that may not be readily apparent. These include increased peripheral blood flow to bone secondary to autonomic neuropathy, metabolic abnormalities that tend to weaken bone, renal failure and transplantation, steroid-induced osteoporosis, decreased cartilage growth activity, and possibly the nonenzymatic glycosylation of bone proteins and extra-articular soft tissues (Fig. 16-2).

The relationship that exists between certain lesions of the spinal cord and the peripheral

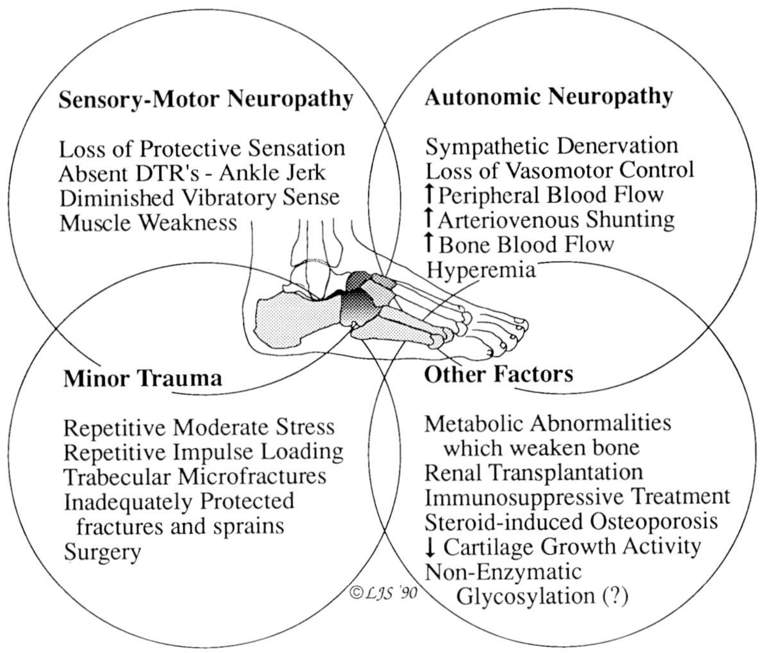

Fig. 16-2. Pathogenesis of diabetic neuropathic osteoarthropathy (Charcot joint).

nerves, and the subsequent development of neuropathic joints has been well documented.[1-4,9-11,26,27,34,35,38,51-54] The presence of peripheral sensory-motor neuropathy characterized by loss of protective sensation, absent deep tendon reflexes, diminished vibratory perception, and muscle weakness sets into motion a series of events that eventually result in the development of Charcot joint. The following discussion will be directed at understanding the neurovascular etiology of DNOAP as well as the possible roles of other important factors, which may be less well known.

Increased Blood Flow To Bone

Autonomic nervous system dysfunction has been noted by various authors as an associated finding in patients with neuropathic osteoarthropathy.[1,5,20,55-59] Support for the hypothesis that increased blood flow and active bone resorption are responsible for the development of Charcot joint is evidenced by several case reports and experimental data.[5,8-10,39,49-51,58-61] Schwarz and colleagues described the case of a 61-year-old diabetic patient who developed severe whittling down of the metatarsal bones and proximal phalanges following a left lumbar sympathectomy 22 years earlier.[39] Edelman and associates reported three cases where neuropathic osteoarthropathy developed within 2 to 5 years following successful lower extremity revascularization.[59] Lippman and colleagues suggested that excess local arterial flow can be a contributing factor to osseous breakdown under stress.[49]

A neurally initiated vascular reflex leading to increased blood flow and active bone resorption has been proposed as an important etiologic factor in the development of bone and joint destruction in neuropathic patients.[5,8-10,59] Wartenberg noted a possible role of the sympathetic nervous system in the manifestations of tabes dorsalis and in the production of tabetic joints.[5] He observed local disturbances in sympathetic vessel innervation in unilateral tabetic arthropathies, in proximity to the affected joints. "The following pathologic disturbances were found: elevation of the local temperature, rise in the arterial and venous blood pressure, increase in the oscillometric index, anomalies of the sweat secretion and disturbances in the pilomotor reflex."[5]

Palpable pedal pulses with no impairment of circulation have consistently been reported in diabetic patients with neuropathic osteoarthropathy.[11,13,36,56] "Pedal pulses in most of our patients were accentuated. The feet were warm with bounding dorsalis pedis and posterior tibial pulses."[13] The existence of autonomic neuropathy in patients with diabetic neuropathic arthropathies has likewise been reported with regularity.[20,39,51,56] M.M. Martin noted disturbances of vasomotor function to be so common in diabetic patients that (autonomic) nerve involvement of some degree should be regarded as common "even in the absence of symptoms and signs of (peripheral) nerve involvement."[51]

Experimental evidence exists that autonomic neuropathy with sympathetic denervation resulting in high peripheral blood flow is common in patients with diabetes mellitus.[54,57,58,60–64] Archer and colleagues, at the King's College Hospital, measured resting foot blood flow in 22 diabetic patients with severe sensory neuropathy, using mercury strain gauge plethysmography and Doppler sonogram techniques. They found blood flow to be increased on the average five times above normal at 20° to 22°C. They also noted that foot skin temperature was also elevated in these patients, reflecting the increased circulation.[57]

Edmonds and colleagues, also from King's College Hospital, studied the uptake of ^{99m} technetium-labeled methylene diphosphonate in 13 neuropathic diabetic patients and eight nondiabetic controls.[61] Five diabetic patients had radiographically proven osteoarthropathy. Eleven patients had a history of plantar ulceration, healed for 1 year before the start of the study. Bone scans were performed, and uptake of radiopharmaceutical was monitored in three phases. Uptake in all three phases (2 minutes after injection, at 4 minutes, and at 4 hours) was markedly elevated and confined to the feet in all neuropathic subjects. Increased uptake at 2 and 4 minutes indicated increased blood flow. These investigators concluded that the most likely explanation for their findings was increased bony blood flow secondary to sympathetic denervation. Other studies of the circulation in neuropathic diabetic feet have shown that blood flow is increased owing to arteriovenous shunting.[63,64]

Boulton and associates found the mean venous PO_2 in the feet of neuropathic patients with ulcers to be significantly higher than in controls.[64] They frequently observed the presence of prominent pedal arteries and distended dorsal foot veins in their diabetic patients who had noninfected neuropathic foot ulcers. These observations led them to believe that arteriovenous (A-V) shunting with increased venous oxygenation was important in the pathogenesis of ulceration.

Edmonds noted that severely abnormal autonomic function occurs in association with neuropathic ulceration.[61] High blood flow, vasodilatation, and arteriovenous shunting, which result from sympathetic denervation, could lead to abnormal venous pooling.[60]

Mechanical Factors

Mechanical factors have long been recognized in the etiology of osteoarthritis. Any situation that imposes chronically increased stress on articular cartilage can act as the inciting primary cause. The repetitive mechanical stress of ambulation with impulsive loading of bone, applied to a foot that has lost protective sensation, results in soft tissue injury (ulcers) and tensile fatigue of cartilage and bone. Trabecular microfractures in the subchondral cancellous bone are the earliest ultrastructural evidence of cartilage damage.[65] The result of healing of these microfractures and remodeling is an increase in the stiffness of the subchondral bone,[29] which reduces the bones normal resilience and ability to absorb shock. Total collapse of the neuropathic foot may occur over a short period of time and may be evidenced clinically by depression of the medial longitudinal arch and complaints by the patient that "my arch has fallen."[66]

It should be apparent that any disturbance of the bones and joints of the neuropathic foot that results in a change in shape, bony deformity, or alteration of normal foot mechanics has the potential for causing soft tissue and skeletal lesions. The consequence of increased vertical force and shear stress directed on the soft tissues overlying prominent bone is ulceration followed by infection and further collapse of the foot. The degree of injury is often determined by the extent of sensory loss, amount of stress on the joint, duration of the inflammatory process, and the patient's persistent ambulation despite the swelling, redness, and deformity.

Fractures

In the majority of the 118 cases of neuroarthropathy reported by Johnson, fractures of significant magnitude were responsible for initiating or increasing joint changes.[27] He concluded that "the behavior of the bones and joints in neuroarthropathy can be explained on the basis of the usual responses of these tissues to trauma modified by the presence of decreased protective sensation." Lack of attentive recognition and a cavalier attitude with regard to protection of fractures, sprains, and effusions sustain the atrophic phase and results in bone and joint destruction. As long as resorption outpaces new bone formation, this destructive cycle continues.

Spontaneous fractures and dislocations were seen in 11 percent of the cases reported by Newman and presented the greatest therapeutic problems compared to other noninfective diseases of bone.[45] Newman stressed the importance of recognizing these conditions and distinguishing them from osteomyelitis.

Increased blood flow to bone secondary to autonomic neuropathy with loss of vasomotor control, combined with an inflammatory hyperemia of the soft tissues results in resorption of bone with further weakening. Atrophic bone is easily fractured or fragmented. Frequent spontaneous fractures in neuropathic patients have led some authors to believe that intrinsic bone disease may be an etiologic factor.[67]

Decreased Cartilage Growth Activity

Insulin deficiency has been reported to affect skeletal integrity through its effect on insulinlike growth factor 1 (IGF-1). IGF-1, also known as somatomedin C, is synthesized in response to growth hormone influence and acts directly to produce cartilage proliferation and skeletal growth. Evidence suggests that IGF-1 serves as a mitogenic signal to cause mitosis of newly differentiated chondrocytes.[68] The induction of streptozocin-induced diabetes in rats has been shown to result in a significant decrease in serum somatomedin and cartilage growth activity.[69]

Renal Transplantation and Steroids

The association between renal transplantation with long-term steroid or other immunosuppressive treatment and the subsequent development of neuropathic osteoarthropathy has been noted in isolated reports.[16] These reviews show that following renal transplantation, diabetic patients have a much higher incidence of neurotrophic joint disease than the normal diabetic population. Clohisy and associates reported on 18 patients with juvenile onset diabetes and severe neuropathic arthropathy of the ankle and tarsus. Fourteen of these patients had received a renal transplant before the fracture was diagnosed, and none had a history of major trauma.[16]

It remains unclear whether steroid-induced osteoporosis or some other metabolic abnormality, which tends to weaken bone, was the underlying factor responsible for the development of bone and joint destruction in these patients. Further discussion of this subject will follow in the section on anatomic patterns of bone and joint destruction, pattern V.

Nonenzymatic Glycosylation of Collagen

Another possible factor in the development of DNOAP may be the synthesis of abnormal collagen types not usually found in cartilage, bone, ligaments, or other soft tissues. Nonenzymatic glycosylation of proteins associated with chronic hyperglycemia, in particular hemaglobin and dermal collagen, has been reported in several publications.[70–74] Digital sclerosis and joint contractures were found affecting the hands in 18 percent of children with insulin-dependent diabetes mellitus.[73] Biopsies of patients with limited joint mobility have shown increased cross-linking and glycosylation of collagen.[72] Limited subtalar joint mobility has been observed in neuropathic diabetics, compared to an age-matched nondiabetic control group (L.J. Sanders, unpublished data).

Small amounts of abnormal (type 1) collagen have reportedly been found by immunohistochemical assays in the immediate vicinity of chondrocytes in osteoarthritic cartilage.[74] Diminution of chondroitin sulfate content relative to the collagen

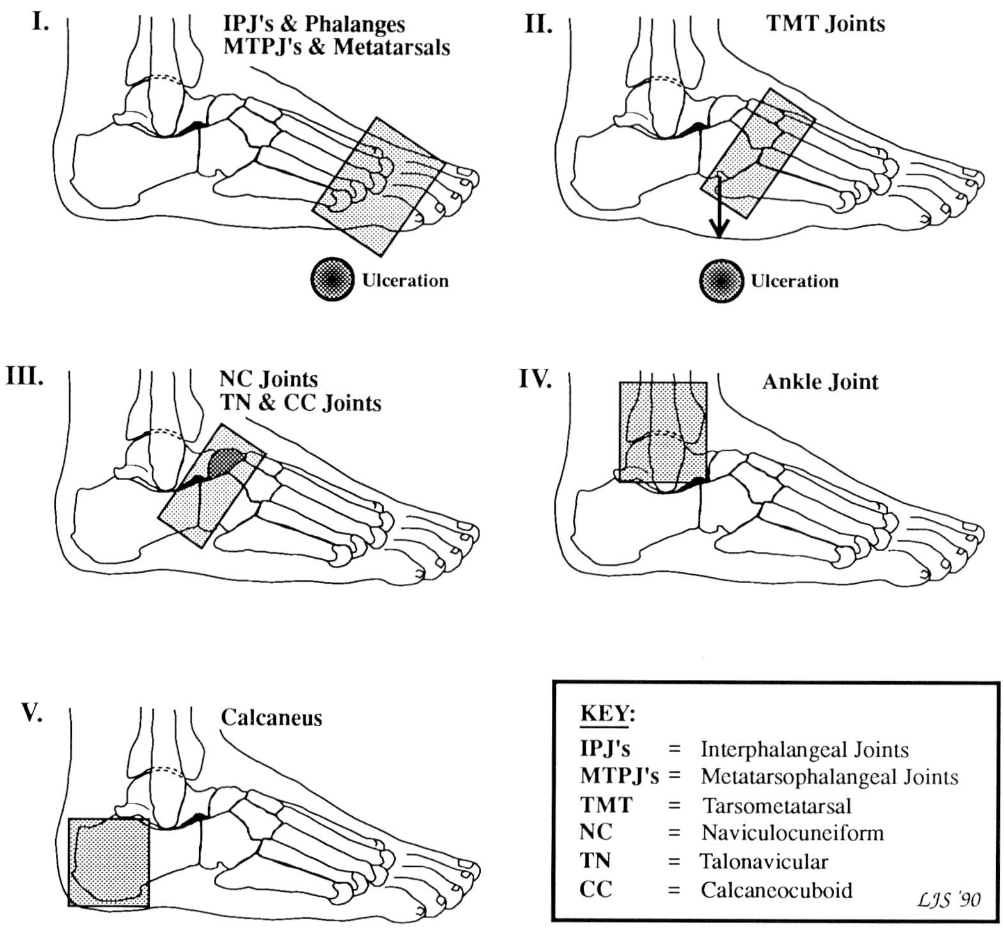

Fig. 16-3. Five anatomic patterns of bone and joint destruction commonly reported in patients with diabetic neuropathic osteoarthropathy of the foot and ankle. Patterns I and II are frequently associated with bony deformity and ulceration. The most frequent joint involvement is seen in patterns I, II, and III, with the most severe structural deformity and functional instability associated with patterns II and IV.

matrix is a feature common to osteoarthritic alteration of joint cartilage. Hough and Sokoloff suggest that this change might alter the material properties of cartilage with respect to wear and tear.[74]

ANATOMIC PATTERNS OF BONE AND JOINT DESTRUCTION

Five characteristic anatomic patterns of bone and joint destruction have been observed to occur in diabetic patients with neuropathic osteoarthropathy. Sanders and Mrdjenovich[18] have described these patterns as follows: pattern I—the forefoot; pattern II—the tarsometatarsal joints; pattern III—the naviculocuneiform, talonavicular, and calcaneocuboid joints; pattern IV—the ankle joint; and pattern V—the calcaneus (posterior pillar). Two of these patterns, I and II, are frequently associated with bony deformity and ulceration. The most frequent joint involvement is seen in patterns I, II, and III, with the most severe structural deformity and functional instability seen in patterns II and IV. Pattern V osteopathy is the least common and may be seen as an isolated fracture of the calcaneus or in association with involvement of other tarsal bones (Fig. 16-3 and Table 16-4).

Table 16-4. Reported Distribution of Bone and Joint Involvement in Patients with Diabetic Neuropathic Osteoarthropathy

Reference	*Tarsal*	*TMTJ*	*MTPJ*	*IPJ*	*Ankle*	*Observations*
Miller and Lichtman[20] 17 cases 21joints	4.8% 1/21 **47.7%**	42.9% 9/21	38.1% 8/21	9.5% 2/21	4.8% 1/21	Described three cases of "a peculiar deformity" of the foot characterized by a "rocker sole." Multiple joint involvement occurred in several cases. The authors noted autonomic nervous system involvement. Destruction of the ankle joint in one case followed surgical intervention for a fractured medial malleolus. Radiography disclosed two main types of osseous changes: (1) the atrophic type with dissolution of joints and absorption of bone, and (2) the hypertrophic type (seen most frequently).
Sinha et al[13] 101 cases 127 sites	37% 47/127 **63.8%**	26.8% 34/127	26.8% 34/127	Not reported	9.4% 12/127	Bony deformity was most common in the TMT group. There were nine "rocker" soles, and each of these patients walked with a limp. Callus formation and ulceration were most common in the MTPJ group.
Cofield et al.[15] 96 cases 116 extremities	17.2% 20/116 33%	15.5% 18/116	67% 78/116 includes phalangeal involvement	Not reported	Not reported	Noted three patterns of bone and joint involvement: (1) at the level of the phalanges and MTPJs, (2) metatarsalcuneiform destruction, and (3) anterior pillar-medial column destruction. Ninety-one % of patients with radiographic evidence of metatarsophalangeal joint involvement had underlying ulcers. Only 3% of patients with midfoot or hindfoot involvement had ulcers adjacent to the affected bone or joint. Cartilage loss, metaphyseal osteosclerosis, osteophytes, juxta-articular bone or calcific debris were more common in feet without ulcers or infection than in those with ulcers. Pain was often an associated feature.
Sanders and Mrdjenovich[18] 28 cases 66 sites	31.8% 21/66 **66.7%**	34.8% 23/66	25.8% 17/66	4.5% 3/66	3% 2/66	Noted five patterns of neuropathic osteoarthropathy: (1) at the level of the MTPJs and IPJs, (2) TMTJs, (3) midtarsal joint and naviculocuneiform joints, (4) ankle joint, and (5) calcaneus. TMTJ involvement was noted in 61% of the patients (17/28). MTPJ involvement occured in 57% (16/28), while IPJ involvement was seen in only 7.1% (2/28). Twelve patients (42.9%) presented with rocker sole deformity of 14 feet.

Abbreviations: TMTJ, tarsometatarsal joint; MTPJ, metatarsophalangeal joint; IPJ, interphalangeal joint.

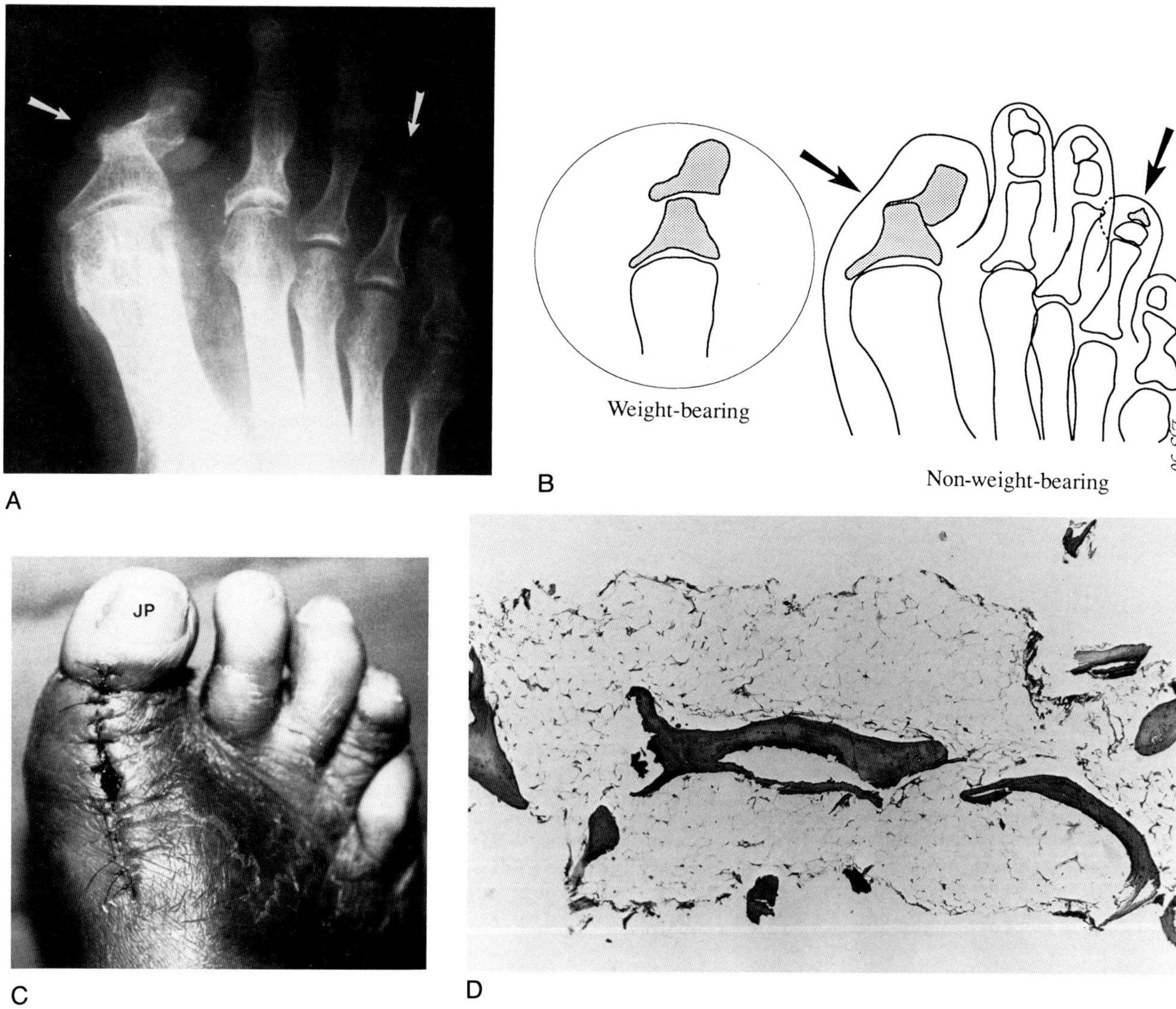

Fig. 16-4. (**A**) Osteolytic destruction of the interphalangeal joint (IPJ) of the right hallux and distal phalanx of the fourth toe (arrows). There is a flexion deformity of the hallux IPJ. (**B**) Graphic illustration of the radiograph showing the appearance of the IPJ extended in a weight-bearing attitude. (**C**) Clinical photograph of the right foot following bone biopsy from the IPJ. Note the characteristic shortening of the hallux and fourth toe. (**D**) Photomicrograph of bone reveals extensive resorption of bone, characterized by thin, widely separated trabeculae.

Pattern I: The Forefoot

Pattern I osteoarthropathy is characterized by involvement of the forefoot, that is, the interphalangeal joints, phalanges, metatarsophalangeal joints (MTPJ), or distal metatarsal bones. The radiographic findings in this location are typically atrophic and destructive in nature characterized by osteopenia, osteolysis, juxta-articular cortical bone defects, subluxation, and destruction. Pattern I involvement has been reported to occur in from 26 to 67 percent of all affected sites.[13,15,18,20] In Miller and Lichtman's study 47.6 percent of the affected joints (10/21) involved the metatarsophalangeal and interphalangeal joints.[20] Sanders and Mrdjenovich found pattern I involvement in 30

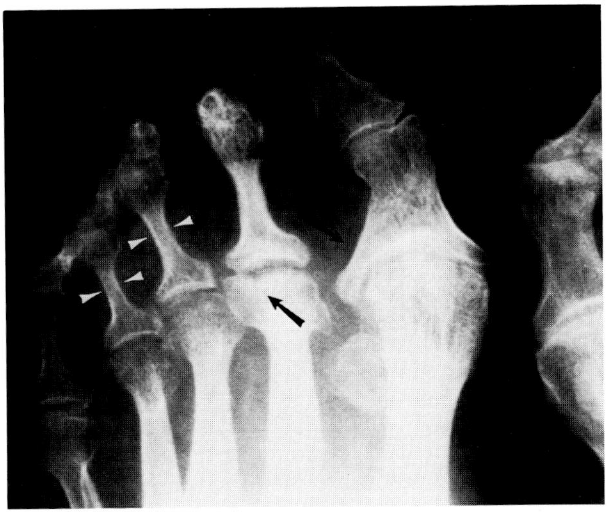

A

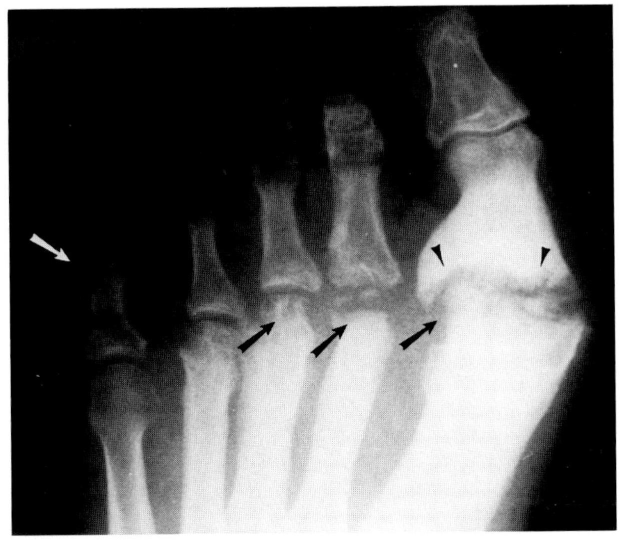

B

Fig. 16-5. (**A**) Concentric resorption of bone involving the proximal phalangeal shafts of the lesser toes (white arrowheads). Note the "hourglass" appearance of the phalanges. Black arrows point to proliferative changes evidenced by fragmentation of the second metatarsal head and broadening of the phalangeal bases of the hallux and second toe. (**B**) Destructive changes are noted involving the first, second, and third metatarsophalangeal joints (MTPJs). Ulceration and infection had previously involved the second and third MTPJs; however, the first MTPJ was unaffected. Also shown are severe osteoarthritic joint changes, "osteoarthritis with a vengeance," affecting the first MTPJ (black arrowheads).

percent of affected sites (20/66)[18]; Cofield and associates reported metatarsophalangeal and interphalangeal joint involvement in 67 percent of 116 affected extremities.[15] Sinha and colleagues reported metatarsophalangeal joint involvement in 26.8 percent (34/127) of all affected sites.[13]

Plantar ulceration is often associated with osteopathy of the forefoot. Cofield and associates reported that 91 percent of their patients with radiographic evidence of MTPJ involvement had underlying ulcers.[15] It may not be readily apparent whether the bone and joint changes preceded or developed as a result of the ulceration. The presence of neuropathic plantar ulceration should be considered a serious finding that may lead to major disability. "A penetrating ulcer is not to be treated lightly but as a potential destroyer of the foot."[31] This finding may in fact be a representative cutaneous marker for DNOAP.

Figure 16-4 demonstrates osteolysis of the interphalangeal joint of the right great toe and the distal phalanx of the fourth toe in a 62-year-old neuropathic type 2 diabetic man. Shortening of the hallux and fourth toes occurred as a result of the osteolysis. Bone biopsy was performed to rule out an infectious cause. Histologic examination revealed extensive resorption of bone, characterized by thin widely separated trabeculae and a fatty infiltration of the marrow. There were no inflammatory changes seen, and the findings were consistent with osteoporosis (Fig. 16-4D). Culture reports were negative.

Concentric resorption of bone may be seen to affect the phalangeal diaphyses with a characteristic *hourglass* picture. Broadening of the bases of the proximal phalanges occurs, with the formation of a *cup* around the metatarsal head[39,75] (Fig. 16-5A). Osteoarthritic changes in the first metatarsal phalangeal joint may be extensive and have been referred to as osteoarthritis "with a vengeance"[8] (Fig. 16-5B).

Resorption of the distal metatarsal bones and phalanges is characteristic of atrophic, destructive diabetic osteopathy. This is evidenced, on anteroposterior radiographs, as a *pencil-like* tapering of the metatarsal bones with a *licked peppermint stick* or *sucked candy* appearance. The histopathologic picture reveals erosion of articular cartilage, peri-

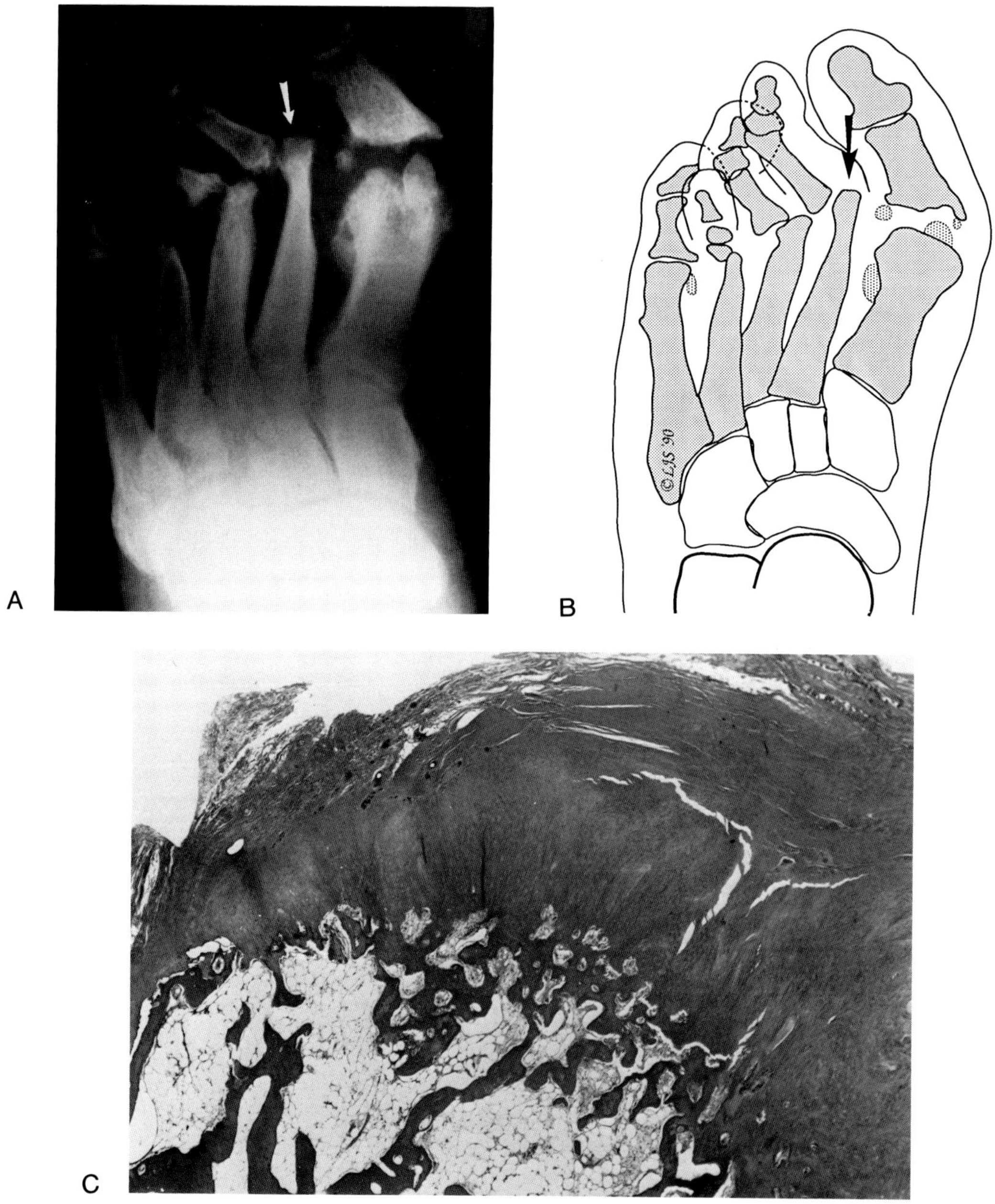

Fig. 16-6. (**A**) Anteroposterior radiograph reveals extensive destruction of all metatarsophalangeal joints (MTPJs) in this 61-year-old type 2 diabetic man. There is extensive osteolytic destruction of the MTPJs with "pencil-like" tapering of the metatarsal shafts, resembling "sucked candy" or a "licked peppermint stick." Arrow points to the site of bone biopsy. (**B**) Graphic representation of the radiographic findings. (**C**) Photomicrograph of bone from the second metatarsal head demonstrates erosion of the articular cartilage, irregular periarticular fibrosis, disorganization and resorption of subchondral bone. The bone is very reactive with evidence of active resorption, new bone formation, and remodeling, as seen with higher magnification. *(Figure continues.)*

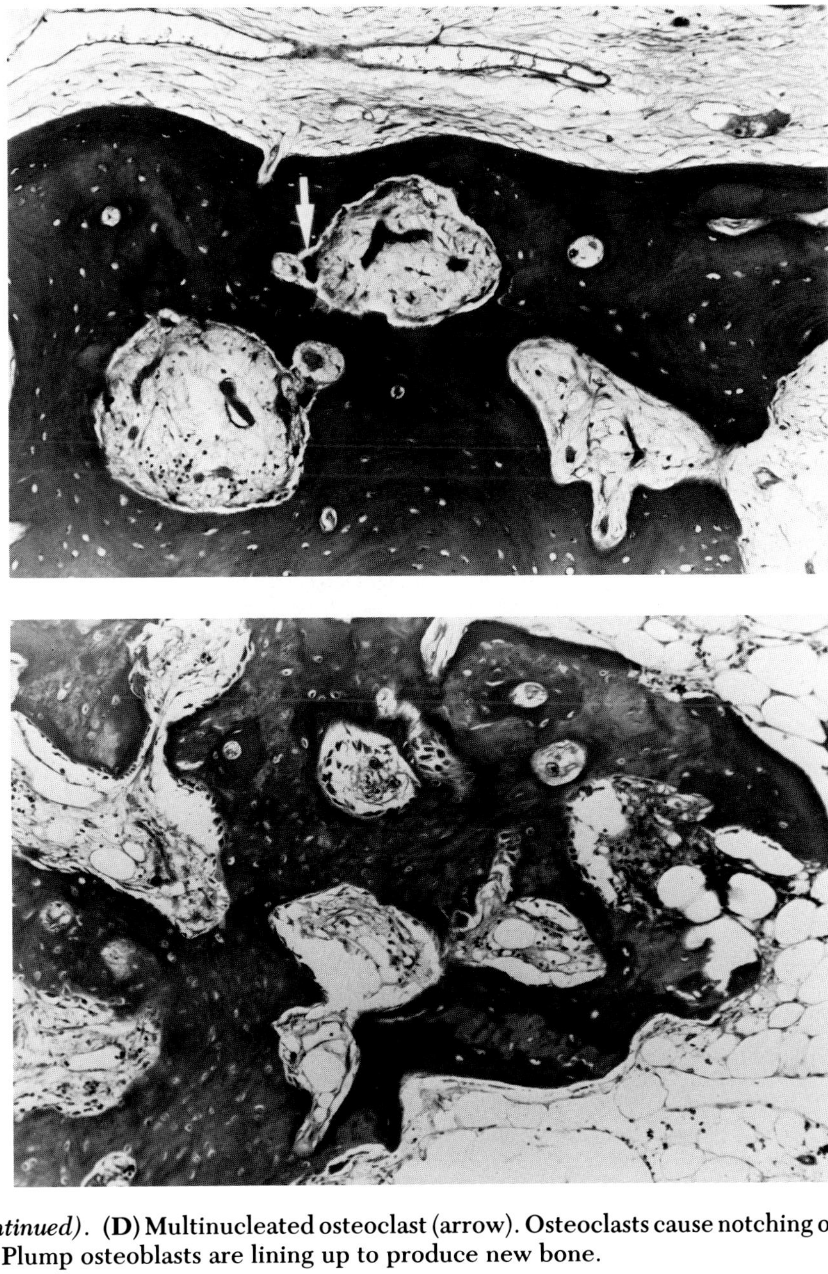

D

E

Fig. 16-6 *(Continued)*. **(D)** Multinucleated osteoclast (arrow). Osteoclasts cause notching or "scalloping" of the bone. **(E)** Plump osteoblasts are lining up to produce new bone.

articular fibrosis, increased vascularity, synchronous resorption of bone and new bone formation. There is disorganization of subchondral bone with bony resorption and a fatty marrow (Fig. 16-6). Chronic ulceration and infection may be associated with these changes.

Osteolysis of the metatarsal head or base of the proximal phalanx may develop rapidly with destruction of the MTPJ, as illustrated in the following case. A 49-year-old white man with a 13-year history of diabetes mellitus developed an ulcer beneath the left second metatarsal head. The ulcer was accompanied by redness, moderate swelling, and infection of the foot. Radiographs of the left foot revealed osteolysis of the second MTPJ with juxta-articular cortical bone defects affecting the second metatarsal head and phalangeal base. Periosteal elevation of the proximal phalangeal diaphysis was also apparent. Osteopenia of the fourth and fifth metatarsal heads was noted as an incidental finding. This patient was treated conservatively by his family medical doctor with resolution of the infection and ulceration. Review of follow-up radiographs of the same foot in January 1989 revealed complete restitution of the integrity, "restitutio ad integrum," of the second metatarsophalangeal joint with proliferation and cupping of the phalangeal base around the enlarged metatarsal head. There was no evidence of osteosclerosis or sequestrum, findings suggestive of chronic osteomyelitis. Another remarkable radiographic finding was the complete disappearance of the fifth metatarsal head with partial resorption of the fourth. There were no cutaneous lesions or soft-tissue infection proximate to these metatarsals (Fig. 16-7).

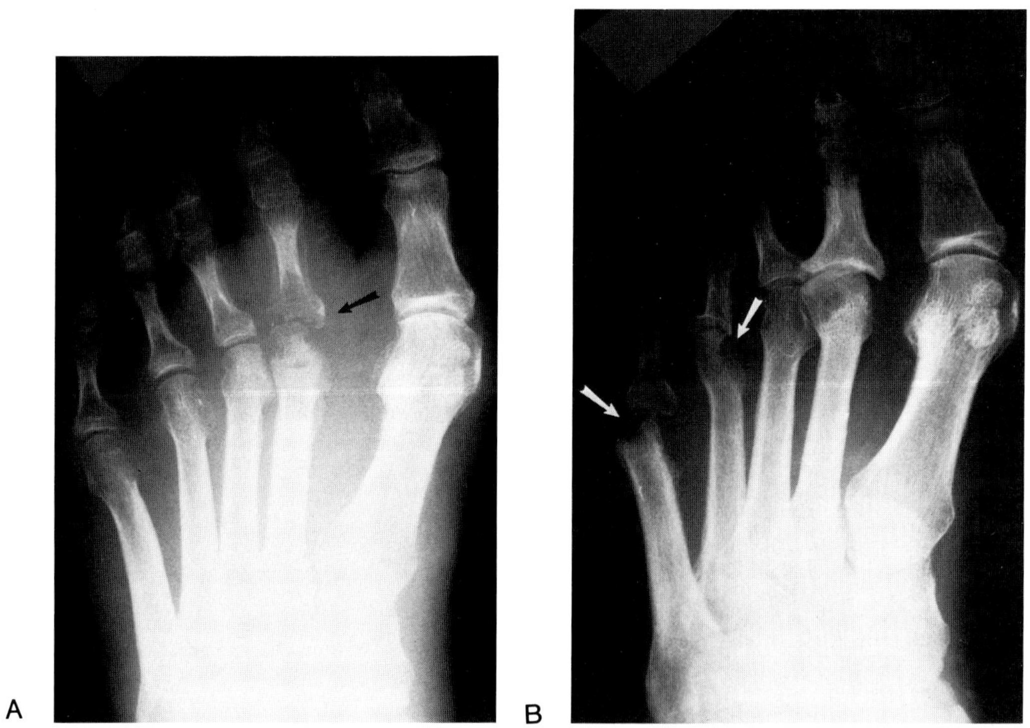

Fig. 16-7. (**A**) Osteolytic destruction of the second metatarsophalangeal joint (MTPJ) (black arrow). Ulceration was present beneath the second metatarsal head. Mild osteopenia is noted affecting the fourth and fifth metatarsal heads. (**B**) "Restitutio ad integrum." Radiograph taken four years later shows complete restoration of the integrity of the second MTPJ with enlargement of the metatarsal head and broadening of the proximal phalangeal base. White arrows point to spontaneous disappearance of the fifth metatarsal head and partial resorption of the fourth.

Pattern II: Tarsometatarsal (TMT) Joints

Pattern II osteoarthropathy is distinguished by affection of the tarsometatarsal (Lisfranc's) joints and is often associated with plantar ulceration at the apex of the collapsed cuneiforms or cuboid. TMT involvement has been reported to occur in from 15 to 43 percent of the cases of DNOAP.[13,15,28,20] This pattern of osteoarthropathy occurs spontaneously and with greater frequency in diabetic patients than in those with leprosy. The *cuneiform-metatarsal base pattern* associated with Hansen's disease has been reported to be "nearly always caused by definite violence."[31]

Early changes in the TMT joints may be subtle, and consistent with incipient osteoarthritis, there may be slight dorsal prominence of the metatarsal bases with local swelling and increased skin temperature on the dorsum of the foot. Late changes reveal degenerative arthritis with fragmentation and subluxation of the cuneiform bones and the metatarsal bases. The metatarsal bases often override the cuneiforms. There may be evidence of total disintegration of the cuneiforms with collapse of the midfoot and a resultant *rocker bottom* foot deformity (Fig. 16-8A & B).

The normal anatomic relationships of the tarsometatarsal joints are illustrated in Figure 16-9. The second metatarsal base is securely recessed in the intercuneiform mortise. This tenon-in-mortise relationship creates a very stable keystone for the midfoot. Disturbance of this relationship weakens the foot and allows for dorsolateral displacement of the metatarsal bones of the lesser tarsus followed by architectural collapse of the cuneiforms and cuboid.

A fracture at the base of the second metatarsal, in the absence of major trauma, may be the harbinger of collapse of the tarsometatarsal joints, as seen in the following case. A 66-year-old neuropathic diabetic man presented in September 1982 with mild swelling and erythema along the dorsum of his right foot, following a fall in his kitchen. Radiographs revealed a laterally displaced fracture of the second metatarsal base (Fig. 16-10). The patient was placed in a plaster cast, non-weight-bearing, with crutches for 6 weeks. During this time he proved to be poorly compliant and refused further immobilization. Within 8 months the patient developed total collapse of his midfoot.

Patients may present acutely with an erythematous, hot, painful, swollen foot, but with no history of trauma. The clinical picture may be nonspecific, resembling an acute gouty arthritis, septic arthritis, or cellulitis. Patients are usually afebrile with no clinical or laboratory evidence of infection. The radiographic picture, however, is quite remarkable, revealing subluxation or fracture dislocation of Lisfranc's joint. The base of the second metatarsal is laterally displaced from its normal recessed position in the intercuneiform mortise, and all the metatarsals are shifted laterally on the lesser tarsus.

Another case represents a classic presentation of acute neuropathic osteoarthropathy affecting the tarsometatarsal articulations. The patient, a 63-year-old white neuropathic diabetic man with a 15-year history of diabetes mellitus, poorly controlled with insulin, presented to the emergency room with acute erythema, swelling, increased skin temperature, and deformity of the right foot. He reported having mild pain and no history of trauma. The patient was afebrile with an elevated blood sugar of 447 mg/dl. He was a unilateral amputee, having undergone a left below the knee amputation 2 years earlier. An anteroposterior radiograph revealed a tarsometatarsal joint (Lisfranc's) dislocation with all the metatarsal bases shifted laterally on the lesser tarsus. The lateral radiograph revealed plantar dislocation of the cuneiforms and navicular, with dorsal displacement of the metatarsal bases. Erosion (osteolysis) of the neck and body of the talus was also noted. The patient was admitted to the hospital for conservative management of the right foot and control of diabetes mellitus. Despite efforts to immobilize the extremity and to limit weight bearing, this unilateral amputee continued to walk on his right lower extremity. Within 6 months total collapse of the foot ensued with extrusion of the medial cuneiform. Ulceration developed medially over the prominent medial cuneiform and plantarly at the apex of the collapsed midfoot. Extensive soft tissue infection, necrosis, and swelling developed, resulting in a below the knee amputation of the right lower extremity (Fig. 16-11).

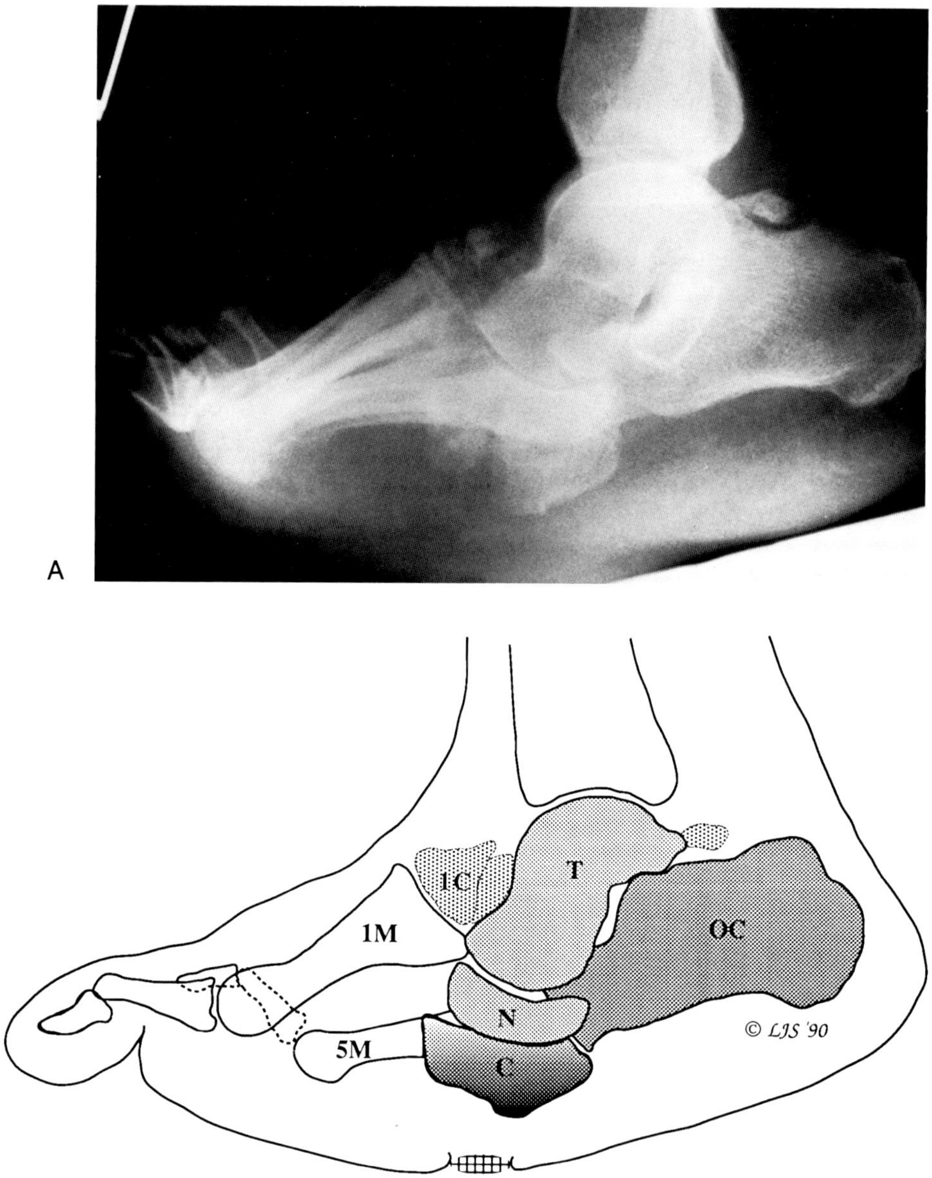

Fig. 16-8. (**A**) Lateral radiograph of a "rocker bottom" foot demonstrating collapse of the tarsometatarsal, naviculocuneiform, talonavicular, and calcaneocuboid joints. Soft tissue ulceration is present at the apex of the rocker. (**B**) Graphic illustration of radiographic findings with identification of involved structures. C, cuboid; N, navicular; T, talus, OC, calcaneus; 1C, medial cuneiform; 1M, first metatarsal; 5M, fifth metatarsal. *(Figure continues.)*

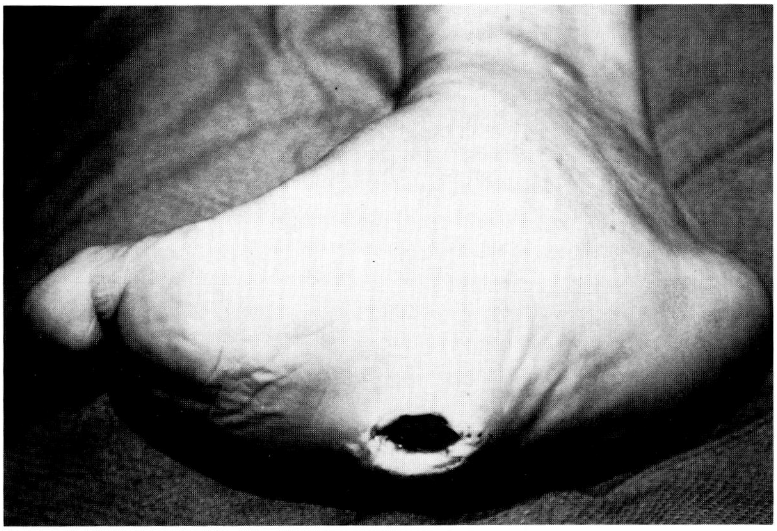

Fig. 16-8 *(Continued)*. (C) Clinical photograph depicting a broad, deformed foot with large plantar ulcer.

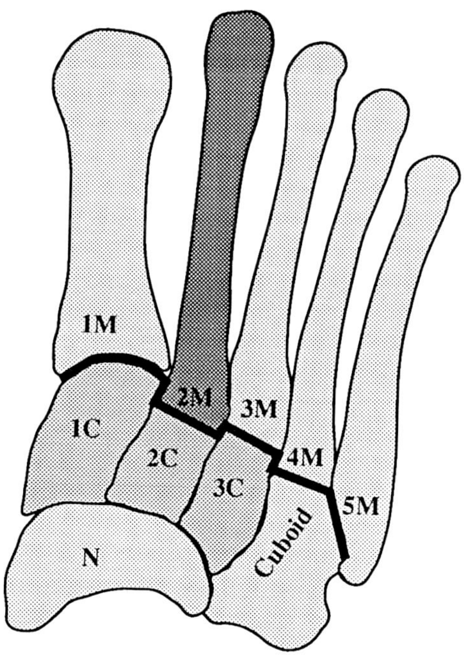

Fig. 16-9. Normal anatomy of the tarsometatarsal (Lisfranc's) joints. Note the recessed position of the second metatarsal base (tenon) in the intercuneiform mortise. M, metatarsal; C, cuneiform; N, navicular.

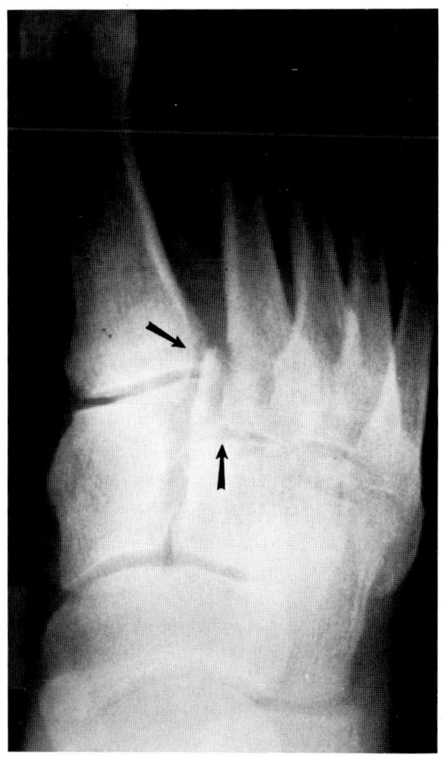

Fig. 16-10. Laterally displaced fracture of the second metatarsal base (arrows).

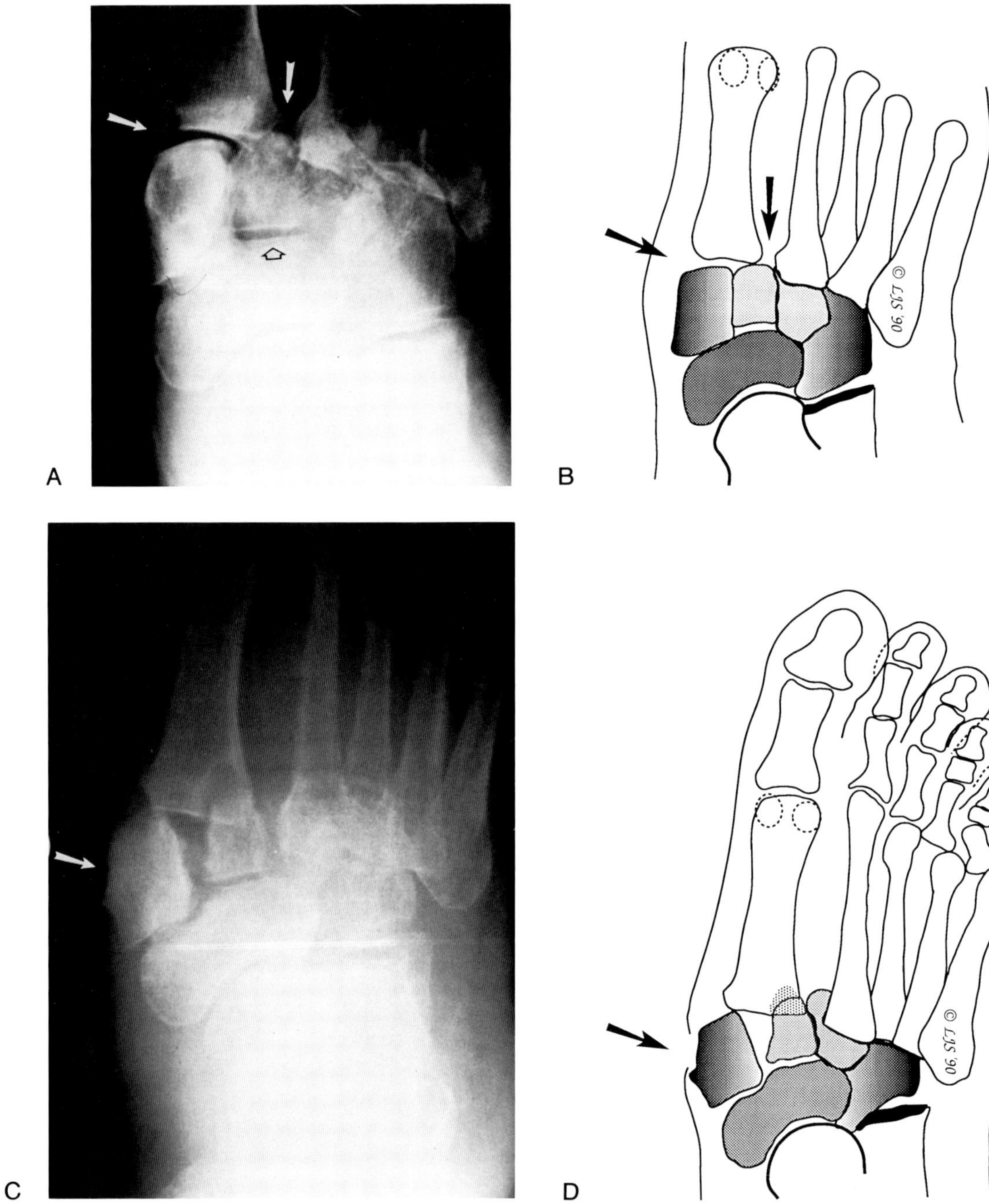

Fig. 16-11. (**A**) Anteroposterior radiograph reveals dislocation of the tarsometatarsal joints with lateral displacement of the metatarsal bases on the cuneiforms and cuboid. The second metatarsal base is completely displaced from the intercuneiform mortise, with the first metatarsal base articulating with the medial half of the second cuneiform (white arrows). The open arrow points to distal migration of the second cuneiform. (**B**) Graphic illustration of the radiographic findings. (**C**) Anteroposterior radiograph taken 6 months after initial presentation. There has been extensive deterioration of the tarsometatarsal, navicular cuneiform, and midtarsal joints. White arrow points to extrusion of the medial cuneiform. The second cuneiform has eroded its way into the plantar-lateral aspect of the first metatarsal base. (**D**) Graphic illustration of the radiographic findings. *(Figure continues.)*

E

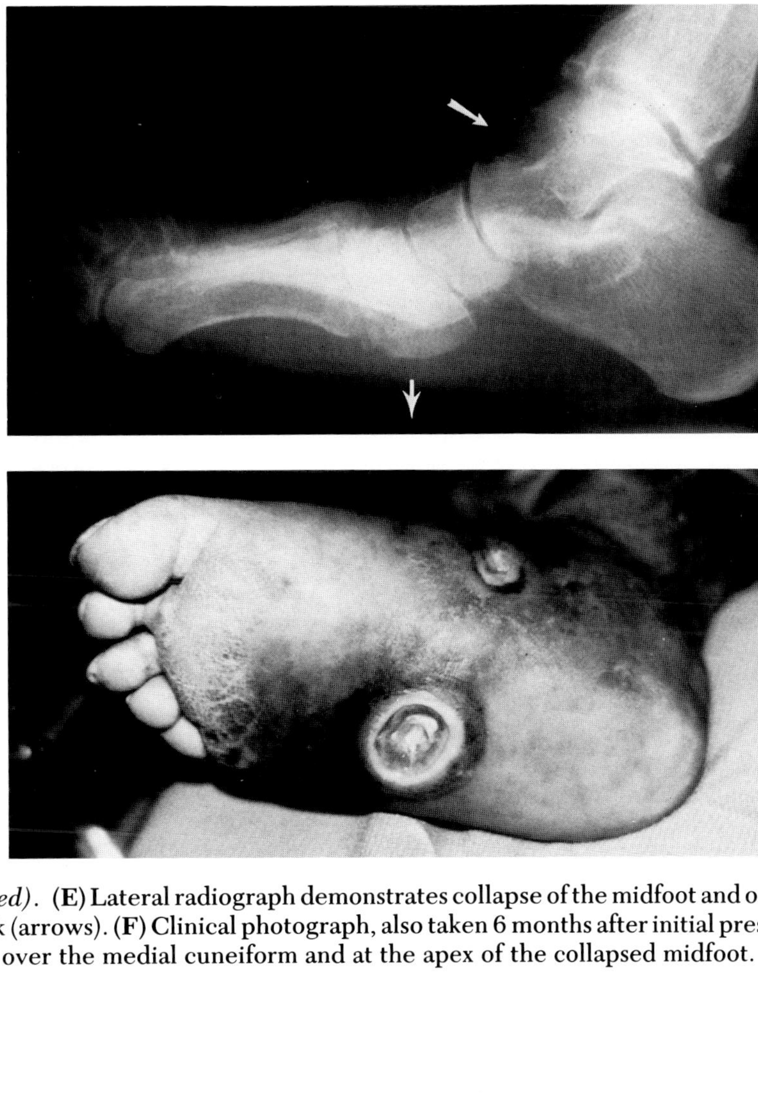

F

Fig. 16-11 *(Continued)*. **(E)** Lateral radiograph demonstrates collapse of the midfoot and osteolytic destruction of the talar neck (arrows). **(F)** Clinical photograph, also taken 6 months after initial presentation, reveals necrotic ulceration over the medial cuneiform and at the apex of the collapsed midfoot.

Pattern III: Naviculocuneiform, Talonavicular, and Calcaneocuboid Joints

Pattern III osteoarthropathy involves the naviculocuneiform and midtarsal joints. This pattern is frequently characterized by dislocation of the navicular or by disintegration of the naviculocuneiform joints. Sanders and Mrdjenovich found naviculocuneiform, talonavicular, or calcaneocuboid involvement in approximately 32 percent of the affected joints (21/66 sites) in 28 cases.[18] Very early radiographic changes of impending Charcot joint destruction may be evidenced by osteolysis of the naviculocuneiform joints. Typical fragmentation, osteolysis, and sharply defined osseous debris are visible on the lateral radiograph (Fig. 16-12). Observation of this finding should signal the need for immediate non-weight-bearing cast immobilization of the foot. Ignoring this finding will result in progressive deterioration of the lesser tarsal bones and ultimately in collapse of the midfoot with *rocker bottom* deformity.

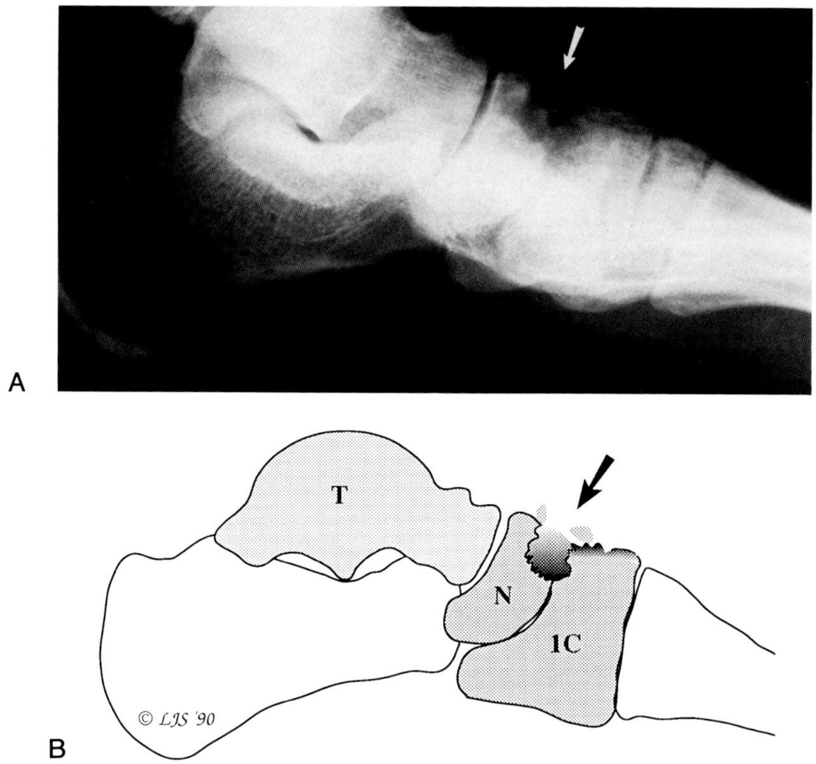

Fig. 16-12. (**A**) Osteolytic destruction of the naviculocuneiform joints (arrow). Fragmentation, osteolysis, and sharply defined osseous debris are noted. (**B**) Graphic illustration of radiographic findings. T, talus; N, navicular; 1C, medial cuneiform.

Isolated midtarsal joint dislocations associated with neuropathic diabetes have been reported by several authors.[27,40,43] Lesko and Maurer reported their experience with eight talonavicular dislocations, in which dislocations of the navicular were described as inferomedial, mediodorsal, or medial.[43] Fragmentation of bone frequently accompanies these dislocations. Talonavicular dislocation may be seen alone or in association with involvement of the naviculocuneiform joints, disintegration of the cuneiform bones, or with deterioration of the head and neck of the talus (Fig. 16-13).

Pattern IV: The Ankle Joint

Pattern IV neuropathic osteoarthropathy affects the ankle joint and accounts for only 3 to 10 percent of the reported cases.[13,15,18,20] This pattern of involvement almost always results in severe structural deformity and functional instability of the ankle joint. Charcot joint may develop rapidly "without any appreciable external cause," with sudden spontaneous swelling and localized redness of the foot and ankle. Patients will initially notice swelling and deformity of the affected ankle, with little pain. They often continue to walk on the affected limb until the collateral ligaments stretch or tear, and there is erosion of bone and cartilage with collapse of the joint. Steindler's observations of foot and ankle fractures in patients with tabetic joints caused him to conclude that "the greatest pathological changes correspond to the maximum of mechanical stress . . . in the direction of the greatest weight-bearing."[35] He noted two types of destruction: one in the direction of the long axis of the leg, breaking down the talus and calcaneus; the other evidenced by collapse of the forefoot and tarsus. Free bodies were seen in the ankle joint in 8 of 21 cases.

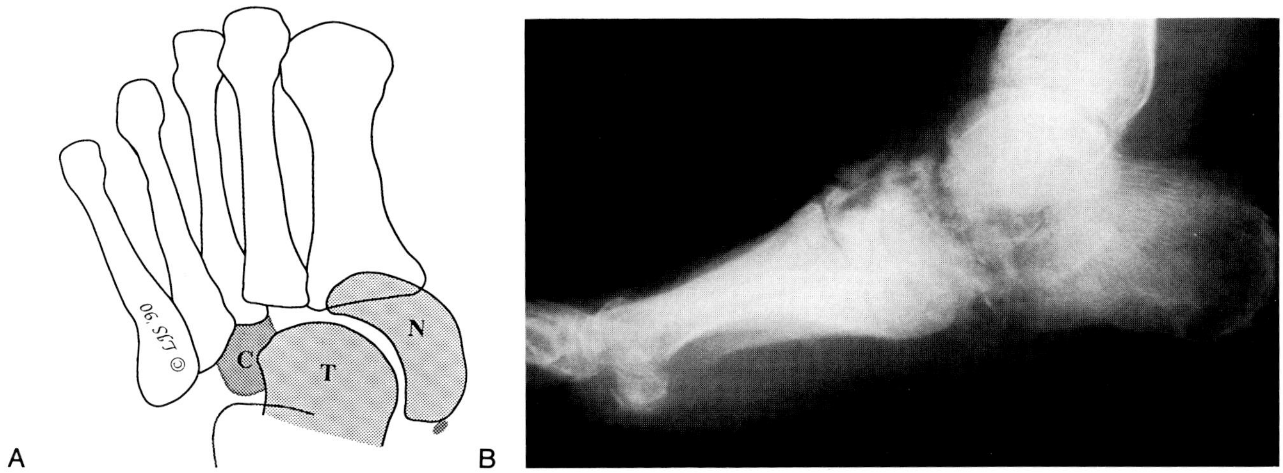

Fig. 16-13. (**A**) Graphic illustration of talonavicular dislocation with inferomedial displacement of the navicular. C, cuboid; T, talus; N, navicular. (**B**) Lateral radiograph of another patient reveals disintegration of the talonavicular and calcaneocuboid joints.

Harris and Brand elaborated on Steindler's pathomechanical theory of tabetic joints noting that if during weight bearing "the posture of the foot is disturbed by external forces or abnormal paralysis an abnormal position results, and the new weight stream will cross the trabecular lines so that minor fractures occur more readily and ligaments may rupture."[31] Therefore, even trivial trauma associated with an ankle sprain or a relatively minor fracture may result in instability of the ankle joint with resultant collapse and disintegration.[20,27,31] Miller and Lichtman described a case in which total destruction of the ankle joint resulted following surgical intervention for a fractured medial malleolus.[20] Johnson reported the case of a 55-year-old woman who 8 weeks following a sprained left ankle developed complete displacement of the medial malleolus with grinding away of one-half of the talus and part of the distal end of the tibia.[27]

Harris and Brand graphically described "a relatively rapid and catastrophic disintegration of the proximal tarsal bones allowing the tibia to grind its way through the foot to the ground, or to become dislocated to one side and rest on the ground with the foot attached as an appendage."[31]

Horowitz focused attention on the striking pathologic feature of bone and cartilage debris (detritus) ground into the synovial membrane, subsynovial tissue, and articular cartilage of the ankle joint, which may help to establish the diagnosis of neuroarthropathy even in its earliest phases. He points out that these findings may be present before any radiographic and clinical evidence is demonstrable.[76]

Rapid and catastrophic disintegration of the ankle joint is illustrated in the following case, where sepsis appears to have played a role in the pathogenesis. A 59-year-old neuropathic woman with a 15-year history of diabetes mellitus presented with the chief complaint of pain, redness, and swelling of her left foot and ankle of 1-week duration. She reported no history of trauma; however, she had been recently treated by her family doctor for an "infected blister" on her left fifth toe. Infection resolved promptly, but shortly thereafter pain and swelling developed over the lateral aspect of her foot and ankle. She had bounding pedal pulses and extensive peripheral neuropathy. Radiographs revealed osteopenia of the tarsal bones with evidence of osteoarthritis of the tarsometatarsal joints. Radionucleotide scan with ^{99m} technetium-labeled methylene diphosphonate revealed very high uptake in the left ankle and tarsal bones as well as marked uptake in the asymptomatic right ankle. Blood cultures and ankle joint aspirate obtained on admission grew *Staphylococcus aureus*. The infectious disease consultant presumed that a septic arthritis was overlying a diabetic neuro-

A 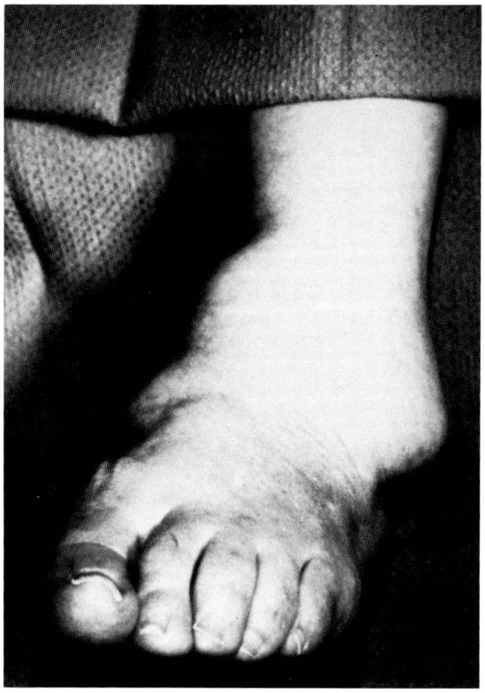

B 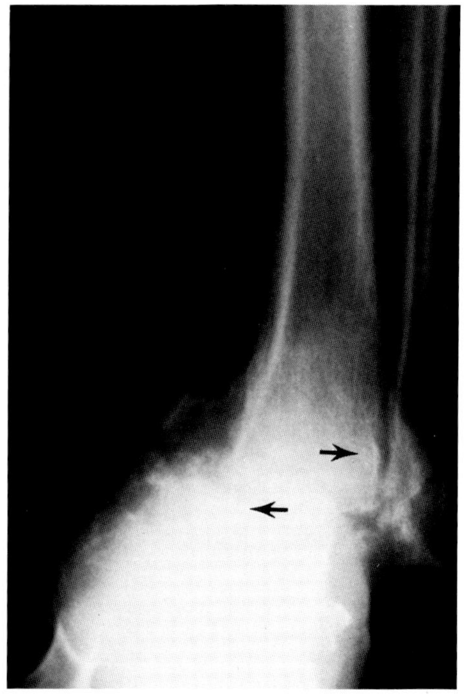

Fig. 16-14. (**A**) Clinical photograph of an unstable neuropathic left ankle, with lateral bulging. (**B**) Anteroposterior radiograph reveals extensive joint destruction with fragmentation of bone. Arrows represent dislocation of the joint with the foot displaced to the medial side of the leg.

pathic arthropathy.[77] Despite appropriate treatment with parenteral antibiotics, bed rest, elevation of the limb, and non-weight-bearing casts, progressive deformity of the left ankle ensued. The clinical picture was characterized by lateral bulging and instability of the ankle, with medial displacement of the foot and fragmentation of bone. Radiographs and clinical photographs revealed progressive and extensive joint destruction with dislocation of the foot to the medial side of the leg (Fig. 16-14).

Another case revealed extensive and rapid destruction of the ankle joint in a 54-year-old neuropathic diabetic man, following a fracture of the fibular malleolus. There was extensive erosion of the calcaneus with collapse of the talus and fragmentation of bone just anterior to the distal tibia. The tibia was grinding its way through the foot to the ground. The onset of osteoarthropathy began when the patient was allowed to ambulate in a short-leg walking cast. Early recognition of the destructive process and strict enforcement of non-weight-bearing would have prevented the severe progression of this Charcot ankle (Fig. 16-15).

Pattern V: The Calcaneus (Posterior Pillar)

Pattern V osteopathy involves fractures of the calcaneus, often with avulsion of the posterior tubercle.[16,67,78] It is the least frequently reported pattern of bone destruction seen in neuropathic diabetes. In their paper on patterns of tarsal disintegration associated with Hansen's disease, Harris and Brand used the positional designation "posterior pillar" to describe calcaneal fractures.[31] They attributed increased vulnerability of the calcaneus in an insensitive foot to (1) increased force on the heel caused by the patient's landing more heavily on an insensitive foot, (2) continued walking on a fractured bone, and (3) previous or concurrent ulceration "which may have weakened the bone by hyperaemic decalcification or may allow infection

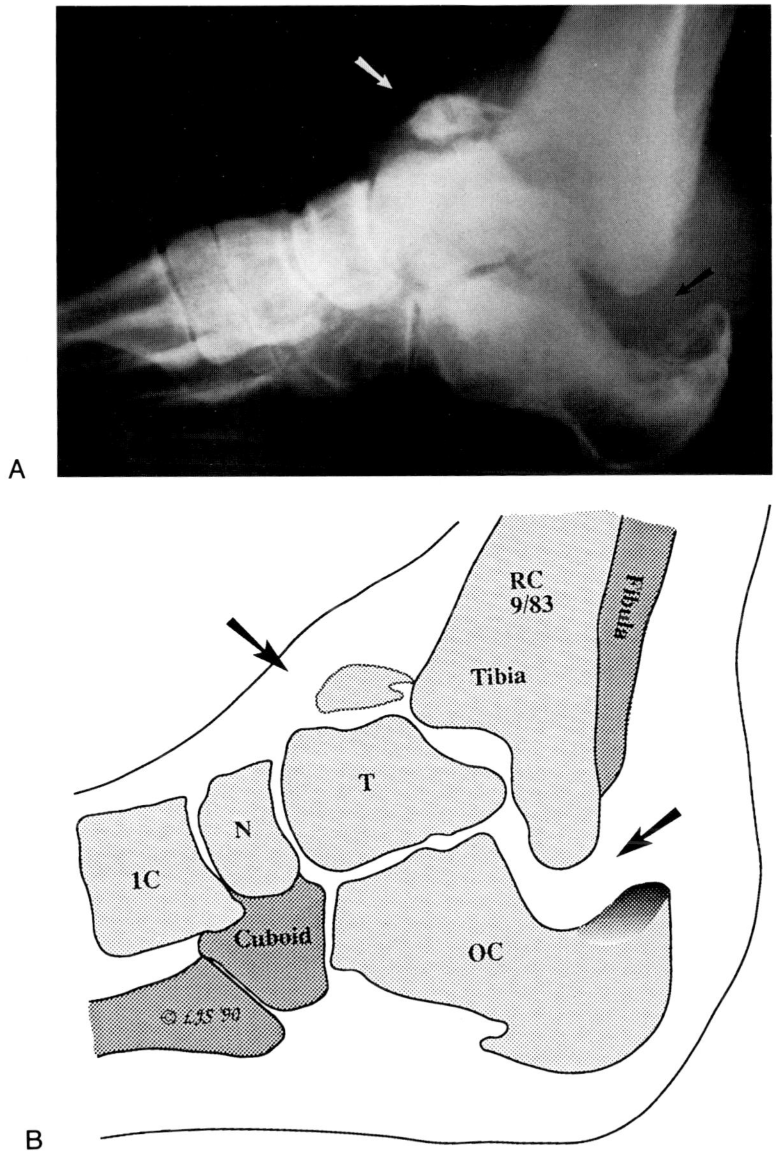

Fig. 16-15. (**A**) Lateral radiograph reveals extensive disintegration of the ankle joint, with the tibia grinding its way through the foot to the ground. Note the extensive erosion of the calcaneus (black arrow) with collapse of the talus and fragmentation of bone (white arrow). (**B**) Graphic illustration of radiographic findings. 1C, medial cuneiform; N, navicular; T, talus; OC, calcaneus.

and osteomyelitis to complicate the fracture."[31] Steroid-induced osteoporosis or postmenopausal osteoporosis, superimposed on the skeletal tissues of a neuropathic diabetic patient may predispose the calcaneus and other tarsal bones to fracture.

Coventry and Rothacker reported a bilateral calcaneal fracture in a 45-year-old neuropathic woman with juvenile-onset diabetes.[78] El-Khoury and Kathol reported on four patients with spontaneous, unusual avulsion fractures of the posterior tubercle of the calcaneus, "where the avulsed fragment migrated superiorly due to the constant pull of the achilles tendon."[67] These patients had diminished pain and vibratory perception. Clohisy and Thompson reported 19 calcaneal fractures in 18 neuropathic juvenile-onset diabetic patients who had no history of major trauma to their extremities. Five of these patients had bilateral calcaneal fractures. In 17 extremities the calcaneal fractures were seen together with fractures of more than one other tarsal bone. Fourteen of the patients in this study underwent renal transplant surgery before the fracture was diagnosed.[16]

In a retrospective review of 55 neuropathic kidney transplant patients at the University of Minnesota, Thompson and associates found a 20 percent incidence of skeletal disease among diabetic patients, with the highest incidence occurring in the third and fourth years after transplantation.[79] They reported seeing three calcaneal fractures in 11 patients with neurotrophic joint disease. The initial manifestation in all patients was a pathologic fracture, usually in a metaphyseal area near a joint. Only later did they see actual joint destruction that seemed to result from the subchondral collapse associated with the initial fracture.

An avulsion fracture of the posterior tubercle of the right calcaneus occurred spontaneously in an active 53-year-old white neuropathic diabetic woman with a 5-year history of diabetes mellitus. She reported hearing a loud crack and feeling a sharp pain in the back of her right heel while walking in the hallway at work. Physical examination revealed a broadened heel with mild swelling, erythema, and elevated skin temperature over the medial and lateral aspects of the heel. Lateral radiographs revealed posterior and superior displacement of the posterior process of the calcaneus (Fig. 16-16). The anteroposterior radiograph of the asymptomatic left foot revealed concentric resorption of the proximal phalanges, a cup-shaped proximal phalangeal base of the hallux, and fragmentation of the second metatarsal head (Fig. 16-5A).

DIAGNOSTIC STUDIES

The diagnosis of DNOAP is primarily dependent on the physician's clinical suspicion of the disease. Medical history, clinical presentation, and radiographic findings should help to narrow down the differential diagnosis. This disorder should be suspected when bone and joint pathology is found in a diabetic patient with loss of protective sensation,

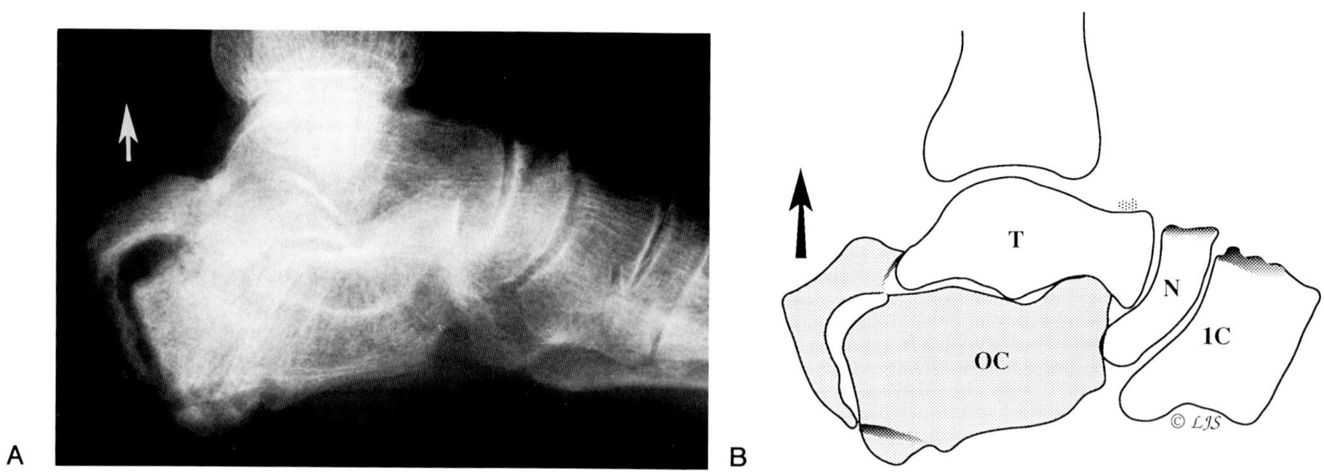

Fig. 16-16. (**A**) Lateral radiograph demonstrates an avulsion fracture of the posterior tubercle of the calcaneus. The arrow points in the direction of pull of the tendo achilles. Early osteolytic changes are seen to affect the naviculocuneiform joint. (**B**) Graphic illustration of radiographic findings. OC, calcaneus; T, talus; N, navicular; 1C, medial cuneiform.

absent deep tendon reflexes, and diminished vibratory sense.

The most specific diagnostic tools for distinguishing between DNOAP and osteomyelitis in the diabetic foot are careful clinical and radiographic examinations, followed by bone biopsy, bone cultures, and histopathologic examination. Positive technetium and gallium bone scans may be seen with osteomyelitis, but they may also be false positive owing to neuropathic bone disease.[66] As noted earlier in our discussion of the pathogenesis of DNOAP, Edmonds and associates demonstrated marked elevation of radiopharmaceutical in all three phases of the ^{99m}technetium-labeled methylene diphosphonate bone scan in neuropathic diabetic patients who had no plantar ulceration or infection.[61] Diffuse and focal uptake of technetium has been reported in neuropathic feet by several authors,[80–83] in areas of active bone turnover and increased bony blood flow, as seen in patients with osteoarthropathy. Positive scans have been reported to sometimes precede radiographic changes.[80] Gallium-67 citrate, which accumulates in sites of infection, has also been reported to localize in noninfected neuropathic bone.[82,84,85]

Indium-111 labeled white blood cell scintigraphy, however, has been shown to have a high specificity as well as a very high negative predictive value for osteomyelitis.[86–91] Keenan and associates reported that using this technique the sensitivity for diagnosis of osteomyelitis is equivalent to that of three-phase bone scintigraphy (100 percent sensitivity).[88] The specificity for osteomyelitis with indium-111 has been reported to be from 78 to 89 percent,[87–89] compared with 38 to 75 percent for three-phase bone scans.[88,91] Schauwecker and associates found that in the absence of infection, indium-111 leukocytes do not accumulate in neuropathic bone.[86,87] In diabetic patients with osteoarthropathy complicated by suspected osteomyelitis, Maurer and colleagues found leukocyte imaging to have an 89 percent specificity for bone infection.[89]

When osteomyelitis is suspected in a patient with active osteoarthropathy, the most specific diagnostic technique, next to bone biopsy, appears to be the indium-111 white blood cell scan, which if negative, reliably excludes the presence of osteomyelitis. When positive, it should be combined with a bone scan, using Shauwecker's protocol to accurately localize the site of infection to either bone or soft tissue.[86] This should then be followed by appropriate bone cultures.

THERAPEUTIC STRATEGIES

Appropriate management of the Charcot foot should be based on the acuteness of symptoms, the anatomic pattern of bone and joint destruction, the degree of involvement (e.g., deformity, fractures, bone fragmentation, and instability), and presence of infection. Lesko and Maurer at the University of California, San Francisco, have outlined an objective rationale of treatment based on the chronicity of injury, anatomic alignment, and associated degree of deformity.[43] For acute injuries with acceptable alignment, they suggest immobilization and protective weight bearing to prevent further progression of neuropathic joint destruction. For acute dislocation with marked deformity and little bone fragmentation, reduction and surgical arthrodesis may be indicated. For chronic dislocation, with severe deformity and bone fragmentation, they suggest custom-molded shoes with stiff rocker soles and patellar tendon weight-bearing braces. In this last category, surgical treatment is recommended only as a last resort if soft tissue breakdown cannot be prevented by therapeutic footwear and bracing. Lesko and Maurer emphasized that surgical reduction and arthrodesis should be reserved for the acute dislocation and for correction of deformities so severe that soft tissue breakdown cannot be prevented by footwear and bracing alone.[43]

Patients who present with acute symptoms of DNOAP, as evidenced by erythema, swelling, and bone/joint destruction, are best treated by early hospitalization, bed rest, non-weight-bearing and cast immobilization. Surgical intervention during the atrophic phase should be avoided, as it will only accelerate the destructive process. If the acute injury goes unnoticed and unprotected, then luxation, fragmentation, architectural collapse, hypertrophic bone formation, and deformity will follow.

The aim of treatment should be to *obtain stability* of the foot with no excessive pressure on the skin from a bony prominence.[21,27,40] The key to treatment is *prevention,* with avoidance of further trauma and inflammation until the soft tissues heal. "Short of complete rest in bed nothing less than immobilization in a plaster boot is adequate."[31]

Contrary to prevailing opinion, progressive destruction of the neuropathic foot can be halted if recognized early enough.[31,49] The appropriate way to treat the Charcot foot is first to prevent its occurrence. Careful history and physical examination directed toward risk assessment and stratification will help to identify/prioritize those patients at greatest risk. Patients in their fifth and sixth decade who have been diabetic for more than 10 years, and who demonstrate peripheral neuropathy with loss of protective sensation are prime candidates for the development of neuropathic osteoarthropathy. Added risk factors include the presence of nephropathy and retinopathy. Patients with triopathy are probably at greatest risk.[13,16]

Early recognition of DNOAP with a *high index of suspicion* is vitally important. It is paramount that the physician and patient look for areas of mild swelling, increased skin temperature, deformity or instability of the foot and ankle. *Local temperature assessment* is valuable for monitoring tissue damage in the insensitive foot. Areas of increased warmth felt by the patient or family member correspond to areas of inflammation in the insensitive limb that are at risk for bony resorption and ulceration. A hand-held infrared digital thermometer is a useful tool for the physician to monitor the inflammatory response in insensate patients. Any increase in skin temperature greater than 2°C should be considered a significant finding indicating impending osteoarthropathy or preulcerative inflammation.[66] Degenerative changes in any foot with proven peripheral sensory impairment are indicative of neuropathic arthropathy.[47]

In contrast to Charcot's classic description of a painless arthropathy, *pain* is often an associated feature, but it appears to be less severe than would normally be expected in view of the pathologic changes present. Elevation of the limb to reduce edema, cessation of weight bearing, prolonged cast immobilization, and comprehensive patient education are basic components of effective treatment.

Cast Immobilization — For How Long?

The duration of cast immobilization should be determined by the skin temperature as well as the radiographic evidence of consolidation of fractures and fragmented bone. Warmth of the skin indicates persistent inflammation that requires continued immobilization. This period may be as short as 2 to 3 months, or perhaps as long as 4 to 6 months, depending on the extent of involvement. Attention should be directed to the "asymptomatic" limb with respect to the development of bilateral osteoarthropathy. Clohisy and Thompson observed that when an affected extremity was prevented from weight bearing, involvement of the contralateral limb became evident after an average of 4.5 months. They therefore recommend prophylactic immobilization of the contralateral extremity with a protective cast or orthosis.[16]

Braces, Total Contact Orthoses, and Shoes

A patella tendon weight-bearing brace (PTB),[16,43] used together with therapeutic shoes may effectively decrease load on the foot. Clohisy and Thompson suggest short-term prophylactic protection of the "uninvolved" extremity with a patella weight-bearing cast or orthosis during the period of cast immobilization of the involved extremity. For long-term protection of the affected extremity they institute a calf-containment patellar tendon-bearing orthosis.[16] These braces are expensive and must be custom made. Patient compliance with the PTB may be somewhat less than desired, as patients often find them to be "inconvenient" or "awkward" to put on. Total contact orthoses are less expensive, well-tolerated by the patient, and effective in evenly distributing pressure across the bottom of the foot. Custom-molded accommodative orthoses should be individually fabricated for each patient. The thickness of materials used is determined by the degree of foot deformity as well as by the intended application, for example, for use in a healing shoe, super extra-depth shoe, or custom-molded shoe. Various combinations of materials are well suited for the purposes of molding, shock absorption, and retention of original shape (memory). Medium density Plastazote, a closed-cell cross-linked polyethylene, molded to the foot and laminated to PPT (Professional Protective Technology, Inc., a subsidiary of the Langer Biomechanics Group, Inc., Deer Park, NY) is a functional and cost effective combination of materials that should be considered when prescribing orthoses for patients with DNOAP.

Therapeutic shoes are essential to the management of patients with DNOAP, both for prevention and for maintenance therapy. Shoes should be used only after adequate medical or surgical management with crutch-assisted non-weight-bearing immobilization of the extremity. Ulcers should be healed or very shallow before allowing ambulation in shoes. An interim healing shoe can be fabricated using a custom-molded orthosis in a surgical shoe.[22-25]

Prescription footwear and orthoses should be considered essential for the management of diabetic patients with loss of protective sensation. Cavanagh and associates have reported a significant reduction in the incidence of plantar lesions following the provision of special footwear to a group of high risk neuropathic patients.[92] Extra-depth, super extra-depth, and thermal moldable shoes, with soft leather uppers and well-molded insoles, represent a cost-effective approach to management of patients with mild to moderate deformity. Custom-molded shoes, which are much more expensive, are required when there is moderate to severe deformity that precludes the use of other types of commercially available footwear.[22,24]

SURGICAL MANAGEMENT

Once the acute inflammatory stage has subsided, deformities that predispose to shearing stress and ulceration should be corrected. When surgery is attempted during the early stages of Charcot joint development, the operative trauma further contributes to the process and is destined to fail.[22,44,93] Most reports advise surgical intervention only if the deformity is severe, the foot/ankle is unstable, or weight bearing is difficult.[20,27,44,93] In Johnson's series, surgery on the feet was limited to excision of bony prominences, except in one patient in whom two unsuccessful attempts at midtarsal fusion were made.[27] In Newman's series it was found that there was always an adequate blood supply to allow simple operations to be undertaken. He recommends prolonged immobilization during the active phase of the disease followed by "removing of the lump," ensuring that there is no excessive pressure on the underlying skin.[79]

Surgical Techniques

The techniques employed for the treatment of chronic neuropathic plantar ulceration generally involve excision of bony prominences through either a plantar or medial-lateral approach. Decompression of the ulcer is often sufficient to prevent recurrence even when there is residual deformity of the foot. The surgeon should consider excision of the ulcer, resection of underlying bony prominence, and primary closure of the wound as a rational and successful method of treatment associated with minimal morbidity.[94]

Patients are admitted to the hospital for bed rest, medical management, local wound care, and non-weight-bearing for several days before surgery. The initial approach to treatment should be directed at metabolic control, reduction of both the size of the ulcer and peripheral edema, as well as treatment of possible infection. Daily debridement of the wound and saline wet-to-dry dressing changes will help to maximize the condition of the wound before surgery. Appropriate wound cultures should be performed, with Gram stain to assist in the selection of antibiotics. Intravenous cefuroxime and ampicillin-sulbactam are reasonable choices for prophylaxis and should be started preoperatively on the day of surgery. A fusiform excision of the ulcer is carried out in the direction of the long axis of the foot, with the length approximately 3.5 times the width, and approximately a 30° angle at the apices. The incision is then directed in a longitudinal manner through the plantar fascia, directly over the bony prominence. The bone is widely exposed with a periosteal elevator and generously resected with power instrumentation. A power burr is helpful to make the bone smooth and concave. Resected bone should be sent for culture and for histopathologic examination. The wound

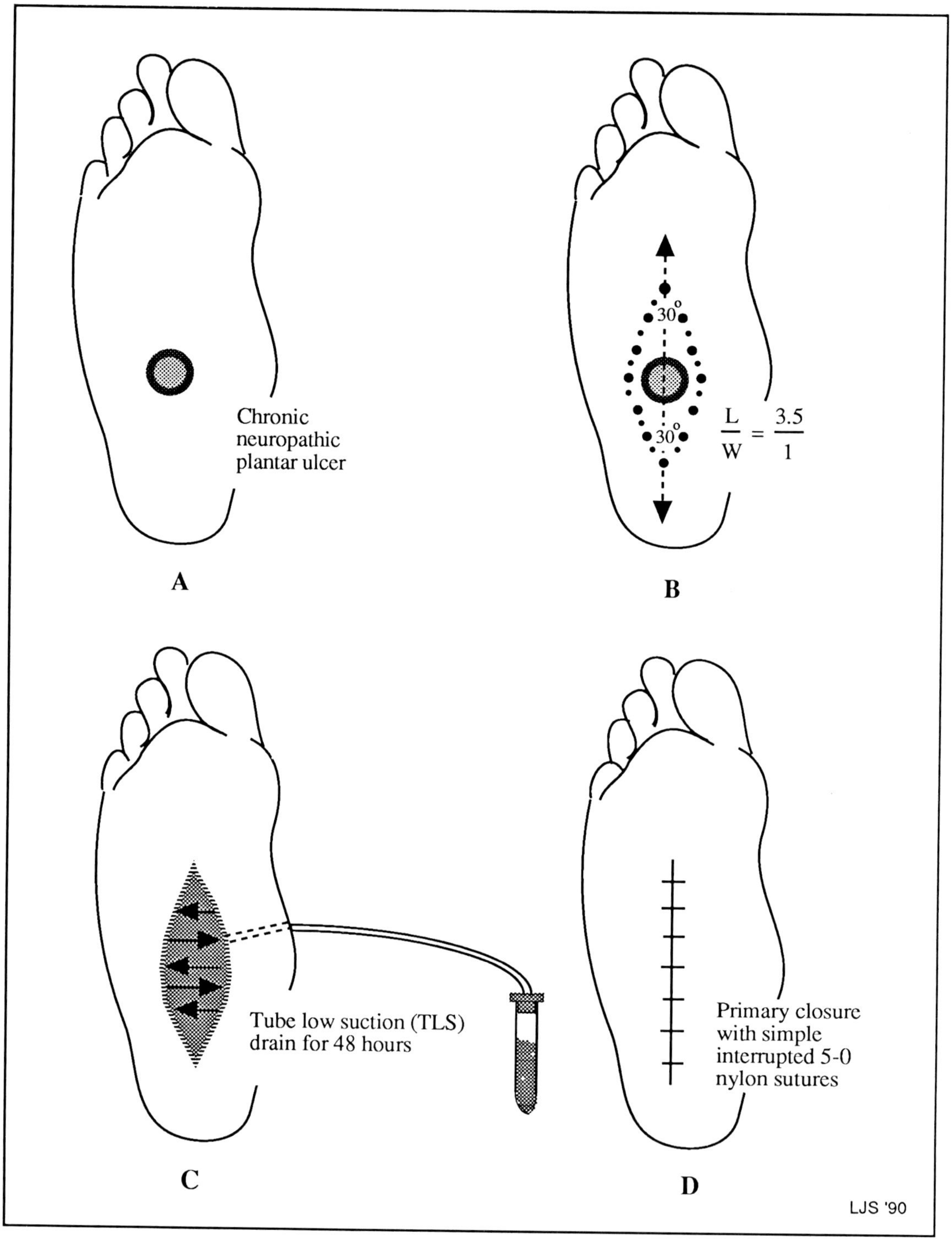

Fig. 16-17. (**A–D**) Illustrated technique for the surgical management of chronic plantar ulceration associated with diabetic neuropathic osteoarthropathy. (Refer to the text and Fig. 16-18 for description.)

should be inspected carefully for fragments/spicules of bone and irrigated thoroughly. The wound is cultured and then closed primarily, in layers, over a tube low-suction drain. The skin should not be undermined, as this will result in sloughing of the skin edges and delayed healing. The patient is placed in a well-padded, non-weight-bearing posterior splint for 2 weeks, or until sutures are removed (Figs. 16-17 to 16-19). Cast immobilization is then required for a minimum of 8 to 12 weeks, until all warmth has subsided and there is radiographic evidence of consolidation of bone. If hyperemia persists, then an additional period of immobilization is required. At the second cast change an orthotist should be available to make plaster impressions of the feet for custom-molded shoes. Appropriate timing for the making of plaster impressions of the feet is important, as it often requires a minimum of 6 to 8 weeks for manufacture of the shoes. Therapeutic shoes should be available for the patient to wear on removal of the final cast. If, however, shoes are not available, an interim healing shoe can be fabricated from a surgical shoe with a custom-molded insole.[22]

A medial or lateral surgical approach can also be employed for access to bony prominences, as illustrated in the case of a patient in whom a chronic neuropathic plantar ulcer was present beneath the medial cuneiform and first metatarsal base of the right foot. The lateral radiograph revealed collapse of the medial arch with a rocker bottom deformity of the foot. Fragmentation of bone was seen on the dorsum of the foot at the level of the talonavicular, naviculocuneiform, and tarsometatarsal articulations. Surgery was performed in this case after satisfactory healing of the ulcer with non-weight-bearing and local wound care. A direct medial longitudinal approach was carried out over the first metatarsal-cuneiform joint, and the prominent plantar bone was resected with an osteotome (Fig. 16-20).

Stabilization of Neuropathic Joints

The results of surgical therapy directed at stabilizing neuropathic joints have been uniformly poor despite the use of acceptable surgical and technical operative procedures.[44,78] Attempts at open reduction and rigid internal fixation of subluxed/dislocated joints, especially the tarsometatarsal joints and ankle joint should be approached with caution. This is often met with failure, as evidenced by increased destruction of bone, redislocation, delayed union, and altered foot mechanics that result in subluxation or disintegration of more proximal articulations.[27,40] Contrary to most reports, Banks and McGlamry state that in their experience "arthrodesis in the Charcot patient rarely fails."[95] However, they do indicate in their case presentation that following "arthrodesis of the tarsometatarsal and lesser tarsal areas" the patient returned to the operating room on two separate occasions, for arthrodesis of the talonavicular joint and then the naviculocuneiform joints.

Achieving anatomic reduction of spontaneous TMT dislocations in the neuropathic diabetic patient is not as critical as it is in the case of non-neuropathic individuals who sustain violent trauma to the foot. In the latter case, incomplete reduction of the fracture or dislocation will frequently result in permanent disability in the form of chronic pain, deformity, and difficulty with wearing shoes.[96] With respect to the surgical management of pattern II osteoarthropathy, the risk-to-benefit ratio is far greater than in the nondiabetic patient. Painful arthritis is generally not a problem, and a reasonable amount of deformity can be accommodated with a well-constructed custom-molded shoe.

Transmetatarsal amputation should be considered for definitive surgical management of chronic, intractable plantar ulceration and infection associated with pattern I neuropathic osteoarthropathy. This operation has a low morbidity and results in a structurally sound stump that is functional, cosmetically acceptable and easy to fit in a shoe.[97]

Complications of Surgery

A common complication of ablative foot surgery, notably metatarsal head resection, ray resection, or partial amputation of the forefoot (toes and rays), is the shifting of plantar pressure and shear stress to adjacent weight-bearing structures with the development of transfer ulceration[97] and/or pathologic fractures. The development of pathologic fractures will be briefly illustrated in the following two cases.

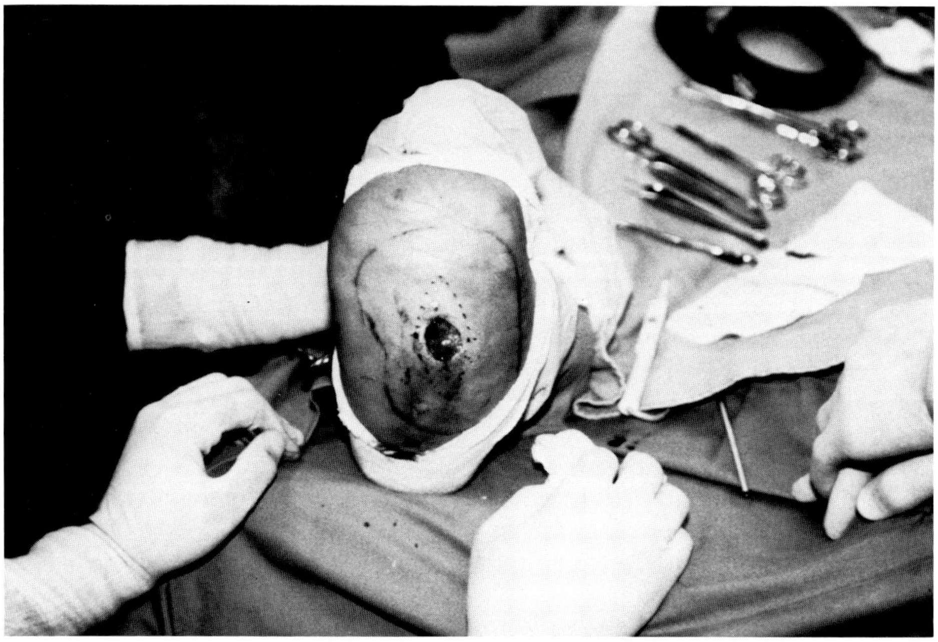

A

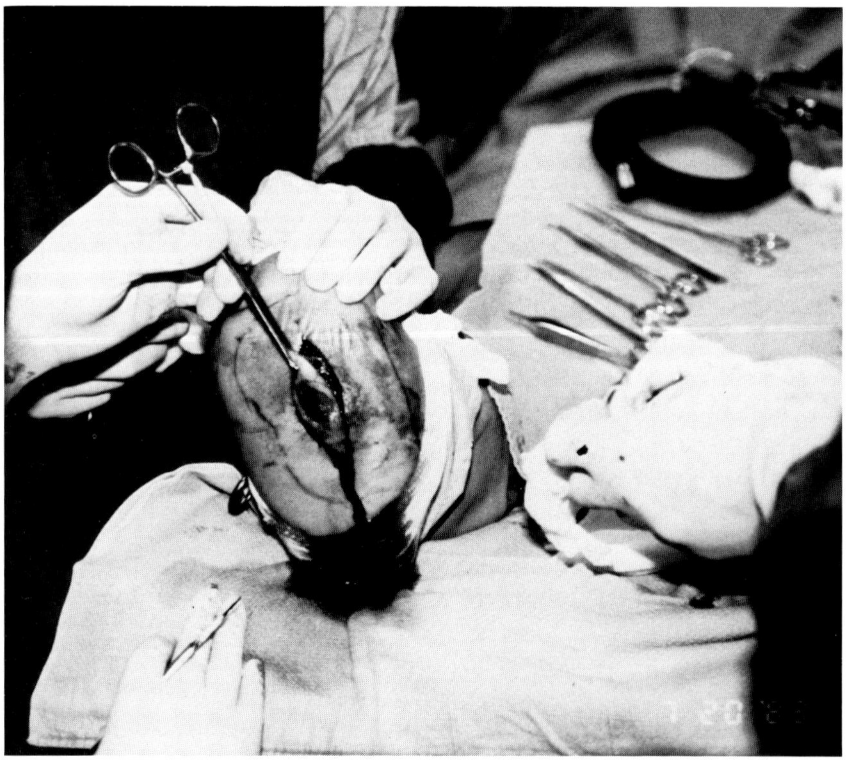

B

Fig. 16-18. Operative technique. (**A**) A fusiform skin incision surrounding the plantar ulcer is planned with a skin marker. The length of the ellipse is approximately 3.5 times the width. (**B**) The incision is carried down to the level of the subcutaneous tissue, and the skin and ulcer are excised. *(Figure continues.)*

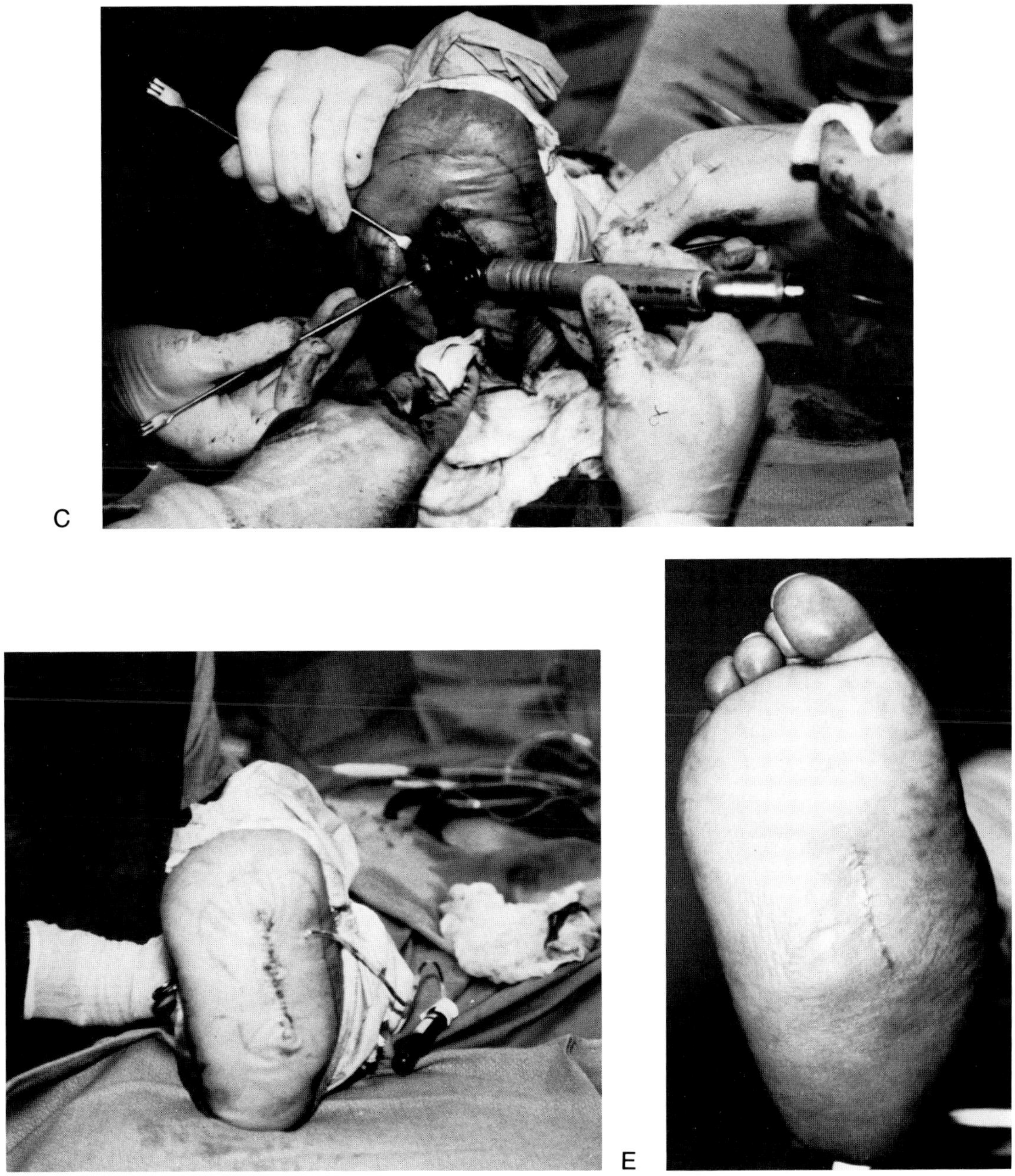

Fig. 16-18 *(Continued)*. (**C**) The incision is carried down to bone, and the prominent bone is resected with power instruments. (**D**) The wound is closed primarily over a tube low-suction drain. (**E**) Appearance of the left foot 4 months postoperatively. There is a well-healed incision with no recurrence of ulceration.

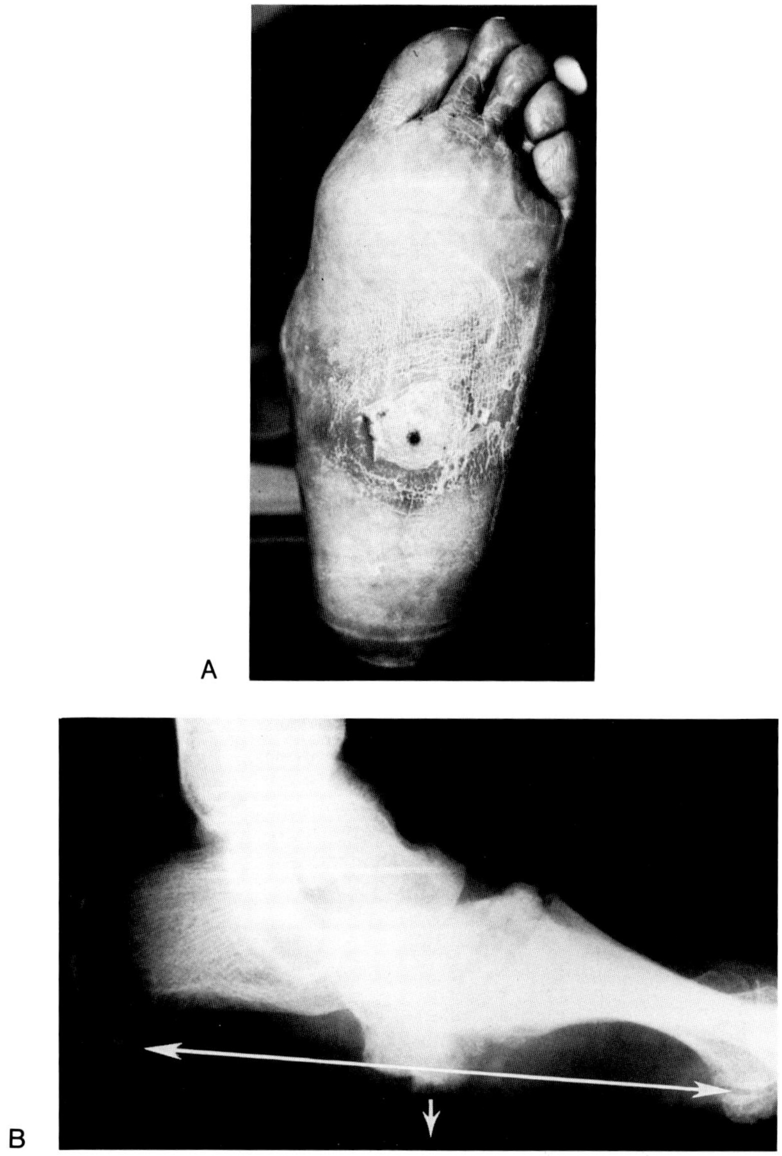

Fig. 16-19. **(A)** Preoperative photograph revealing site of recurrent plantar ulceration. **(B)** Preoperative non-weight-bearing lateral radiograph of same patient reveals prominence of the cuboid, corresponding to the location of plantar ulceration. Cuboid projects down (downward arrow), below the level of the heel and ball of the foot (horizontal line), creating a rocker bottom deformity with increased vertical force and shear stress at the apex of the rocker. *(Figure continues.)*

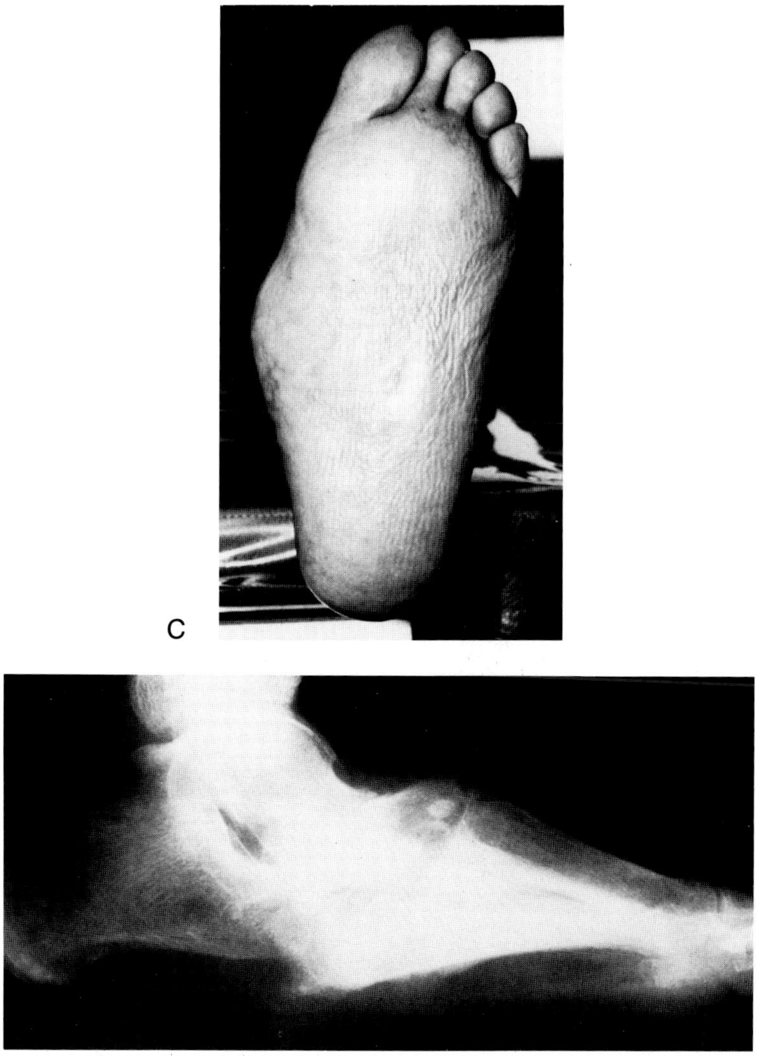

C

D

Fig. 16-19 *(Continued)*. **(C)** Appearance of the patient's left foot, 4 months postoperatively. All swelling has resolved and the patient has returned to full weight-bearing in custom-molded shoes. The plantar incision is barely visible. **(D)** Lateral radiograph, also taken 4 months postoperatively, reveals coalescence and reconstruction of bone, with remodeling of the midfoot. The amount of resected plantar bone can be appreciated when compared with the preoperative radiograph.

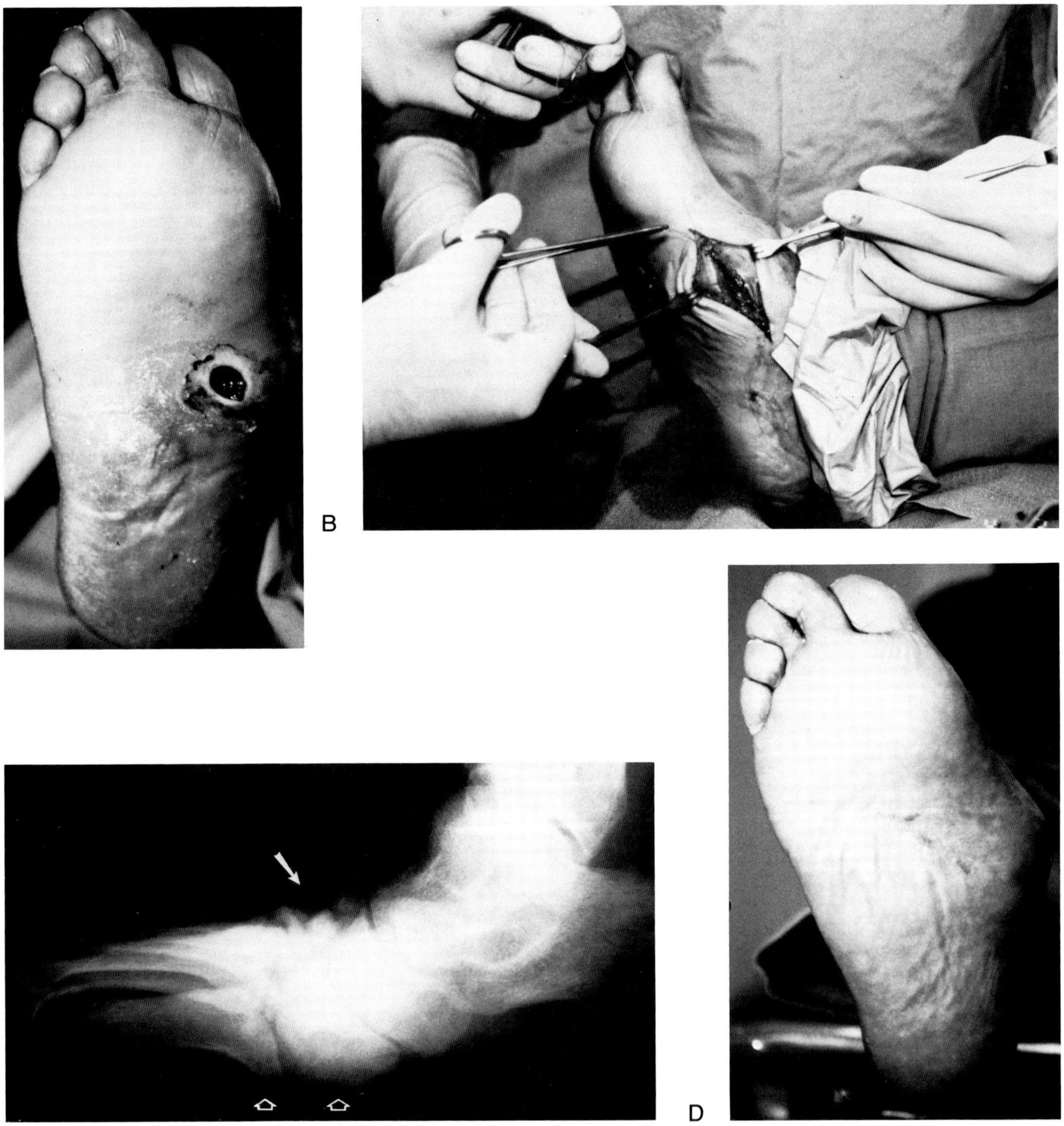

A B C D

Fig. 16-20. Medial surgical approach for the treatment of plantar ulceration in the Charcot foot. (**A**) Neuropathic plantar ulceration beneath the medial cuneiform-first metatarsal base. (**B**) Intraoperative photograph demonstrating a direct medial approach over the first metatarsal-cuneiform joint. Prominent bone was resected with an osteotome. (**C**) Postoperative lateral radiograph. Open arrows point to the site of resected bone. White arrow points to fragmentation of bone on the dorsum of the foot. (**D**) Clinical photograph taken almost 3 years postoperatively. The patient has remained lesion free.

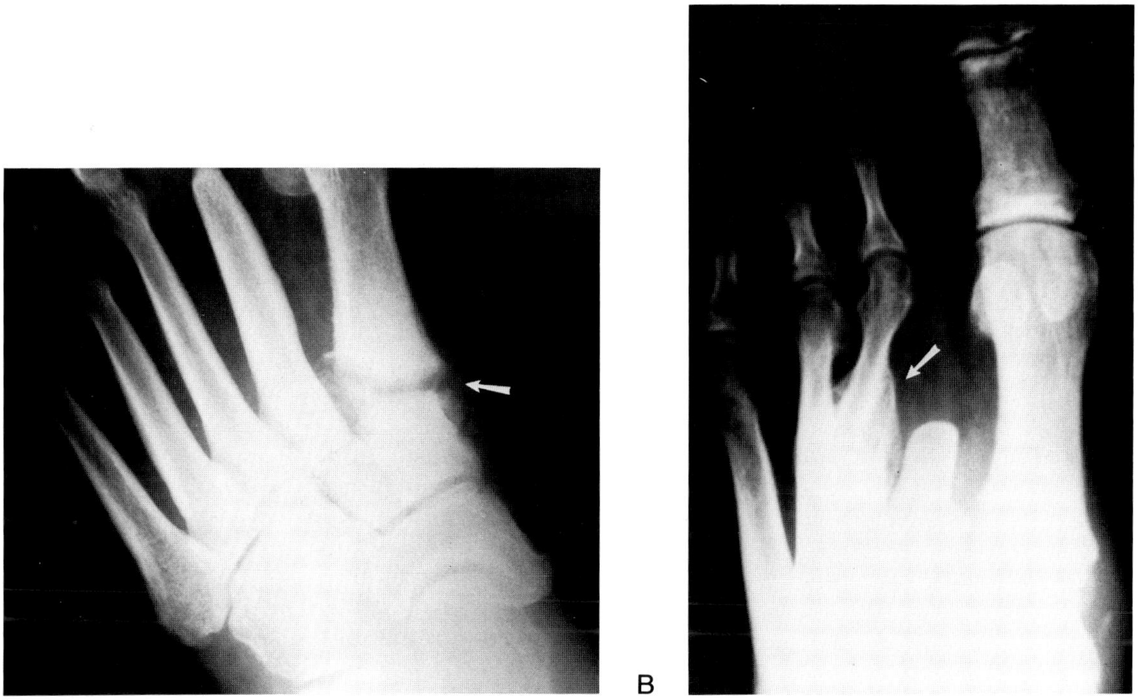

A B

Fig. 16-21. Pathologic fractures resulting from surgical alteration of the forefoot. (**A**) Fracture at the base of the first metatarsal following resection of the second metatarsal head. (**B**) Healing fracture of the third metatarsal shaft following partial resection of the second ray.

A 35-year-old black, neuropathic type 1 diabetic man developed a fracture at the base of his left first metatarsal within 16 months of the resection of his second metatarsophalangeal joint for treatment of osteomyelitis associated with chronic plantar ulceration. The second patient developed a pathologic fracture of the third metatarsal shaft following partial resection of the second ray (Fig. 16-21).

Structural or functional alteration of the neuropathic foot, resulting in limited joint mobility, mechanical instability, decreased weight-bearing surface area, or bony deformity has the potential for causing soft tissue disruption and pathologic fractures. Surgical fusion of the tarsometatarsal joints may result in increased stress on the naviculocuneiform, midtarsal, subtalar, and ankle joints, perhaps owing to the effect of a longer, more rigid lever arm. The proximal tarsal joints may demonstrate acute destructive changes within a short period of time following resumption of full weight-bearing and daily activities. Without addressing the underlying etiologic factors responsible for the structural collapse of the foot, arthrodesis is at best a stopgap measure, which should be reserved for acute, unstable dislocations of the foot.

Postoperative infection is one of the greatest hazards following surgery on any neuropathic joint.[27] It can result in further destruction of bone followed by total collapse of the foot/ankle, and ultimately in loss of limb. Surgical technique, extent of dissection, length of operation, and use of internal fixation devices all affect postoperative morbidity.

ACKNOWLEDGMENTS

The authors wish to express their appreciation to Georges A. Hoché, M.D., Chief, Surgical Service, Department of Veterans Affairs Medical Center, Lebanon, PA, for his assistance in translating J.M. Charcot's original paper on neuropathic arthropathies. Mack Sexton, M.D., Department of Anatomic Pathology, The Milton S. Hershey Medical Center, Hershey, PA, graciously assisted in the preparation of the photomicrographs used in this chapter. Special recognition is extended to Mrs. Roxanne Felli, library technician, and Mrs. Barbara E. Deaven, medical librarian, Department of Veterans Affairs Medical Center, Lebanon, PA, for their invaluable assistance in reviewing the medical literature.

REFERENCES

1. Charcot JM: Lectures on the diseases of the nervous system: Lecture IV, On some visceral derangements in locomotor ataxia. Arthropathies of ataxic patients. Sigeison G (ed and trans). The New Sydenham Society, London, 1881
2. Charcot JM: Sur quelques arthropathies qui paraissent dépendre d'une lésion du cerveau ou de la moelle épiniére. Arch Physiol Norm et Pathol 1:161, 1868
3. Charcot JM: On certain arthropathies apparently related to a lesion of the brain or spinal cord. Hoché GA, Sanders LJ (eds and trans). 1990 (in press)
4. Guillain G: J. M. Charcot 1825–1893 His Life—His Work. Bailey P (ed and trans). Paul B. Hoeber, New York, 1959
5. Wartenberg R: Neuropathic joint disease. JAMA 111:2044, 1938
6. Mitchell JK: On a new practice in acute and chronic rheumatism. Am J Med Sci 8:55, 1831
7. Delano PJ: The pathogenesis of Charcot's joint. Am J Roentgen 56:189, 1946
8. Brower AC, Allman RM: Neuropathic osteoarthropathy in the adult. p. 1. In Taveras JM, Ferrucci JT (eds): Radiology: Diagnosis-Imaging-Intervention. Vol. 5, Skeletal Radiology. JB Lippincott, Philadelphia, 1989
9. Brower AC, Allman RM: Pathogenesis of the neurotrophic joint: neurotraumatic vs. neurovascular. Radiology 139:349, 1981
10. Brower AC, Allman RM: The neuropathic joint: a neurovascular bone disorder. Radiol Clin North Am 19:571, 1981
11. Jordan WR: Neuritic manifestations in diabetes mellitus. Arch Intern Med 57:307, 1936
12. Clouse ME, Gramm HF, Legg M, Flood T: Diabetic osteoarthropathy: clinical and roentgenographic observations in 90 cases. Am J Roent 121: 22, 1974
13. Sinha S, Munichoodappa C, Kozak GP: Neuroarthropathy (Charcot joints) in diabetes mellitus. Clinical study of 101 cases. Medicine 52:191, 1972
14. Forgács S: Clinical picture of diabetic osteoarthropathy. Acta Diabet Latina 13:111, 1976
15. Cofield RH, Morison MJ, Beabout JW: Diabetic neuroarthropathy in the foot: patient characteristics and patterns of radiographic change. Foot Ankle 4:15, 1983
16. Clohisy DR, Thompson RC: Fractures associated with neuropathic arthropathy in adults who have juvenile-onset diabetes. J Bone Joint Surg 70A: 1192, 1988
17. Classen JN: Neuropathic arthropathy with ulceration. Ann Surgery 159:891, 1964
18. Sanders LJ, Mrdjenovich D: Diabetic neuropathic osteoarthropathy: an analysis of 28 cases. (in press)
19. Soto-Hall R, Haldeman KO: The diagnosis of neuropathic joint disease (Charcot joint): an analysis of 40 cases. JAMA 114:2076, 1940
20. Miller DS, Lichtman WF: Diabetic neuropathic arthropathy of feet. Arch Surg 70:513, 1955
21. Norman A, Robbins H, Milgram JE: The acute neuropathic arthropathy—a rapid, severely disorganizing form of arthritis. Radiology 90:1159, 1968
22. Frykberg RG, Kozak GP: Neuropathic arthropathy in the diabetic foot. Am Fam Physician 17:105, 1978
23. Frykberg RG: The diabetic Charcot foot. Arch Podiatric Med Foot Surgery 4:15, 1978
24. Frykberg RG: Diabetic osteoarthropathy. p. 75. In Brenner MA (ed): Management of the Diabetic Foot. Williams & Wilkins, Baltimore, 1987
25. Frykberg RG: Osteoarthropathy. Clin Podiatr Med Surg 4:351, 1987
26. Bruckner FE, Howell A: Neuropathic joints. Semin Arthritis Rheum 2:47, 1972
27. Johnson JTH: Neuropathic fractures and joint injuries. Pathogenesis and rationale of prevention and treatment. J Bone Joint Surg 49A:1, 1967
28. Resnick D: Neuroarthropathy. p. 2422. In Resnick D, Niwayama G (eds): Diagnosis Of Bone and Joint Disorders with Emphasis on Articular Abnormalities. Vol. 3. WB Saunders, Philadelphia, 1981
29. Rodnan GP: Neuropathic joint disease (Charcot joints). p. 1095. In Hollander JL et al (eds): Arthritis and Allied Conditions. Lea & Febiger, Philadelphia, 1985
30. Ellman MH: Neuropathic joint disease (Charcot joints). p. 1255. In McCarty DJ (ed): Arthritis and Allied Conditions. A Textbook of Rheumatology. Lea & Febiger, Philadelphia, 1989
31. Harris JR, Brand PW: Patterns of disintegration of

the tarsus in the anesthetic foot. J Bone Joint Surg 48B: 4,1966
32. Wastie ML: Radiological changes in serial x-rays of the foot and tarsus in leprosy. Clin Radiol 26:285, 1975
33. Bjorkengren AG, Weisman M, Pathria MN, et al: Neuroarthropathy associated with chronic alcoholism. Am J Radiol 151:743, 1988
34. Kernwein G, Lyon WF: Neuropathic arthropathy of the ankle joint resulting from complete severance of the sciatic nerve. Ann Surg 115:267, 1942
35. Steindler A: The tabetic arthropathies. JAMA 96:250, 1931
36. Bailey CC, Root HF: Neuropathic foot lesions in diabetes mellitus. N Engl J Med 236:397, 1947
37. Pogonowska MJ, Collins LC, Dobson HL: Diabetic osteopathy. Radiology 89:265, 1967
38. Knaggs RL: Charcot joints. p. 105. In: Inflammatory and Toxic Diseases of Bone. John Wright, Bristol, UK, 1926
39. Schwarz GS, Berenyi MR, Siegel MW: Atrophic arthropathy and diabetic neuritis. Am J Roentgenol 106:523, 1969
40. Newman JH: Spontaneous dislocation in diabetic neuropathy. J Bone Joint Surg 61B: 484, 1979
41. Friedman SA, Rakow RB: Osseous lesions of the foot in diabetic neuropathy. Diabetes 20:302, 1971
42. Zlatkin MB, Pathria M, Sartoris DJ, Resnick D: The diabetic foot. Radiol Clin North Am 25:1095, 1987
43. Lesko P, Maurer RC: Talonavicular dislocations and midfoot arthropathy in neuropathic diabetic feet: natural course and principles of treatment. Clin Orthop 240:226, 1989
44. Eichenholtz SN: Charcot Joints. Charles C Thomas, Springfield, IL, 1966
45. Newman JH: Non-infective disease of the diabetic foot. J Bone Joint Surg 63B:593, 1981
46. Aegerter E, Kirkpatrick JA: Metabolic diseases of bone. p. 33. In Aegerter E, Kirkpatrick JA (eds.): Orthopedic Diseases. WB Saunders, Philadelphia, 1983
47. Kelly PJ, Coventry MB: Neurotrophic ulcers of the feet: review of forty-seven cases. JAMA 168:388, 1958
48. Treves F: Treatment of perforating ulcer of the foot. Lancet 2:949, 1884
49. Lippman HI, Perotto A, Farrar R: The neuropathic foot of the diabetic. Bull N Y Acad Med 52:1159, 1976
50. Martin MM: Charcot joints in diabetes mellitus. Proc R Soc Med 45:503, 1952
51. Martin MM: Diabetic neuropathy. A clinical study of 150 cases. Brain 76:594, 1953
52. Eloesser L: On the nature of neuropathic affections of the joints. Ann Surg 66:201, 1917
53. Shands AR: Neuropathies of the bones and joints. Report of a case of an arthropathy of the ankle due to a peripheral nerve lesion. Arch Surg 20:614, 1930
54. Brooks AP: The neuropathic foot in diabetes. Part II: Charcot's neuroarthropathy. Diabetic Medicine 3:116, 1986
55. Lister J, Maudsley RH: Charcot joints in diabetic neuropathy. Lancet 2:1110, 1951
56. Foster DB, Bassett RC: Neurogenic arthropathy (Charcot joint) associated with diabetic neuropathy. Report of two cases. Archives Neurology and Psychiatry 57:173, 1947
57. Archer AG, Roberts VC, Watkins PJ: Blood flow patterns in diabetic neuropathy. Diabetologia 27:563, 1984
58. Edmonds ME, Nicolaides KH, Watkins PJ: Autonomic neuropathy and diabetic foot ulceration. Diabetic Medicine 3:56, 1986
59. Edelman SV, Kosofsky EM, Paul RA, Kozak GP: Neuro-osteoarthropathy (Charcot's joints) in diabetes mellitus following revascularization surgery: three case reports and a review of the literature. Arch Intern Med 147:1504, 1987
60. Watkins PJ, Edmonds ME: Sympathetic nerve failure in diabetes. Diabetologia 25:73, 1983
61. Edmonds ME, Clarke MB, Newton S, Barrett J: Increased uptake of bone radiopharmaceutical in diabetic neuropathy. Q J Med 57:843, 1985
62. Cundy TF, Edmonds ME, Watkins PJ: Osteopenia and metatarsal fractures in diabetic neuropathy. Diabetic Medicine 2:461, 1985
63. Edmonds ME: The neuropathic foot in diabetes. Part I: Blood flow. Diabetic Medicine 3:111, 1986
64. Boulton AJM, Scarpello JHB, Ward JD: Venous oxygenation in the diabetic neuropathic foot: evidence of arteriovenous shunting? Diabetologia 22:6, 1982
65. Radin EL: Mechanical aspects of osteoarthrosis. Bull Rheum Dis 26:862, 1976
66. Sanders LJ, Murray-Leisure K: Infections of the diabetic foot. In Abramson C, McCarthy (eds): Infectious Diseases of The Lower Extremity. Williams & Wilkins, Baltimore, 1991
67. El-Khoury GY, Kathol MH: Neuropathic fractures in patients with diabetes mellitus. Radiology 134:313, 1980
68. Schwartz ER: Chondrocyte structure and function. p. 289. In McCarty DJ (ed.): Arthritis and Allied Conditions. A Textbook Of Rheumatology. Lea & Febiger, Philadelphia, 1989
69. Levin ME: Diabetes and bone. Compr Ther 4:63, 1978

70. Monnier VM, Vishwanath V, Frank KE et al: Relation between complications of type I diabetes mellitus and collagen-linked fluorescence. N Engl J Med 314:403, 1986
71. Brownlee M, Cerami A, Vlassara H: Advanced glycosylation end products in tissue and the biochemical basis of diabetic complications. N Engl J Med 318:1315, 1988
72. Brink SJ: Limited joint mobility as a risk factor for diabetes complications. Clinical Diabetes 5:122, 1987
73. Buckinham BA, Uitto J, Sanborg C et al: Scleroderma-like changes in insulin-dependent diabetes mellitus: clinical and biochemical studies. Diabetes Care 7:163, 1984
74. Hough AJ, Sokoloff L: Pathology of osteoarthritis. p. 1571. In McCarty DJ (ed): Arthritis and Allied Conditions. Lea & Febiger, Philadelphia, 1989
75. Kraft E, Spyropoulos E, Finby N: Neurogenic disorders of the foot in diabetes mellitus. Am J Roentgenol 124:17, 1975
76. Horwitz T: Bone and cartilage debris in the synovial membrane: its significance in the early diagnosis of neuro-arthropathy. J Bone Joint Surg 30A: 3, 579, 1948
77. Rubinow A, Spark EC, Canoso JJ: Septic arthritis in a Charcot joint. Clin Orthop 147:203, 1980
78. Coventry MB, Rothacker GW: Bilateral calcaneal fracture in a diabetic patient. J Bone Joint Surg 61A:462, 1979
79. Thompson RC, Havel P, Goetz F: Presumed neurotrophic skeletal disease in diabetic kidney transplant recipients. JAMA 249:1317, 1983
80. Eymont MJ, Alavi A, Dalinka MK, Kyle GC: Bone scintigraphy in diabetic osteoarthropathy. Radiology 140:475, 1981
81. Hart TJ, Healey K: Diabetic osteoarthropathy versus diabetic osteomyelitis. J Foot Surg 25:464, 1986
82. Hetherington VJ: Technetium and combined gallium and technetium scans in the neurotrophic foot. J Am Podiatr Med Assoc 72:458, 1982
83. Edmonds ME, Morrison N, Laws JW, Watkins PJ: Medial arterial calcification and diabetic neuropathy. Br Med J 284:938, 1982
84. Glynn TP: Marked gallium accumulation in neuropathic arthropathy. J Nucl Med 22:1016, 1981
85. Hartshorne MF, Peters V: Nuclear medicine applications for the diabetic foot. Clin Pod Med Surg 4:361, 1987
86. Schauwecker DS, Park HM, Burt RW et al: Combined bone scintigraphy and indium-111 leukocyte scans in neuropathic foot disease. J Nucl Med 29:1651, 1988
87. Schauwecker DS: Osteomyelitis: diagnosis with In-111-labeled leukocytes. Radiology 171:141, 1989
88. Keenan AM, Tindel NL, Alavi A: Diagnosis of pedal osteomyelitis in diabetic patients using current scintigraphic techniques. Arch Intern Med 149:2262, 1989
89. Maurer AH, Millmond SH, Knight LC et al: Infection in diabetic osteoarthropathy: use of indium-111 labeled leukocytes for diagnosis. Radiology 161:221, 1986
90. Zeiger LS, Fox IM: Use of indium-111 labeled white blood cells in the diagnosis of diabetic foot infections. J Foot Surg 29:46, 1990
91. Rosenblatt S: Principles of evaluation and treatment of osteomyelitis in the diabetic foot. Clin Diabetes Sept/Oct:85, 1989
92. Cavanagh PR, Sanders LJ, Sims DS: The role of pressure distribution measurement in diabetic foot care. Rehabilitation R&D Progress Reports 1987. J Rehabil R D 25:53, 1988
93. Kidd JG: The Charcot joint: some pathologic and pathogenetic considerations. Southern Med J 67:597, 1974
94. Leventen EO: Charcot foot—a technique for treatment of chronic plantar ulcer by saucerization and primary closure. Foot & Ankle 6:295, 1986
95. Banks AS, McGlamry ED: Charcot foot. J Am Podiatr Med Assoc 79:213, 1989
96. Arntz CT, Veith RG, Hansen ST: Fractures and fracture-dislocations of the tarsometatarsal joint. J Bone Joint Surg 70A:173, 1988
97. Sanders LJ: Amputations in the diabetic foot. p. 481 In Harkless LB, Kendrick JD (eds): The Diabetic Foot. Clinics in Podiatric Medicine and Surgery. Williams & Wilkins, Baltimore, 1987

17

Lower Extremity Amputations

F. William Wagner, Jr., M.D.

There are nearly one-half million amputees in the United States.[1-3,5,6] Each year nearly 40,000 new amputations are performed. Approximately 85 percent of these are major lower extremity amputations. Dysvascular complications account for approximately 85 percent of the amputations in the lower extremity and well over half of these are in the diabetic patient.[4-6] This is despite the fact that only 5 percent of the population of the United States is diabetic or has some alteration of carbohydrate metabolism. As noted in Chapters 13 to 15, vascular evaluation and vascular surgery have gone a long way in aiding the healing of diabetic lesions and in allowing more distal areas of amputation.

With the entry of the bioengineer as a member of the amputation team, with the appearance of lightweight prosthetic materials, with the total contact concept, and with better gait analysis, far more versatile prosthetic designs are now being produced. Even more important has been the renewed interest in amputation surgery and prosthetics by physicians, physical therapists, and prosthetists. Much of the information presented in this chapter is a reflection of that interest. Some of the procedures may represent departures from previous management techniques. The improvement in overall patient care we hope will continue to evolve well through the balance of this century.

Amputation centers continue to receive many patients for rehabilitation whose residual limbs are not suitable for the use of prostheses. The operating surgeon has violated many of the rules of fashioning the residual limb. The surgeon is charged with providing a suitable interface between the patient and his or her new environment, the prosthesis. The prosthetist cannot fashion an artificial limb to correct surgical mistakes.

The surgical procedure is but one part of the rehabilitation process. A team approach has been shown to be superior in the total care of the amputee.[7-11] The psychic trauma of a major amputation can be devastating. Support along the way must be afforded by all members of the team and rehabilitation must start well before the operation itself.

Each amputee will be facing a different set of problems with home, family, and occupation. Thus it is obvious that in addition to the medical staff, other parts of the team will be valuable in providing some part of the solution of this multifaceted problem. The team will obviously vary from institution to institution, but the basic concept is the same. The team must obviously compromise nurses, prosthetists, physical and occupational therapists, social workers, psychologists, psychiatrists, vocational counselors, as well as the surgical staff. Goal setting is thus more realistic. Input from each member of the team aids in formation of a treatment plan. For example, above knee prostheses are not prescribed for elderly diabetic patients with minimal cardiopulmonary reserves. Extended periods of training are avoided when it appears that the goal of prosthetic ambulation is not attainable.

SURGICAL TECHNIQUES

There are relatively few new surgical principles which must be followed to achieve optimum results. Tissues must be handled gently. All dead, potentially nonviable, or infected tissues must be removed from the wound. For all amputations, but especially those performed in geriatric and dysvascular patients, the skin must be closed with plastic surgical techniques. The skin edges should not be crushed with forceps or clamps. For wounds that are grossly infected or contaminated, guillotine amputation followed by skin graft is archaic. Preparatory guillotine amputation is performed to remove infection, and once the infection has cleared, a formal primary amputation at the planned level should be performed. In many settings amputation surgery is performed by the least experienced members of the surgical staff. It is my view that optimum results in amputation surgery can be obtained if an experienced surgeon is involved in all amputations and attention is paid to meticulous surgical detail. The diabetic patient requires even more exacting techniques than those used in young healthy patients.

SPECIFIC TECHNIQUES

General Anesthesia

Coordination is essential among the surgeon, the internist, and the anesthesiologist when considering anesthesia for diabetic patients. The surgeon generally will not be responsible for control of the diabetic state or choosing the anesthetic agents. However, on occasion an emergent situation may arise. Chapter 15 gives some excellent information on indications for anesthesia. In addition, two articles may be consulted to assist in diabetic control of the surgical patient.[12,13]

Local Anesthesia

If there are any questions as to cardiopulmonary status or ability to withstand a general anesthetic, local or regional anesthesia can be used for virtually any level of lower extremity surgery. Preanesthetic agents are used in quantities dictated by the patient's age, weight, and general condition. Atropine sulfate or glycopyrrolate are given to provide cardiac stimulation, to reduce gastric secretion and acidity, and to provide vagal suppression as necessary. Lidocaine has been found to be relatively rapid in onset and is shorter in duration of action. Bupivicaine has been found to be less rapid in action but provides longer-lasting anesthesia. Its use with the intravenous Bier block has allowed release of the tourniquet with sufficient anesthesia remaining for hemostasis control and closure of the wound. Care must be taken not to release the tourniquet before fixation of the agent in the tissues is complete. Bupivicaine appears to be more toxic to the cardiovascular system.

Regional blocking of the femoral, sciatic, and obturator nerves will provide anesthesia suitable for the whole limb except for hip disarticulation. Supplementing these nerve blocks with skin anesthesia in the proposed incisional sites has been satisfactory.

Tourniquet control is possible with regional anesthesia with performance of a ring block of the circumference of the limb at the level of the tourniquet. Vasoconstrictors are usually not used in the anesthetic solutions. They have not been found necessary for hemostasis and there appears to be greater cardiovascular toxicity in diabetic and cardiac patients. Local and regional infiltrations are performed before the surgical team scrubs. Adequate anesthesia is usually present by the time the patient's skin has been prepared and draping is complete. On very few occasions small additional injections may be necessary at local sites during the procedure.

Above Knee Amputation
Local skin blockage of the skin, muscle, bone, and nerve is adequate. A tourniquet is not used in above knee amputations in our institution. The patient is placed on the side opposite the limb to be amputated. This allows rotation of the leg at the hip so that all sides are available, both for injection and for surgical approach. The incisional lines are drawn on the skin and infiltrated. At the apex of the fishmouth flap a longer needle is used to reach the femur. Anesthetic agent is infiltrated into the peri-

osteum around the femur, into the musculature, and into the subsartorial canal. Aspiration is performed before each injection to be sure that the anesthetic agent is not injected into the major circulation. When the artery and vein are exposed in the subsartorial canal, they are clamped and divided. The distal femur is then divided and pulled anteriorly with a bone hook. The sciatic nerve then is dissected out readily. It is injected with a small volume of local anesthetic under direct vision. It is then clamped and divided after the anesthetic has had time to set.

Through Knee Amputation
Local anesthesia is well tolerated in the through knee amputation. Many of the patients for whom this level is indicated will not be prosthetic candidates and their general health is usually so poor that general anesthesia is poorly tolerated. Thirty milliliters of half-strength local anesthetic is injected into the knee joint. Full-strength anesthetic solution is used to infiltrate the skin incisional lines. The subcutaneous tissues are infiltrated down to the bone. The medial and lateral joint capsules and hamstring tendons are injected. The surgical technique is then carried out as described in the section on through knee amputation. When common peroneal and posterior tibial nerves are exposed during the procedure, they are injected directly. This allows division of the nerve without pain. If an irrigation system is used, it may be necessary to raise a small skin wheal at the site for introduction of the drain, as it may be proximal to the level of anesthesia.

Below Knee Amputation
The skin flaps are outlined on the skin. The skin, underlying muscle, and bone are then infiltrated directly. The arteries and veins are dissected out bluntly, clamped, and divided. Posterior tibial nerve and anterior tibial nerve are infiltrated under direct vision. When posterior anesthesia has been achieved, section of the posterior flap is then completed.

Syme Amputation and Foot Procedures
The posterior tibial, superficial peroneal, and sural nerves are blocked above the ankle joint. The ankle joint is injected and distended with anesthetic solution. If a tourniquet is necessary, the skin is infiltrated circumferentially just above the nerve block area. An Esmarch or Martin bandage is wrapped from the toes upward and then wrapped around the leg and tied above the ankle. About 100 mmHg of pressure is produced with each turn. The distal portion of the bandage is then unwrapped, leaving the tourniquet tied above to provide hemostasis. With the release of the tourniquet sufficient anesthetic remains to secure hemostasis and to close the wound.

Toe Procedures
Infiltration at the base of the toes will permit either amputation or disarticulation to be performed. A small Penrose drain can be wrapped from distal to proximal and tied at the base for hemostasis.

Use of Tourniquet

Because of reports of postoperative problems after tourniquet use,[14–17] a series of tests was performed at Rancho Los Amigos Medical Center to determine any long-term complication from the use of a tourniquet. Amputations were performed both with and without tourniquets in approximately 50 patients at each level of foot, ankle, knee, and thigh. No complications could be ascribed to the tourniquet in any of the levels except the above knee level. It was postulated that patients requiring above knee amputations had more diffuse dysvascularity, were older, and were actually sicker than the other patients. It was thus felt that the residual limb had less ability to heal. Since this test was performed, we have used tourniquets at all levels except the above knee amputation level.

SPECIFIC TISSUE TREATMENT

Skin

The skin must be treated as in the most delicate hand and plastic procedures. With total contact prostheses, the location of the scar is of less importance than previously. The scar should be nonadherent, thin, pliable, not directly over bone, and contain no neuromas. In weight-bearing areas the flaps should be covered with normal full thickness skin and subcutaneous tissue with as complete sensation as possible. Completely insensitive skin is susceptible to breakdown. However, with careful prosthetic fit and careful attention to skin hygiene, even patients with Hansen's disease and diabetes mellitus do amazingly well with incomplete or complete loss of sensation.

Skin grafts do not usually wear well over weight-bearing areas. Split thickness or full thickness grafts may be used away from weight-bearing areas. Pedicle grafts are of value, as they provide subcutaneous tissue, but still suffer from sensory loss. The newer free grafts transferred by microsurgical techniques to both vessels and nerves show great promise for resurfacing pressure-bearing areas with sensitive skin, subcutaneous tissue, and virtually normal blood supply. Dermal overgrafting is a useful procedure that can save a surface in which the skin graft is thin, lacks pliability, and has developed recurrent ulceration. The area is dermabraded to a depth of a few thousandths of an inch and then a second split thickness graft is applied over the abraded area. I have used this procedure several times and have been pleased to see a thicker, more pliable, and pressure-resistant covering develop.[18]

Muscle

A divided muscle does not have a resistance point against which to pull. It will still be able to contract but will frequently produce pain and spasm with the unresisted contraction. Various myodesing techniques have been advocated for many years. If the amputation is through a tendinous area, the tendon may be fixed to bone relatively easily. A pair of drill holes will accept the tendon and it may be tied back upon itself. When muscle bellies are cut, fixation is more difficult. Mattress sutures may be placed through the central tendon and aponeurosis and then tied through drill holes in the bone to stabilize the muscle ends. A "satisfied" muscle is one which has some point to pull against and appears to provide a pain-free stump with greater proprioception, greater circulation, and greater strength.

Fixation of the calf musculature to the tibia has been satisfactory when performed through suturing of fascia, muscle, and tendon and aponeurosis of the posterior flap to the periosteum of the anterior tibia. The use of drill holes in the anteromedial tibia has been abandoned by us because each drill hole had a capacity to heal with an exostosis or spike of bone that could be markedly painful under a prosthesis.

The tension under which to place a myodesis is still impossible to measure exactly during surgery. It is often said that the tension should be "physiological." A simple rule to follow is that after myodesis or myoplasty it must be possible to put the joint above through a full range of motion so that no contracture has been produced by the myodesis.

Nerves

One of the most important aspects of management of the nerve in amputation surgery is to allow the cut nerve to retract out of the healing wound. Axons will grow distally if within a Schwann tubule. Following amputation the tubules are absent and the axons grow in an irregular manner in the scar formed by the perineural or glial tissue. Thus the amputation nerve bulb is a combination neuroma and glioma. If it exists at a pressure or traction point, it can produce virtually unbearable pain and has been implicated in the production of phantom pain. Many procedures have been proposed to lessen neuroma formation. Cups made of silicone rubber, tantulum, and other materials have been placed over the nerve ends. Local treatment with chemicals, heat, and cold have been advocated. The nerve ends have been placed in holes drilled in the bone, buried in adjoining muscle, sutured to adjacent muscles, and tied back upon themselves. Each of these methods has been proposed and then abandoned by many of the centers trying them. My personal preference is to pull the nerve down gently, crush it at the point of division, use a ligature through the crushed area to control the vasa nervorum, divide the nerve just below the ligature, and then allow it to retract to an area where it will not undergo pressure. Too vigorous traction may strip the nerve of some of its blood supply and contribute to an ischemic or traction neuritis.

Post-Tourniquet Reaction Time

An intraoperative aid to supplement any preoperative vascular tests has been the post-tourniquet reaction time. With the use of a tourniquet most parts to be amputated have been removed within 20 minutes and the tourniquet has then been released after clamping and ligation of the major vessels. It has thus been inflated a relatively short time, which might account for the fact that no complications have been seen with a tourniquet at those sites distal to the above knee level. Timing is begun at release of the tourniquet. When bleeding appears in the distalmost skin edge, the time is noted. When the distal skin bleeds almost immediately, the healing rate is usually over 95 percent. If the distalmost skin bleeds by 3 minutes there is greater than 80 percent chance that the wound will heal. If there is no bleeding by 5 minutes, strong consideration should be given to moving to the next higher level.

Blood Vessels

Hemostasis is good surgical technique in amputation surgery as well as in other surgical procedures. Hematoma formation can lead to pressure on adjacent vessels sufficient to cause death of tissue. In addition, accumulation of blood makes an excellent culture medium for bacterial growth. Smaller accumulations can also act as "bruises" which further increase the need for healing potential of the residual limb. Large arteries should be doubly closed with suture ligatures. Simple ligation may fail when the pulse pressures are strong enough to roll the suture down and off the end of the vessel. Smaller arteries and large veins are ligated with absorbable ties. The type and size of ligature are determined by the surgeon's experience and preference. The smallest vessels are electrocoagulated using a needle tip.

Sutures

There are no hard and fast rules that govern the type of suture material to be used. The surgeon's preference and local ground rules will obviously be the final determinants. Absorbable material such as plain gut, chromicized gut, and polyglycolic acid are used in fascia, tendon, and muscle. The most often used sizes are 00 and 000. Myoplasty, myodesis, and fixation of patellar tendons to cruciate ligaments may require nonabsorbable sutures. The skin is closed with wire, nylon, polypropylene, polyethylene, skin staples, or similar nonabsorbable materials.

Drains

Drainage of surgically created cavities and evacuation of hematomas are well recognized surgical procedures. Their usage should be individualized to each case. The following principles are followed in private practice, and at Rancho Los Amigos Hospital in diabetic patients:

1. Penrose drains are no longer used through the suture lines. We have noted infection in drainage tracts following removal of such drains. Many of these wounds required local revision of the drainage tract.
2. All drains or irrigation tubes are brought into the wound through a separate stab incision at some distance from the surgical incision.
3. Disarticulations at the hip, knee, and ankle are treated with a double-lumen tube for irrigation and gravity drainage because of the larger dead spaces formed. The two-lumen Shirley abdominal sump drain is modified by using the air intake tube to bring in fluid to lavage the cavity and using the suction tube for gravity drainage to a collecting bag. The irrigating fluid is a physiologic solution such as Hartman's or Ringer's solution for noninfected cases. Antibiotics such as Bacitracin, Kantrex, Polymixin, or Neomycin are added for infected cases. Care must be taken that ototoxic or nephrotoxic levels are not reached. Hearing function is monitored, serum creatinine levels are followed, and peak and trough serum antibiotic levels are measured. The outflow tube is clamped every 2 to 3 hours for several minutes to be sure that all areas of the cavity are lavaged. Irrigation is continued for 48 to 72 hours at a rate of 1 L/24 h. The tube is removed aseptically when the irrigating fluid is

clear. The tip is cut off and sent to the laboratory for culture and sensitivity testing. This system has been used for over 20 years and the results have been quite satisfactory.

4. Amputation through muscle masses and those with large areas of open bone are treated with soft plastic suction tubes for 24 to 48 hours. Separate tubes may be used for each layer that appears to need drainage. If the wound is dry at closure, no drains are used.
5. Smaller foot amputations are irrigated by the system described by Kritter.[19] A small plastic tube is brought into the wound through a separate stab incision. Major incisions are usually closed through skin and subcutaneous tissue only. Rarely one or two stabilizing sutures are needed in the deep fascia. The tube is placed next to bone and the fluid exits between the sutures. It carries out debris, diluted hematoma, and probable residual bacteria. Irrigation is continued at 500 to 1,000 ml/24 h for 72 to 96 hours. The duration of the irrigation is determined by the status of the wound preoperatively. At the conclusion of irrigation the tip is removed aseptically and cultured for presence of bacteria.

Bone

The residual bone must continue to provide a stable framework for the soft tissues. It must provide leverage, mobility, and transmission of forces. It must be cut at such a length that the soft tissues can be closed without tension. The distal ends must be shaped so that no areas of high pressure are formed. Trial closure of the flaps is done manually before suturing is begun. If closure is not possible without tension, more bone must be removed or the flaps must be rotated or lengthened. Any open areas produced by such rotation or lengthening may be skin-grafted. The rotation is fashioned so that skin graft is not in a weight-bearing position.

Treatment of the periosteum has varied over the years. Some have advocated removal of one-half inch or more above the end of the bone. We have found this to provide an avascular end of the bone which may become a ring sequestrum. Some have advocated forming a distal cuff of periosteum to seal the open end of the tubular bone. On occasion we have found that this will devascularize the periosteum and lead to death of the tissue and subsequent drainage. The simplest procedure is to divide the periosteum at the bone division line. Periosteum is not elevated except for the small distance necessary to allow rounding of the bone edges.

Wound Closure

General surgical principles apply also to amputation surgery. Hemostasis is made as complete as possible. Cavities and dead spaces are eliminated or drained if not closed. Drainage systems are placed in bone and muscle layers for possible hematoma accumulation. Fascial layers are closed edge to edge and special care is taken not to strangulate tissue edges. Suture material should be of the finest size consistent with strength needed in that area. Absorbable sutures are usually used in the deeper layers except when tenodesis or myodesis is performed. In areas where the thickness of the subcutaneous fat is uneven from one side to the other, the sutures are placed so that the skin edges are level. Healing of skin probably predicts healing of the surgical procedure more so than any other tissue. Forceps should not be used directly on the skin. Large gaps of exposed subcutaneous fat should not be allowed between the sutures. Checks should be made for blanching of the skin margins after closure is complete and the sutures should be loosened if necessary. If blanching still appears, the skin sutures should be removed and fine subcutaneous suture material substituted. Final closure of the skin can then be performed with plastic tape strips.

Antibiotic Coverage

Postamputation infections usually result in higher levels of amputation. This then leads to a subsequent decrease of rehabilitation potential. When wounds have been opened prior to amputation, there is a great likelihood that the infection will involve multiple organisms. Appropriate antibiotic coverage will frequently include three antibiotics. Preoperative cultures and sensitivity testing will usually indicate the specific antibiotic therapy for the infection present. During surgery the amputation wound is cultured just before closure. Results of this testing will aid greatly in the postoperative antibiotic coverage. Continuation of antibiotic coverage will depend upon the intraoperative cultures and the clinical course of the patient.

Guillotine Amputation

The guillotine amputation had its greatest application as a preliminary debriding operation to remove an infecting source. There now appears to be little indication for its use as the single operative procedure. When skin traction was used previously, there would be granulation and scarring. The guillotine amputation is now used as a preparative operation to aid definitive amputation at a higher level. There appears to be a statistically lower rate of subsequent stump infections when patients have guillotine amputations prior to a definitive amputation.[20] At Rancho Los Amigos the experience with a two-stage Syme amputation would tend to support the same statistics. However, the first-stage Syme amputation is closed over drainage tubes and therefore cannot be truly considered a guillotine amputation. Nevertheless the removal of the infected material has raised the success rate in Syme amputation to a higher level. In addition, our use of the Kritter irrigation system has permitted salvage of infected feet when the ischemic index indicated that local healing was possible. We have also had a higher healing rate with closure than with open wounds that were allowed to heal by granulation, as has been reported by others.[21]

Postoperative Treatment

The surgeon's experience will dictate the postoperative treatment of the residual limb.

Conventional Soft Dressings

Conventional soft wrappings are used if there has been no experience with immediate postsurgical casting. The patient is then ambulated early with mobility aids. Prosthetic fitting is begun as rapidly as the wound allows.

Rigid Dressings

Patient comfort is greater with a plaster dressing applied over suitable padding. This procedure has its greatest applicability in the below knee amputation. It aids in edema control, prevents the wound from being injured, prevents knee flexion contractures, and allows early mobilization with aids such as crutches and walker.

Immediate Postoperative Prosthetic Ambulation

A plaster cast is applied with stronger walls than for plaster dressings. A pylon and prosthetic foot are fastened to the cast. The patient is then ambulated with walking aids. This must be done with care in the dysvascular amputee, as it may actually delay healing if used too early or too vigorously. In those centers where it has been used, immediate postoperative prosthetic fitting has been found to achieve the best rehabilitation results. I would suggest, however, that unless the surgeon or prosthetist has sufficient experience with this procedure, the results for immediate postoperative prosthesis quoted in the literature may be unduly optimistic for the diabetic patient.

Postoperative Rehabilitation

It is extremely important to continue the rehabilitation process the morning after surgery. Patients should continue physical therapy for upper and lower extremity strengthening with walking between parallel bars and general reconditioning exercises as soon as possible. There is information to suggest that deterioration occurs in muscular function from bed rest alone.[22] Care in a rehabilitation setting markedly increases the function of elderly lower extremity amputees.[23]

Selection of Level

At one time 80 percent of amputations for lower extremity gangrene and infection were performed at the above knee level. Now 80 percent are performed below the knee, and in some centers as many or more Syme amputations are performed as at the below knee level. Many years ago the teaching was "not to whittle." A patient with a black toe received an above knee amputation because everyone knew it would heal. Research at Rancho Los Amigos Hospital and other centers has emphasized the value of saving the knee. The gait laboratory under the direction of Jacqueline Perry and Robert Waters has provided measurements that show why very few of the above knee dysvascular amputees walk with a prosthesis after the age of 55.[24] A series of normal individuals, a series of dysvascular amputees, and a series of young traumatic amputees were compared. Oxygen consumption was measured. Stride length, cadence, and gait velocity were measured from heel switch signals as the subjects walked on a measured track. The superiority of the Syme level in all of the variables measured was evident. Measurement of the oxygen consumption per meter traveled revealed a major increase for the above knee level. Patients with a Syme level report a feeling of stability and a sense of knowing where their limb is in three-dimensional space. Patients with a below knee on one side and a Syme on the other side report a wish to have had both sides at the Syme level.

Bilateral Amputees

A fairly large number of diabetic and other dysvascular patients will become bilateral amputees. This incidence has been reported from 9 to 28 percent. Goldner has shown that 23 percent of patients who have had amputation for gangrene will have a lesion of the opposite extremity within 1 year.[25] Thirty-eight percent more will have a lesion by the second year and only 6 percent will have an intact opposite limb at 5 years. Whitehouse found in a similar study that approximately five times more patients died than went on to a second amputation.[26] Studies of the rehabilitation potential of bilateral lower extremity amputees show that there is even a greater importance to save the knee in a dysvascular patient.[27] Of 44 patients with bilateral below knee amputations, 52 percent used a prosthesis for community ambulation, 27 percent used a prosthesis for household ambulation, and 20 percent required a wheelchair. Of the 37 bilateral above knee amputees, 2 were of traumatic origin. Only one of these became a limited community ambulator with prostheses and crutches. Of 21 patients with above knee and below knee combinations, 5 used prostheses in some manner daily, 10 were wheelchair users, and 6 were bedridden. Thus success for rehabilitation of the above knee/below knee amputee is significantly greater than for the bilateral above knee amputee. Again, the importance of saving even a single knee joint must be emphasized.

Open Amputation

With the use of antibiotics and better level selection through the use of vascular indices, we have rarely found the open amputation to be indicated. It may be used to control a spreading infection that has not yet localized and is not yet responding to antibiotic treatment. The presence of gas in the tissues does not always indicate the presence of clostridia.[28] Gram-negative and anaerobic organisms frequently will produce gas. Local debriding procedures should be attempted before high amputations are performed if clostridia have not been proven by culture.

SPECIFIC AMPUTATION TECHNIQUES

Amputation of the Toes

Amputation of a toe or toes is usually performed for infection or gangrene. Use of Doppler ultrasound will allow evaluation of circulation at the base of the toes. The amputation level is then determined by the presence of infection or gangrene and the availability of skin for closure. Individual toes may be amputated at any level. Surgical incisions may be of any type as long as the flap is not too long for the width at the base. A one-to-one ratio has worked best in our hands. Fishmouth flaps may be used mediolaterally or anteroposteriorly. Long plantar flaps, long dorsal flaps, longer medial flaps, or longer lateral flaps can all be used successfully. Disarticulations do well at all joints including the metatarsophalangeal. We have not found it necessary to remove cartilage from the remaining articu-

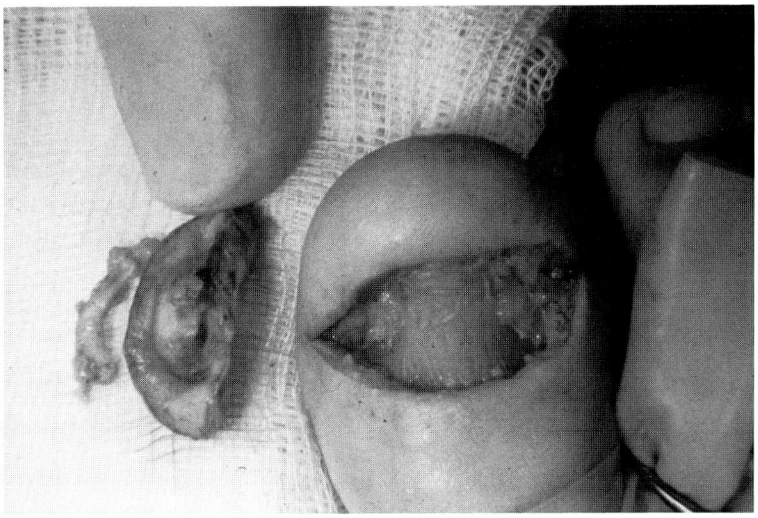

Fig. 17-1. Elliptical incision to remove nail, matrix, and tissue in nail groove. Penrose drain used as tourniquet.

lar surfaces. However, sharp edges may be removed from the condyles if they are palpable through the flaps.

Syme Terminal Amputation

The indications for a Syme terminal amputation is failure of lesser techniques to control recurrent infection of the toenail.

Procedure

The toe is usually prepared by avulsing the toenail under local anesthesia. When all signs of infection have disappeared and the toe has remained quiescent for 6 weeks, the operation is performed under local anesthesia. The steps in the procedure are as follows:

1. The residual nail and matrix are outlined elliptically. Care is taken not to sever the insertion of the extensor tendon when the matrix is removed (Fig. 17-1).
2. The distal tuft of the phalanx is outlined subperiosteally and sharply. Enough bone is removed to allow closure of the distal flap.
3. The tourniquet is released and hemostasis is secured with electrocoagulation.

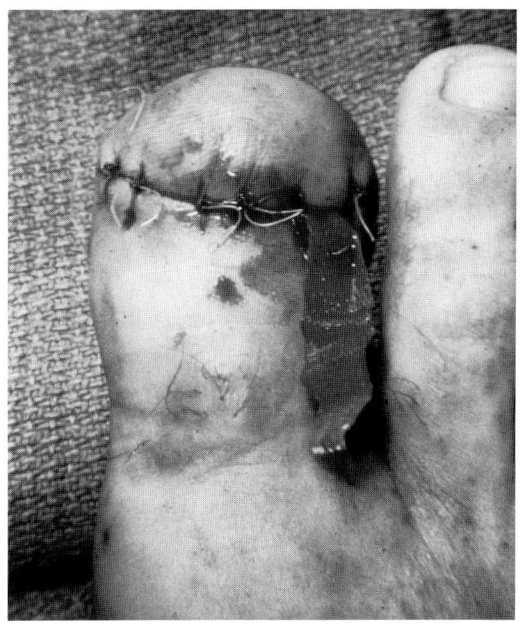

Fig. 17-2. Closure of flap with iodoform wick for drainage.

4. Iodoform gauze is used as a wick to aid in drainage of hematoma. The skin only is closed. No deep sutures are necessary (Fig. 17-2).

Postoperative Care

Light compression dressings are applied. The patient is allowed to walk in a postoperative shoe. Oral antibiotics are prescribed for 3 to 4 days. When healing is complete protective footwear is indicated based on any deformities of the residual toes and feet.

Virtually no function is lost. No prosthesis or orthotic device is required.

Amputation of Metatarsal Heads

The feet shown in Figure 17-3 represent the "foot at risk." This patient has had previous ulceration as evidenced by the scarring at the first metatarsal heads. The ulcers healed with walking cast treatment. Pressure at other metatarsal heads is evident from the incipient keratoses. The patient asked specifically for a definitive treatment for long-term relief of pressures. Procedures ranging

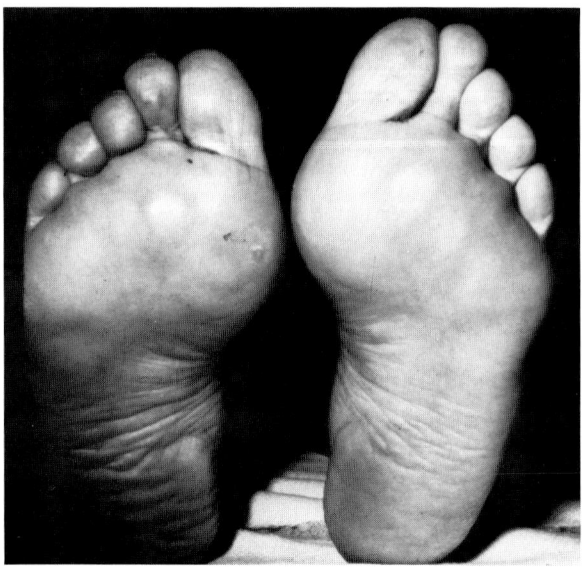

Fig. 17-3. Plantar view of 64-year-old diabetic woman. She has had several episodes of ulcerations that healed with serial casting. Note prominence of metatarsal heads.

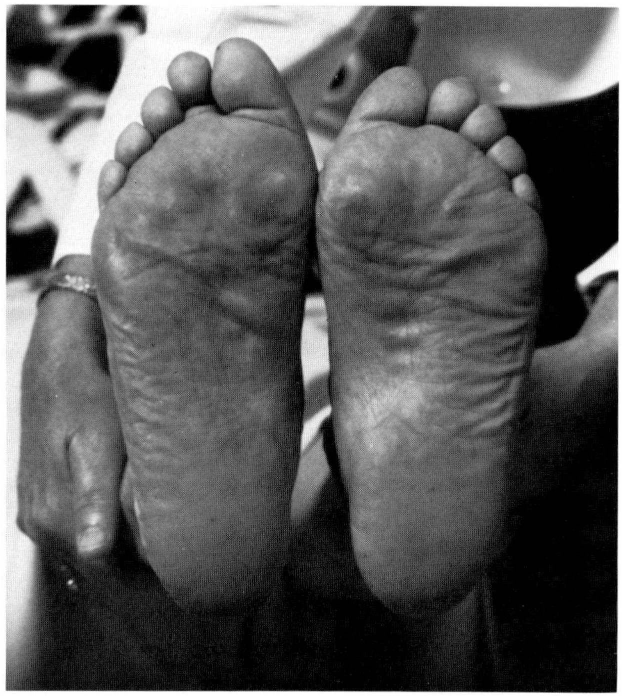

Fig. 17-4. Plantar view of patient in Fig. 17-3 after Hoffman-Clayton removal of metatarsal heads. Note lack of pressure areas.

from clawtoe procedures, tendon releases and transfers, metatarsal osteotomites, and metatarsal head amputations were discussed at length. She asked for the last procedure as she felt that it would be the most definitive. A full Hoffman-Clayton resection arthroplasty was performed on both feet. The plantar surfaces were shown postoperatively at 6 months (Fig. 17-4). The release of pressure is evident when compared with the previous figure.

The foot shown in Figure 17-5 is that of a diabetic patient who had severe infection of the great toe of her right foot previously. Evacuation of the infected bone and soft tissues allowed healing of the residual foot. Despite protective footwear she developed an ulcer under the second metatarsal head. The deformity was secondary to changes in the joint that appear to be Charcot breakdown.

Amputation of the remaining metatarsal heads was performed through a dorsal incision (Fig. 17-6). The paddle screw designed by Hampar Kelikian is a useful tool for removing the metatarsal heads. It is screwed down the metatarsal neck into

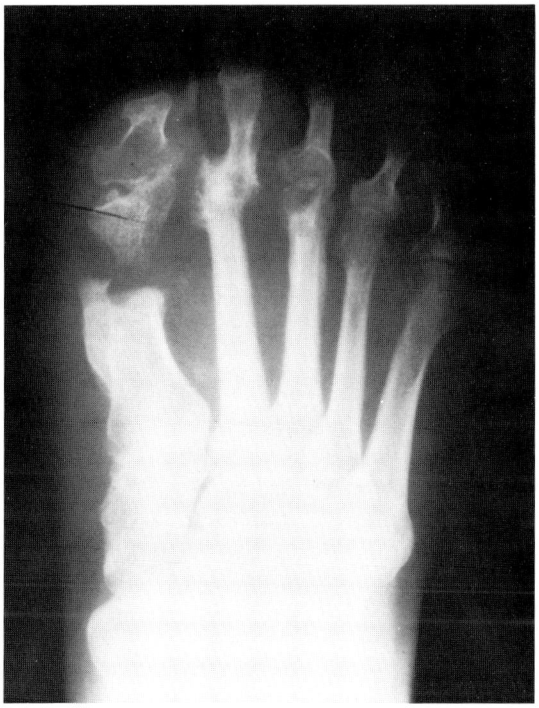

Fig. 17-5. Radiographic evidence of resection of first metatarsophalangeal joint for infection and Charcot destruction of second and third joints.

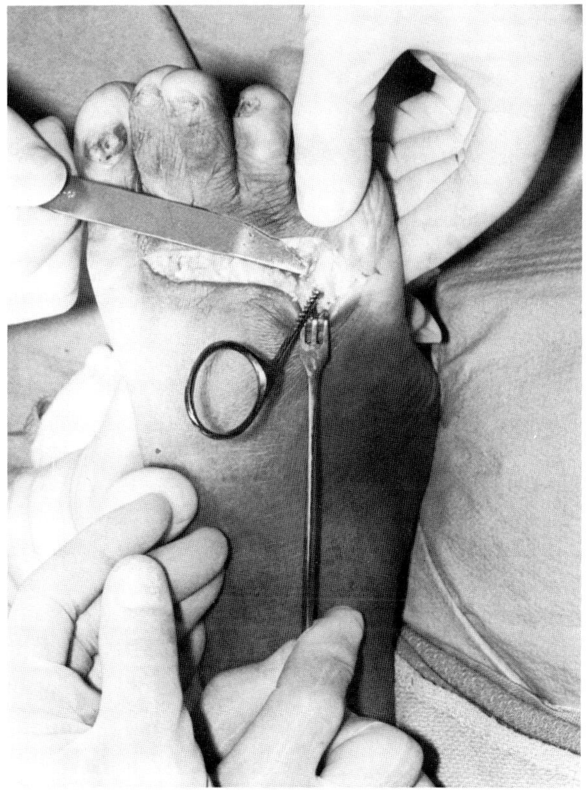

Fig. 17-6. Resection of fifth metatarsal head with use of screw device to control distal head and neck during removal.

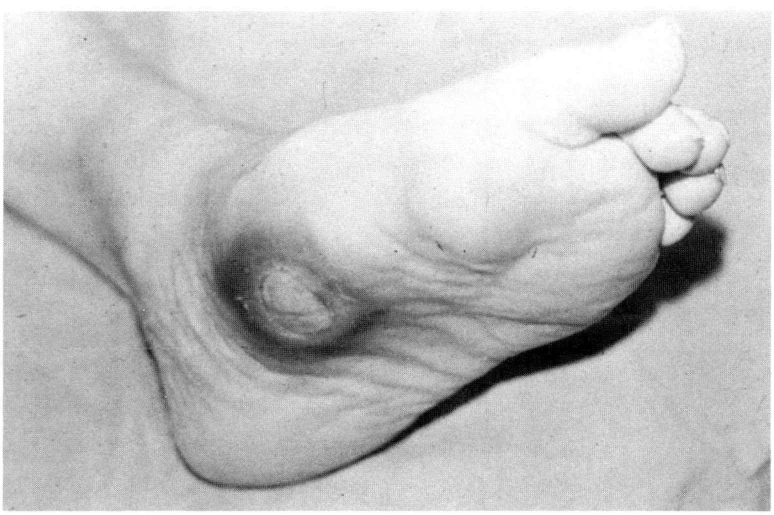

Fig. 17-7. Diabetic Charcot breakdown with ulceration under talonavicular prominence.

the head. The head is then levered out easily and the capsule and ligamentous structures cut under direct vision. The final result is a foot free of pressure points.

Amputation of Bony Prominences

Midfoot breakdown is the most common deformity seen from Charcot arthropathy. Ulceration will usually regress and frequently heal with cast protection. Circulation is virtually always adequate for healing if internal bony pressure is relieved. The site of incision is at a distance so that the ulcer heals by rapid filling and epitheliazation. In Figure 17-7 the typical depression and medial displacement of the talonavicular complex are shown. The patient has been in a walking cast for several weeks. There is no surrounding cellulitis and granulation tissue is abundant. Incision should be made 3 to 4 cm superior to the ulcer and deeply to bone without development of any tissue layers. Sufficient bone is removed to smooth the contours and decompress the ulcer. A Kritter drain is used to irrigate the wound. The patient is allowed to bear weight in a cast at 2 weeks. The rapidity of healing will be seen at 2 weeks when the granulation tissue is already being covered with epithelium from the edges. With complete coverage of the ulcer with epithelium the patient is placed in protective orthoses or shoes depending upon the degree of bone healing.

Toe Amputation and Disarticulation

Amputation of the Tip

The longer second toe frequently is flexed at the tip and is subject to abnormal pressures, ulceration, and osteomyelitis. The thickening and drainage of the second toe are virtually pathognomonic of osteomyelitis (Fig. 17-8). Removal of the toe surgically is far more "conservative" than attempting to treat this lesion with incision, drainage, and antibiotics. Under local anesthesia and with a Penrose drain as a tourniquet, the tip is outlined with a longer plantar flap. The condyles in this instance were quite sharp and would have led to further pressure points. They were removed with bone-biting forceps. The flap is palpated before closure to be sure no bony prominences remain. Nonabsorbable sutures are used after the tourniquet is released and hemostasis is secured with electrocoagulation.

Great Toe Disarticulation

Figure 17-9 represents disarticulation of the great toe with fishmouth incision. Again, closure is tested manually before sutures are added. A Kritter irrigation is also used in this type of amputation.

Toe and Ray Resection

In cases representing obvious infection and osteomyelitis of the lesser toes, the toe is disarticulated through a fishmouth incision. Upon examining the residual metatarsal head, if it is obvious that there is already osteomyelitis in the head, it is removed with an oblique osteotomy that then allows complete closure of the flaps. The Kritter drain is then used.

Complete amputation of the lesser toes and rays leaves a remarkably functional foot. Patients who have a residual great toe on one side and who have had a transmetatarsal amputation on the other side relate that the residual great toe gives them greater stability and greater takeoff and rolloff power.

In toe and ray amputations, sufficient bone must be removed from the heads and shafts of the metatarsals to gain soft tissue for closure. At one time these wounds were left open and treated with healing casts until they closed spontaneously. Approximately 85 percent eventually healed. Later procedures with primary closures over the Kritter irrigation system have provided virtually 100 percent healing. It is postulated that all open wounds are colonized or infected and multiple bacteria can usually be cultured. Removal of all infected and gangrenous tissues, resection of sufficient bone to allow closure of the wound, and use of an irrigation system to dilute the infecting bacteria aid in primary healing of these difficult wounds. Ecker and Jacobs report only 2 of 18 closed wounds failed, whereas 16 of 36 open wounds failed.[29]

Postoperative Care

Soft compression dressings are used until the Kritter tube is removed. The residual portion of the foot is allowed to dry for one day. A nonwalking

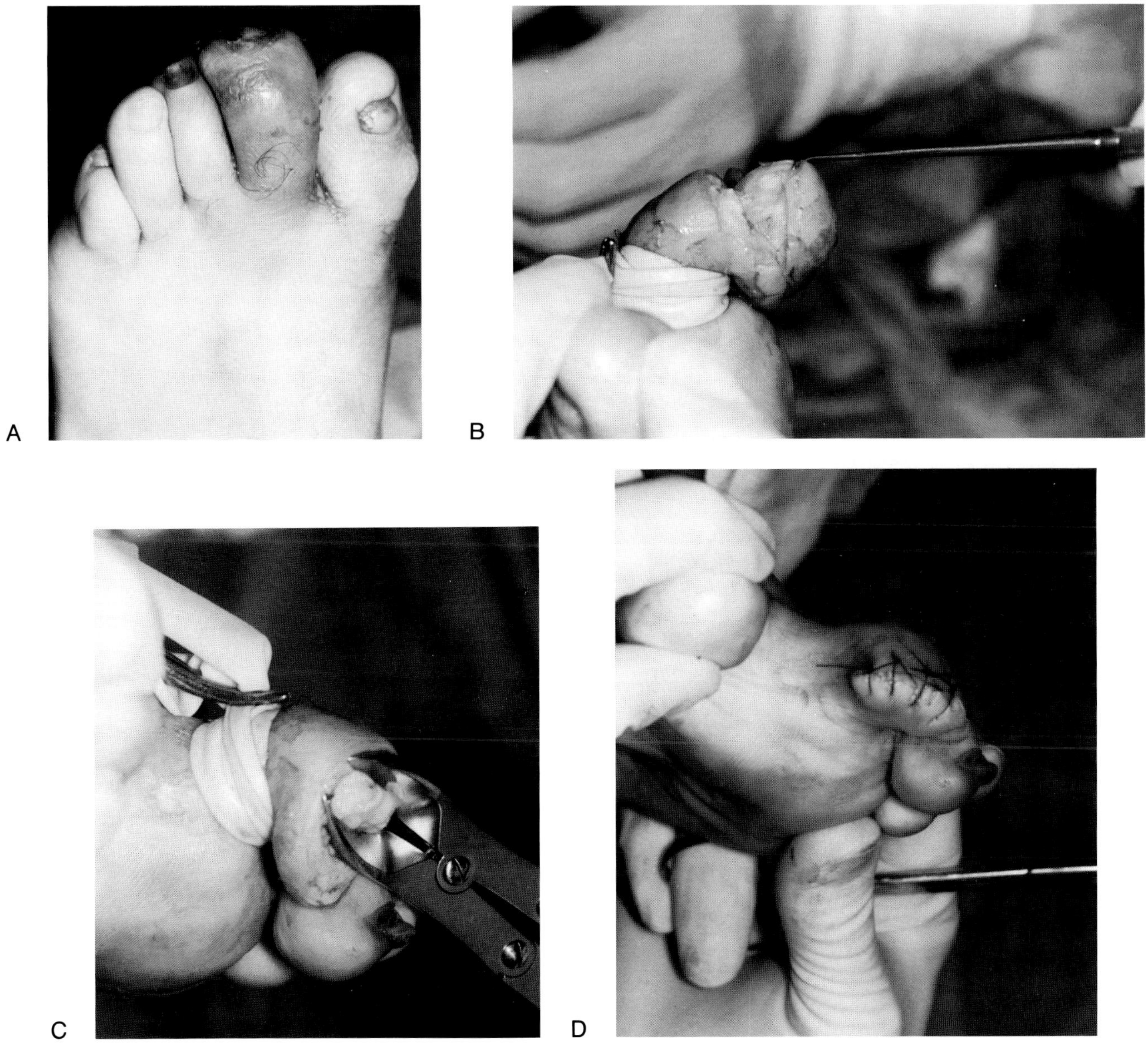

Fig. 17-8. (A) Second toe infected at tip from hammertoe deformity. (B) Resection of infected tip through incision with long plantar flap. (C) Resection of head of middle phalanx to remove sharp condyles. (D) Closure of flap produces weight-bearing skin at tip of residual toe.

cast is applied and the patient is started on assisted ambulation. Parallel bars, pickup walkers, or crutches are used as indicated. At 10 to 14 days the patient is started in a walking cast. When the tissues have matured, a shoe with heat-formed plastic inserts is fitted. Prosthetic foot parts are rarely indicated except for cosmesis.

Transmetatarsal Amputation

McKittrick and co-workers reported success with transmetatarsal amputations in diabetic patients in 1949.[30] The criteria they developed then are still valuable today. Some protective sensation should be present at the level of resection. Infec-

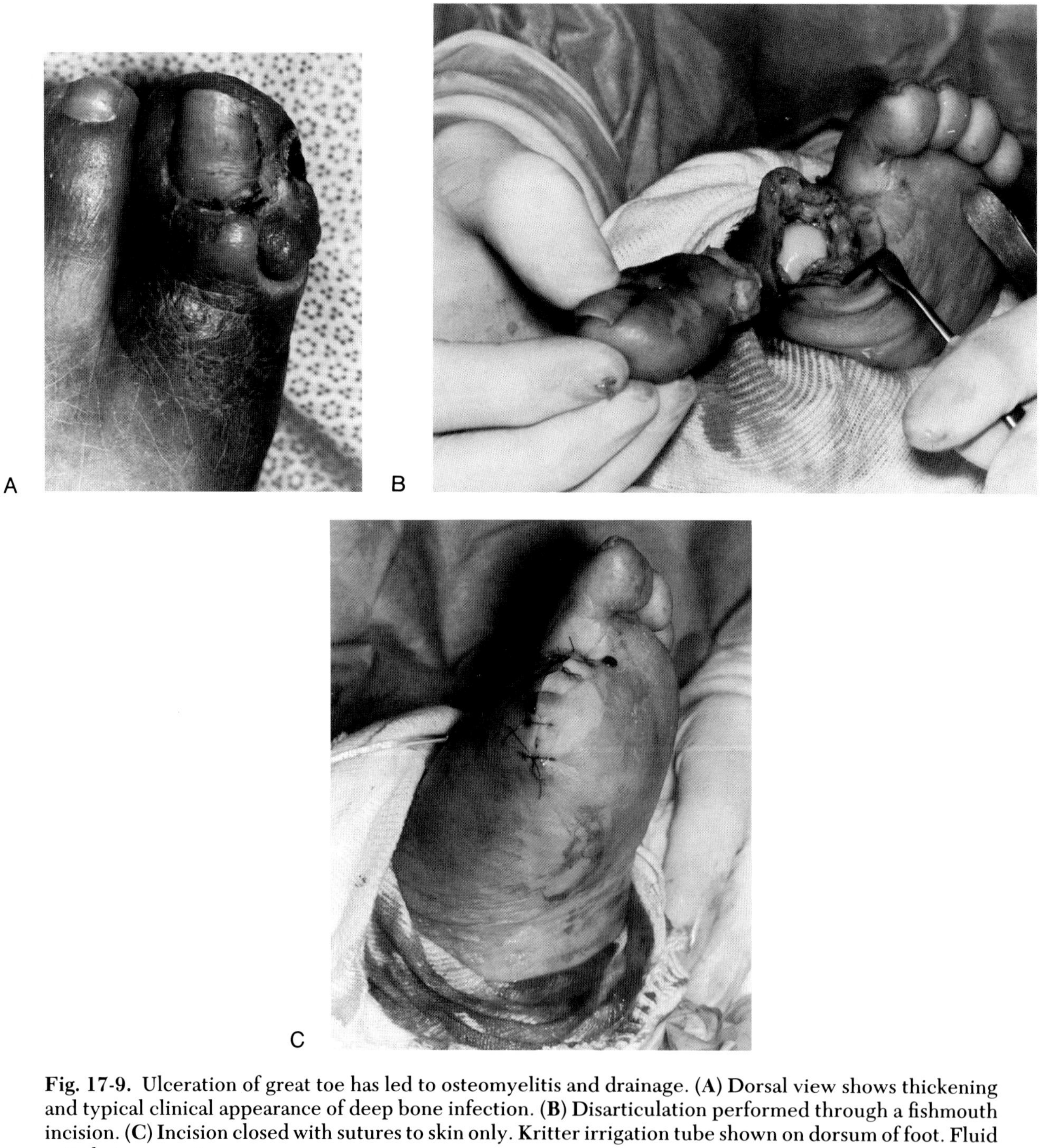

Fig. 17-9. Ulceration of great toe has led to osteomyelitis and drainage. (**A**) Dorsal view shows thickening and typical clinical appearance of deep bone infection. (**B**) Disarticulation performed through a fishmouth incision. (**C**) Incision closed with sutures to skin only. Kritter irrigation tube shown on dorsum of foot. Fluid exits between sutures.

tion should be controlled and should not extend proximal to the base of the toes. Diabetes mellitus should be under control. The foot should be warm. With evaluation now by Doppler index or other vascular tests, the success rate is well over 90 percent and there are very few late breakdowns.

Technique

The incision traverses the dorsum of the foot obliquely at the level of the metatarsal necks (Fig. 17-10). It is slanted posteriorly to the lateral side approximately 15° to correspond to the break of the shoe and the articulation angle of the metatar-

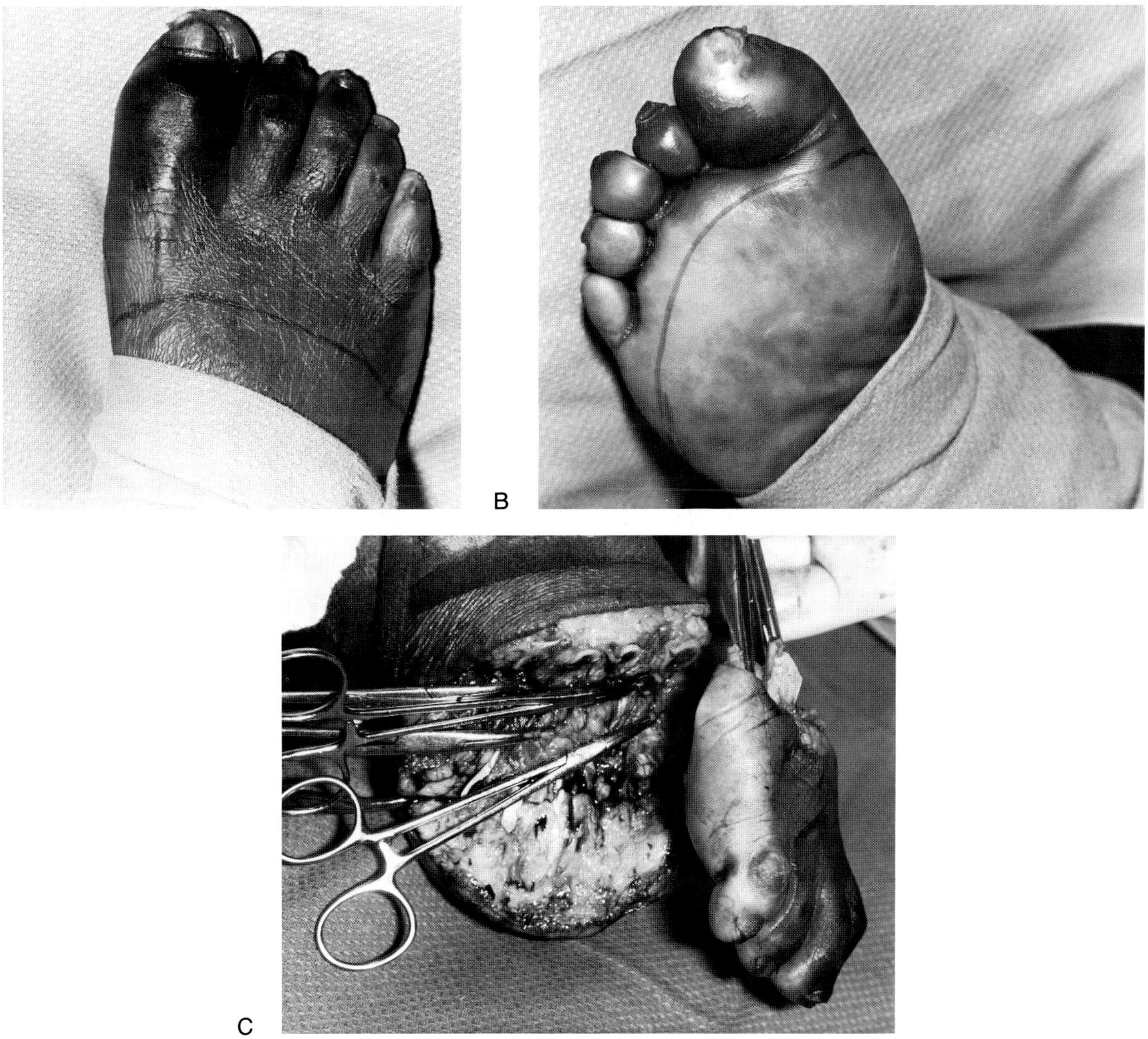

A B C

Fig. 17-10. (**A**) Dorsal incision for transmetatarsal amputation. (**B**) Plantar incision for transmetatarsal amputation. (**C**) Removal of distal toes from plantar flap. Note bleeding at removal of tourniquet.

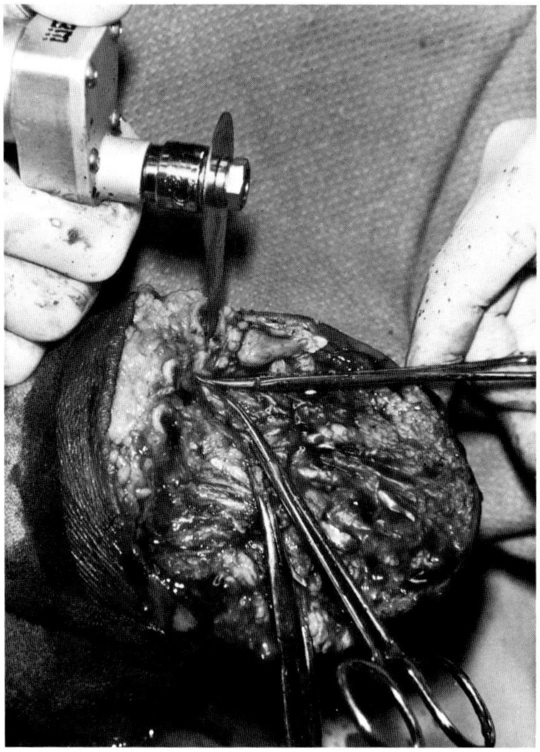

A

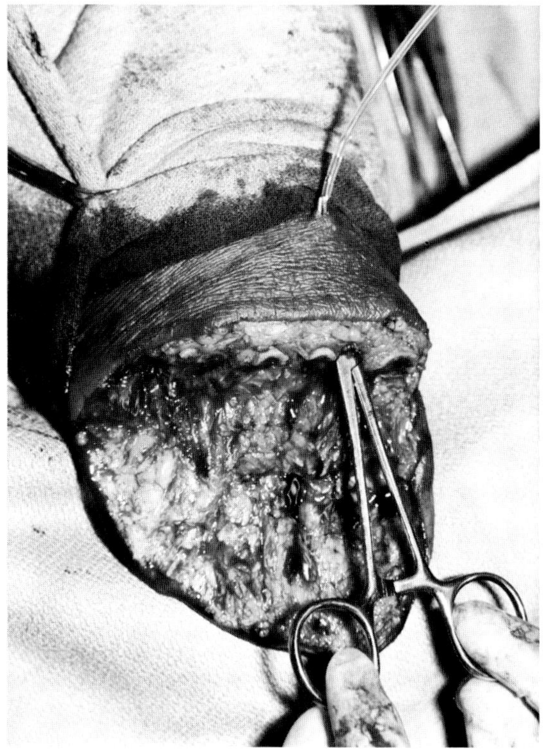

B

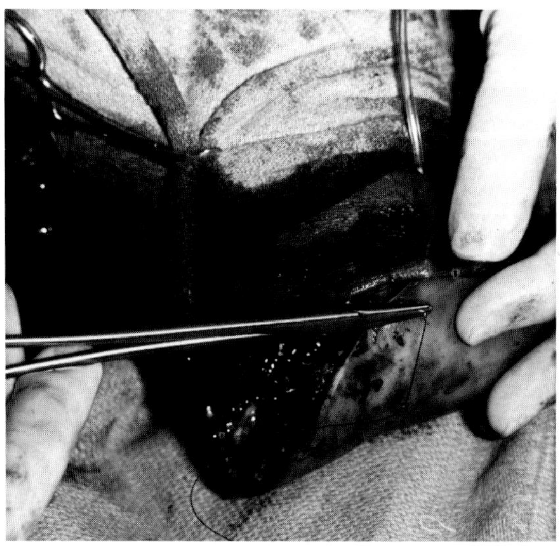

C

Fig. 17-11. (**A**) Beveling of the inferior edge of the residual metatarsal shafts removes pressure points. (**B**) Introduction of Kritter irrigation tube. Note rounded plantar edges of residual metatarsal shafts. (**C**) Closure of flap with single layer of sutures through skin and subcutaneous tissues.

sophalangeal joints. It continues to one-half the thickness of the foot on the medial and lateral sides. It then slopes distally to the plantar surface and across the foot just proximal to the base of the toes. The incision is carried sharply to bone in all areas. The metatarsals are divided at the proximal level of the incision. The distal foot is then raised dorsally and divided from the plantar flap. The inferior edges of the metatarsal shafts are beveled to remove any pressure points from the plantar surface (Fig. 17-11). The wound is irrigated thoroughly, removing all minor bits of debris. A Kritter drain is then introduced into the wound from a separate stab incision. The flap is then closed with a single layer of nonabsorbable sutures. A light compression dressing is applied.

Postoperative Function

Following removal of the Kritter drain and use of a walking cast at 2 weeks, the residual foot heals rapidly. Some patients are able to use an ordinary shoe. Others develop a pressure point under the residual metatarsal shaft that can be accentuated by the lever arm of the distal portion of the shoe. In these cases the sole must be thickened, stiffened, and rockered. This will then imitate the action of the rolloff at the metatarsophalangeal joint.

Lisfranc and Chopart Amputations

Lisfranc and Chopart amputations were designed before anesthesia, antibiotics, and blood transfusions were available. They were planned as disarticulations to be performed as rapidly as possible with soft tissue instruments alone without the need for cutting bone. Late complications of equinus deformity and ulceration are common, and both levels are infrequently used now, although there are still indications for their use with some modifications.[31] Some of the late problems can be prevented by transfer of the peroneus brevis tendon to the cuboid, transfer of the anterior tibial tendon to the neck of the talus, and lengthening of the Achilles tendon. However, when performing these amputations in an infected gangrenous foot it is not wise to attempt tendon transfers at the same time. Stabilization can usually be performed at a later date. Jacobs has reported success at these levels by including subcutaneous tenotomy of the Achilles tendon with the subsequent use of a polypropylene ankle/foot orthosis.[32] A further technique has been developed at Rancho Los Amigos that involves leaving the bases of the fourth and fifth metatarsals in place and thus saving the function of the peroneus brevis. The anterior tibial tendon is drawn down and incorporated in the skin closure so that it is also attached to the plantar fascia.

Technique

The incision passes over the dorsum of the foot at the base of the metatarsals. The plantar incision is kept long enough so that all infected material is removed, but the flap can be tailored to cover the ends of the bone. The tarsometatarsal joints are then disarticulated at the first, second, and third metatarsal bases. The fourth and fifth metatarsal bases are cut through with motorized saw and left in place. The residual foot is then dissected away from the plantar surface at the level of the short flexor muscles (Fig. 17-12). The residual flap is then checked further for infectious material and tailored to close without tension. A Kritter tube is used to irrigate the wound postoperatively. A light compression dressing is applied.

Irrigation is continued for 24 to 72 hours, depending upon the severity of preoperative infection. Cultures and sensitivities are tested from swabs taken during the procedure. When the tube is removed the foot is allowed to dry for approximately 1 day. It is then placed in a nonwalking cast. At 2 weeks the patient is allowed to ambulate in a plaster cast. The residual foot is shorter than that of a transmetatarsal and occasionally an ankle/foot orthosis is necessary (Fig. 17-13).

Chopart's amputation is a disarticulation through the talonavicular and calcaneocuboid joints. Surgical technique is quite similar to that of the Lisfranc amputation. The plantar flap is beveled distally to the skin edge. Any bony ridges that are palpable through the flap are rongeured smooth to prevent secondary pressure points. Kritter irrigation tubes are used and the flap is closed in one layer.

The residual foot is much shorter. Ankle/foot orthoses are frequently necessary for stability. If any deformity develops when healing is complete, tendon transfers and releases can correct such problems.

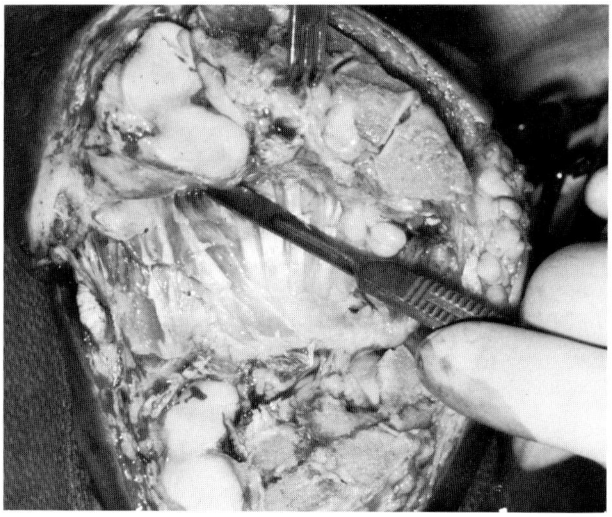

Fig. 17-12. Lisfranc amputation. Removal of distal foot from residual foot. Note cancellous bone through bases of fourth and fifth metatarsals.

The Syme Amputation

James Syme first performed his disarticulation at the ankle in 1842 and published a description in 1843. Syme recognized the superior function of the longer lever arm and the weight-bearing heel pad[33]:

> The advantages promised by amputation at the ankle joint instead of near the knee are: First, that the risk to life will be smaller; second, that a more comfortable stump will be afforded; and third, that the limb will be more seemly and useful for progressive motion. . . . On these grounds I think amputation at the ankle joint may be advantageously introduced into the practice of surgery. I regret having cut off many limbs that might have been saved by it and shall be glad if what has been said here in its favor encourages others to its performance.

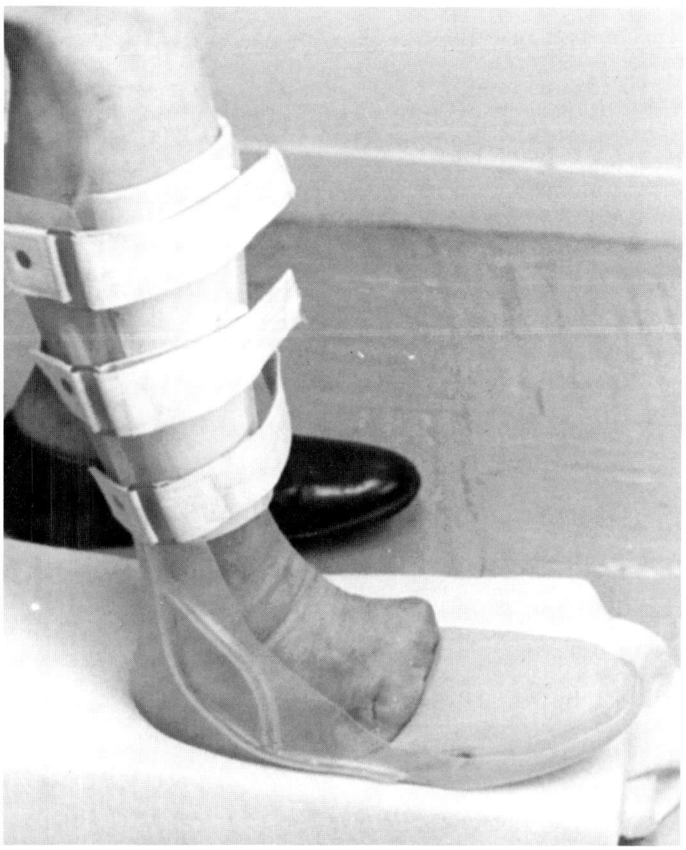

Fig. 17-13. Polypropylene orthosis used for very short transmetatarsal or modified Chopart amputation.

With the development of anesthesia, blood transfusions, antiseptics, bacteriostasis, and antibiosis, the risk to life is no longer as important a factor in limb amputation as it was in Syme's time. However, his amputation has its chief merit in that the limb is more seemly and useful for progressive motion. Around the world it has had varied acceptance in young vigorous patients but even more spotty acceptance in dysvascular patients. Canadian acceptance of the amputation has been greater than in most countries. R. I. Harris of Toronto has written two erudite articles on the history, development, and technique of this procedure, which remain classics.[34,35] Spittler et al. reported Hulnick's two-stage method in 1954.[36] In the Korean War it had been found that when the regular Syme amputation was performed for severely infected forefeet, virtually all of the residual limbs became infected. However, when ankle disarticulation alone was performed, the wounds healed. The definitive amputation was then performed 6 to 8 weeks later with virtually 100 percent healing of the definitive amputation.

The two-stage procedure was introduced at Los Angeles County Hospital in 1954 for infected diabetic foot problems. Early success was at 50 percent in these difficult feet. As experience grew, it rose to 70 percent. Addition of the post-tourniquet reaction time increased success to over 80 percent. In 1969 the Ortho/Diabetic Service was started at Rancho Los Amigos Medical Center for care of diabetic patients from the Los Angeles County Hospital system. Experience with the two-stage procedure continued. In 1975 the Doppler ultrasound flowmeter was introduced and the ischemic index developed further. With this procedure the success rate has risen to over 90 percent.[37] The two-stage method is used in all infected cases. The classical single-stage procedure is still used for traumatic and noninfected cases. Nearly 800 procedures have now been performed. Patient acceptance has been excellent in both men and women. The amputation is long lasting, and once the second stage is healed virtually none have required late higher amputation. The few late failures have been as a result of vascular occlusion.

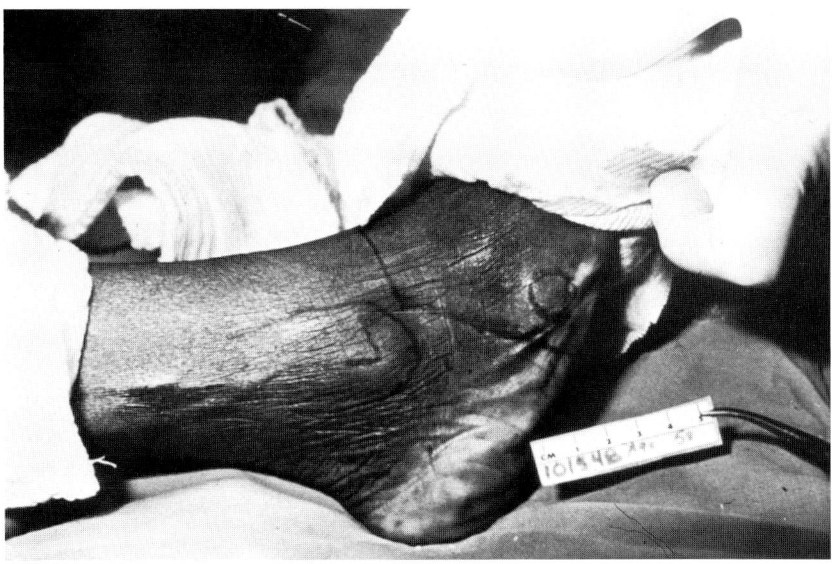

Fig. 17-14. Incision for Syme first stage of two-stage amputation technique. Incision leaves longer distal flap to cover the malleoli that remain.

In some patients, especially those with Charcot arthropathy, loose pads have developed. These pads have been stabilized by resecting the synovial clefts that have formed. Excess tissue is resected through wedges that allow the pad to be shifted to a normal position. It is then anchored to the tibia and fibula through drill holes in the bone.

Surgical Technique

The incision begins 1 cm below and 1 cm anterior to the distal tips of the malleoli (Fig. 17-14). This allows a slightly longer pad that will cover the retained malleoli without tension. Dorsally the incision goes just below the anterior edge of the tibia at the ankle joint. Medially and laterally the incisions go straight to the sole and across. In all areas the incision goes directly to bone without dissection of tissue planes. Dorsally the tendons are exposed, pulled down, divided, and allowed to retract. The superficial peroneal nerve is pulled down gently, divided, and allowed to retract. Entering the joint capsule exposes the dome of the talus (Fig. 17-15). The medial and lateral collateral ligaments are divided close to the malleoli. They are divided as the foot is manipulated side to side to expose and tighten the ligaments. A bone hook is driven into the talus as it begins to sublux from the joint. This aids in distal traction and provides control of the foot as the dissection proceeds. Care is taken on the medial side not to divide the posterior tibial nerve and artery as they course just behind and beneath the medial malleolus. When the lateral side is completely freed, subperiosteal dissection is begun. Carrying the dissection over the posterior dorsal surface exposes the tendon of the flexor hallucis longus almost directly in the center of the joint (Fig. 17-16). The tendon is just lateral to the neurovascular bundle and aids in its identification and protection. Subperiosteal dissection of the os calcis is continued medially, carrying the nerve and artery away from the bone. The flexor hallucis longus tendon is carefully dissected from under the sustentaculum tali, which frees the foot from the nerve and artery. Continued sharp and subperiosteal dissection then delivers the os calcis from the fat pad and the Achilles tendon. There is always a ridge of bone on the posterior aspect of the os calcis at the insertion of the Achilles tendon. The retrocalcaneal bursa is reflected plantarward to expose the tendon. When dissecting the Achilles tendon from the os calcis, care must be taken as the ridge of bone can deflect the knife blade and thus cut the posterior skin. Dissection of the attachment of the Achilles tendon and plantar aponeurosis completes the removal of the foot. The tourniquet is released and timing of appearance of bleeding to the distal-

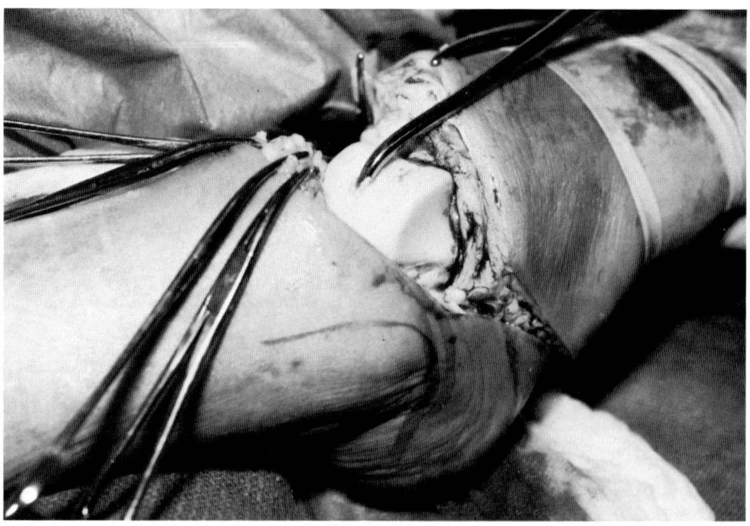

Fig. 17-15. Bone hook in talus aids in control of the distal foot. Collateral ligaments have been partially cut to allow subluxation of the talus.

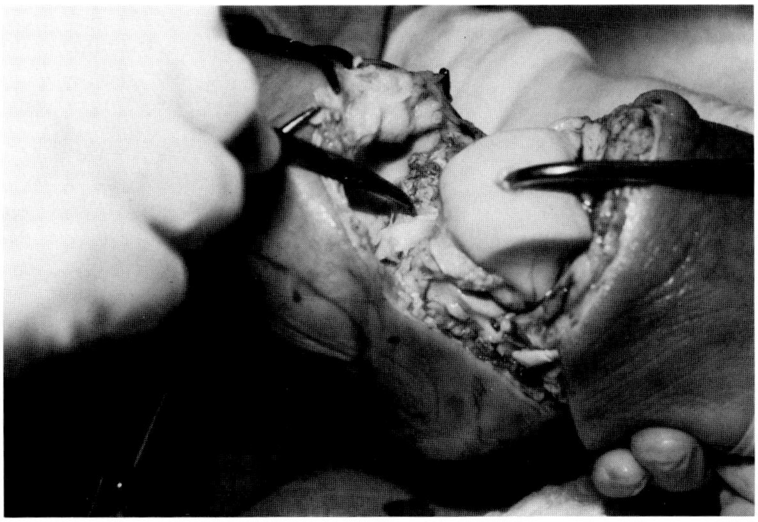

Fig. 17-16. Forceps indicates flexor hallucis longus tendon in center of ankle joint. The neurovascular bundle lies medially.

most skin is started (Fig. 17-17). If any of the preoperative vascular indicators have been at the lower limits and bleeding does not return by 5 minutes, serious consideration should be given to continuing the surgery at the below knee level. After release of the tourniquet, hemostasis is secured with ligatures and pinpoint electrocoagulation. There is always a nutrient vessel in the Achilles tendon that supplies the posterior os calcis. This can lead to troublesome bleeding if it is not found and coagulated. Tags of fascia and muscle are tidied up. The posterior tibial and peroneal tendons are pulled distally, excised, and allowed to retract. Any fascia that appears devitalized is excised.

For postoperative drainage a modified Shirley drain is brought in through a separate stab incision. Irrigation is started with an antibiotic in Ringer's lactate solution. If the pad is pushed to one side or the other by one of the malleoli, slits can be made in the deep fascia and the fat pad so that one or more of the malleoli will nest in the slits. This is tested before closure is begun. Closure is started by bringing the aponeurosis to the periosteum and deep fascia overlying the distal tibia. The deep fascia of the pad is sutured to the deep fascia of the anterior tissue just above the joint. Subcutaneous fat is closed with sutures that are placed so as to level the skin edges. Nonabsorbable sutures or skin

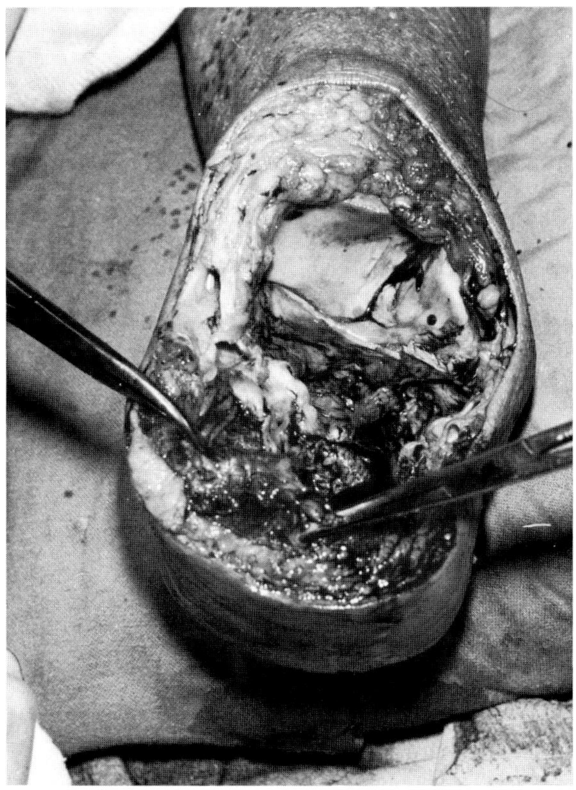

Fig. 17-17. Plantar flap after removal of os calcis 40 seconds after release of tourniquet that had been inflated 23 minutes. Note bleeding along distal skin edges.

staples are used in the skin. No attempt should be made to "tidy up" the dog-ears. They will be excised at the second stage. A light compression dressing is applied and wrapped with bias-cut stockinette. Care should be taken not to pull the dog-ears back upon themselves or this will jeopardize the circulation. A thin posterior splint of plaster of paris is used to support the pad from the effects of gravity and to take stress from the suture line.

Postoperative Care

Irrigation is continued into the cavity of the heel pad. The outflow tube is connected to gravity drainage. Irrigation is continued for 48 to 96 hours depending upon the character of the drainage fluid. If it is still cloudy or bloody, the irrigation system is continued until the fluid clears. The tube is removed aseptically and the tip is sent for culture and sensitivity studies. Following one day of drying out of the wound, a short leg nonwalking cast is applied. At 10 days a walking cast is applied and the patient started on crutch- or walker-assisted ambulation. Medical conditions may contraindicate this phase until the patient becomes systemically stronger. Reconditioning exercises can be performed in bed if necessary. The patient is then discharged to be followed in the clinic for cast changes, suture removal, and control of further medical problems. At 6 to 10 weeks the patient is readmitted for the second stage if the first stage has healed.

Second-Stage Technique

The second stage is the definitive amputation. The procedure has been modified so that the complete amputation need not be redone. Dog-ears are removed through elliptical incisions. The approach is carried through all layers down to bone. The wedge of tissue removed approximates the volume of the malleolus removed. The malleoli are further outlined by sharp dissection close to bone. With the osteotome, the malleoli are removed flush with the plafond. The medial and lateral flares are smoothed to prevent pressure points (Fig. 17-18). The deep fascia of the pad is then approximated to the periosteum of the tibia and fibula and held with a clamp or towel clip. The pad is tested. If it is not loose, the deep fascia is then sutured to the periosteum. If the pad is loose, soft tissue is removed until the pad is tightened. Drill holes are made in the tibia and fibula. The deep fascia of the pad is sutured through these drill holes to bone. The plafond is not denuded of cartilage. The subcutaneous fat and skin are closed. The completed amputation has a narrowed diameter and no bony prominences. A light compression dressing is applied. A short leg walking cast is used for ambulation at 1 week. The limb is ready for a definitive prosthesis at about 8 to 12 weeks.

Classical One-Stage Technique

In most cases without infection the amputation is begun at the tips of the malleoli. The dorsum and plantar incisions are similar but more proximal than in the two-stage technique. The procedure then follows the two-stage method down to the removal of the foot. After removal of the foot the anterior and posterior tibia and both malleoli are outlined sharply to 1 cm above the plafond. With an amputation saw or motorized saw, the tibia and fibula are removed at such a level that approximately 2.5 cm of articular cartilage remains in the dome of the ankle joint. The cut is at right angles to the weight-bearing line. All sharp edges are smoothed. The heel pad is then closed manually and the edges of the bone palpated through the pad. Any remaining sharp edges are smoothed. Since the distal flare provides suspension for the prosthesis, care is taken not to destroy the flare by removing too much bone. The flap is tested again, and if it is still loose, some of the distal soft tissue is removed. If it is too tight, further bone must be removed.

After release of the tourniquet and completion of hemostasis, a Shirley drain is brought into the wound. Drill holes are made in the edges of the tibia and fibula. The wound is irrigated thoroughly. The pad is then sutured through the drill holes into the tibia and fibula.[38] The skin edges are leveled by sutures in the subcutaneous tissue. The skin is closed. No attempt is made to tidy up the dog-ears, as they will flatten with time and stump wrapping. A cast is applied after removal of the irrigating system. Weight bearing is begun at 7 to 10 days. A definitive prosthesis is prescribed at 8 to 12 weeks.

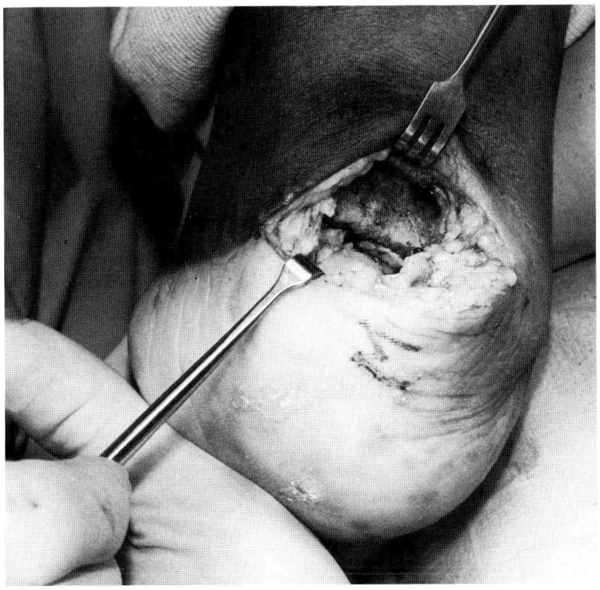

A

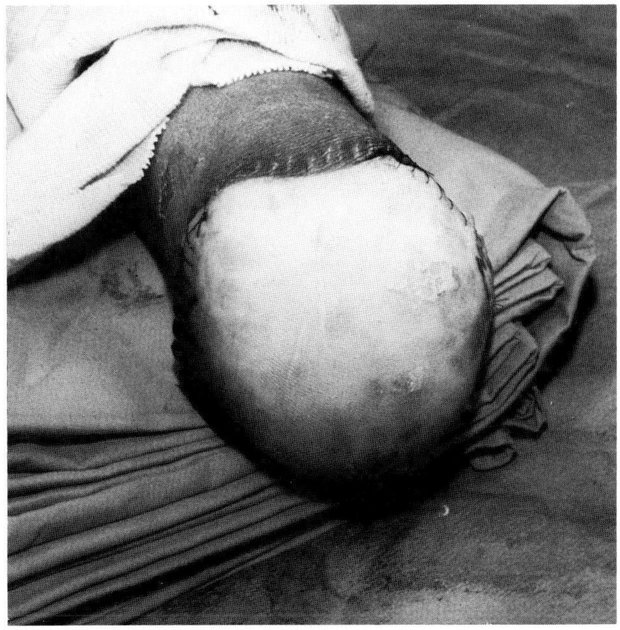

B

Fig. 17-18. (**A**) Second-stage Syme amputation. Medial malleolus removed flush with plafond. Flare of distal tibia removed to prevent pressure area. Note residual articular cartilage remaining on tibia. (**B**) With removal of the "dog-ears" and the malleoli, the residual stump is narrowed and there are no bony prominences.

Prosthetic Replacement for the Syme Amputation

A prosthesis must replace as much as possible of the form and function lost through amputation. The Syme amputee retains the full length of the shin and the weight-bearing heel pad while losing the height of the talus and calcaneus as well as foot and ankle function. Many prosthetic designs have been tried in attempt to provide support during stance phase, to provide suspension during swing phase, and to provide the equivalent of ankle and foot function. Bioengineering is now providing answers through laboratory analysis for some of the problems that were previously approached only through the "cut and try" methods of the workbench. Radcliffe has aided markedly in the understanding of the biomechanics of the Syme prosthesis through work at the Biomechanics Laboratory at University of California, San Francisco and Berkeley.[39]

Plastic laminates with fiberglass roving and epoxy resins have largely replaced the steel-reinforced leather sockets, willow sockets, and aluminum sockets that were used in the previous 145 years. The bulbous end of the residual limb provides suspension of the prosthesis. Various methods have been used to allow its passage into the prosthesis. In an artificial limb with a laced leather corset, the bulbous end passes easily when the laces are loosened. Tightness of the corset can be adjusted for comfort and variations in tissue fluids. In plastic molded prostheses medial or posterior windows allow passage of the pad and the cover provides suspension when reattached. The disadvantages of a removable part are that it may be lost and the straps and buckles are unsightly. The double-wall socket has a more bulbous ankle area but has no straps, buckles, or windows (Fig. 17-19). It is also stronger, since there is no break in the outer cylindrical walls. The elastic panel in the liner socket expands to allow passage of the heel pad. Contraction of the elastic provides suspension of the prosthesis. There is a posterior rubber heel wedge cushion that simulates ankle flexion after

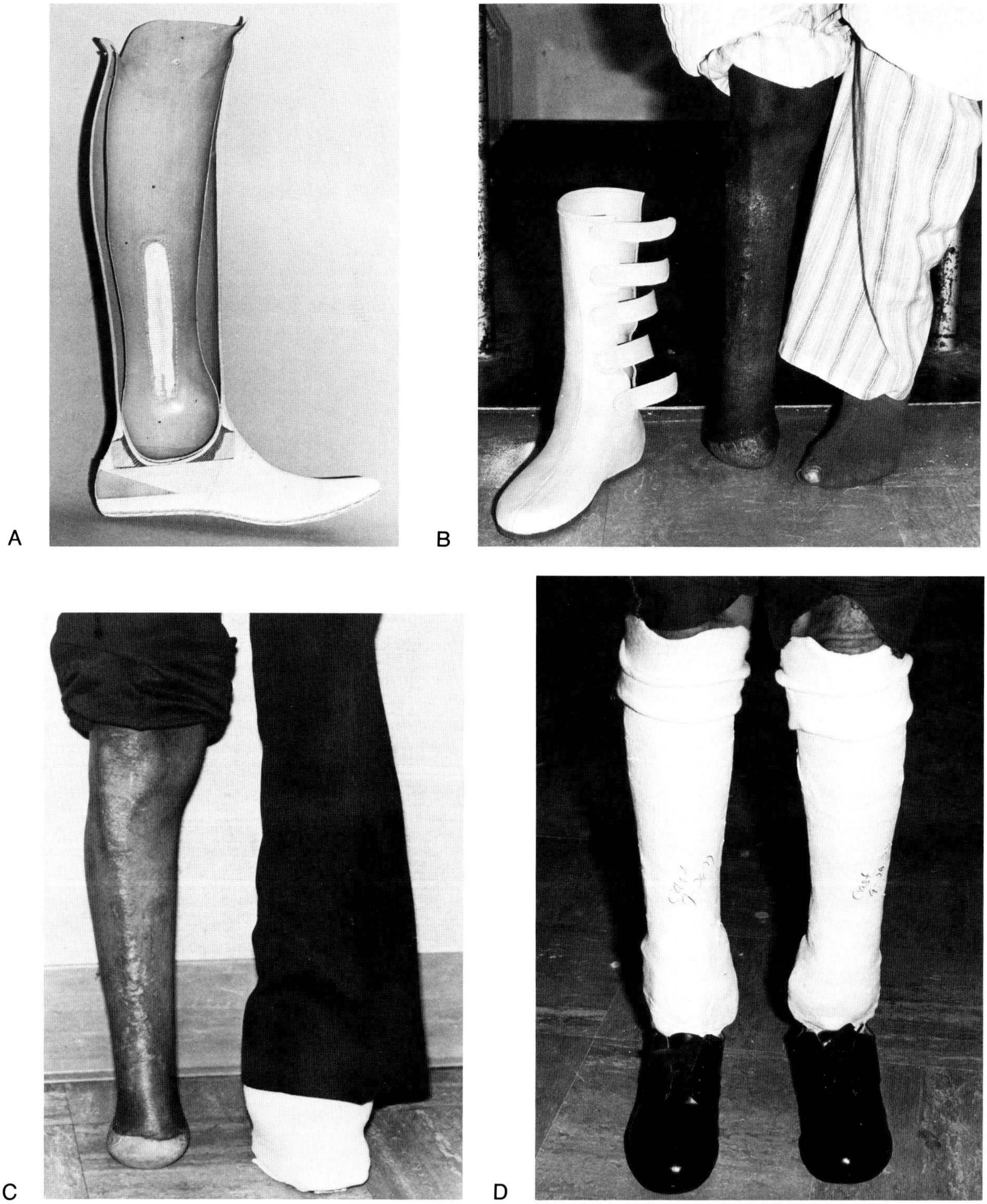

Fig. 17-19. (**A**) Syme prosthesis with double walls. Note elastic panel, which allows passage of bulbous end, rocker bottom forefoot for rolloff, and posterior cushion heel, which imitates ankle motion and cushions heel strike. (**B**) Plastic prosthesis for Syme amputee for limited household transfers and ambulation. (**C**) A walking cast is used following the second-stage Syme amputation. This aids markedly in rapidity of rehabilitation. (**D**) Walking casts fitted with feet to simulate the finished prosthesis. Height adjustment is relatively easy because of bilaterality.

heel strike. Elasticity and contour of the distal artificial foot allow virtually normal rolloff.

On occasion patients who will not be community ambulators may need a prosthetic device for passage from wheelchair to bed, bath, toilet, chair, and table. Such a device can be formed over a plaster mold. Thus protection is provided against foreign objects and against any weight bearing on a hard floor.

Rehabilitation of the Syme Amputee
Between the first and second stages the patient is usually discharged in a walking cast. Following the second stage a similar cast is used. Transition from the walking cast with a rubber heel or with an artificial foot to a prosthesis requires the least training and practice for the Syme amputee when compared with higher amputations. Assistive devices such as canes, crutches, and walkers are rarely needed except with bilateral amputees. As strength, endurance, and agility are regained, the need for assistive devices decreases. Most Syme amputees consider their loss an annoyance rather than a major disability. After a few lessons in donning and doffing the prosthesis, the average amputee says, "It will take me a week or two to get used to the new leg."

Below Knee Amputation

The procedure for determination of length of the below knee residual limb is not well described in most articles on amputation. Statements that the bone should be 5 to 7 inches in length actually help very little. A 5-inch stump in a 6½-foot person is short. A 7-inch stump in a 5-foot person is long. Cutting at the thickest part of the calf wastes a good portion of the available lever arm. Articles relating function to length of stump invariably show that a longer stump is more efficient.[40,41] Consultations with many prosthetists have failed to raise any objection to a longer below knee stump. A system has been devised for determining length of residual bone that is based upon the length of the limb (Fig. 17-20). If gangrene, ulceration, or infection extend into the proposed area, the flaps and lengths will have to be adapted to the tissue available. A simple test to determine if the limb is too short can be performed during surgery. The flaps are closed manually and the knee is bent. If no shelf is formed posteriorly, the residual limb is then too short to hold a prosthesis in place. In younger patients skin grafting and flap rotation may save a useable stump. This is rarely feasible in the older patient.

The site of tibial division is determined by dividing the distance from the tibial plateau to the musculotendinous junction into four parts. Bone division is performed at the distal three quarters. The skin incision begins ½-inch distal to the bone line. It slants backward to the tibial division line at the posterior third of the leg. From there it curves distally and rises ½-inch to accommodate the bulge of the calf. It then courses distally on the posterior calf to a point that makes the flap equal to two-thirds of the diameter of the leg. Since the last cut is bevel across the cone of the calf, the shape of the flap approximates the anterior triangular contour of the leg. After a little practice in drawing these incisions there is seldom any need to trim the flaps before closure. The skin incision is completed around the leg and the tissues allowed to retract. The anterolateral compartment muscles are divided at the retracted skin line. The anterior tibial artery and vein are clamped. The fibula is exposed approximately 2 cm above the line for tibial division (Fig. 17-21). It is then divided with a Gigli or motorized saw. The tibia is exposed subperiosteally to the limit of the anterior curve that is proposed. The contour of this tibial cut is drawn onto the bone with a marking pen. The mark is more easily followed with a Gigli saw. After bone division, the distal tibia and fibula are raised anteriorly with a bone hook. The posterior musculature is cut to one-half its thickness and the blade of the amputation knife is then turned distally to follow the line of the skin flap. The large vessels are clamped and the tourniquet released. This portion usually takes 15 to 20 minutes. Hemostasis is then completed with ligatures and electrocoagulation. The flap is brought anteriorly and the tibia and fibula are palpated through the soft tissues. The final shape of the crest of the tibia is contoured with osteotome and smoothed with bone file. If the fibula is too prominent, it is rounded or shortened until it feels satisfactory to the surgeon. The flap is again tested and adjusted or trimmed as necessary. On occasion the posterior musculature may be too thick for clo-

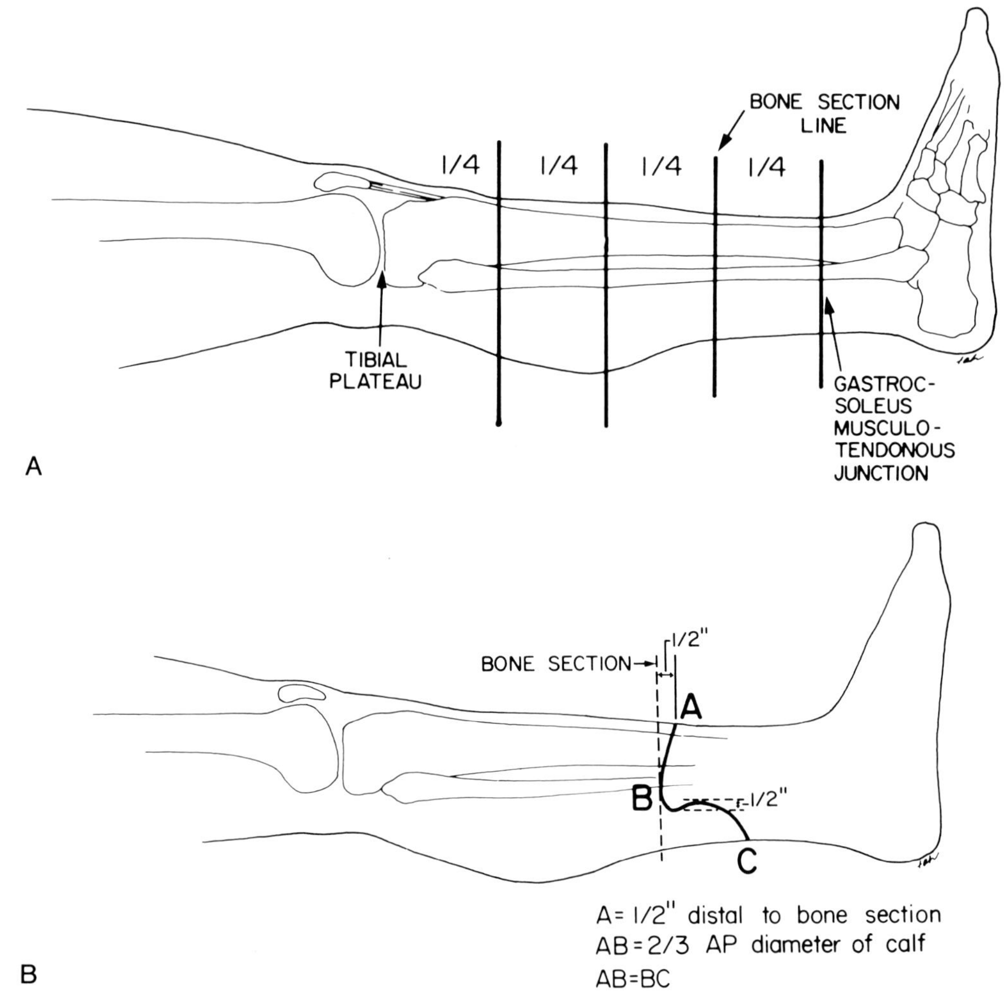

Fig. 17-20. (**A**) Below knee amputation. Measurements are to determine stump length based on body proportions. (**B**) Outline of incision to produce flap shape that will match shape of calf.

sure and more or all of the soleus must be removed. The wound is irrigated to remove minor bits of debris. Drains are used as indicated. The posterior flap is folded up to the tibia. The tendon and aponeurosis of the gastrocnemius are sutured to the anterior periosteum of the tibia. The anterolateral muscles have been sutured to the posterior surface and aponeurosis of the posterior muscles. The deep fascia is sutured around the periphery of the wound. The subcutaneous fat is leveled with interrupted horizontal mattress sutures. The skin is closed with nonabsorbable sutures.

Postoperative Care

A soft compression dressing is applied over the wound and wrapped with bias-cut stockinette. A plaster cast is applied over suitable padding. Care is taken to relieve pressure over the patella (Fig. 17-22). We no longer use immediate pylons and weight bearing in the dysvascular patient. The wound is inspected, and at 14 days a pylon is applied if sufficient healing has taken place. As the wound matures a temporary prosthesis is applied. A definitive prosthesis is prescribed at 8 to 12 weeks. Primary healing and prosthetic use occur in

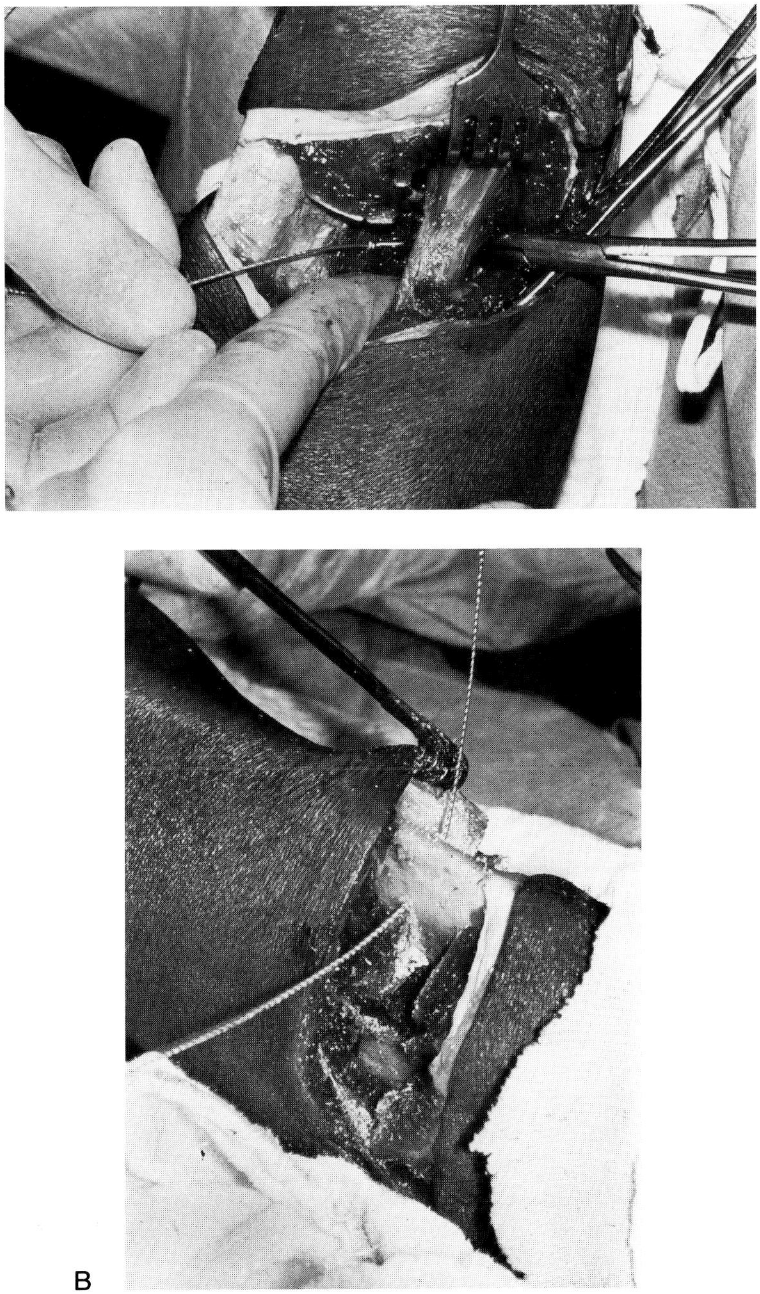

A

B

Fig. 17-21. (**A**) Below knee amputation. Division of the fibula with Gigli saw. (**B**) Note beginning of curved osteotomy. *(Figure continues.)*

C
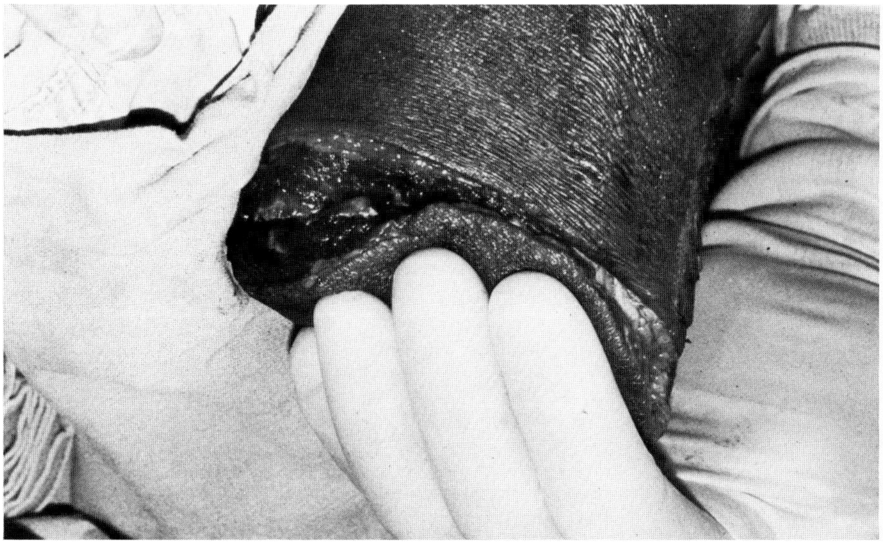

Fig. 17-21 *(Continued)*. **(C)** Manual closing of flaps and palpation tests for bony prominences and closure of flap without tension. Note shape of flap similar to shape of calf.

a high percentage of the patients at this level.[42] Complications and revisions are still somewhat more frequent than at the Syme level.

Side to Side Flaps

Equal medial and lateral flaps have been advocated for the below knee level.[43] Length is determined for bone division as described earlier. The flap length is equal to one-half the diameter of the leg at the bone division line. Tibial and fibular division are the same as for the long posterior flap. The shape of the residual limb is slightly more conical. Healing and prosthetic use are the same as in the long posterior flap amputation. The major usage has been in patients whose skin is not suitable for the long posterior flap procedure.

Ertl Procedure (Tibial-Fibular Stabilization)

Since most patients are being operated on for infection and gangrene, additional elective bony or soft tissue procedures should not be performed at the time of the initial amputation. For such complications as recurrent ulcers, pressure problems over the fibular head, pistoning in the prosthesis, and feelings of instability, the patient should be considered for the Ertl procedure (Fig. 17-23). This is performed as a secondary procedure. The primary stabilization as described by Ertl is done with osteoperiosteal flaps at the time of amputation in noninfected cases.[44] Secondary stabilization is provided between the tibia and fibula by developing a graft from the lateral side of the tibia and swinging it over to the fibula. It is felt that weight bearing on the conical stump pressing into a conical socket produces motion of the fibula as the limb is pressed into the socket. In many patients this results in additional shear pressure on the skin. Stabilizing the fibula to the tibia stops this motion.

Surgical Procedure

The healed incision over the anterior tibia is entered sharply and developed through the subcutaneous tissue to bone. The periosteum over the tibia is incised and the anterolateral surface is exposed subperiosteally. The muscle is divided longitudinally to expose the fibula. A 2 by 4 cm graft is cut with a fine saw on the lateral surface of the tibia. It is raised from its bed and fashioned to fit between the tibia and fibula. The end of the fibula is notched to hold the graft. Sutures of polyglycolic acid and/or wire are placed through drill holes in the graft and the tibia and fibula. The graft is then tied in place. Cancellous chips from the interior of the tibia are packed around the graft sites. Divided

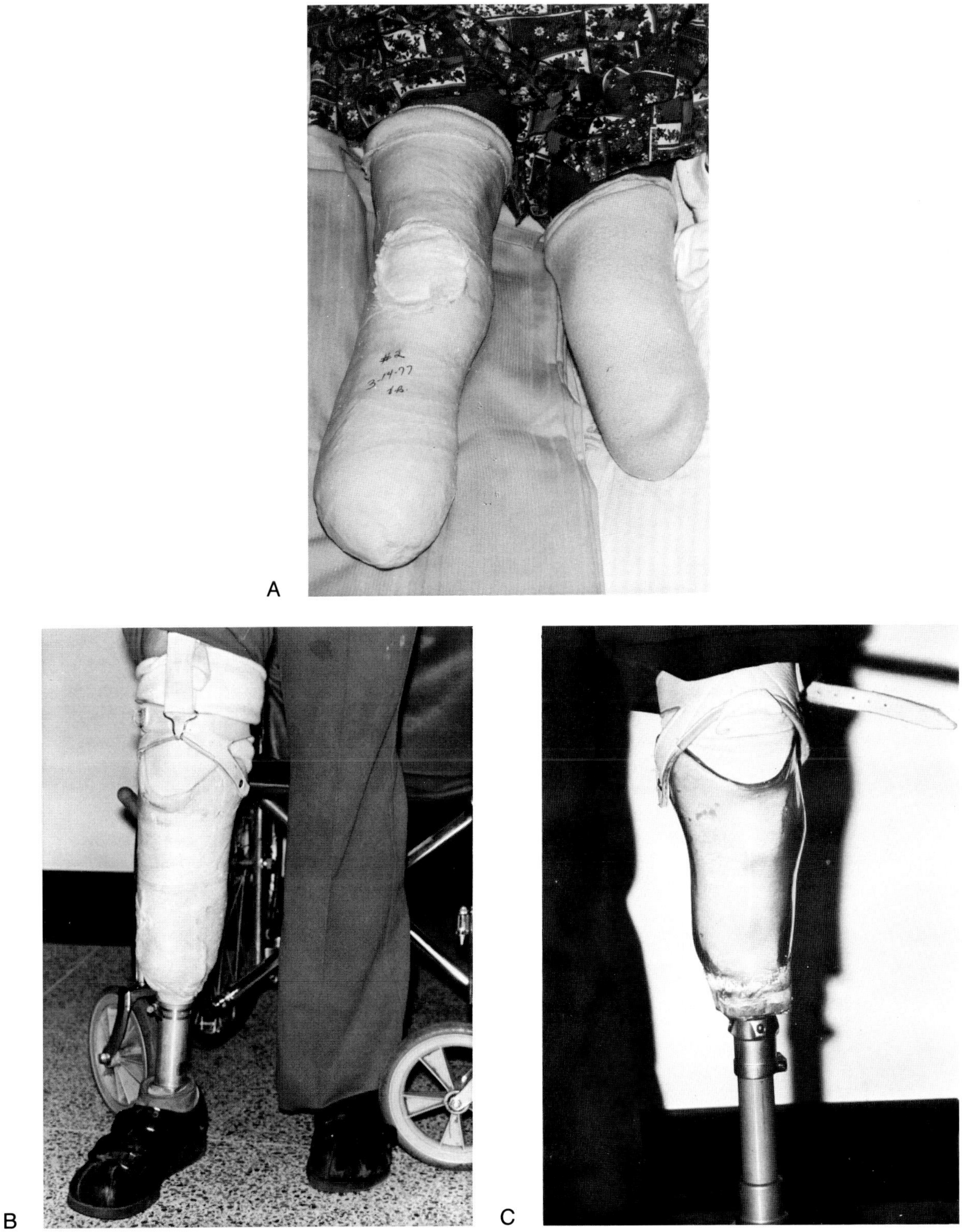

Fig. 17-22. (**A**) Below knee amputation. Protective cast applied at surgery. Note cutout over patella to prevent pressure. (**B**) Pylon attached to cast to provide ambulation during maturation phase of healing. (**C**) Temporary prosthesis with test socket to allow planning of final definitive limb.

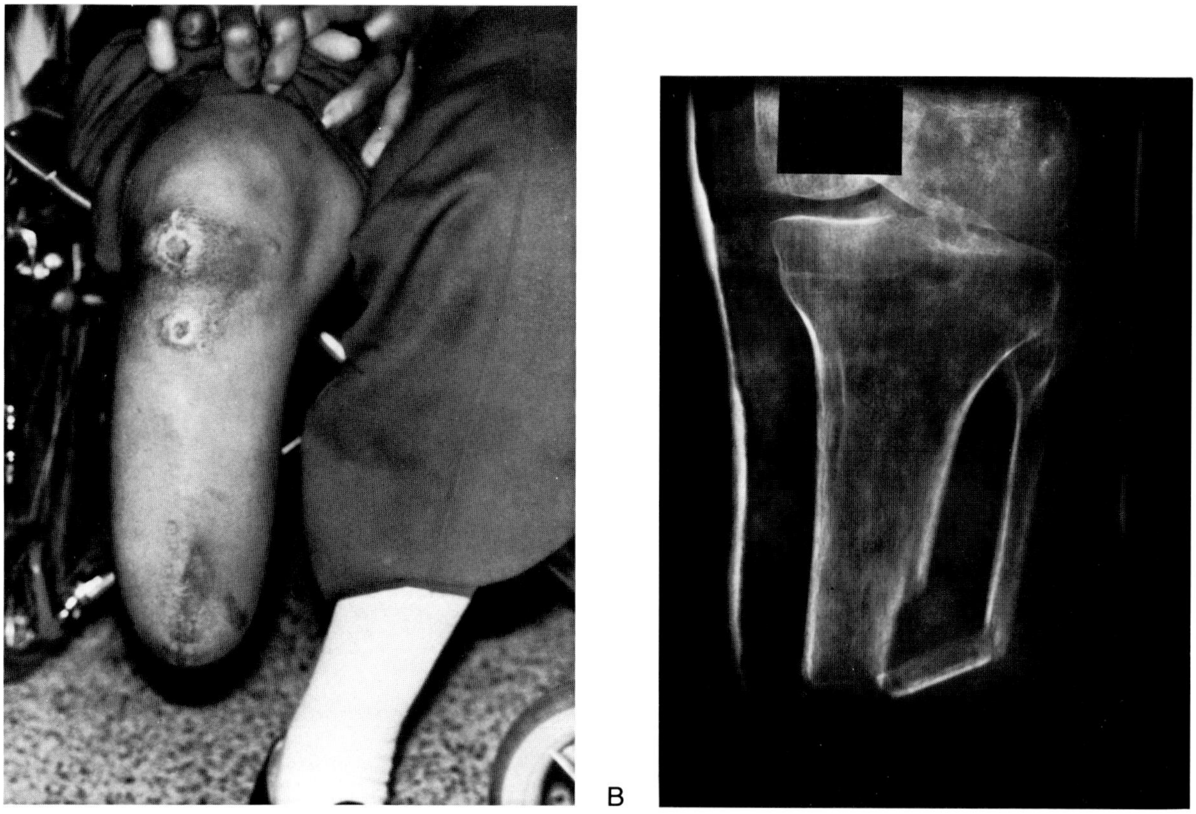

A B

Fig. 17-23. (A) Below knee amputation. Multiple pressure areas on residual limb from mobile fibula and pistoning in the prosthesis. Note also the sagittal incision. (B) Below knee amputation with secondary Ertl (tibiofibular) stabilization. Note defect in tibia at graft site and drill holes in graft.

musculature is sutured over the graft. The posterior muscles are sutured to the anterior periosteum as the flap is closed in layers. A plaster cast is applied over suitable padding. A walking pylon is used at 3 weeks. A definitive prosthesis can be prescribed at 8 to 12 weeks. Patients report an immediate feeling of stability, cessation of pressure sores, and even an ability for partial end bearing. Excellent maturation of the graft has been the usual result.

Prosthetic Replacement for Below Knee Amputations

Saving of the knee has probably been the most important advance in amputation surgery for the ischemic lower limb. With this level there is increased prosthetic control. With this increased control there is also increased activity and the demands on the prosthesis are increased. There are also increased demands on the weight-bearing surfaces that cannot be end bearing with the usual amputation techniques. With plastic laminates the socket is formed to closer tolerances. The plaster model of the stump is modified to provide areas of relief from pressure, with resulting comfort as well as stability. The socket can be lined with materials of varied resiliency depending upon the patient's needs. Suspension can be provided by socket brim design, suprapatellar straps, condylar wedges, and waist belts. The prescription is modified for individual requirements. Special additions provide closer to natural function. A multiaxis ankle allows greater mobility on rough ground and relieves stress at the hip and knee joints. A transverse rotation device can be fitted above the ankle. It is frequently indicated for patients with skin problems.

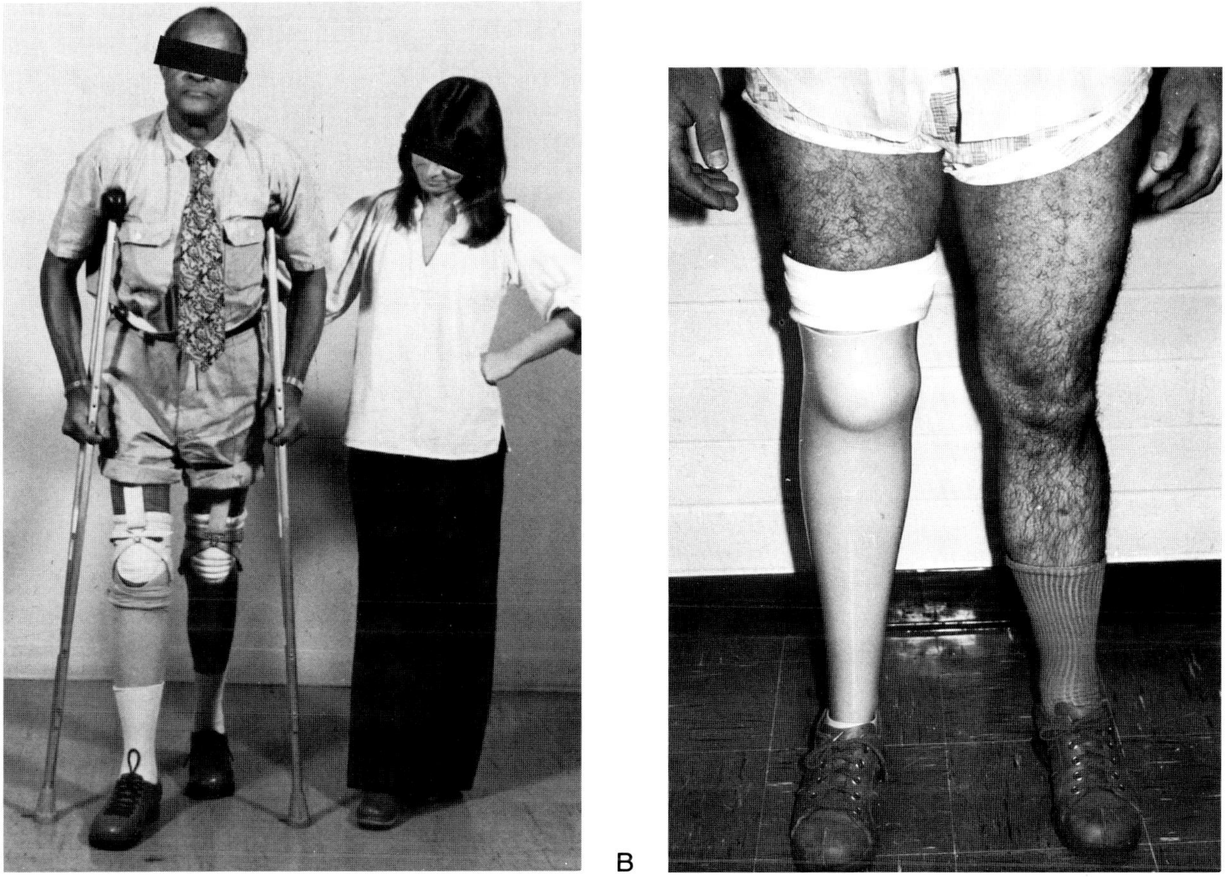

A B

Fig. 17-24. (**A**) Below knee prosthesis with patellar tendon bearing (PTB) brim, suprapatellar strap, and pelvic belt suspension. These additions are frequently necessary in obese and heavy patients to help absorb stress to the residual limb and knee joint. (**B**) Below knee prosthesis with suprapatellar brim at patella, which provides excellent suspension.

Suspension devices of various types are available, including the following: patellar tendon bearing brim with suprapatellar strap and pelvic belt (Fig. 17-24); patellar tendon bearing brim with knee joints, thigh lacer, and pelvic belt; patellar tendon bearing socket with suprapatellar brim and cuff suspension (the support is endoskeletal and is covered with a cosmetic cover); suprapatellar brim with suspension provided against the flares of the femur, in which knee stability in the mediolateral plane is excellent; and the suprapatellar brim with removable section, which is used when the femoral condyles are wider than usual. The most commonly used foot and ankle combination is the solid ankle cushioned heel (SACH foot), as seen in the Syme prosthesis. Addition of a spring keel either of plastic or metal is a new development that has promised additional function. At present it is indicated usually in younger, more vigorous amputees. Older patients relate that they must actually push the prosthesis down to get the value of the spring and at times this can be tiring for them.

Rehabilitation for Below Knee Amputees

The training begun upon admission to the hospital is continued postsurgically as soon as medical conditions permit. Pain must be minimized by adequate analgesia and immobilization. Flexion contractures must not be allowed to occur. Edema must be reduced by bandaging and use of pylons or temporary prostheses. Joint motion is encouraged, as are progressive resistance exercises for both upper and lower extremities.

Ambulation is a learned activity that becomes automatic early in life. For many patients the stress of walking with a pylon or prosthesis is near the extreme of their physical ability. As with any other physical skill, practice is essential. Training usually begins between bars, progresses to crutches or a walker, then to a single cane, and finally to no mobility aids.

Through Knee Amputation

Nathan Smith first reported amputation at the knee joint in the American literature in 1825.[45] It had been reported sporadically in the world literature as far back as the 1600s. In comparison with other lower extremity levels, relatively few reports have been made. During the Civil War 211 cases were reported from the records of the Union Army. The mortality rate was much lower than amputations through the thigh or calf. Occasionally authors relate antipathy of limb makers to end-bearing stumps as a major cause of disinterest among surgeons.

Many standard textbooks have ignored this level; it is mentioned but not recommended in others, and even discouraged in some. The most enthusiastic modern advocate, Rogers, does not feel it should be performed in patients with peripheral vascular disease.[46] Our success rate with diabetic patients has been over 90 percent.

The through knee amputation has many similarities to the Syme amputation: (1) it is end-bearing, (2) the lever arm of the entire bone is preserved, (3) the end is bulbous and aids in prosthetic suspension, (4) limb makers have reported difficulty in producing a satisfactory prosthesis, (5) indications for the procedure have changed as dysvascular patients have become more numerous.

Following a below knee amputation, hip and knee contractures are common in patients who do not become prosthetic users. These deformities can interfere markedly with hygiene and sleeping positions. Amputation through the knee is an eminently satisfactory procedure for the nonambulatory patient. For the severely ill patient, a careful preoperative assessment must be made to determine the potential level of postamputation activities. If sufficient blood supply is indicated by vascular examination, the knee is saved in most instances except in those in which the patient was not ambulatory preoperatively.

Experience at Rancho Los Amigos Medical Center has shown the through knee amputation to be an excellent level from the surgical standpoint. It can be performed rapidly, local anesthesia can be used, there is minimal blood loss, no bone is transected, and fewer muscle masses are divided. The long anterior flap as described in most texts was used in our early cases. Frequent pressure ulcerations were noted (Fig. 17-25), incisions healed slowly, and there was a high revision rate. It was postulated that sectioning of the geniculate arteries, thinner skin in the anterior flap, and increased pressure from the femoral condyles predisposed to these problems.

Side to side flaps were designed to include the geniculate arteries. Gastrocnemius muscle bellies

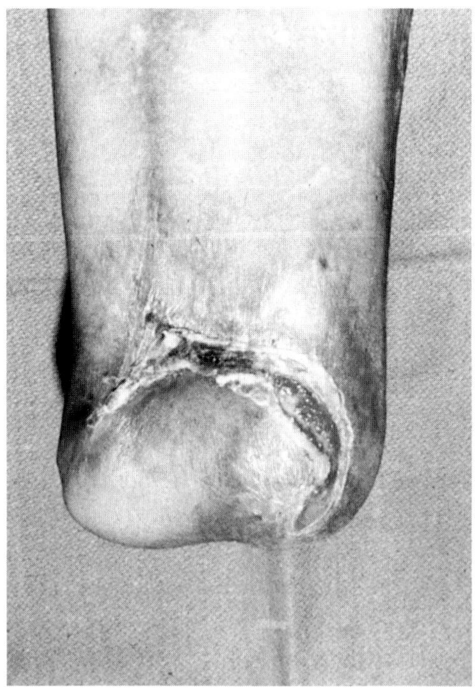

Fig. 17-25. Through knee amputation performed with long anterior flap with typical slow healing and ulceration over the femoral condyles.

were beveled and folded back over the femoral condyles for padding. The increased thickness of the subcutaneous tissue and increased vascularity were evident immediately. In addition, the resulting skin closure produced a midline posterior scar between the femoral condyles. There was thus no direct pressure on the scar. With the development and use of the side to side flaps and the muscle padding, the complication and revision rate dropped from 27 to 3 percent. Further revisions have been proposed to narrow and shorten the femoral condyles to provide room for knee control mechanisms. Mazet narrows the condyles and resects the posterior portion.[47] Burgess resects the distal 1.5 cm of the condyles and resurfaces the residual bone to gently rounded shape.[48] From further review of the world literature, the origin of the sagittal posterior closure appears to have first been described by Delpoe in 1830. Approximately one-half of the articles reviewed mention the use of the gastrocnemius muscles for padding the femoral condyles.

Surgical Technique

The medial and lateral incisions start at the midpoint of the infrapatellar tendon and end in the popliteal fossa at a point exactly opposite the starting point. The incisions curve medially and laterally below the tibial plateau and the flaps are equal in length to one-half the diameter of the leg at the plateau. The flaps are mobilized bluntly upward over the deep fascia and aponeurosis of the leg muscles. The patellar ligament is incised on either side and dissected from the tibial tubercle. The patellar tendon is reflected upward and the joint is entered above the infrapatellar fat pad. The hip and knee are now flexed and the cruciate ligaments sectioned at their tibial attachments. A bone hook is driven into the tibia and is used for traction and control of the distal leg. The joint capsule is incised just above the menisci that remain with the tibia. When cutting the posterior capsule, the scalpel is directed upward to protect the popliteal artery. With complete freeing of the capsule, the popliteal vessels can be dissected under direct vision, clamped, divided, and ligated. The hamstrings are divided at the tibial attachments. The posterior tibial and common peroneal nerves are divided above the femoral condyles. The gastrocnemius heads are beveled distally with an amputation knife to such a length that they will fold over and cover the femoral condyles (Fig. 17-26). Hemostasis is completed with suture ligatures to the major vessels and fine ligature and electrocoagulation to the lesser vessels. The flaps are tested for closure. Trimming and alterations are usually not necessary. A Shirley drain is drawn into the cavity through a lateral stab incision. Closure is begun by suturing the patellar tendon to the cruciate ligaments so that the inferior edge of the patella is level with the femoral condyles. The gastrocnemius heads are sutured to the remnants of the joint capsule along the superior and lateral margins. The hamstring tendons are sutured to the aponeurosis of the gastrocnemius.

Subcutaneous fat is closed with interrupted absorbable sutures. This is performed so that the skin edges are level. The skin is closed with staples or continuous or interrupted nonabsorbable sutures. A light compression dressing is wrapped on with bias-cut stockinette. Irrigating fluid is continued for approximately 48 hours when the drain is removed. The patient is started on mobilization as soon as practicable and uses crutches or walker until the wound is secure enough for a temporary prosthesis.

Postoperative Rehabilitation for Through Knee Amputees

For those patients who will have to be content with a wheelchair existence, all efforts are directed toward making them as independent as possible. Transfers from chair to bed and from chair to toilet are emphasized. Rehabilitation of the patient who can use a prosthesis is limited by loss of the knee joint. As with other levels, the rehabilitation potential depends upon the state of general health and the preoperative ambulatory activities.[49]

Through Knee Prosthesis

Because of the highly functional end-bearing characteristics of the residual limb, continued demand has been made on the prosthetic profession to produce an artificial limb capable of enhancing these characteristics. The objections of the prosthetists to the length and bulbous shape are disappearing. This had paralleled the acceptance by most prosthetists of the Syme amputation with its bulbous end. A four-bar linkage is placed mainly in the

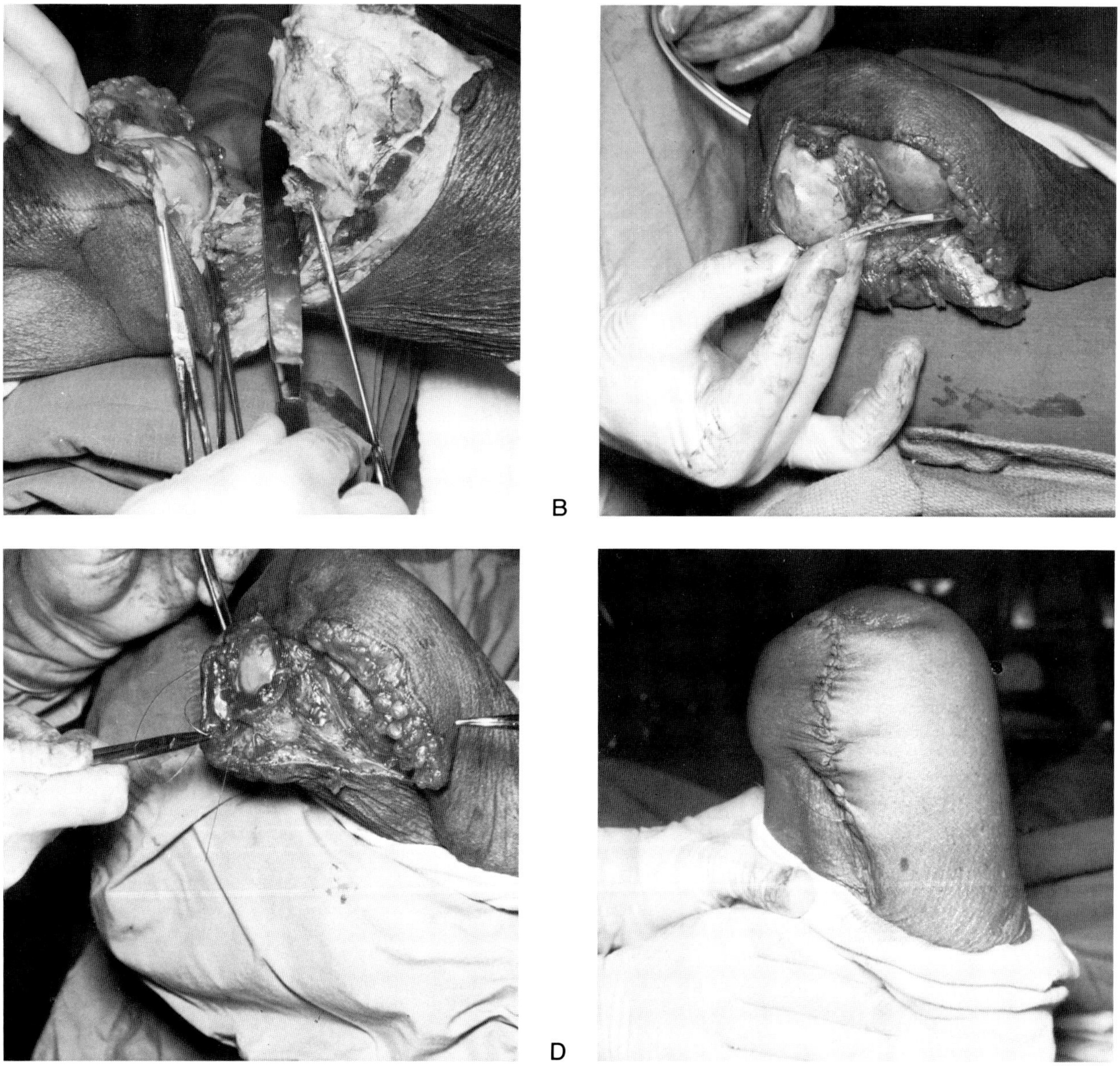

A B C D

Fig. 17-26. (**A**) Through knee amputation. The amputation knife is used to bevel the gastrocnemius heads parallel to the skin incision. (**B**) A Shirley two-lumen tube is drawn into the cavity through a separate stab incision. The white tube instills an antibiotic solution. The clear tube carries the effluent to gravity drainage. (**C**) The heads of the gastrocnemius muscle are sutured to the rim of joint capsule at the edges of the knee joint. (**D**) Closure of the skin results in a posterior midline incision not susceptible to pressure problems.

shank and allows articulation as well as control in swing and stance phase. Modifications and variations are available from many equipment suppliers. Surgical narrowing of the condyles allows room in the prosthesis for other types of control with hydraulic or pneumatic components.[47,48]

The socket design has several variations. For older patients who will be household ambulators only, a polypropylene anterior-opening socket can be fastened to the lower limb through steel side bars. Closure with Velcro straps allows for change in volume of the residual limb, which can occur daily. This socket also has the advantage of being donned in a lying or sitting position. This is of great help in older, less agile patients and in bilateral amputees. To allow entry of the bulbous end from above, an anterior cutout can be made in a molded socket. This cutout then can be laced shut. Expandable inner liners are now being made in a double-wall design such as in the Syme socket. An inner socket can be made of polyurethane foam that will provide total contact. The outer shell is of laminated plastic.

Above Knee Amputation

In the diabetic dysvascular patient the blood supply to the whole lower limb is markedly disturbed whenever an above knee amputation is indicated. For this reason tendoplastic procedures are generally avoided. Development of fascial planes will frequently lead to devascularization and death of some part of the fascial layers. This inevitably leads to major revision or to reamputation at a higher level. Because of their advanced age and general debility, relatively few of these patients become full prosthetic users. It is therefore important that the amputation be carried out at a level where primary healing is virtually guaranteed. The use of the Doppler flowmeter and the avoidance of tourniquet at this level has led to virtually 100 percent healing at Rancho Los Amigos Medical Center and in private practice.

Surgical Technique

The choice of incision is usually dictated by local considerations. The fleshy bulk of the thigh allows virtually any orientation of incision. If skin necrosis and/or infection do not permit standard flaps, there is no contraindication to asymmetric flaps of all shapes. Again, basic surgical criteria require that the flap length be cut not more than 1 to $1\frac{1}{2}$ times the base length. Side to side flaps work very well at this level. The bone is sectioned at such a length so as to allow closure without tension. This is usually at the apex of the fishmouth incision. Outlining the flaps on the skin obviates the necessity of trimming during the procedure (Fig. 17-27). The anterior musculature is divided with an amputation knife parallel to the skin flap to provide a tapered muscle flap. The femur is cut with a Gigli saw so that the anterior edge is rounded (Fig. 17-28). This detail has prevented protrusion of the bone by relieving the sharp edge that can literally saw through the atrophic soft tissues. Such protrusion has been a frequent problem with elderly nonambulatory patients who develop hip flexion contractures and do not have some type of myodesis. After rounding of the femur, the distal portion is then lifted anteriorly with a bone hook and the posterior musculature is beveled distally with the amputation knife.

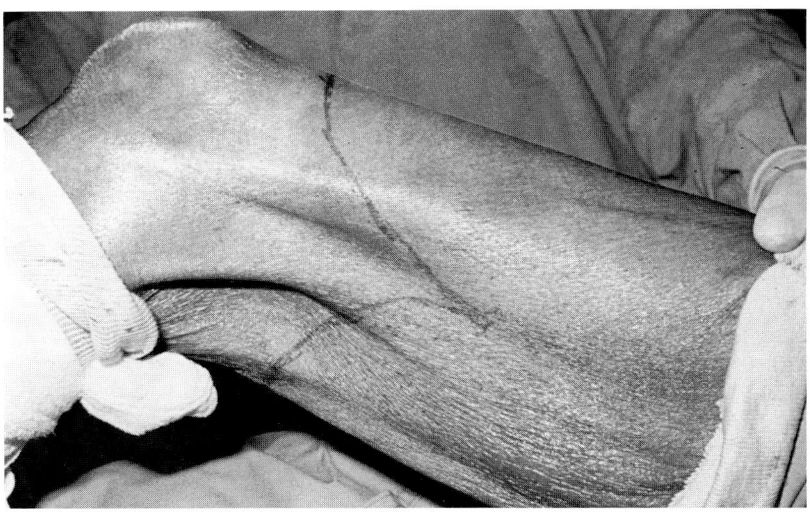

Fig. 17-27. Above knee amputation. Outline of fishmouth incision. This is typical appearance of elderly patient with gangrene of foot and not amenable to vascular surgical reconstruction.

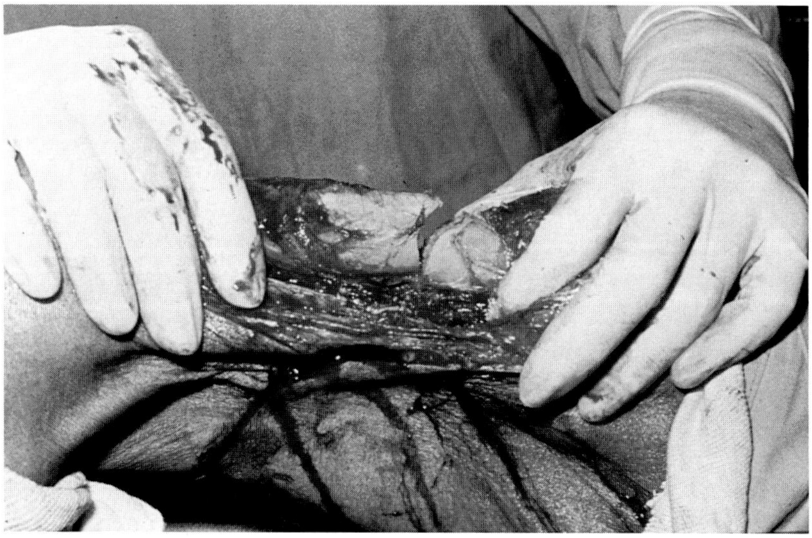

Fig. 17-28. Above knee amputation. The femur has been cut in a rounded fashion with the Gigli saw. The anterior edge is smoothed with osteotome and file. The knee is to the left.

The vascular structures are readily dissected in the subsartorial canal. Most often the superficial femoral artery is completely occluded. Bleeding vessels are clamped, divided, and ligated as indicated. After removal of the distal femur the sciatic nerve is dissected out, drawn gently, and ligated to control the large vasa nervorum. If there is strong pulsatile flow, the vessel is doubly ligated. The edges of the femur are smoothed with a file. Four drill holes are placed 90° apart. The wound is irrigated to remove bone dust and minor bits of debris. Hemostasis is completed with electrocoagulation and fine ligatures. If additional bone or muscle bleeding is expected, a soft plastic suction drain is placed through a separate stab incision.

In closing the wound the quadriceps bellies are myodesed to the anterior medial and lateral drill holes (Fig. 17-29). The needle is passed through the bone, the medullary canal, and the muscle to the aponeurosis. It is moved 1 cm and then back to the edge of the femur where the suture is then tied. Similar sutures are placed through the hamstrings through the medial, inferior, and lateral holes. The anterior muscles are tied first and the thigh brought to neutral to be sure that a hip contracture has not been produced. The posterior muscles are then sutured. The ends are brought over the quadriceps and sutured to the aponeurosis. The subcutaneous layer is closed so as to level the skin edges. The skin is then closed with a continuous or interrupted nonabsorbable suture or skin staples. A soft compression dressing is applied and stabilized with a hip spica wrapping and then stabilized further with elastic adhesive tape.

Postoperative Care

Early activity with emphasis on transfers and self-care is begun as soon as the medical condition permits. Drains are removed at 24 to 72 hours as indicated by the amount of aspirated blood. Stump wrappings are easily dislodged and sometimes must be reinforced with stump shrinkers or similar stockings held on with belt suspension. The above knee level is more difficult to treat with immediate-fit temporary prosthesis. They are indicated only in the younger active patients. The belt and shoulder suspension harnesses are poorly tolerated in the elderly.

Prosthetic Management

The reader is referred to the American Academy of Orthopaedic Surgeons' *Atlas of Limb Prosthetics* for detailed discussions.[50] The problems with above knee prostheses serve only to remind us to save the knee if at all possible. Since most patients are in the geriatric group, their needs are for a

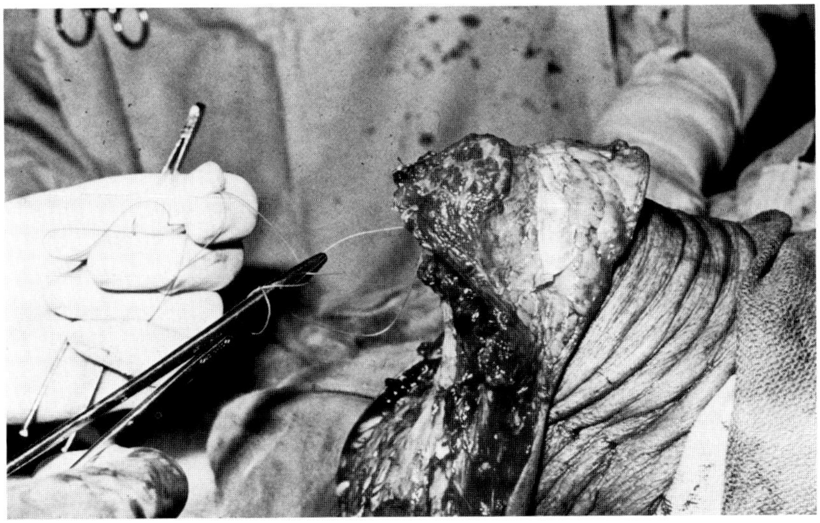

Fig. 17-29. Above knee amputation. Myodesis of quadriceps muscle to end of femur.

stable knee. They do not want a prosthesis that allows the knee to buckle. Stance phase is thus probably more important than swing phase. All knee units obtain knee flexion from the patient's forward motion and hip flexion. The amount of knee flexion is controlled by different knee mechanisms.

Friction Knee

The constant-friction knee is controlled by use of an adjustable screw or rubber pad that applies enough friction to dampen the swing, similar to that of the opposite limb. Stability in stance is obtained through alignment only. It cannot be used for infirm patients or those with joint deformities. The variable-friction knee has staggered friction pads that allow a cadenced response. It has more parts and requires almost constant adjustment.

Safety Knee (Weight-Activated Friction)

The safety knee acts as a constant-friction device during swing phase but will lock during stance phase from full extension to about 20° of flexion. A housing presses against the knee mechanism and prevents further flexion. The amount of weight necessary can be adjusted to meet the patient's bodily habitus. It is of most use in geriatric patients. It requires occasional adjustment and does not provide response to different cadence.

Polycentric Linkage

Several mechanisms are available that change the instantaneous center of rotation as the thigh and shin move on each other. Increased flexion can be provided, and this is a distinct advantage in through knee and long above knee amputations. Stability can be provided by locating the center behind the weight-bearing line at heel strike. A major disadvantage is the increased weight and bulk.

Hydraulic Mechanisms

Hydraulic units are quite responsive to cadence changes. Fluid is passed from one cylinder to another during motion of the knee. As the knee flexes, a piston forces oil through a bypass channel, past the check valve, into the cylinder above the piston. Because of the additional weight and muscular control needed in this mechanism, it is not indicated in the older diabetic patient.

Pneumatic Mechanisms

The pneumatic unit uses compressible air as a "spring" to store energy during knee flexion. This energy is returned to help extend the knee during swing phase. Adjustments can be made in the valve and its travel to regulate the flow of air and thus the resistance to knee flexion and the amount of energy returned. Again, this device requires frequent adjustment and probably is not indicated in the older diabetic patient.

When choosing a knee mechanism, multiple factors must be considered such as age, strength, agility, coordination, and other deformities and medical conditions. The first consideration must be stability (safety), next is function, then cosmesis, and finally ease of maintenance and durability. Probably more development and research has gone into the knee mechanism than all other phases of prosthetic manufacture combined.

Hip Disarticulation

At Rancho Los Amigos Medical Center, hip disarticulations have been life-saving for diabetic patients with proximal progression of infection and gangrene. When surgery will result in a femoral shaft shorter than 5 cm, a hip disarticulation is usually preferred. Short femoral shafts with the lesser trochanter and iliopsoas tendon still intact tend to develop marked contractures that may be painful and produce pressure sores and protrusion of the femur anteriorly. Short residual limbs are difficult to keep in a socket and the power transmitted by such a short lever is usually insufficient to operate a prosthesis. These patients usually should be treated as a hip disarticulation.

Surgical Technique

Boyd minimized blood lost by dividing muscles either at the origins or insertions.[51] Flaps may be fishmouth, long anterior, long posterior, and racquet-shaped. We have found the fishmouth to be quite successful (Fig. 17-30). The incision starts at the greater trochanter and ends at a point just opposite on the medial side. The flap length is one-half the anteroposterior diameter of the thigh at the level of incision. The femoral canal is entered and the femoral vessels and nerves are clamped, divided, and ligated. The sartorius and tensor fascia femoris muscles are divided at the anterior superior spine. The thigh is flexed and held by an assistant and the posterior incision is made in skin and subcutaneous fat. The gluteus medius and minimus are divided at the greater trochanter. This leaves excellent padding over the hollow of the hip and lateral pelvic wall. The anterior and posterior muscles are then divided on an oblique line from inward toward the skin. This detaches the gluteus maximus from the linea aspera. With adduction of the leg, the neck of the femur is exposed and the capsule divided at the edge of the acetabulum. The leg is externally rotated to expose the medial capsule and iliopsoas tendon. These are divided along with the adductors and pectineus. With external rotation, the short external rotators are exposed and divided. The hip is then dislocated and the

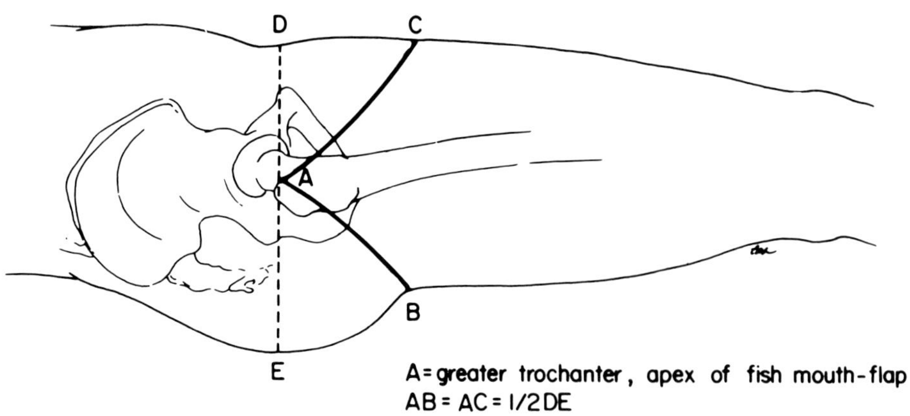

Fig. 17-30. Outline of hip disarticulation incision.

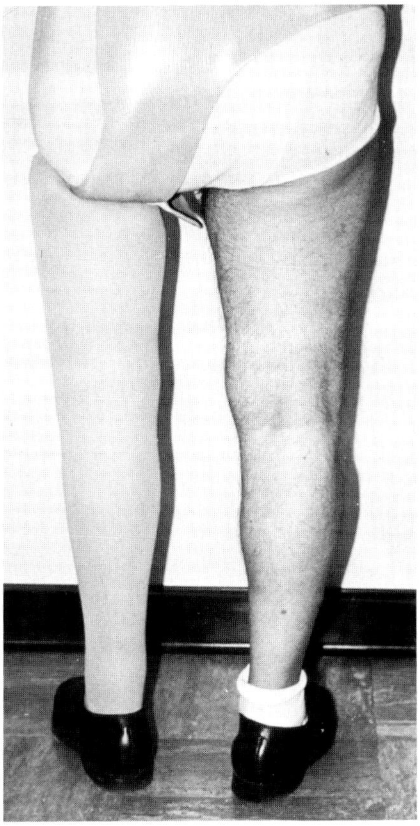

Fig. 17-31. Hip disarticulation prosthesis. This prosthesis is worn over a prosthetic gluteal pad for a patient with hemipelvectomy.

ligamentum teres cut. It usually must be ligated, since the vessel in the ligament is almost always patent. The hamstrings and quadratus femoris are separated from the ischeum. The sciatic nerve and superior gluteal vessels are identified at the sciatic notch, then clamped, divided, and ligated.

There is a relatively small amount of divided muscle and this does tend to ooze. Some form of drainage is necessary. We use a Shirley drain in the acetabulum for irrigation and gravity drainage. A second soft plastic drain is placed above the muscle layer and connected to suction. The wound is closed in layers. The anterior and posterior muscles are closed over the acetabulum. The subcutaneous tissue is closed with interrupted absorbable sutures. The skin is closed with interrupted or running nonabsorbable sutures or skin staples. A hip spica type of dressing is wrapped with bias-cut stockinette. This is reinforced with elastic adhesive. The drains are continued until the fluid is clear.

Virtually no elderly dysvascular patient will use a hip disarticulation prosthesis. If one is indicated, a Canadian type of hip disarticulation prosthesis is prescribed (Fig. 17-31).

Hind Quarter or Hemipelvectomy Amputations

Hind quarter or hemipelvectomy amputations are usually performed only for malignancy, and then in centers specializing in such procedures. They are rarely indicated in the elderly diabetic patient. The average surgeon will almost never have occasion to perform the operation. The reader is referred to articles by Gordon-Taylor and Munro[52] and Lazarri and Rock[53] for indications and details of the surgical technique.

REFERENCES

1. Glattly HW: A statistical study of 12,000 new amputees. South Med J 57:1371, 1964
2. LeBlanc MA: Patient population and other estimates of prosthetics and orthotics in the USA. Orthot Prosthet 27:38, 1973
3. Vital and Health Statistics Series 13, No. 32 DHHS Pub No (P&S) 85-1743. Public Health Service, Washington, DC, US Government Printing Office, March 1985
4. Report of the National Diabetic Advisory Board, NIH Publication No. 81-2284. p. 25. Bethesda, MD, November 1980
5. Most RS, Sinnock P: The epidemiology of lower extremity amputations in diabetic individuals. Diabetes Care 6:87, 1983
6. Division of Diabetic Control Center for Prevention Service: A plan for the prevention of lower extremity amputation in persons with diabetes. Centers for Disease Control, Atlanta, November 1986
7. Jacobs RL, Karmody AM: The team approach in salvage of the diabetic foot. Surg Annu 9:231, 1977
8. Wagner FW, Jr: Orthopedic rehabilitation of the dysvascular lower limb. Orthop Clin North Am A:325, 1978
9. Wagner FW, Jr: A classification and treatment pro-

gram for diabetic, neuropathic and dysvascular foot problems. p. 143. In AAOS Instructional Course Lectures. Vol. 28. CV Mosby, St. Louis, 1979
10. Wagner FW, Jr: The dysvascular lower limb. p. 291. In Nickel VL (ed): Orthopedic Rehabilitation. Churchill Livingstone, New York, 1982
11. Goodman J, Bessman AN, Teget B, Wagner FW Jr: Risk factors in local surgical procedures for diabetic gangrene. Surg Gynecol Obstet 143:587, 1976
12. Bessman AN: Management of the diabetic surgical patient. Compr Ther 5:57, 1979
13. Rossini AA, Hare JW: How to control the blood glucose level in the surgical diabetic patient. Arch Surg 111:945, 1976
14. Giannestras NJ, Kranley JJ, Lentz M: Occlusion of the tibial artery after a foot operation under tourniquet. A case report. J Bone Joint Surg 59A:682, 1977
15. Love BRT: The tourniquet and its complications. Proceedings of the Australian Orthopaedic Association. J Bone Joint Surg 61B:239, 1979
16. Moldaver J: Tourniquet paralysis syndrome. Arch Surg 68:136, 1954
17. Shaw JA, Murray DG: The relationship between tourniquet pressure and underlying soft tissue pressure in the thigh. J Bone Joint Surg 64A:1148, 1982
18. Webster GV, Peterson RA, Stein HL: Dermal overgrafting of the leg. J Bone Joint Surg 40A:796, 1958
19. Kritter, AE: A technique for salvage of the infected diabetic gangrenous foot. Orthop Clin North Am 4:21, 1973
20. Moore, TJ: Amputation of the lower extremities. p. 606. In Chapman MW (ed): Operative Orthopaedics. JB Lippincott, Philadelphia, 1988
21. Ecker MD, Jacobs BS: Lower extremity amputations in diabetic patients. Diabetes 19:189, 1970
22. Wills CA, Caiozzo VJ, Jasukawa DI et al: Effects of immobilization on human skeletal muscle. Orthop Rev 11:57, 1982
23. Malone JM, Moore WS, Leal JM, Childers SJ: Rehabilitation for lower extremity amputation. Arch Surg 116:93, 1981
24. Waters RL, Perry J, Antonelli D, Hislop H: Energy costs of walking of amputees. The influence of level of amputation. J Bone Joint Surg 58A:42, 1976
25. Goldner MG: The fate of the second leg in the diabetic amputee. Diabetes 9:100, 1960
26. Whitehouse FW, Jurgensen C, Block MA: The later life of the diabetic amputee, another look at the fate of the second leg. Diabetes 17:520, 1968
27. Volpicelli KJ, Chambers RB, Wagner FW, Jr: Ambulation levels of bilateral lower extremity amputees: An analysis of 103 cases. J Bone Joint Surg 65A:599, 1983
28. Bessman AN, Wagner FW, Jr: Nonclostridial gas gangrene: report of 48 cases and review of the literature. J Am Med Assoc 233:958, 1975
29. Ecker MD, Jacobs BS: Lower extremity amputations in diabetic patients. Diabetes 19:189, 1970
30. McKittrick LS, McKittrick JB, Risley TS: Transmetatarsal amputation for infection or gangrene in patients with diabetic mellitus. Ann Surg 130:826, 1949
31. Roach JJ, McFarlane DS: Midfoot amputations: application of pioneer procedures in a new age. Contemp Orthop 18:517, 1989
32. Jacobs RL, Karmody AM: Diabetic neurotrophic foot: diagnosis and treatment. p. 141. In AAOS Instructional Course Lectures. Vol. 28. CV Mosby, St. Louis, 1979
33. Syme J: Amputation at the ankle joint. London and Edinburgh Monthly Journal of Medical Science 2:93, 1843
34. Harris RI: Syme's amputation. The technical details essential for success. J Bone Joint Surg 388:614, 1956
35. Harris RI: The history and development of Syme's amputation. Artif Limb 6:4, 1961
36. Spittler AW, Brennan JJ, Payne JW: Syme amputation performed in two stages. J Bone Joint Surg 36A:37, 1954
37. Wagner FW, Jr: A classification and treatment program for diabetic, neuropathic and dysvascular foot problems. p. 143. In AAOS Instructional Course Lectures. Vol. 28, 1979
38. Wagner FW, Jr: The Syme amputation. p. 326. In Atlas of Limb Prosthetics: Surgical and Prosthetic Principles. CV Mosby, St. Louis, 1981
39. Radcliffe CW: The biomechanics of the Syme prosthesis. Artif Limb 6:76, 1961
40. Gonzales EG, Corcoran PJ, Reyes RL: Energy expenditure in below knee amputees, correlation with stump length. Arch Phys Med Rehabil 55:111, 1974
41. Waters RL, Perry J, Antonelli D, Hislop H: Energy costs of walking of amputees: The influence of level of amputation. J Bone Joint Surg 58A:42, 1976
42. Mooney V, Wagner FW, Jr, Waddell J, Ackerson T: The below knee amputation for vascular disease. J Bone Joint Surg 58A:365, 1976
43. Persson BM: Sagittal incision for below knee amputation in ischemic gangrene. J Bone Joint Surg, 56B:110, 1974
44. Ertl I: Über Amputationsstumpfe. Chirug 20:218, 1949
45. Smith N: Amputation of the knee joint. Am Med Rev and Journal of Original Selected Papers in Medicine and Surgery. 2:370, 1825
46. Rogers SP: Amputation at the knee joint. J Bone Joint Surg 22:973, 1940

47. Mazet R, Hennessy CA: Knee disarticulation: a new technique and a new knee joint mechanism. J Bone Joint Surg 48A:126, 1966
48. Burgess EM: Disarticulation of the knee. Arch Surg 112:1250, 1977
49. Mensch G: Physiotherapy following through-knee amputation. Prosthet Orthot Int 7:79, 1983
50. American Academy of Orthopaedic Surgeons: Atlas of Limb Prosthetics: Surgical and Prosthetic Principles. CV Mosby, St Louis, 1981
51. Boyd HB: Anatomic disarticulation of the hip. Surg Gynecol Obstet 84:346, 1947
52. Gordon-Taylor G, Munro RS: Technique and management of "hind quarter" amputation. J Bone Joint Surg 39A:536, 1952
53. Lazarri JH, Rock FJ: Method of hemipelvectomy with abdominal exploration and temporary ligation of common iliac artery. Ann Surg 133:267, 1951

18

Limb Salvage Techniques

Flair Goldman, D.P.M.
Gary W. Gibbons, M.D.
Ingrid Kruse-Edelman, D.P.M.

HISTORICAL PERSPECTIVE

Gangrene and the subsequent loss of a limb are probably the most feared complications of diabetes. The treatment of lower extremity gangrene caused by peripheral vascular disease or overwhelming infection has presented a major challenge to surgeons for many years. During the first half of this century, the debate centered around the questions of when to amputate and at what level. In 1917, Stern and Adams stated, "Diabetic gangrene presents the peculiarity of a slow and steady advance unless an unusually high amputation be performed. Thus, if the great toe is the site of the beginning of a true diabetic gangrene, amputation through the lower third of the thigh is indicated; otherwise, the prognosis is very bad."[1] Statistics showed a high mortality rate associated with major amputations. Veal, in 1938, reported a mortality rate of 48.5 percent,[2] and Silbert one of 44 percent when he reviewed thigh amputations in diabetics at 22 large metropolitan hospitals.[3] Holden, in 1947, reported that multiple operations increased the mortality rate considerably[4] and McLaughlin and Weidman, in 1950, stressed the importance of early high amputation to avoid reamputation.[5] The high morbidity associated with major amputations is also a well known and documented fact. Silbert, in 1952, published his classic follow-up study of 294 diabetic patients with major amputations for gangrene and demonstrated that 30 percent of them required amputation of the remaining leg within 3 years and 51 percent within 5 years.[6] The potential for rehabilitation is, therefore, very small, since it is rare indeed for the elderly bilateral amputee to learn the use of prostheses.[7] Mere survival of the amputee was the primary goal through the first half of the twentieth century, with little consideration being given to rehabilitation. Once the overall management of the diabetic patient improved and considerations were given to renal and cardiac complications as well as improving blood glucose control, the mortality rate began to decrease. Controlling the infection, both with antibiotics and surgical incision and drainage procedures, was one of the greatest factors in reducing mortality rates.[8] Perlow and Roth, in 1949, showed a decline to 11.7 percent in their mortality rates between 1945 and 1947.[9] McKittrick, in 1946, reported a mortality rate of only 4.7 percent and stated, "Diabetes mellitus is no contraindication to any surgical procedure whose indications are clear, provided always that the medical, surgical and hospital teamwork is set to ensure efficient, cooperative care of the patient's metabolic disturbance."[10] It was during the period of declining mortality that surgeons began to experiment with more distal amputation, such as below knee, transmetatarsal, and single toe.[11,12] It was also during this time that general surgical techniques were improved. By using atraumatic technique in handling skin edges, taking care not to undermine tissues, and improving anesthesia and fluid loss replacement, overall success of the surgical outcome increased.

In the last two decades we have seen tremendous advances in podiatric, vascular, and plastic surgery as well as diagnostic techniques. These have all contributed to a decrease in major amputations and salvage of the diabetic foot has become an attainable goal.

PHILOSOPHY OF LIMB SALVAGE

Many functionally oriented surgeons still do not embrace a limb salvage philosophy. Instead they are guided by the belief that the surgical management of diabetic foot problems should be limited to one definitive operation that will minimize hospitalizations and allow for early return to activity. Such an approach requires not operating in marginal distal areas and areas compromised by infections and/or diminished circulation. Consequently, attention is focused more proximally in healthier areas and major amputations are performed most commonly below the knee. Such an approach does offer two distinct advantages. First, it greatly increases the likelihood of primary wound healing, thus reducing the need for multiple operations, and second, it eliminates the possibility of further problems with the foot that has been removed, again limiting the number of operations on that extremity. These advantages do, however, have real costs. Little has changed over the years as far as the fate of the remaining limb is concerned. Hoskov and Josephsen, in 1980, still found the incidence of contralateral amputation to be 53 percent within a 4-year period after the fist amputation.[13] Others report that after amputation the contralateral leg will have problems within 18 to 36 months in half of the patients.[14] Most and Sinnock report the risk for amputation to be 10 to 20 times that of the general diabetic population in people with previous amputation.[15] The statistics for mortality rates associated with major limb amputation have been reported as being 18 percent with an average hospitalization time of 68 days,[16] while other authors report hospital mortality rates ranging from 8 to 25 percent.[17] The 3-year survival rate for people with diabetes who have undergone lower extremity amputation has been reported to be 50 percent, and 20 percent of patients who had any part of their foot amputated were dead in 2 years.[18] Furthermore, one must also consider that not all high level amputations heal without further complications, including primary wound problems, later stump problems, prosthetic problems, and flexion contracture problems; nor do all amputees gain the same level of functional independence they had prior to their amputation. Finally, reliance on the principle of early high level amputation can promote a defeatist attitude and a dependence on dealing with all complex diabetic foot lesions with an expedient early high level amputation, even when such patients may be candidates for limb salvage.

For these reasons, let us examine the philosophy and principles of limb salvage. The overriding belief in the limb salvage philosophy must be that it is worth the cost in terms of time and effort to attempt to salvage the foot, part of the foot, or the leg. Factors that must be considered in the decision-making process are the patient's general medical condition and functional status, the patient's motivation, the patient's compliance, as well as the obvious local factors of the type and extent of infection or necrosis and the patient's vascular status. When surgeons adopt the limb salvage philosophy, they must realize that they are often pushing the limits and will have to accept a certain number of failures, both long-term and short-term, that would be greater than the number of failures they would experience if early high level amputation was performed. In fact, the old saying that on certain types of bottom fishing, "If you aren't losing a few rigs to snags, you aren't fishing close enough to the bottom," could be modified to apply to limb salvage statistics. If your success rate for primary healing is 100 percent, you probably are not attempting enough limb salvage procedures.

In addition to major revisions or higher level amputations during the same hospitalization, limb salvage often requires that patients undergo multiple staged operations for debridement and delayed closure. Treatment may involve frequent out-patient visits, home care visits, or treatment at an extended care facility at times when patients are too well to be hospitalized but before a healed wound is achieved. Also, patients can be expected to develop secondary problems such as transfer lesions and digital deformities causing ulcerations and infection, thus requiring revision. Progression of peripheral vascular disease can require reoperation as well. In one recent report, follow-up from midfoot amputation in neuropathic or dysvascular feet showed a complication rate of 42 percent, including early wound dehiscence and late reulceration.[19] However, by providing aggressive management and appropriate local revisions, 84 percent of the original group's limbs was salvaged. This study underscored the fact that midfoot amputation requires diligent immediate and long-term follow-up care if acceptable success rates are to be achieved. Another study revealed a 45 percent failure rate with ray resections in the dysvascular foot, with 31 percent good to excellent results and 24 percent classified as poor because of secondary ulcerations in adjacent metatarsals requiring further treatment.[20] Naturally, patients must be made aware of these issues as well. If the greater goal of limb salvage and its benefits is not kept in mind, minor setbacks and major failures can be very discouraging to both the patient and the surgeon. Our experience has been that the overall rewards of attempted limb salvage outweigh the problems associated with it. We are not aware of any good studies that demonstrate the economic verities of attempted limb salvage versus early high level amputation.

OVERVIEW OF LIMB SALVAGE TECHNIQUES

All aspects of limb salvage are of equal importance, and these include patient education, prophylactic care, clinical evaluation, biomechanical management, ulcer management, medical management, and surgical management. That there is room for improvement in limb care is demonstrated by the fact that one study found examination of the foot occurred only in 12.3 percent of visits at a diabetes specialty clinic.[21] Support for the concept that patient education and prophylactic treatment are mainstays of preventive care come from published data showing that the annual number of lower extremity amputations decreased by almost 50 percent when a diabetes unit instituted and integrated in-patient and out-patient services that included a comprehensive podiatry service, nurses, clinicians, and an extensive educational program.[22] The amputation rate declined 44 percent in 2 years in a program that consisted of intensive podiatry when biomechanical care was instituted.[23] Another study showed a 68 percent reduction in hospital days for peripheral vascular disease–related illness and amputation when the frequency of patient clinical contacts and home care visits increased with specially trained nurse practitioners providing care under specified protocols. Finally, one further study showed 85 percent reduction in below the knee amputations over a 4-year period after education and training in foot care was instituted to patients with diabetes.[24] These studies and others[25] certainly reinforce the notion that prevention, when possible, is the best treatment. Chapters 2 and 10 go into greater depth in terms of prevention and program implementation for identification, evaluation and treatment of high risk individuals; Chapters 15, 19, 1, and 17, respectively, discuss at length methods for vascular reconstruction, plastic reconstruction, the medical management of diabetes and the techniques for various amputations for such patients.

The remainder of this chapter will emphasize the early aggressive management of the already infected or necrotic foot, as well as methods for prevention of the recycling of patients through the local amputation, healed wound, new infection, new problem cycle. To accomplish this goal we will first discuss some of the principles involved in the surgical management of the already infected foot and then illustrate these concepts through the use of several case reports.

When facing the infected diabetic foot, one must determine as quickly as possible whether one is dealing with a superficial infection or an established deep space infection (i.e., plantar compartment abscess). An understanding of the anatomy of the compartments of the foot, the clinical appearance and systemic signs of deep space infections, and the surgical approach to such infections are key elements in the management of this problem. These topics are discussed in the following section of this chapter. The issues of antibiotic selection and peripheral vascular examination, while both very important, are only briefly mentioned here; they are discussed in greater detail in other chapters.

Generally speaking, patients in whom pedal pulses are not palpable, or patients with an ankle arm index of less than 0.45 or an absolute systolic pressure of less than 50 mmHg, should be evaluated by a vascular surgeon for peripheral vascular disease (PVD). Arteriograms are generally reserved for patients who are medically considered candidates for vascular reconstruction. If infection is present, it should be cleared surgically and/or medically before an arteriogram is obtained. Clinical impression and experience should not be underestimated. One study found a healing rate of 38 percent in patients for whom systolic pressure indices predicted failure.[26] One must also remember that failure can occur when various laboratory findings point to success. Some key points in antibiotic selection include a recognition that most diabetic infections are polymicrocrobial.[27-29] Furthermore, it must be recognized that although multiple organisms may be cultured from any given diabetic wound, the number of primary pathogens creating clinical infection is probably much smaller. Culture and sensitivity reports are not available at the time of initial antibiotic selection, and clinical judgment is required. This situation allows for two possible approaches to antibiotic use. First, one could treat the patient for all possible pathogens including anaerobic, aerobic, gram-positive, and gram-negative organisms. On the other hand, one could use a broad-spectrum antibiotic covering the majority or organisms and combine this with aggressive surgical management. This is generally our preferred method. Other authors as well have stated their belief that surgical treatment is more important than the selection of proper antibiotic combination.[30] It must be remembered, however, that if a patient is critically ill, "shotgun" therapy with complete coverage may be indicated. Furthermore, the patient's clinical response must be considered in antibiotic management as well as the results of culture and sensitivity testing. In patients who are doing well, if culture results show organisms that are not covered by antibiotics, it is often not necessary to change antibiotic selection. Similarly, patients who are not doing well may require additional antibiotics or a change in antibiotics. Changing the class of antibiotics may be better than changing antibiotics within the same class. If patients are not progressing well, additional surgical intervention should also be considered. Because of poor tissue perfusion, antibiotics may not achieve therapeutic levels in the foot, especially if pockets of pus or necrotic tissue persist. Recommendations for the discontinuance of antibiotic treatment vary; clinical judgment, experience, and the individual patient's need all are important factors. One general recommendation is to continue antibiotic coverage for 7 to 10 days in closed amputations and for as long as 4 weeks after open amputations.[31] The clinical observation of a solid barrier of granulation tissue covering all deep tissues signals the time for discontinuance.

CLINICAL PATTERNS OF INFECTION

Infections of the plantar space account for 75 percent of above the knee and below the knee amputations in diabetic patients.[32] In diabetic foot infections, the clinician must distinguish between superficial and deep infections. This can at times be difficult. Most deep space infections start with infected ulcers on the plantar aspect of the foot (52 percent in one series[30]), interdigital infections, nail problems, or a foreign body in the foot.

Once the deep space infection is established, the foot is often massively swollen, especially in the arch region, which may be obliterated. Ascending cellulitis, lymphangitis, and lymphadenopathy also develop.

In the examination, the foot should be squeezed proximally to distally to determine whether frank pus can be expressed. The foot should also be felt for crepitus within the soft tissue. Ulcers should be probed for sinus tracts. Frank septicemia may be present with spiking fevers, shaking chills, lethargy, anorexia, nausea, and sweats. Blood sugar levels must be checked, since they may be far out of control in the presence of deep space infection. White blood cell count may be increased with a shift to the left, and sedimentation rate is also increased. Blood cultures may be positive. Findings may be obscured because of the diabetic patient's inability to respond in the presence of such infection. Radiographs should be examined for evidence of gas, osteomyelitis, and foreign bodies. Sinograms may be helpful in determining the extent of infection.[33] Recent investigations suggest that computed tomography scans may be helpful in determining location and extent of deep space plantar abscesses[34]; and reports of the use of magnetic resonance imaging for such purposes should be expected.

In one study of major foot infections, 30 percent of the infections started in the nail or nail bed, 60 percent started within the web space, and 10 percent started after direct penetration of the sole. Most cases that proceeded to amputation started as web space infections.[32]

Medial Compartment Infections

Most infections of the medial compartment start from either an ulcer under the first metatarsal head or when associated with a bunion, from an ulcer on the medial side of the first metatarsal head (Fig. 18-1). Medial compartment infections may be accompanied by cellulitis extending into the arch and proximally toward the medial malleolus.

Plantar ulcers must be adequately debrided to check for collections of deep pus. Pus can be expressed by milking the leg, starting proximally

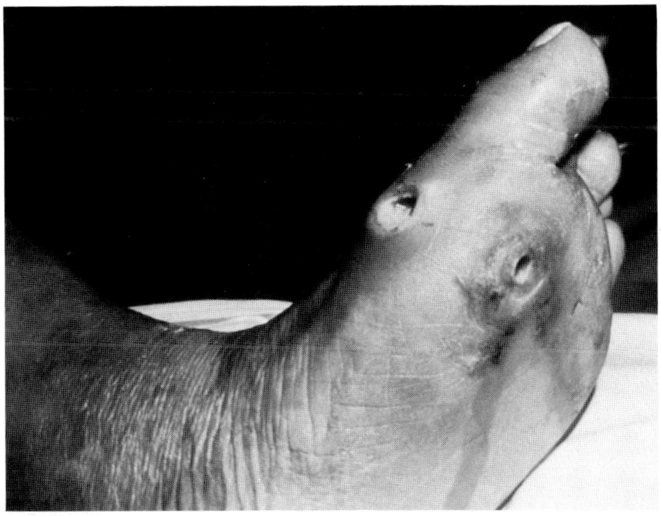

A

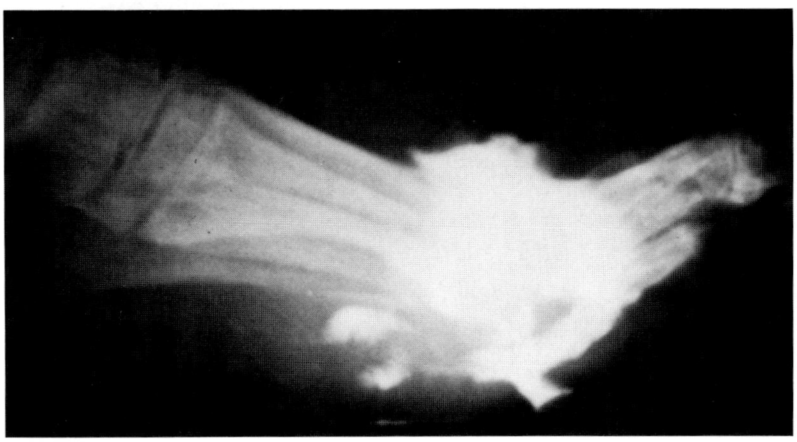

B

Fig. 18-1. (**A**) Classic cause of medial compartment infection: either a plantar or medial ulceration associated with the first metatarsal head. (**B**) Sinogram, lateral view, showing plantar and dorsal extension.

above the malleolus and continuing distally through the arch toward the open draining area. All wounds should be probed for sinus tracts. Radiographs must also be reviewed.

Central Compartment Infections

Infections of the central space have a less favorable prognosis than infections of either the medial or lateral spaces and have been reported to be more common. Most central space infections proceed from ulcers under the central metatarsal heads, from web space infections arising from interdigital corns, from fungal infections, or they may be proximal extension of central toe infections[35–37] (Fig. 18-1A).

A digital infection that has progressed to a deep infection of the central space often shows a funnel-shaped, affected toe with marked edema at the base of the toe, interspace, and base of the foot. As central space infection progresses and pus accumulates, the infection spreads proximally. This spread is sometimes aided by gravity when the foot is elevated and the patient is bedridden. Characteristically, a pointing abscess forms in the midarch region (Fig. 18-2). If left untreated, this abscess decompresses by spontaneous rupture through the plantar skin and by extension into the deep posterior compartment of the leg or peroneal compartment.

Another decompression route would be through the interosseous space and into the dorsal subaponeurotic space of the foot (see Fig. 18-12B & D). Pointing abscesses of the midarch signify advanced infection and its corresponding poor prognosis. When associated with diabetic foot infections, such abscesses constitute a surgical emergency and require prompt surgical attention. Patients often suffer from septicemia at this point. As pus and edema accumulate and compartment pressure is increased, the plantar arterial arch can be compro-

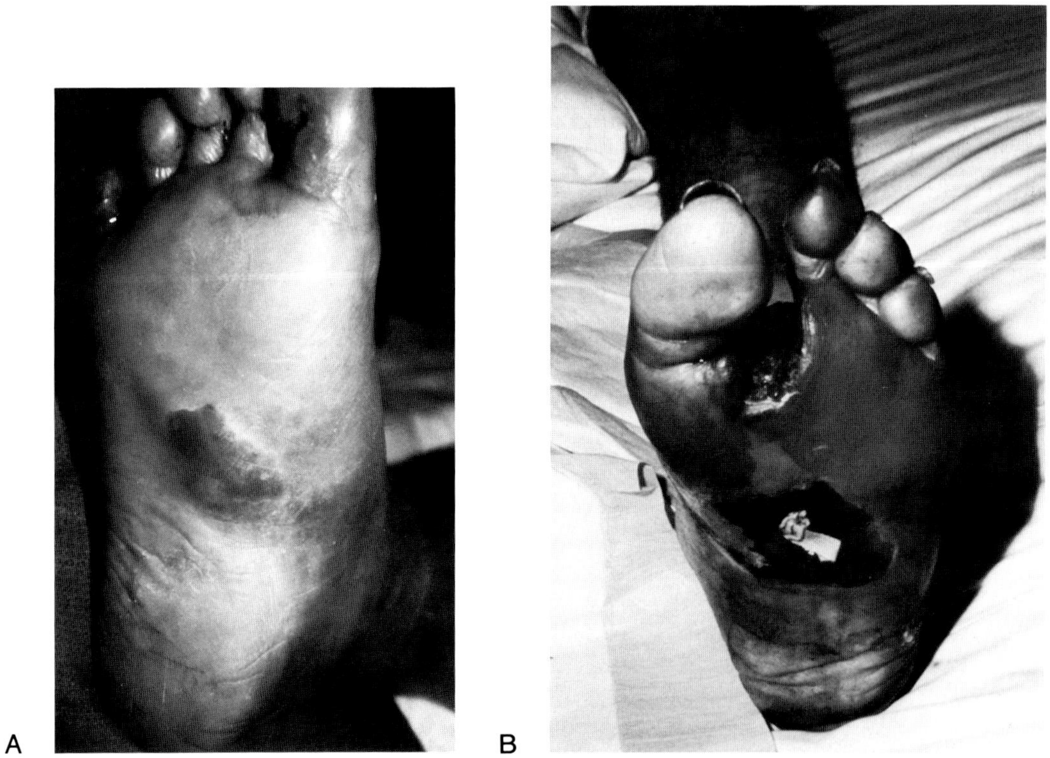

Fig. 18-2. (**A**) Classic advanced central space infection with decompression to plantar aspect of foot. (**B**) Small stab incision used to drain central space infection. This is inappropriate.

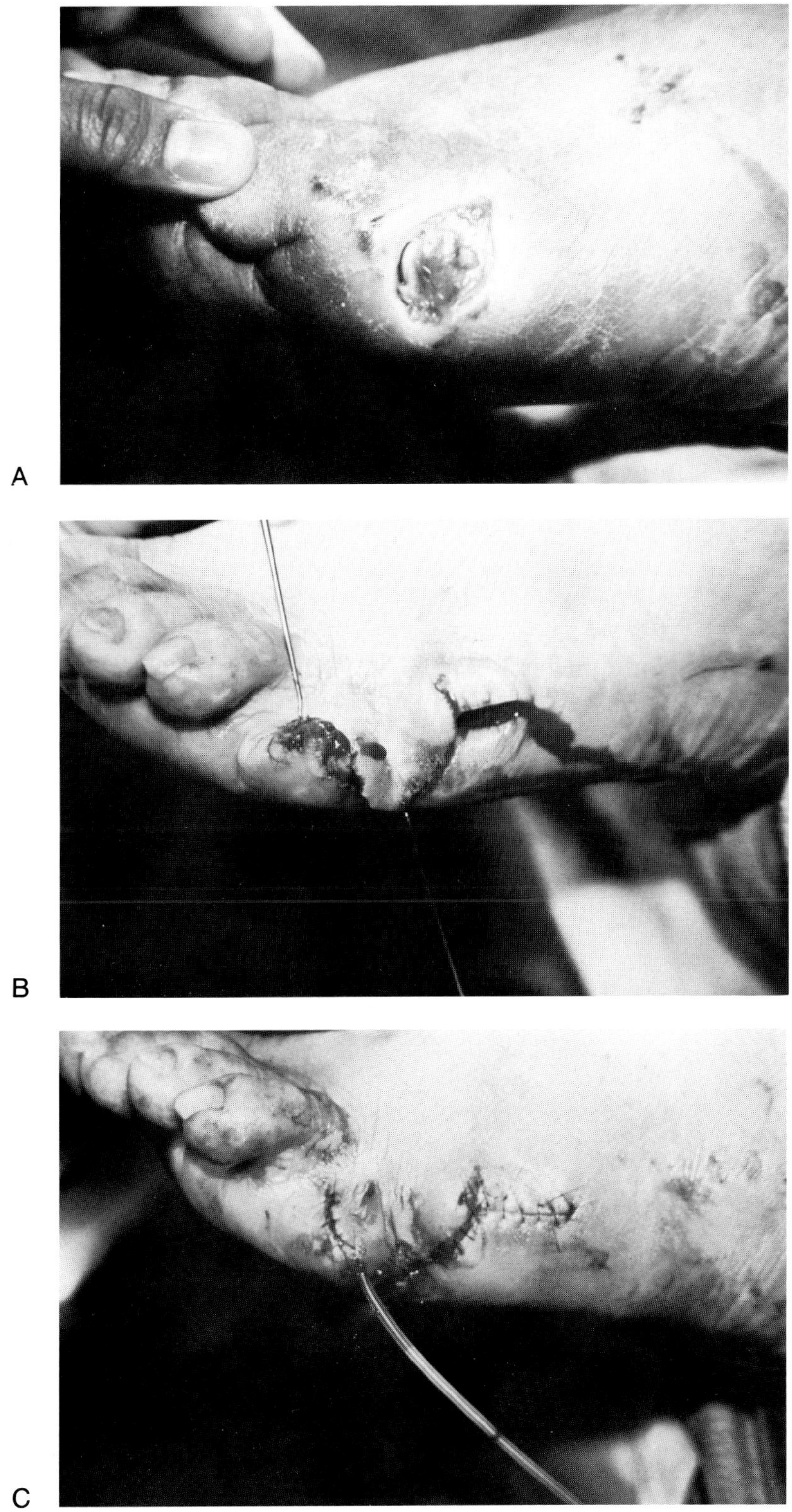

Fig. 18-3. (**A**) Classic source of lateral infection: lesion associated with fifth metatarsal head. Note metatarsal phalangeal joint exposure. (**B**) Fillet of fifth toe to use as durable skin flap. (**C**) Flap in place with drain.

mised, leading to further necrosis of the distal foot and toes.[38]

Lateral Compartment Infections

Infections of the lateral compartment usually start with skin ulcerations associated plantarly or laterally with the fifth metatarsal head (Fig. 18-3). Extension is usually dorsally into the subcutaneous space or medially into the central compartment (Fig. 18-4). Spread into the dorsal space follows closely the pattern described in experimental studies by Feingold and associates.[39] Clinically, cellulitis is present and frank pus often collects dorsally. These infections are usually readily controlled by prompt surgical drainage. Progression to the central compartment usually occurs distally from periarticular infections about the fifth metatarsophalangeal joint, which spread medially and proximally into the central compartment (see Fig. 18-11). In such infections, radiographs must be checked for osteomyelitis of the fifth metatarsal head as well as of the fourth metatarsal head. Spread can also occur proximally into the peroneal compartment (see Fig. 18-12E & F).

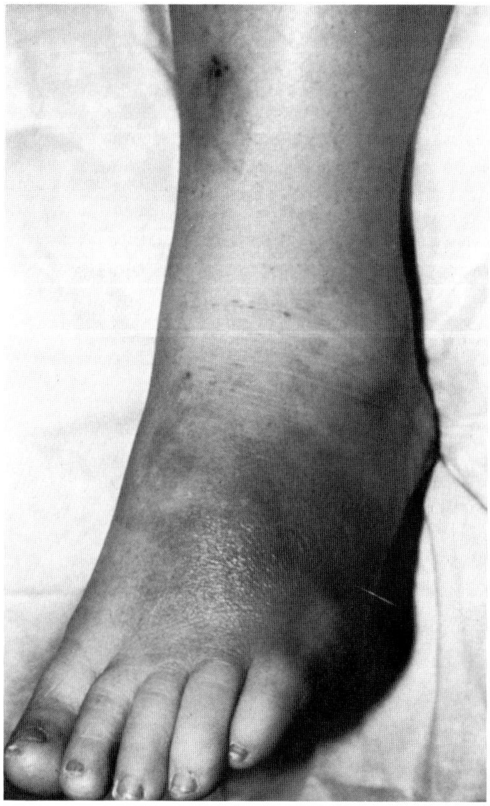

Fig. 18-4. Classic appearance of dorsal compression of lateral space infection. Note dorsolateral erythema.

SURGICAL MANAGEMENT OF DEEP SPACE INFECTIONS

Anatomy Overview

Most serious deep space infections of the foot occur on the plantar aspect. A working knowledge of the anatomy of the plantar aspect of the foot is helpful in the management of such lesions. For a more thorough review of this topic, see Goldman.[40] Although anatomists do differ as to the exact boundaries of the compartment of the foot, they generally agree that the plantar aspect of the foot contains three compartments: central, medial, and lateral (Fig. 18-5). Likewise, experiments using injection studies of methyl methacrylate, paraffin, and gelatin do differ some degree on the various locations of *breaches* and communications within these compartments.[39,41,42] All studies, however, do confirm that communication does exist between the three compartments on the plantar surface of the foot. Similarly, communication exists between the plantar compartments of the foot and the dorsal subaponeurotic space, as well as between the plantar aspect of the foot and the deep posterior and peroneal compartments of the leg. The medial compartment communicates with the central compartment through the flexor digitorum longus, peroneus longus, and adductor hallucis tendons. The web spaces may have ready access to the deep central space through the digital nerves, lumbrical muscles, and flexor digitorum longus tendons. Also, subcutaneous interspaces communicate with the subaponeurotic space on the dorsum of the foot. For this reason, a dorsal pointing abscess on the foot may be the result of a deep plantar infection, and whenever a dorsal abscess is noted, one should look for a plantar source. The lateral compartment of the foot communicates with the central

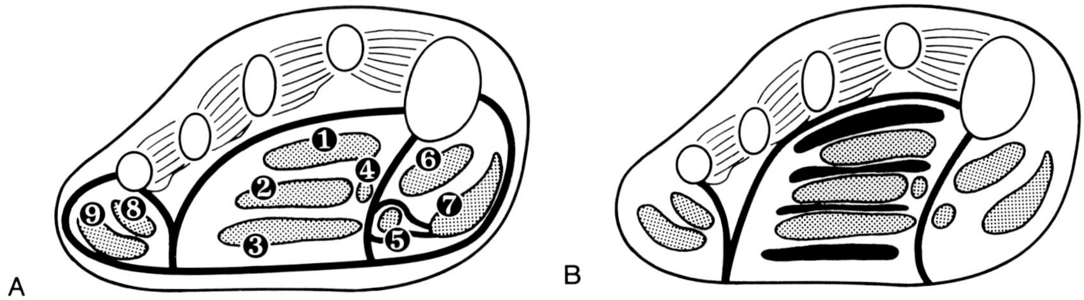

Fig. 18-5. (A) Diagrammatic representations of plantar compartments of the foot. (1) Adductor hallucis; (2) quadratus plantae; (3) flexor digitorum brevis; (4) flexor digitorum longus; (5) flexor hallucis longus; (6) flexor hallucis brevis; (7) abductor hallucis; (8) flexor digiti minimi brevis; (9) abductor digiti minimi. **(B)** Fascial spaces of the central compartment as described by M. Grodinsky.[41]

compartment through the flexor tendons to the fifth toe, the lateral plantar neurovascular structures, and several tendons. One must also consider that when infection is present, it may spread along various courses that are atypical as tissue is necrosed.

SURGICAL INCISION AND DRAINAGE

Incision, drainage, and debridement should be accomplished as soon as a deep space infection is recognized and the patient is medically stable. Often however, the patient cannot be stabilized until incision and drainage and amputation is accomplished. Small stab incisions are inadequate and therefore inappropriate for the management of deep central space infections. Thorough incision, drainage, and debridement are necessary, and at times amputation of the toe, ray, forefoot, entire foot, or below the knee is necessary to stabilize the patient. It is our belief, which is shared by others,[30] that surgical treatment is more important than the selection of the proper antibiotic combination. Furthermore, wound closure under unfavorable circumstances can re-establish an environment fostering infection and necrosis that cannot be overcome by antimicrobial agents. Survival and stump healing are favorably affected when the wound is left open after the initial procedure. The open wound is extremely resistant to infection and this has been known for centuries.[43] Sizer and Wheelock reported a successful healing rate of 54 percent in patients operated on for control of sepsis.[31] Wounds were left open with later conversions to transmetatarsal amputations. Only 4 patients out of 50 had a palpable pedal pulse. They concluded that even in these patients one should not immediately perform a major amputation, since more than 50 percent would not be indicated. They also reported a 94 percent healing rate with definitive toe–partial ray resection when surgery was for a more stable chronic condition (i.e., osteomyelitis, ulceration, necrosis). No mention of follow-up or recurrence was noted. Scher and Steele reported 71.4 percent rate of successful healing of partial foot amputations with aggressive local debridement followed by revision or grafting.[30]

Incision and Drainage Technique

Medial Space

The medial space is best drained from a plantar medial incision extending proximally as far as necessary toward the posteroinferior aspect of the medial malleolus and above it as required. This approach also gives adequate exposure to the hallux and first metatarsophalangeal joint as well as the first ray as needed; the approach also allows total or subtotal ray resection. Likewise, this incision can easily be combined with hallux amputation or with resection of the first metatarsophalangeal joint (Fig. 18-6).

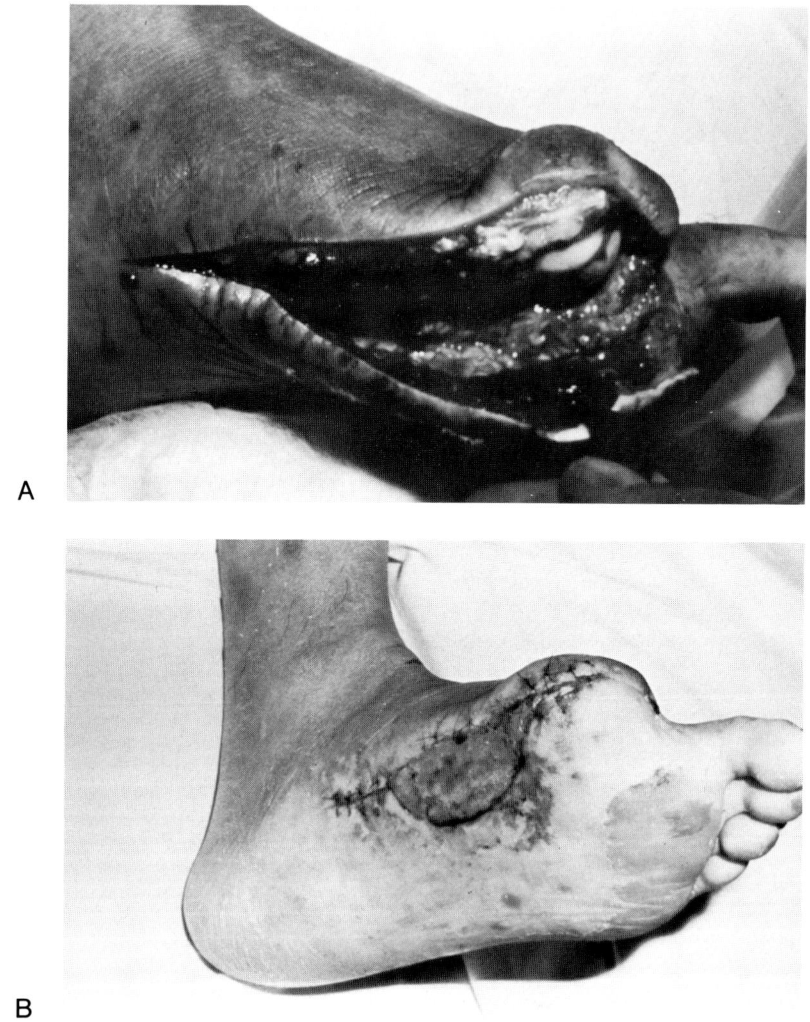

Fig. 18-6. (A) Appearance of medial compartment infection originating with great toe infection. Note: Removal of toe and incision and drainage done from plantar medial approach. (B) Note skin graft in mid-arch area and intact weight-bearing skin under first metatarsal head.

If metatarsal head ulcers are present under the first metatarsal bone, they can be excised and the wound closed or left open to granulate; or an incision can be made, starting plantarly at the ulcer and extending proximally. A plantar medial incision can be inadequate, however, when exposure of the first interspace is necessary. This often occurs when no bony resection of the distal metatarsal or first metatarsophalangeal joint is required and the first interspace is thus inaccessible. A dorsal, plantar, or through-and-through interspace incision may be required in such cases for adequate visualization and drainage of the first interspace. The hallux can sometimes be used as a flap by excising the nail bed and matrix and filleting the phalanges out of the toe, creating a durable flap for plantar coverage. In more chronic cases involving the first metatarsophalangeal joint without proximal plantar extension, a dorsomedial longitudinal incision can be used.

Central Space

In the past, the recommended approach to the central compartment was through a medial incision. The incision is deepened until it reaches the medial intermuscular septum and then is continued through this septum. Because the medial intermuscular septum is common to all fascial spaces in the central compartment, the septum, in theory, provides adequate drainage. The proposed advantage of such an incision is the avoidance of a plantar incision and the resulting scar. Even advocates of such incision state that dorsal or plantar counterincision is often required. We do not recommend such an incision for central space infections in diabetic patients, primarily because drainage is often inadequate and debridement is extremely difficult. Furthermore, since most of these patients are insensate because of diabetic peripheral neuropathy, painful plantar scars are not a consideration. The recommended approach is a plantar incision starting at the site of the affected metatarsal head and extending medially and plantarly toward the tarsal tunnel. The incision should be extended as far proximally as necessary (Fig. 18-7).

For interspace lesions, the incision should start at the affected interspace and may require distal and dorsal extension through the interspace and dorsally on the foot (Fig. 18-8). When a lesser digit is involved, it can be opened distally and the incision carried proximally as previously described.

When a lesser digit is beyond salvage, it can be amputated and the incision carried proximally.

A

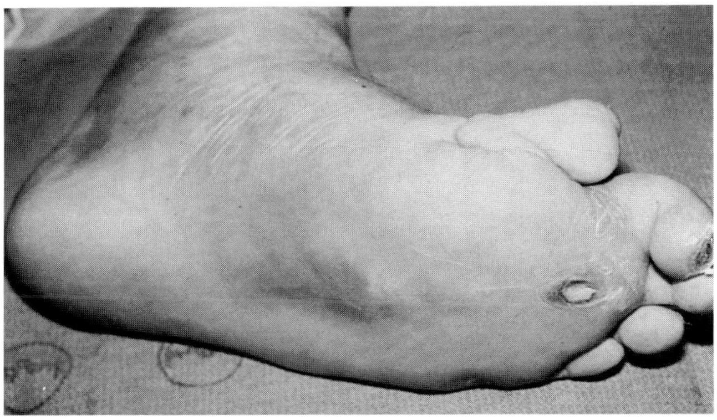

B

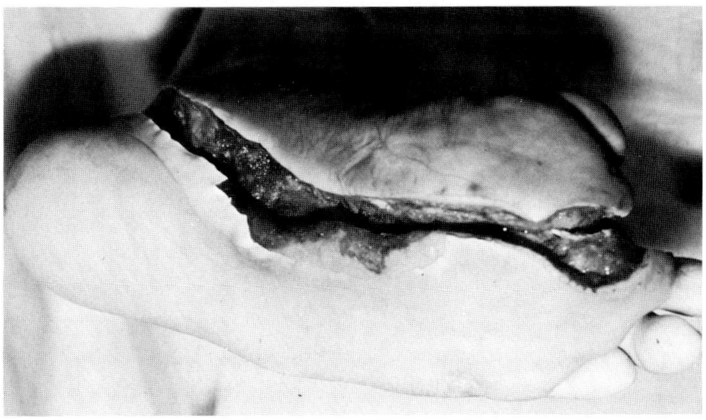

Fig. 18-7. (**A**) Note plantar central space mid-arch abscess formation secondary to second metatarsal head ulceration. (**B**) Note incision and drainage, plantar medial incision, starting at site of infection and tracking along the course of infection through the tarsal tunnel, combined with subtotal second ray resection. *(Figure continues.)*

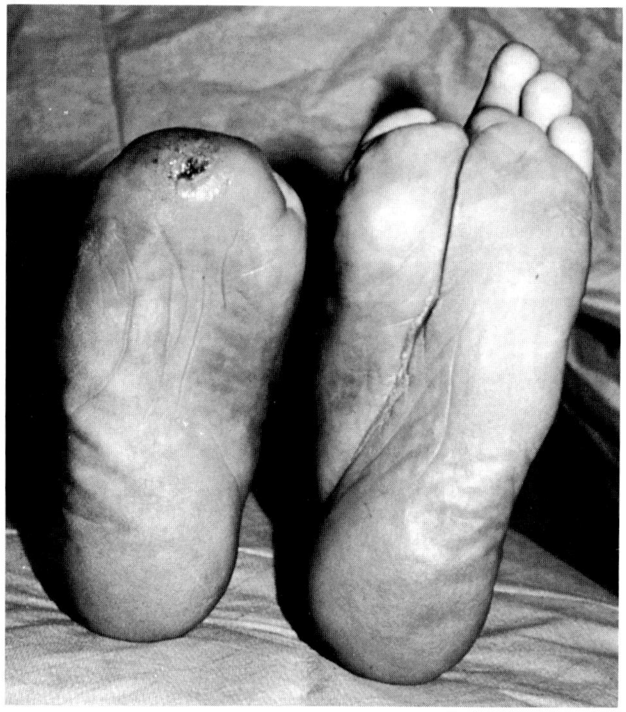

C

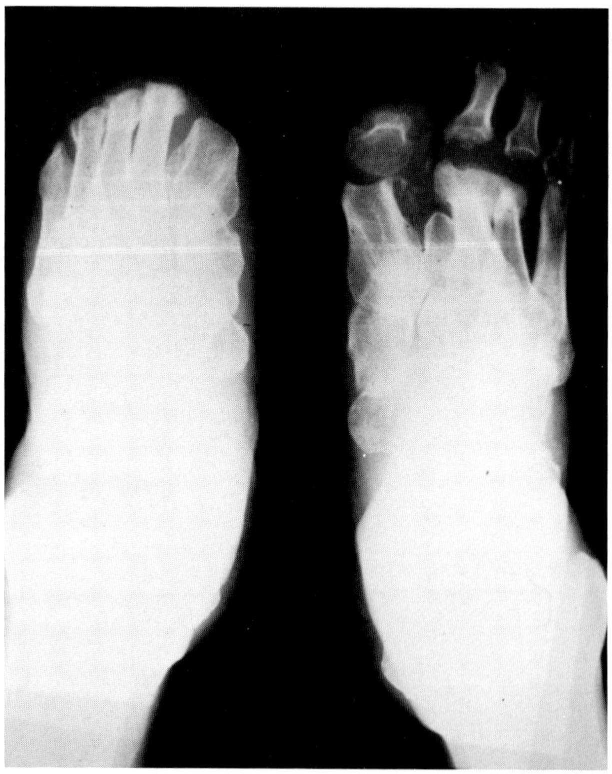

D

Fig. 18-7. *(Continued).* (**C**) Appearance after healing by tertiary intention aided by Steri-Strip closure. (**D**) Anteroposterior radiograph views. Excision of central metatarsal heads to allow for a more normal parabola.

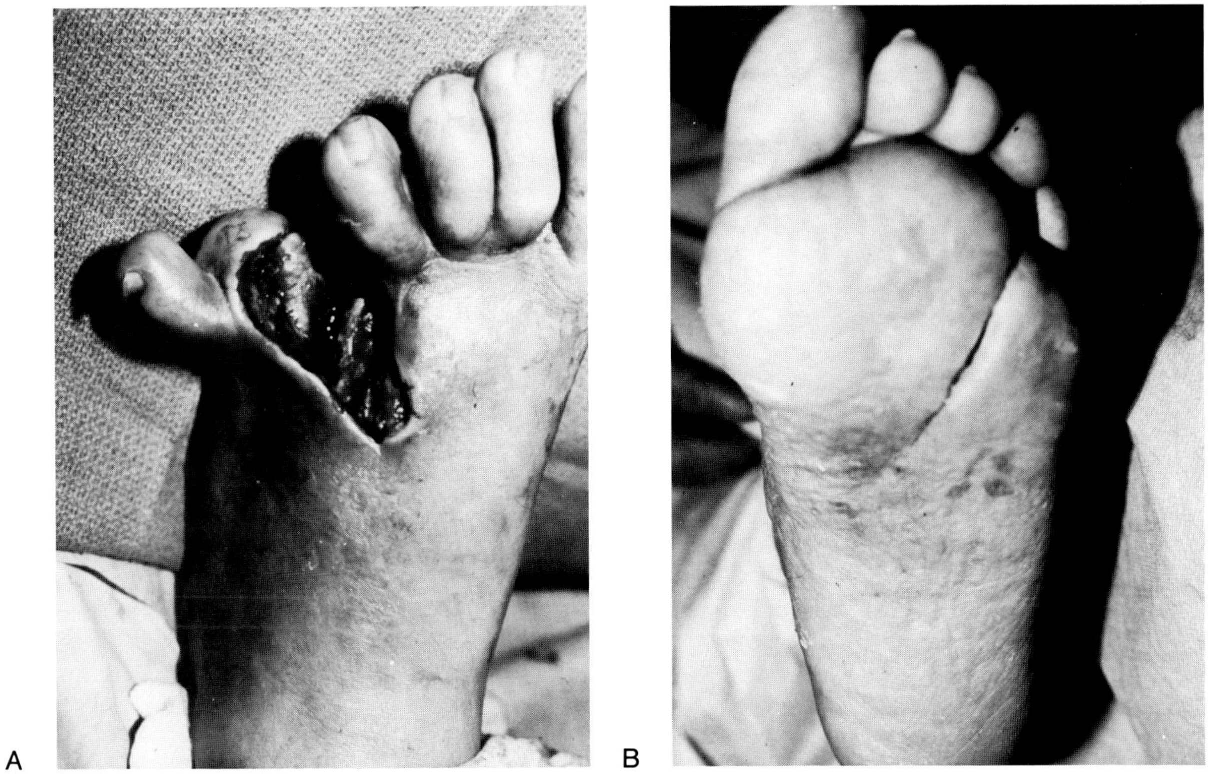

Fig. 18-8. (A) Dorsal view of interspace incision for infection starting with subfourth metatarsal head lesion and extending into the fourth interspace. (B) Plantar view showing medialization of incision as it extends proximally, following course of infection.

When the digit, metatarsophalangeal joint, metatarsal bone, or any combination of these are osteomyelitic (Fig. 18-9), a ray resection or partial ray resection may be carried out. If pus is still present at the proximal reaches of the ray resection, the incision must be carried from this point proximally and directed toward the posteroinferior aspect of the malleolus and then proximally as necessary. Similarly, the metatarsal head and the adjacent base of a lesser digit can be excised without digital amputation.

An alternate approach to the metatarsophalangeal joint is by dorsal incision and plantar counterincision (via ellipse) of the infected ulcer, establishing through and through drainage. However, such an approach is best used in cases that involve *chronic* osteomyelitis of the metatarsal head or metatarsophalangeal joint involvement originating from contiguous skin ulceration and not from acute deep space infection. Transverse incisions at the level of the transverse plantar ligament have been recommended. Such incisions are used for treating interspace infections and are designed to avoid the weight-bearing aspect of the foot. We believe such incisions should be avoided whenever possible because skin necrosis may occur.

Lateral Compartment

Infections of the lateral compartment are best approached by a lateral incision carried as far proximally as necessary. Such incisions usually give adequate exposure to the dorsal compartment, fifth metatarsal bone, and fifth metatarsophalangeal joint. This approach also combines well with amputation of the fifth toe, with excision of the fifth metatarsophalangeal joint, with partial or total fifth ray resection, or with a combination of these procedures (Fig. 18-10). The fifth toe can be used to

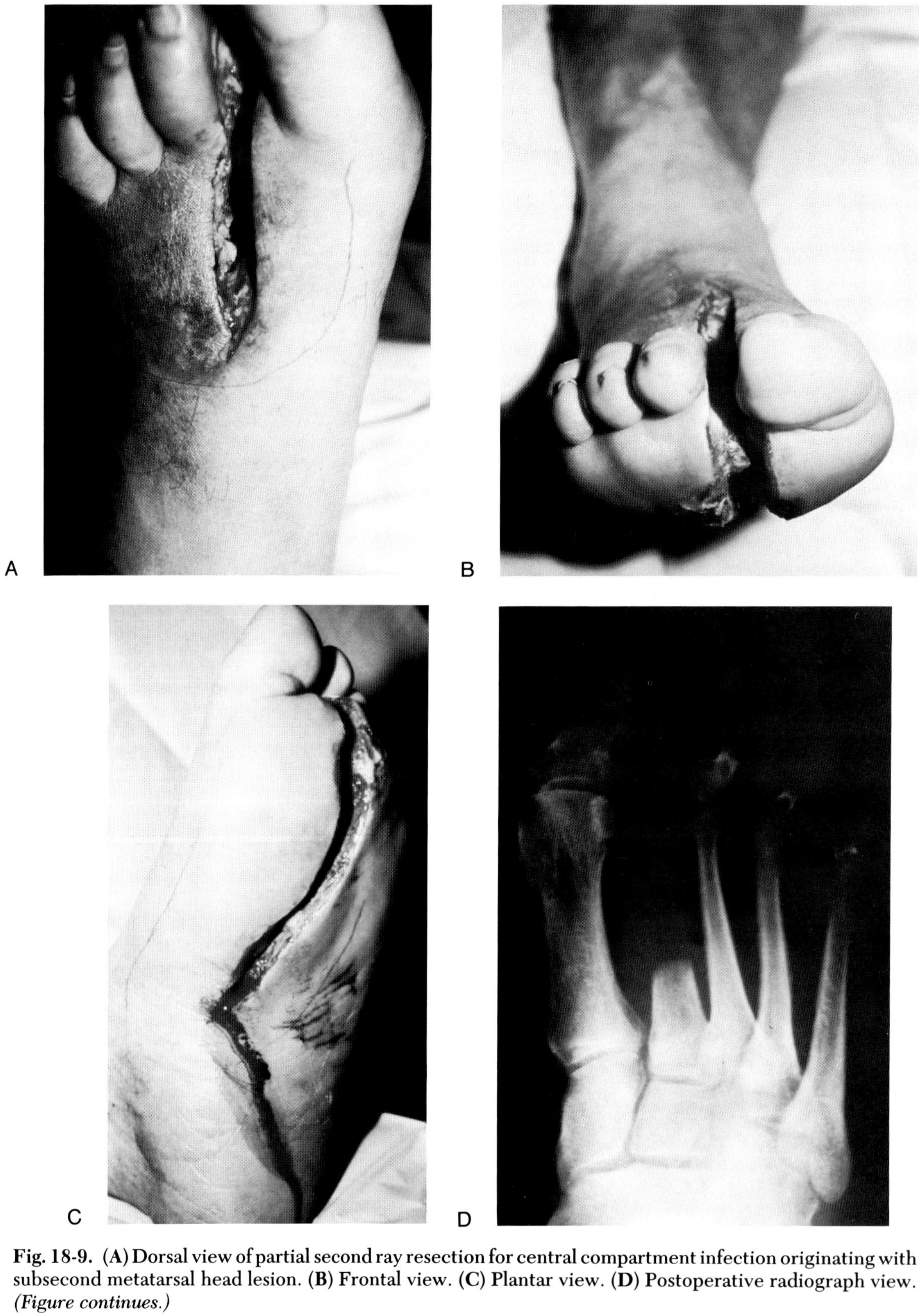

A B C D

Fig. 18-9. (**A**) Dorsal view of partial second ray resection for central compartment infection originating with subsecond metatarsal head lesion. (**B**) Frontal view. (**C**) Plantar view. (**D**) Postoperative radiograph view. *(Figure continues.)*

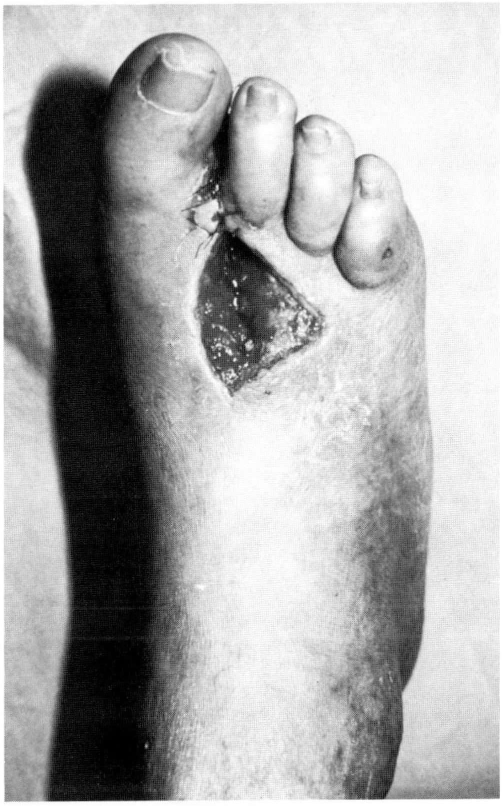

E

Fig. 18-9. *(Continued)*. (E) Dorsal view showing loss of dorsal skin; this healed by tertiary intention.

create a durable flap for defects on the plantar lateral aspect of the foot (Fig. 18-3). This approach may prove to be inadequate for fourth interspace drainage and debridement. When bone resection is unnecessary and the fifth toe does not require amputation, a dorsal, plantar, or interspace incision may be adequate. When primary lateral compartment infections extend to the central space, the plantar lateral incision must extend proximally and medially to provide access to the central plantar compartment (Fig. 18-8). Often such spread is at the metatarsophalangeal joint level (Fig. 18-11).

Dorsal Abscess

Dorsal abscesses are usually well localized and are easily approached from a dorsal incision centered over the pointing abscess. The source of such dorsal abscesses is often a plantar space infection that has decompressed itself to the dorsum of the foot through the interspace. In such cases, the affected plantar compartments must be adequately drained. Often the dorsal lateral skin will necrose and a split thickness graft will aid in closure (Fig. 18-12).

Limb salvage requires aggressive revascularization once sepsis is controlled in patients where ischemia threatens healing.[44] Although vascular reconstruction is detailed in another chapter, certain points deserve emphasis. Most important is to eliminate any notion that diabetic patients have inoperable vascular disease or that it is too risky. Modern arteriographic techniques, routine magnification, and advances in cardiovascular sutures with cardiac cutting needles make it possible for even routine vascular reconstruction of the pedal arteries and branches with excellent initial and long-term success.[45]

SUMMARY

Prevention is the best cure; however, prevention is not always possible. When problems occur, limb salvage is often possible and enhanced by early recognition and aggressive treatment of the acutely infected foot. Surgical management includes thorough debridement, incision, and drainage. Leaving such incision and drainage sites open will often allow salvage at a more distal level, as will vascular consultation when indicated. Limb salvage is not always possible and, when it is, it often involves multiple surgeries with considerable wound care to obtain a closed wound. Once healed, the foot is at risk for developing another limb-threatening problem necessitating ongoing care. Limb salvage requires a long-term commitment from the patient and the doctor and can involve considerable time and effort. These issues need to be appreciated by all involved. Patients need to be educated and compliant. Another author put it this way[31]:

> Some of the people we treat who are at the same time undergoing a rather intensive educational program concerning foot care . . . take this very much to heart and, once they leave the hospital, do very well. Others, as soon as they get well, go home, buy a new pair of boots and hike 20 miles, so I think that it depends more upon the patient and his willingness to care for and protect his feet rather than upon any other particular aspect.

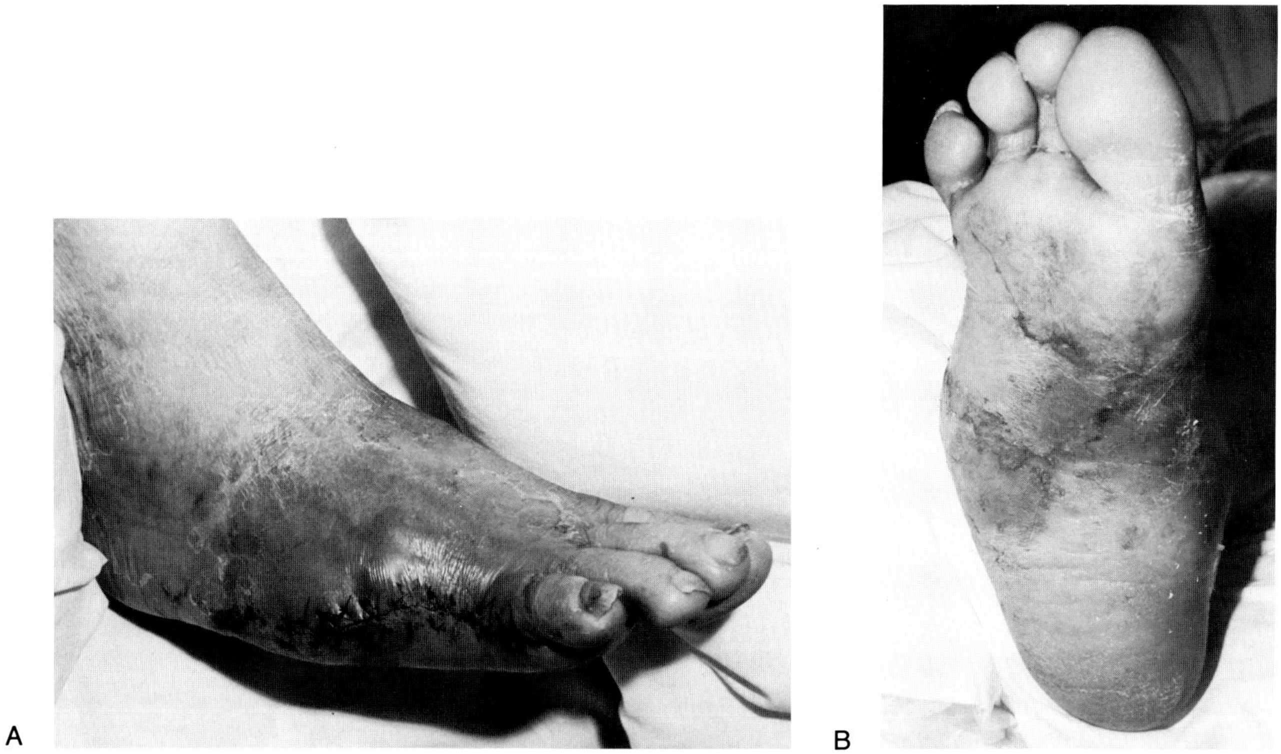

Fig. 18-10. (A) Postoperative view after subtotal, fifth, and fourth ray resection for infection of the lateral and central compartment, originating with a subfifth metatarsal head. (B) Plantar view.

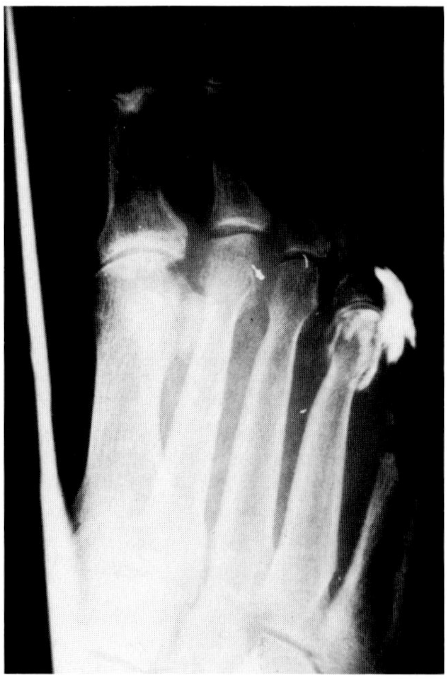

Fig. 18-11. Oblique radiograph view sinogram showing extension from lateral compartment infection after excision of fifth metatarsal head and debridement.

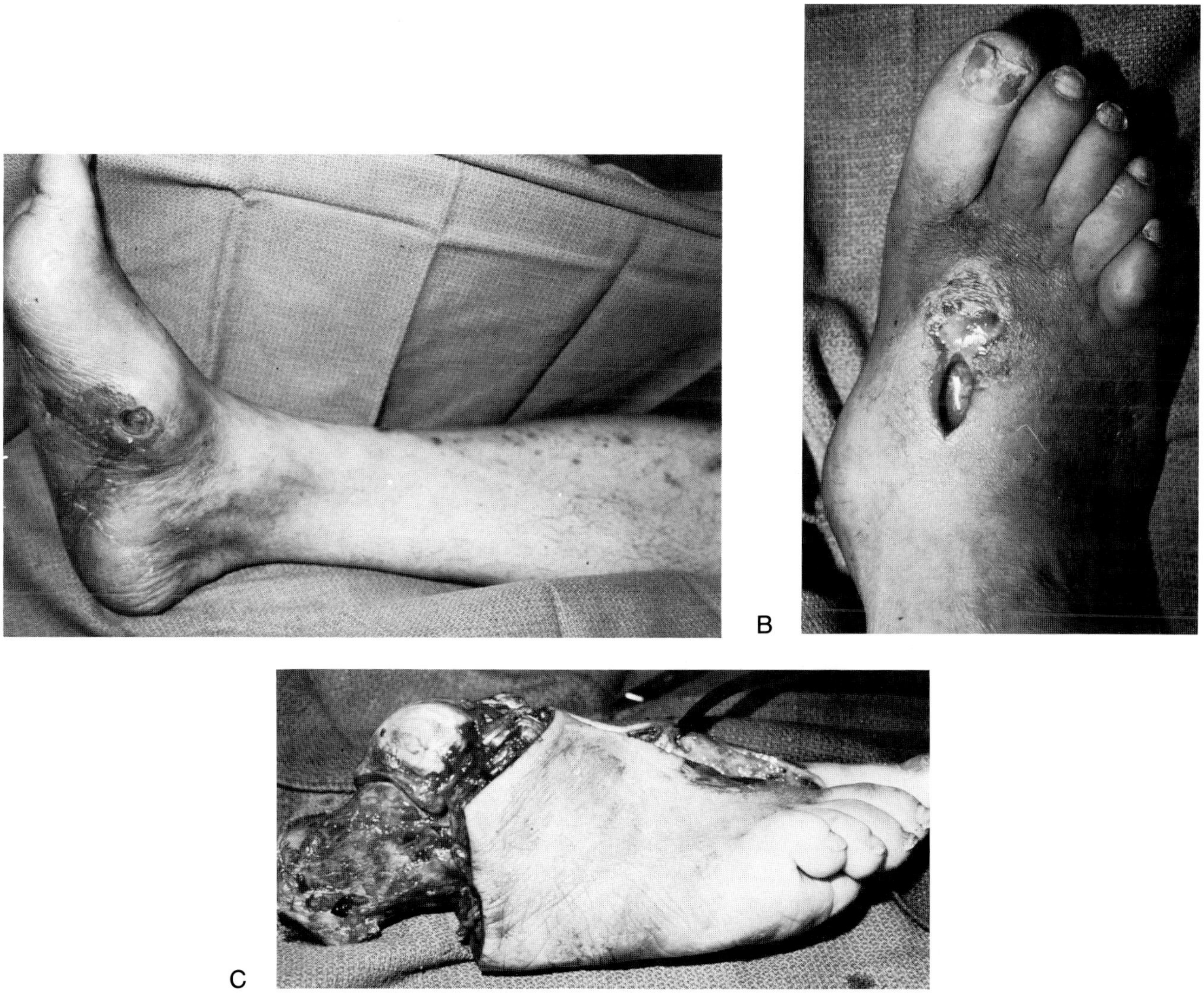

A B C

Fig. 18-12. (**A**) Charcot foot with medial ulceration about medial cunéiform. (**B**) Dorsal view of the same showing spread of infection from medial compartment into central compartment. (**C**) Specimen from Syme amputation. *(Figure continues.)*

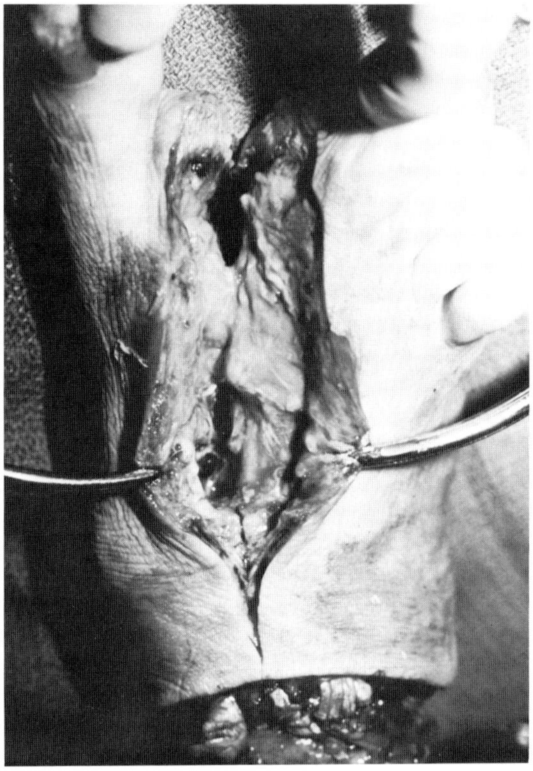

D

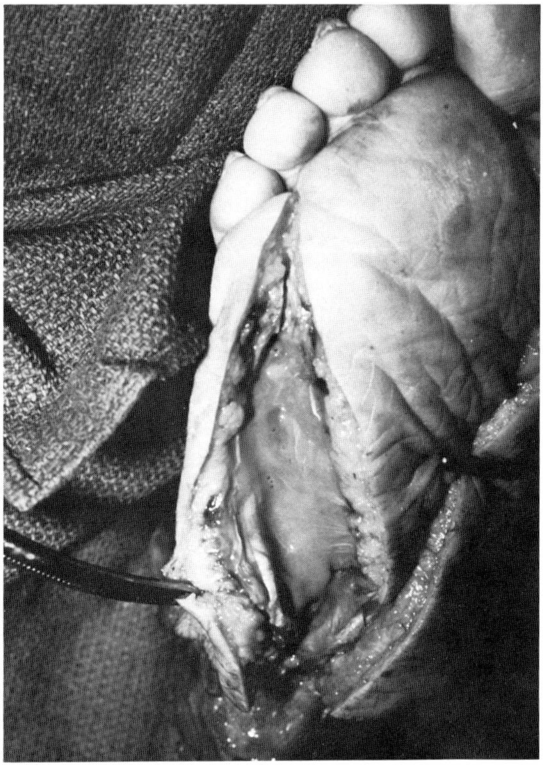

E

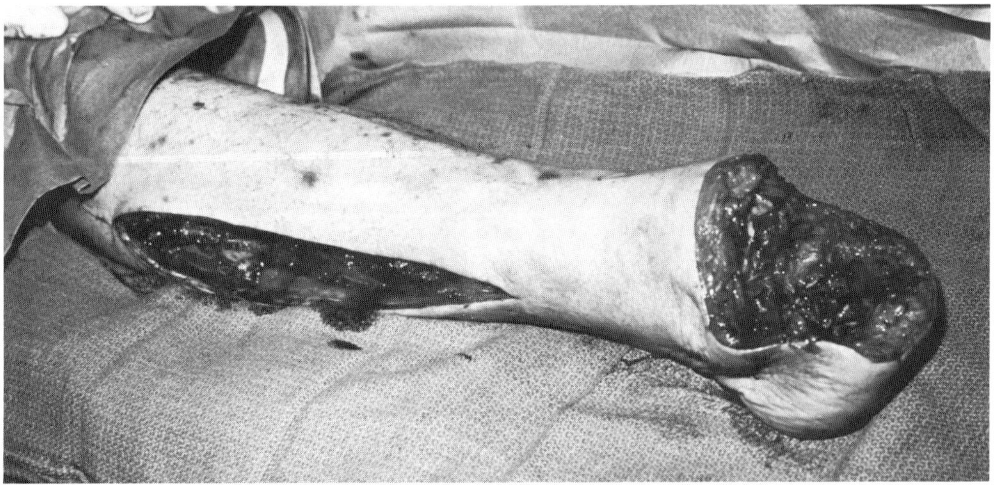

F

Fig. 18-12 *(Continued)*. **(D)** Dissection of amputated specimen shows through-and-through necrosis of the central compartment. **(E)** Dissection of amputated specimen shows infection with pus filling lateral compartment; infection traveled along peroneus longus. **(F)** Intraoperative photograph at time of Syme amputation showing extension of pus up into the lateral compartment of the leg. This was the first stage of a three-stage Syme procedure. The first stage consisted of incision and drainage and leaving the wound open; the second stage, closure of the wounds; and the third stage, remodeling of the malleoli.

Doctors need to resist a defeatist attitude and be informed, experienced, and interested to achieve optimal results.

CASE STUDIES

Case 1

The patient is a 60-year-old white man with a history of insulin-dependent diabetes mellitus of 33 years' duration complicated by peripheral neuropathy and peripheral vascular disease (Fig. 18-7). Initially this patient was admitted with a 2-month history of a nonhealing ulceration on the medial aspect of the first metatarsal head *left* foot on 9/12/86. The cause of the ulcer was a foreign body penetration, and the wound progressively worsened over the course of several months. Radiographs on admission showed osteomyelitis of the first metatarsal head of his left foot and gas in the soft tissues as well as extensive vascular calcification. Culture and sensitivities grew out *Enterobacter aerogenes* and *Enterococcus*. The patient underwent a left first metatarsal phalangeal joint resection for osteomyelitis. Postoperatively he developed Charcot fractures of the second, third, and fourth metatarsals on the left foot, and with time also a chronic ulceration underneath the fifth metatarsal head on his left foot. The patient was admitted again on 12/8/87, this time with wet gangrene of the *right* hallux and a deep space infection. He underwent an open right first ray resection and on 12/28/87 a revision to a right transmetatarsal amputation as well as a left fifth metatarsal head resection for a chronic infected ulcer. On 3/3/88 he had delayed primary closure of his right transmetatarsal amputation site. On 5/10/88 he presented again with an infected ulcer and osteomyelitis of the distal tip of the second digit of his left foot, a deep space infection in the medial arch of his left foot, and a superficial ulcer underneath the fifth metatarsal stump right transmetatarsal amputation site. The patient had an incision and drainage procedure on the left foot with a second ray resection and healed uneventfully. On 2/10/89 he had elective excision of his third and fourth metatarsal heads on the left foot for chronic ulcerations without evidence of infection. Currently all wounds are healed. There is intermittent superficial plantar ulceration distally of his right foot.

Case 2

A 64-year-old white man with a 20-year history of adult-onset diabetes mellitus and severe arteriosclerosis obliterans was admitted on 2/4/85 with rest pain in the right foot and dry gangrene of the distal tip of his right second toe. Other past medical history was significant for hypertension, angina, and anterolateral myocardial infarction (MI) in October of 1984. An arteriogram showed complete occlusion of the right superficial femoral artery and of the posterior tibial artery just above the ankle. The patient underwent a right common femoral to posterior tibial in situ saphenous vein bypass graft and was discharged on 2/13/85 with local wound care. The dry gangrene demarcated and the patient achieved a healed wound. On 9/17/86 the patient was readmitted with the diagnosis of an occluded femoral posterior tibial graft. Arteriography was performed and clot lysis by streptokinase was prescribed. He was discharged on 9/21/86. He presented again on 1/25/89 with complaint of rest pain in his right foot and gangrene of the distal aspect of his right hallux, and second and third toes. On the following day, he had a repeat right femoral to posterior tibial bypass graft using the left saphenous vein. His postoperative course was complicated by an MI and pulmonary edema on postoperative day 1, and he was discharged on 2/2/89 with a palpable posterior tibial pulse on the right foot but gangrenous distal digits. A definitive procedure was delayed because of his impaired cardiac status until 6/19/89, when he underwent a right transmetatarsal amputation for nonhealing chronically infected and painful great and lesser toes. He is fully healed and doing well at the present time (Fig. 18-13).

Case 3

The patient is a 57-year-old Asian man with an 18-year history of adult-onset diabetes mellitus with the complications of peripheral neuropathy and peripheral vascular disease as well as proliferative retinopathy. He presented with a dysvascular

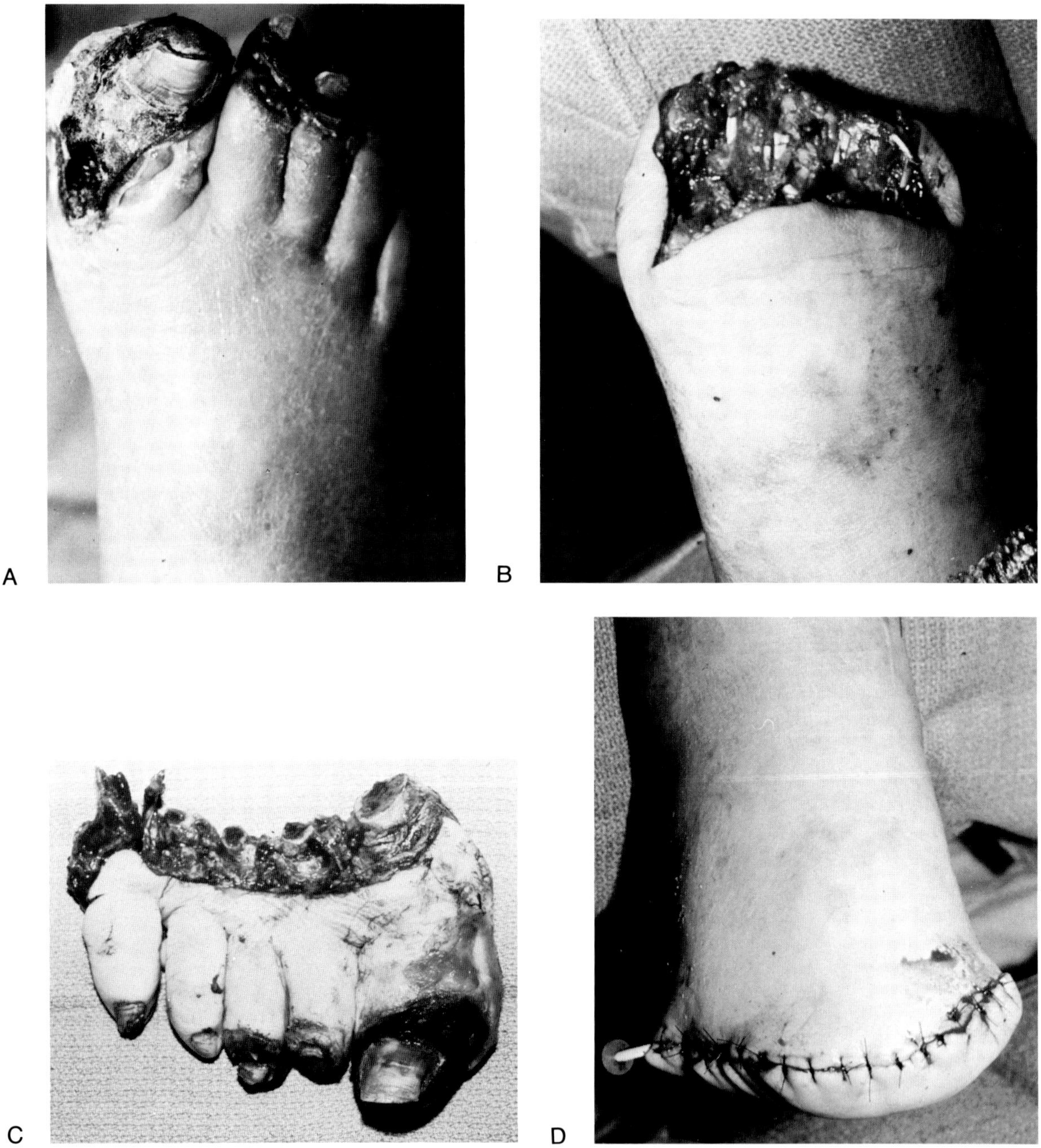

Fig. 18-13. (**A**) Status following lower extremity bypass. (**B**) Transmetatarsal amputation with plantarly based flap. (**C**) En bloc resection of distal forefoot. (**D**) Closed wound with drain in place.

second digit of his left foot and ascending cellulitis on 2/12/84. No evidence of deep infection was found on examination. Culture and sensitivity procedures grew out two strains of *Morganella* as well as *Escherichia coli.* Despite broad-spectrum intravenous antibiotics, the patient continued to spike fevers to 103°, and the cellulitis continued to spread proximally. A femoral arteriogram was obtained, which revealed a complete blockage in the left superficial femoral artery at mid-thigh with poor reconstitution of the leg vessels. The vascular surgeons felt that the patient was not a candidate for bypass surgery. On the fifth day of hospitalization he underwent resection of the second digit, which was revised 4 days later to an *open Syme* amputation. Seven days later the patient had delayed primary closure of the amputation site (second-stage Syme) procedure was discharged on 3/10/84. On 8/9/84 the patient underwent revision of his Syme amputation site (traditional second stage; in this case third-stage Syme) and did well postoperatively. On 5/22/86 he was again admitted with an infected ulcer underneath the fifth metatarsal head of his right foot and was discharged after 2 days of intravenous antibiotics, bed rest, and local wound care. On 9/11/86 he was again admitted with wet gangrene of the second digit of his right foot and ascending cellulitis, fever, and chills. He had a Syme amputation of his right foot performed on 9/25/86 but continued to spike fevers postoperatively. The right leg stump deteriorated with evidence of frank necrosis along the wound margins by 10/14/86. The patient underwent a below knee amputation on 10/21/86, which healed uneventfully. The Syme amputation stump on the left continues to do well and the patient is currently ambulating.

REFERENCES

1. Stern M, Adams E: Surgery with Special Reference to Podiatry. The William G. Hewitt Press, Brooklyn, 1917
2. Veal JR: Factors in the mortality rate of arteriosclerotic gangrene. J Am Med Assoc 110:785, 1938
3. Silbert S: Mid-leg amputations for gangrene in the diabetic. Ann Surg 127:503, 1948
4. Holden WD: Arteriosclerotic ischemic necrosis of the lower extremities. Surgery 22:125, 1947
5. McLaughlin CW, Jr, Weidman JG: Infection and gangrene in the diabetic extremity: critical review of surgical management over 17-year period. Nebraska Med J 35:316, 1950
6. Silbert S: Amputation of the lower extremity in diabetes mellitus: follow up of 294 cases. Diabetes 1:297, 1952
7. McKenzie DS: The elderly amputee. Br Med J 1:153, 1953
8. Samuels SS: Management of Peripheral Arterial Diseases. Oxford University Press, New York, 1950
9. Perlow S, Roth HA: Amputation for gangrene due to occlusive arterial disease. Surgery 25:547, 1949
10. McKittrick LS: Recent advances in care of surgical complications of diabetes mellitus. N Engl J Med 235:929, 1946
11. McKittrick LS, McKittrick JGB, Risley TS: Transmetatarsal amputation for infection or gangrene in patients with diabetes mellitus. Ann Surg 130:826, 1949
12. Silbert S, Haimovici H: Criteria for the selection of the level of amputation for ischemic gangrene. J Am Med Assoc 155:1554, 1954
13. Hoskov H, Josephsen P: Incidence of reamputation and death after gangrene of the lower extremity. Prosthet Orthot Int 4:77, 1980
14. Goldner M: The fate of the other leg in diabetic amputations. Diabetes 9:100, 1960
15. Most RS, Sinnock P: The epidemiology of lower extremity amputation in diabetic individuals. Diabetes Care 6:87, 1983
16. Mandrup-Poulsen T, Steen Jensen J: Mortality after major amputation following gangrene of the lower limb. Acta Orthop Scand 53:879, 1982
17. Kahn O, Wagner W, Bessman AN: Mortality of diabetic patients treated surgically for lower limb infection and/or gangrene. Diabetes 23:287, 1974
18. Scarlet J, Blais M: Statistics on the diabetic foot. J Am Pod Med Assoc 306, 1989
19. Sage R, Pinzur M, Cronin R et al: Complications following midfoot amputation in neuropathic and dysvascular feet. J Am Pod Med Assoc 79:277, 1989
20. Pinzur M, Sage R, Schwaegler P: Ray resection in the dysvascular foot. Clin Orthop Rel Res 191:232, 1984
21. Bailey TS, Yu HM, Rayfield EJ: Patterns of foot examination in a diabetes clinic. Am J Med 78:371, 1985
22. Hobgood E: Conservative therapy of foot abnormalities, infections, and vascular insufficiency. p. 397. In Davidson JK (ed): Clinical Diabetes Mellitus. Thieme, New York, 1986

23. Edmonds ME, Blundell MP, Morris HE et al: The diabetic foot: impact of a foot clinic. Q J Med 232:763, 1986
24. Assal JP, Muhlhauser I, Pernat A et al: Patient education as the basis for diabetes care in clinical practice. Diabetologia 28:602, 1985
25. Bild DE, Selby JV, Sinnock P et al: Lower extremity amputations in people with diabetes: epidemiology and prevention. Diabetes Care 12:24, 1989
26. Gibbons GW, Wheelock FC, Jr, Hoar CS, Jr et al: Predicting success of forefoot amputations in diabetics by noninvasive testing. Arch Surg 114:1034, 1979
27. Wheat LJ, Allen SD, Henry M et al: Diabetic foot infections: bacteriologic analysis. Arch Intern Med 146:1935, 1986
28. Louie TJ, Bartlett JG, Tally FP et al: Aerobic and anaerobic bacteria in diabetic foot ulcers. Ann Intern Med 85:461, 1976
29. Lefrock JL, Joseph WS: Lower extremity infections in diabetes. Infect Surg 5:135, 1986
30. Scher JS, Steele FJ: The septic foot in patients with diabetes. Surgery 104:661, 1988
31. Sizer JS, Wheelock FC: Digital amputations in diabetic patients. Surgery 72:980, 1972
32. Bose K: A surgical approach for the infected diabetic foot. Int Orthop 3:177, 1979
33. Goldman F, Manzi J, Carver A et al: Sinography in diagnosis of foot infections. J Am Pod Assoc 71:497, 1981
34. Sartoris DJ, Devine S, Resnick D et al: Plantar compartmental infection in the diabetic foot: the role of computed tomography. Invest Radiol 20:772, 1985
35. Meade JW, Mueller CB: Major infections of the foot. Med Times 96:154, 1968
36. Karmody AM, Jacobs RL: Salvage of the diabetic foot by vascular reconstruction. Orthop Clin North Am 7:957, 1976
37. Burgess EM, Matsen FA III: Determining amputation levels in peripheral vascular disease. J Bone Joint Surg 63A:1493, 1981
38. Bernhard LM, Bakst M, Coleman W et al: Plantar space abscess in the diabetic foot: diagnosis and treatment. J Foot Surg 232:283, 1984
39. Feingold ML, Resnick D, Niwayama G et al: The plantar compartments of the foot: a roentgen approach. I. Experimental observations. Invest Radiol 12:281, 1977
40. Goldman FD: Deep space infection in the diabetic patient. J Am Pod Med Assoc 77:431, 1987
41. Grodinsky M: A study of the fascial spaces of the foot and their bearing on infections. Surg Gynecol Obstet 49:737, 1929
42. Kamel R, Sakla FB: Anatomical compartments of the sole of the human foot. Anat Rec 140:57, 1961
43. Gottrup F: Delayed primary closure of wounds. Arch Surg 4:171, 1985
44. Gibbons G: Diabetic foot sepsis. p. 412. In Brewster DD (ed): Common Problems in Vascular Surgery. Year Book Medical Publishers, Chicago, 1989
45. Pomposelli FB, Jr, Jepsen SA, Gibbons G et al: Efficacy of the dorsalis pedis bypass for limb salvage in diabetic patients. J Vasc Surg 11:745, 1990

19

Plastic Surgical Approaches to the Diabetic Foot

Lawrence B. Colen, M.D.
Leonard Miller, M.D., F.A.C.S., F.R.C.S. (Edin.)

Many plastic and reconstructive surgeons have found themselves playing a new role in the management of the diabetic patient. Approximately 20 percent of all diabetic patients who enter the hospital are admitted for foot problems,[1] and of the many complications affecting the diabetic patient, none are more devastating than gangrene and the threat of leg amputation. Despite the availability of antibiotics, approximately 50 to 70 percent of the major leg amputations being performed are done in the diabetic population.[2,3] Additionally, there is nearly a 50 percent incidence of a second amputation in the contralateral limb within 2 years of the first amputation.[4,5] More than 40,000 major amputations in diabetic patients take place each year in the United States,[6] and a recent randomized sample of over 700 diabetic patients revealed that only 30 percent were free of diabetic foot symptoms.[7] Of the 10 million Americans who have diabetes mellitus, 15 percent (1.5 million) will develop foot ulcers.[8] The economic and social impact to both the nation and patient is enormous.[9] Surgical intervention can substantially reduce the morbidity in this group of patients.

We have adopted an aggressive surgical approach to the management of plantar ulceration in the diabetic patient, and a recent review of more than 150 of our diabetic patients revealed that 97 percent maintained bipedal ambulation.[10] It is our feeling that debridement and closure of the foot wounds in diabetic patients will substantially decrease the incidence of limb- and life-threatening infection.

OVERVIEW

Because it is increasingly appreciated that plantar ulceration in the patient with diabetes is no longer hopeless, rote amputation has gradually been supplanted by newer salvage procedures. Improved understanding of wound bacteriology and the availability of more effective topical antimicrobial agents have allowed for better control of devastating infection. The routine use of in situ saphenous vein bypass grafting to the pedal vessels and the appearance of newer hemorheologic agents such as pentoxifylline[11] have produced functional improvement in the circulation of the diabetic foot, thereby facilitating successful reconstructive surgery. The numerous advances in free tissue transfer have made possible the reconstruction of extremities previously thought to be unsalvageable.

Evaluation begins with a complete physical examination to determine the location and size of the wound, the status of the peripheral circulation, and the presence or absence of peripheral neuropathy. Radiographs are *not* helpful in diagnosis of bone infection,[12] but do aid in planning the surgical procedure since spurs, prominences, and other deformities are clearly visible on plain films. Radionuclide scans are also inconclusive in the evaluation of the diabetic foot because the presence of neuroarthropathy (seen in 0.1 to 2.5 percent of diabetic patients and in many diabetic patients with plantar ulceration[13–15]) causes increased nuclide uptake.[12] Confirmation of osteomyelitis requires bone biopsy either before or at the time of wound debridement and closure.[12]

In the absence of palpable pulses, vascular surgical consultation and noninvasive vascular laboratory studies should be obtained. Ankle-brachial indices are often elevated in these patients because of the noncompressible nature of their vessels; hence Doppler waveform assessment and duplex imaging become more valuable. Supplemental studies of cutaneous blood flow are particularly important in patients who are marginal candidates for revascularization or who are not candidates at all. Transcutaneous PO_2 measurements, dermal fluorometry, or laser Doppler velocimetry indicate the likelihood of healing after reconstructive surgery.

Since most foot wounds in the diabetic patient are the result of neuropathic changes, it behooves the plastic surgeon to spend some time evaluating the distribution of the sensory loss that these patients exhibit. The loss of sudomotor function causes an anhidrosis and hyperkeratosis that will lead to fissuring of the skin and subsequent infection. The lack of sensibility over bony prominences and between the toes results in delayed detection of breaks in the skin. The motor component of the neuropathy contributes to Charcot deformities as the intrinsic foot musculature atrophies and becomes fibrotic. The resulting metatarsophalangeal extension and interphalangeal flexion produce excessive pressure on the metatarsal heads and the ends of the phalanges. The loss of the transverse arch of the foot further exacerbates the unfavorable weight distribution across the metatarsal heads. Once the longitudinal arch is destroyed, weight is borne on the midfoot with substantial morbidity resulting. If a patient presents with hypoesthesia in the tibial nerve distribution of the foot but has intact sural or peroneal nerve sensibility, one may consider nerve transfer surgery to help restore protective sensation to the weight-bearing sole of the foot. As has been elucidated by other authors, compression neuropathy in the diabetic patient is far more common than in the nondiabetic patient.[16,17] Nerve conduction studies may be helpful to identify neuropathies such as tarsal tunnel syndrome that would be amenable to surgical decompression. The improvement in plantar sensibility after tarsal tunnel release may be substantial enough to prevent ulcer recurrence once reconstructive surgery has been completed.[18]

Basic wound management principles apply to the care of diabetic foot ulcers. If the patient presents with frank infection, it is imperative that he or she be made nonambulatory upon admission to the hospital. Strict bed rest and extremity elevation are essential to eliminate edema and help control infection. Adequate surgical debridement of necrotic tissue and wide drainage of purulent cavities are mandatory. Plantar space infection should be suspected in any patient who presents with cellulitis and a plantar ulcer, especially if palpation reveals tenderness or swelling over the midfoot. Occasionally aspiration with a 3-cc syringe and an 18-gauge needle will help confirm the presence of such a problem. If clinically indicated, bone biopsy should be performed and the patient should be started on broad spectrum antibiotics to combat aerobes, anaerobes, gram-positive, and gram-negative bacteria. Once debridement has been completed, the use of long-acting, broad spectrum topical antibacterials (Silvadene or Sulfamylon) helps to obtain final bacteriologic control of the wound. Patients presenting with ulceration without frank sepsis may be treated a bit differently as a single-stage debridement and closure can usually be performed. Again, culture-specific antibiotics are essential.

Wound closure should be undertaken either in conjunction with the debridement (if there is no gross infection) or 3 to 5 days after adequate debridement and drainage of the infected area. In some patients the debridement process may require serial surgical procedures. Reconstructive options vary with the location of the wound, the vascular status of the foot, and the presence or absence of midfoot neuroarthropathy. In planning the reconstruction it is helpful to consider three distinct regions of the foot: the forefoot (from toes to metatarsal shaft), the midfoot (from metatarsal shaft to the talus), and the hindfoot (from the talonavicular joint to the most posterior aspects of the calcaneus). The surgical options vary from region to region.

FOREFOOT

Wounds in this location are often secondary to both peripheral vascular disease and neuropathy and may range from a simple ischemic toe ulcer to deeper wounds over the metatarsal heads. When infection complicates these wounds, subfascial extension can markedly increase the morbidity of these ulcers.

Surgical management may involve simple toe amputation for the most distal wounds, provided arterial inflow has been optimized. Ray amputation may be required if the process involves the metatarsal as well (Fig. 19-1). When metatarsal head ulceration occurs, skin grafts may be considered for the most shallow wounds although grafts are rarely durable enough to withstand the forces of weight bearing. When indicated, these grafts may be harvested from the non-weight-bearing instep area of the same extremity (Fig. 19-2). The use of "local" tissue has been the mainstay of treatment for these wounds because durable coverage is provided

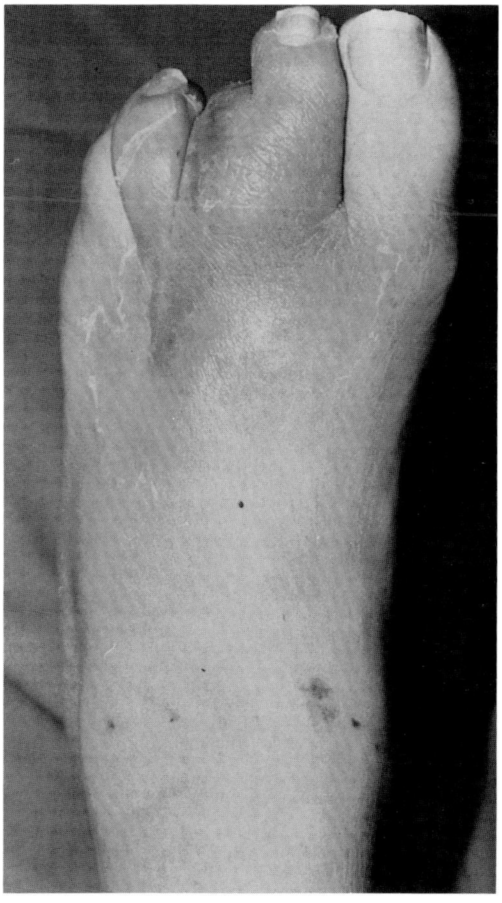

A

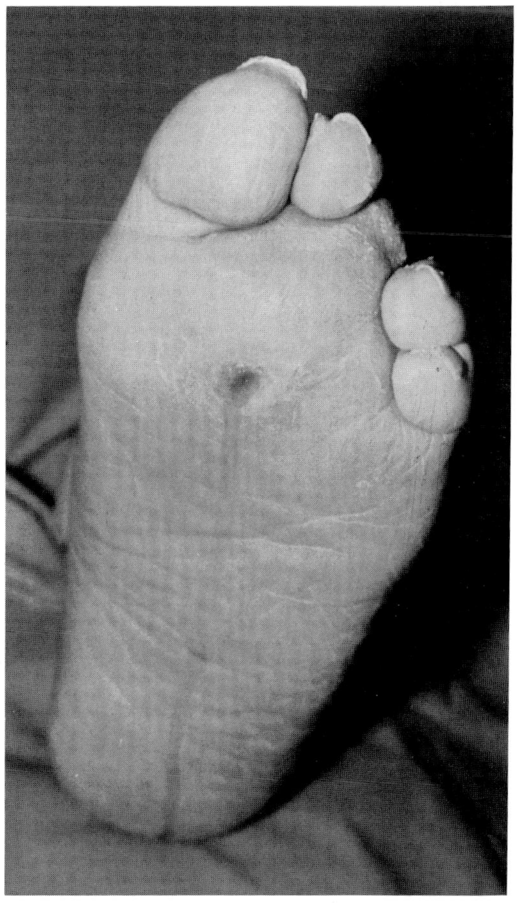

B

Fig. 19-1. (**A**) Forefoot infection status post amputation of the third toe. (**B**) Second metatarsal head ulcer is the etiology of the infection. *(Figure continues.)*

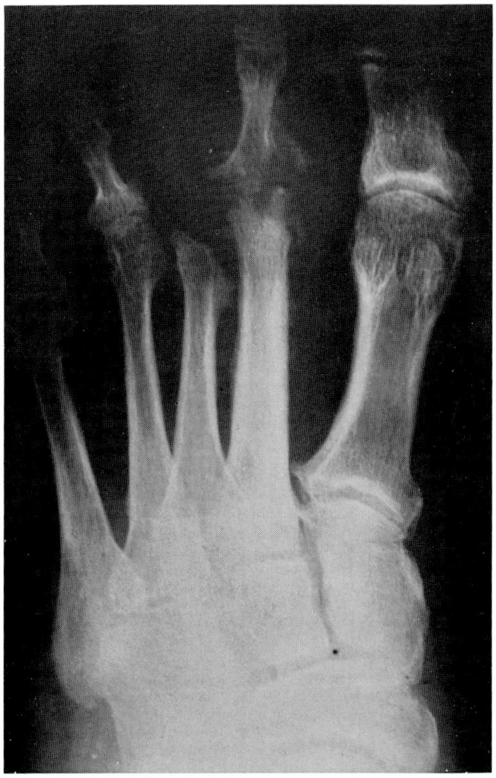

C

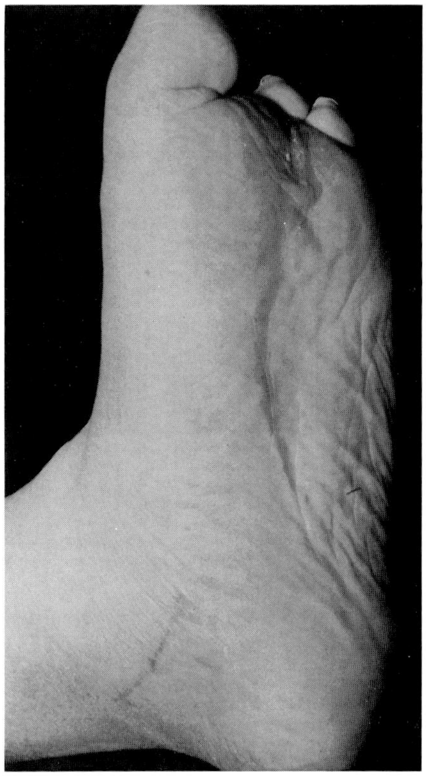

D

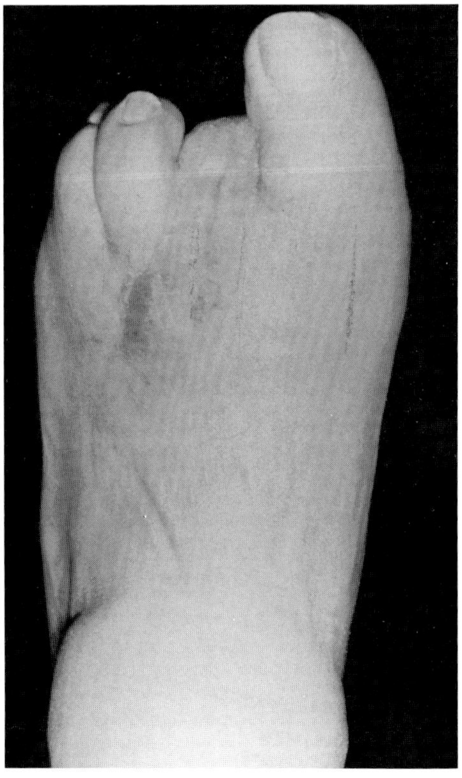

E

Fig. 19-1. *(Continued).* **(C)** Bone biopsy confirmed the radiograph of second metatarsal head infection. **(D & E)** Second ray resection followed by delayed primary closure.

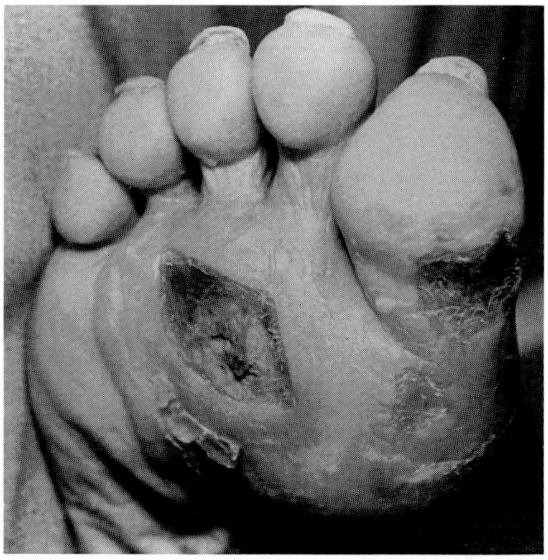

A

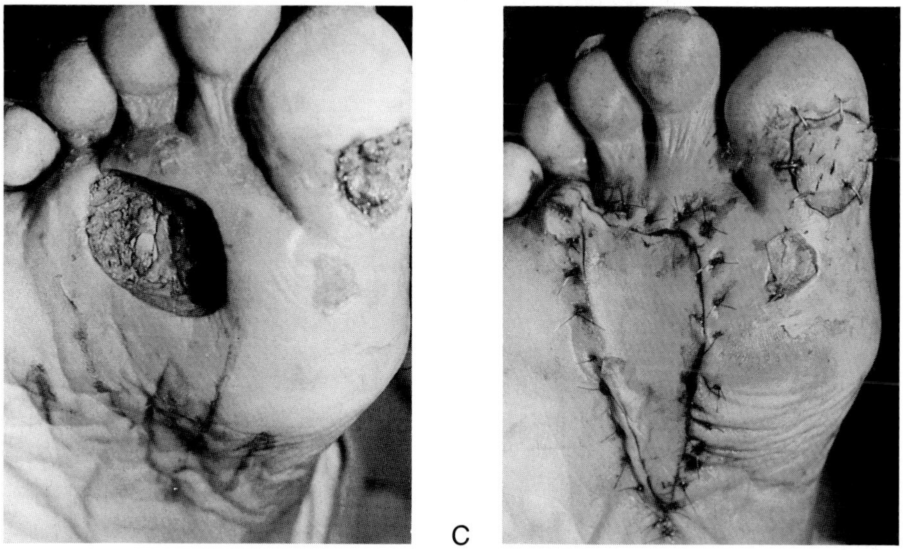

B C

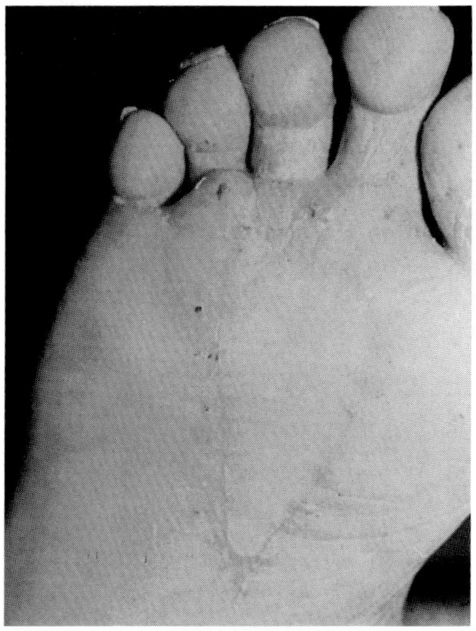

D

Fig. 19-2. (**A**) Forefoot wounds and peripheral vascular disease. (**B**) After femoral-popliteal bypass wounds are debrided. (**C**) V-Y advancement of plantar skin and fascia close the third metatarsal head ulcer. Skin graft is used for the shallower wounds. (**B**) Three months after surgery wounds are well healed.

without sacrificing functional length of the foot. Options include either the use of tissue harvested from the toes or the use of plantar tissue from the forefoot. For coverage of wounds up to 2 cm, the fillet of an adjacent toe may be used, preserving the nutrient neurovascular bundles.[19] Larger defects can be closed with the sacrifice of two or more toes. Use of the neurovascular island flap from the fibular side of the great toe based on either the dorsal or plantar circulation is also an effective means of closing small defects (2 to 3 cm) and does not require toe sacrifice (Fig. 19-3).[20,21] Depending on flap size, the donor site may be closed either directly or with a split-thickness skin graft. Forefoot tissue may be advanced in a V-Y fashion to close small defects as well (Fig. 19-2). If necessary, two

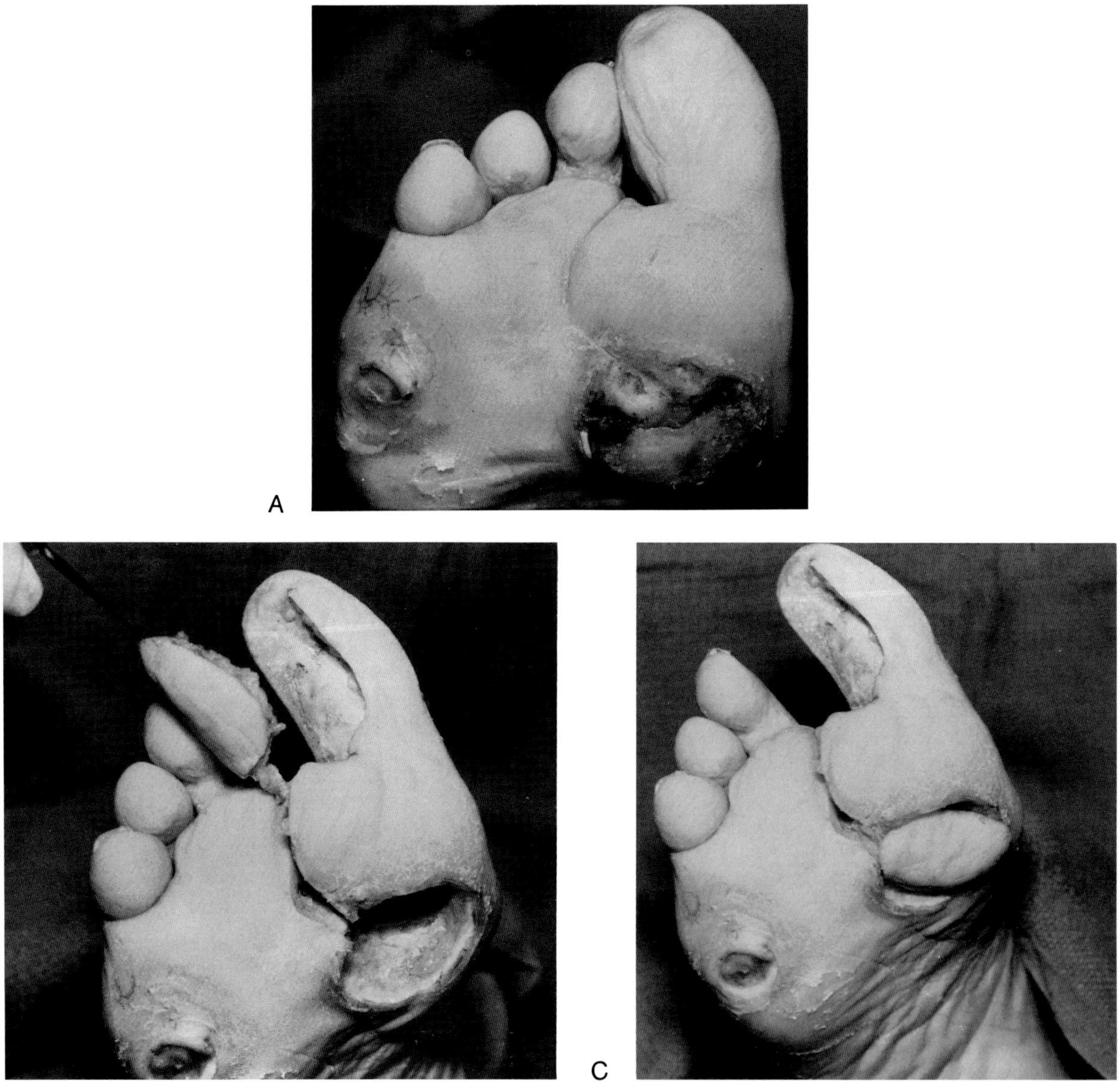

A B C

Fig. 19-3. (A) First and fifth metatarsal head ulcers. (B) Neurovascular island flap elevated on the dorsal circulation. (C) Transposition into the debrided first metatarsal head wound. The fifth metatarsal head ulcer was debrided, the metatarsal head resected, and the wound closed with a V-Y plantar advancement flap.

such flaps can be used to resurface defects of up to 4 cm in diameter (Fig. 19-4).[22] Flap mobilization requires the release of the plantar fascia above the circumference as well as judicious release of the "vertical" slips of fascia that tether the flap to the underlying metatarsals.

Manipulation of the underlying bony architecture appears to help prevent recurrent ulceration.[22] When wounds involve the fifth metatarsal head, resection through the metatarsal neck is recommended. This can be done by a dorsal approach or, if the ulcer penetrates deeply, through the debrided plantar wound. Ulceration associated with the second, third, and fourth metatarsal heads is best treated with a "floating" osteotomy of the prominent metatarsal. Accomplished through a linear dorsal incision, the osteotomy through the metatarsal neck allows the metatarsal head to move into a less prominent position without transferring excessive weight-bearing pressure to the adjacent metatarsal head (Fig. 19-5). The first metatarsal is debrided only if involved with the ulcer base. More

A

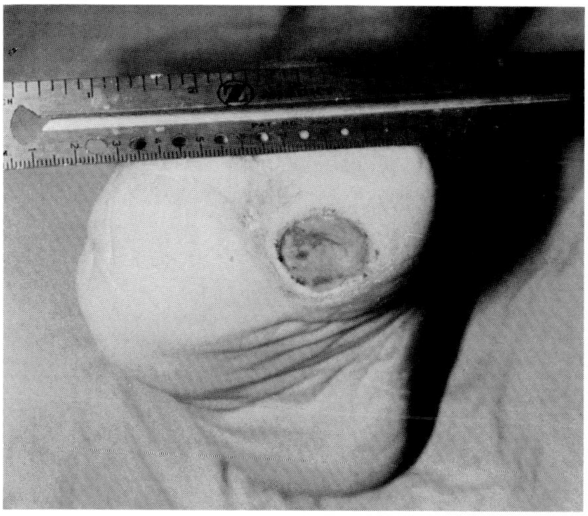

B

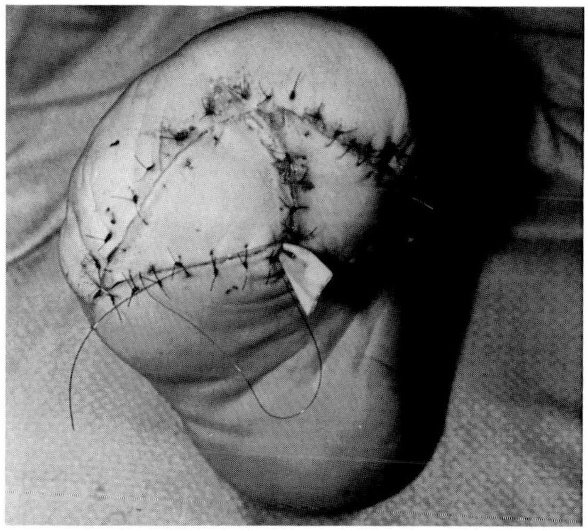

Fig. 19-4. (**A**) Large forefoot ulcer after transmetatarsal amputation. (**B**) Wound managed with two opposing V-Y advancement flaps.

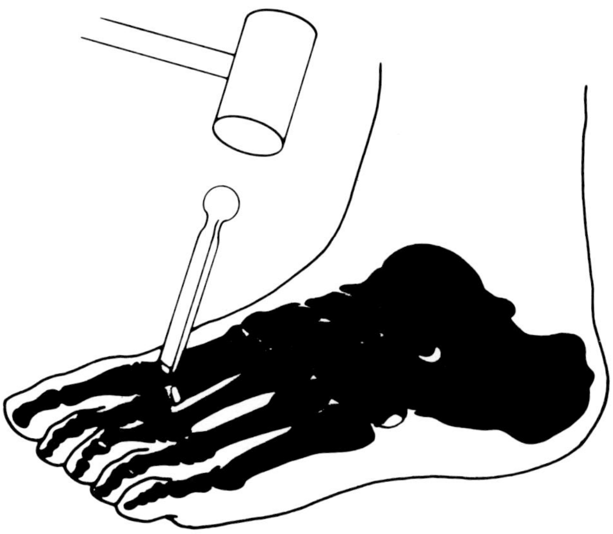

Fig. 19-5. Surgical approach to metatarsal neck "floating" osteotomy. See text for details.

often the source of pressure is from the medial or lateral sesamoid bones, which may be excised at the time of flap closure.

MIDFOOT

Ulceration of the midfoot is almost uniformly the result of the neuroarthropathy associated with diabetes mellitus. The tarsal bones and the tarsometatarsal joints are involved in almost 60 percent of patients with Charcot deformities.[13] In these patients, the midfoot becomes an important component in the distribution of weight during ambulation. The often-seen medial instep wound results from deformity about the first metatarsal base, medial cuneiform, and navicular bones. The most lateral wound occurring in the midfoot region is secondary to prominence of the fifth metatarsal base and cuboid bones. Addressing these bony deformities at the time of wound closure is the key to a successful outcome from reconstructive surgery. Small- to moderate-sized deficits (less than 4 cm) can usually be reconstructed by local tissue techniques. V-Y advancement flaps (Fig. 19-6), neuro-

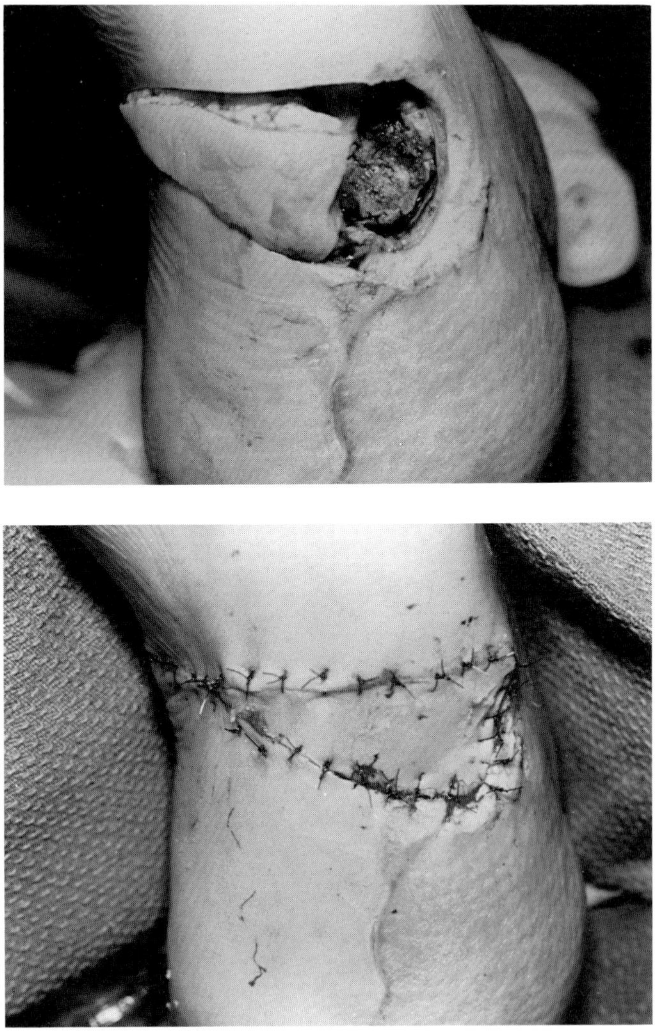

Fig. 19-6. (**A**) Lateral midfoot ulcer. Debrided (including the underlying cuboid) and V-Y plantar flap incised. (**B**) Wound closed with advancement of the flap.

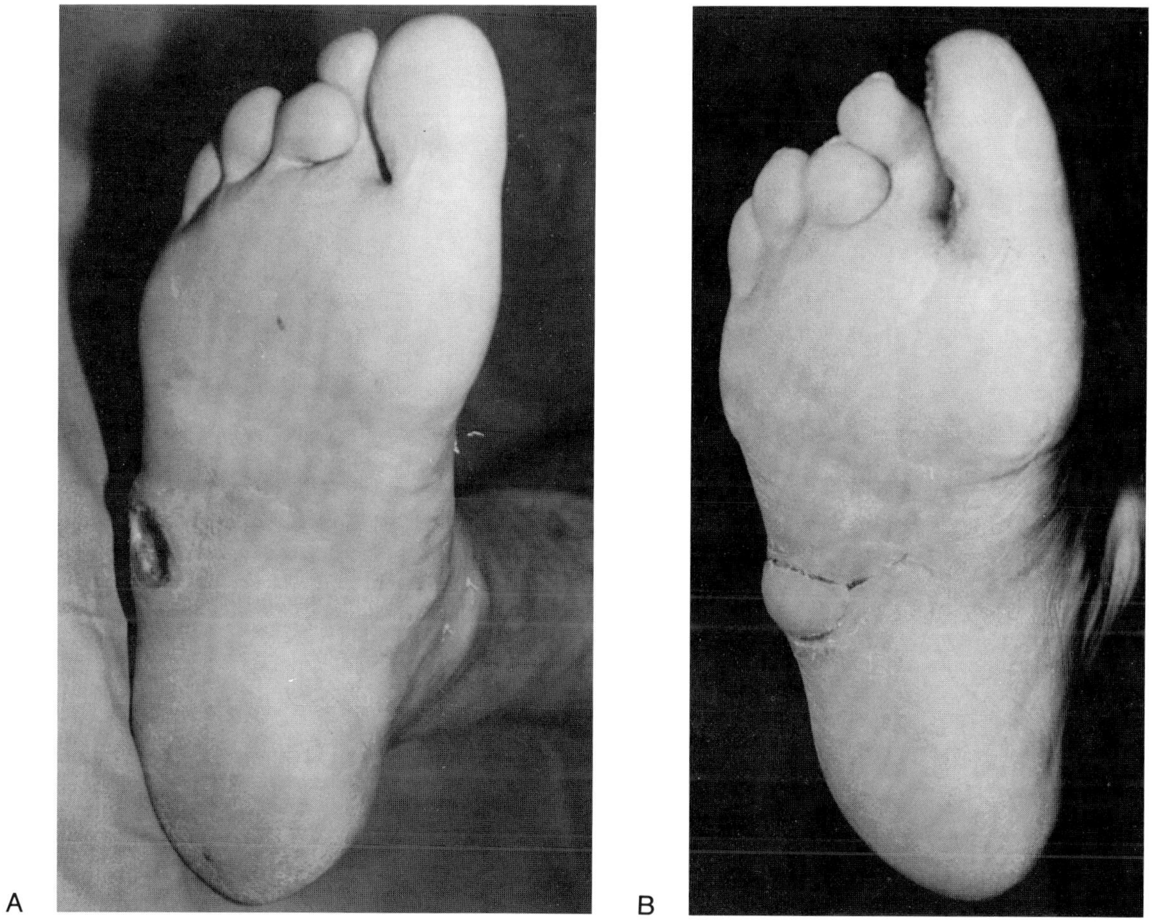

Fig. 19-7. (**A**) Lateral midfoot wound. (**B**) Two months after closure using a neurovascular island flap from the lateral side of the great toe based on the plantar circulation.

vascular island flaps from the fibular side of the great toe (Fig. 19-7), or total toe fillet flaps can be used, as indicated by the size and location of the wound and the patient's history of prior reconstructive surgery. Wound size greater than 4 to 5 cm requires either free flap reconstruction (Fig. 19-8) or amputation revision (Fig. 19-9) to obtain stable coverage. It is important to maintain foot length at the midfoot level (Lisfranc or Chopart) so that simple orthotics rather than prostheses will permit ambulation. As noted previously, bony prominences should be judiciously debrided and limited midfoot fusions should be considered when clinically indicated.[23,24]

HINDFOOT

Ulceration in the hindfoot is most often a result of hypoesthesia resulting from neuropathy. It is often exacerbated by atherosclerosis and frequently involves calcaneal osteomyelitis. Numerous local flaps are available from the foot to provide for wound closure in the hindfoot region.[25] With the exception of the lateral calcaneal artery flap,[26] all of these flaps require patent antegrade flow in the posterior tibial artery and its branches to ensure successful transposition. The lateral calcaneal artery flap is particularly useful for small wounds of

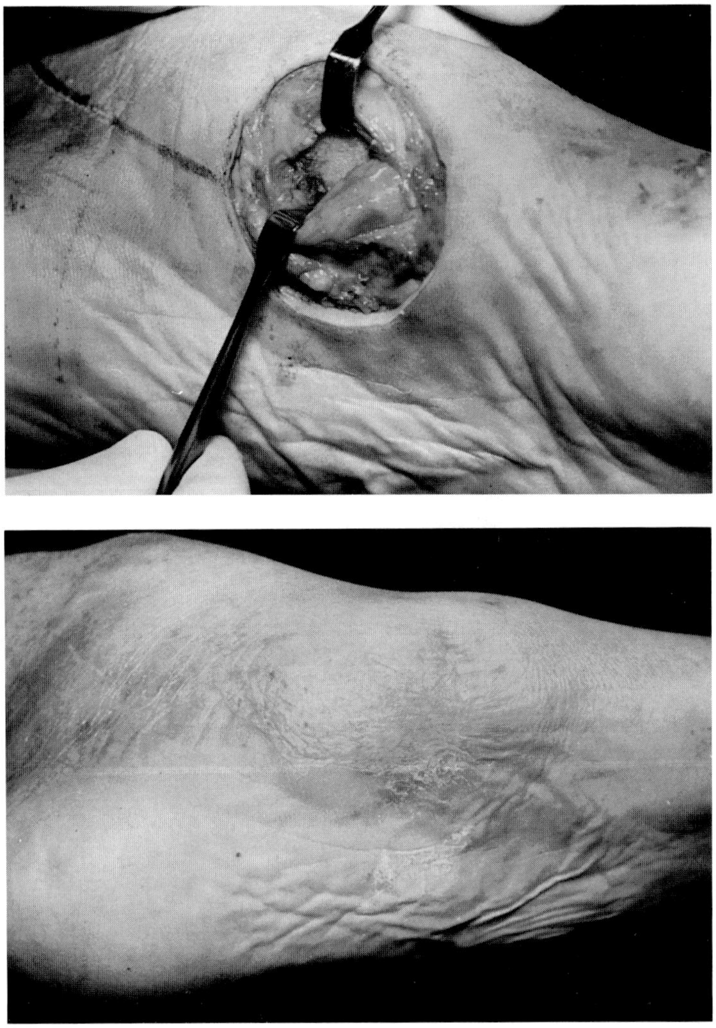

A

B

Fig. 19-8. (**A**) Large instep wound, debrided (including underlying medial cuneiform). (**B**) Three years after rectus abdominus free flap and skin graft.

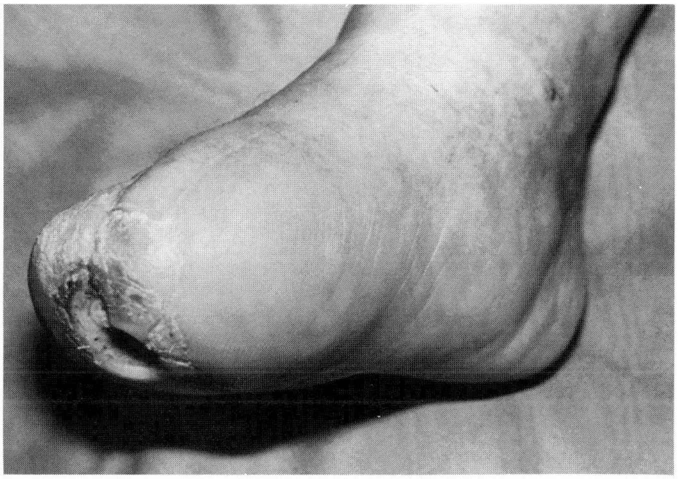

A

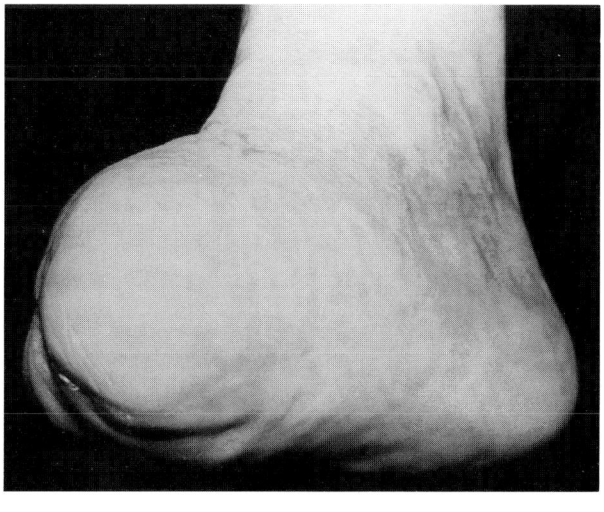

B

Fig. 19-9. (**A**) Recurrent ulceration after transmetatarsal amputation. (**B**) Closure via revison to a Lisfranc level.

A B
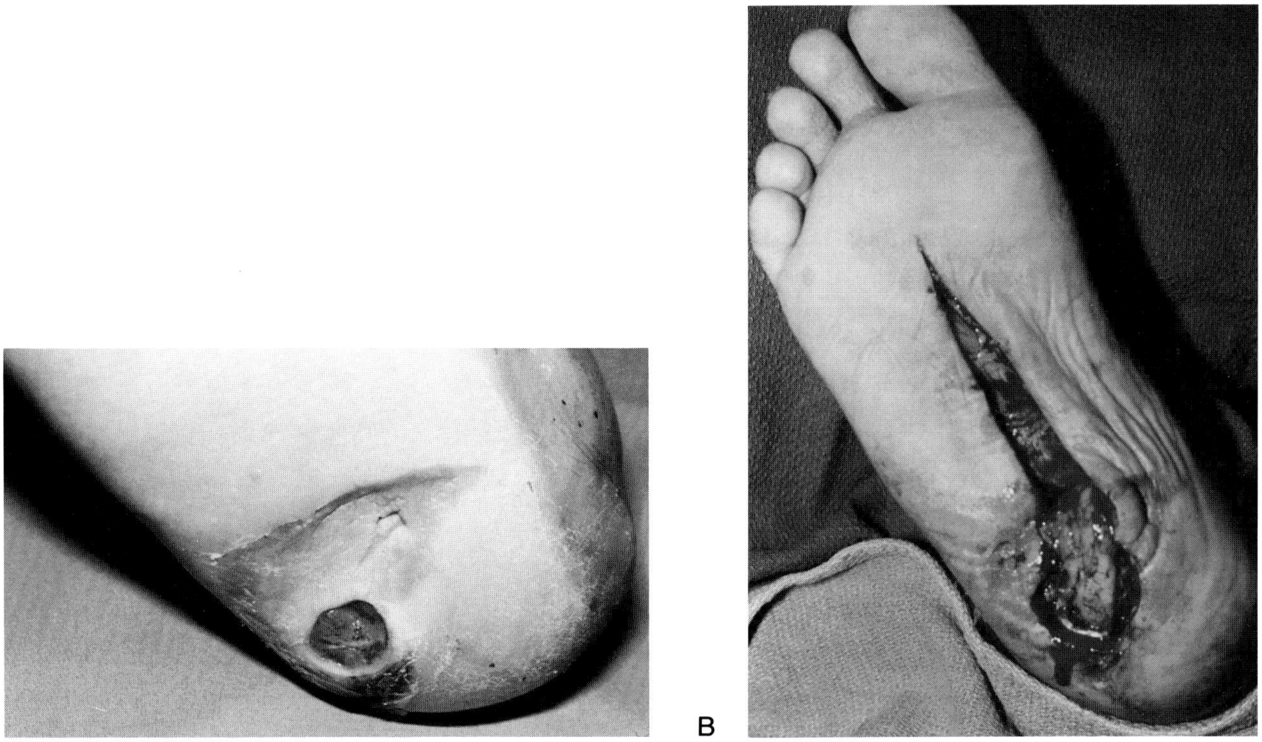

Fig. 19-10. (**A**) Recurrent heel ulceration. (**B**) Flexor digitorum brevis muscle transposed into the debrided wound before donor site closure and skin graft application.

the posterior hindfoot as the "parent" vessel (the peroneal artery) is the last vessel to be affected with atherosclerosis in the patient with diabetes.[27]

The abductor hallucis, abductor digiti minimi and the flexor digitorum brevis muscles are useful for the reconstruction of small deficits (2 to 4 cm) (Fig. 19-10). Wounds located more posteriorly on the plantar heel may be closed with a posterior transposition of the heel pad when elevated suprafascially (Fig. 19-11).[28] The instep fasciocutaneous flap may be used for larger heel defects (4 to 6 cm) and requires skin grafting to the instep donor site (Fig. 19-12).[29,30] Patients with Charcot deformities of the instep may present unique donor site problems, making selection of this flap less advisable. As the instep in these patients is generally a weight-bearing structure, the resultant skin-grafted donor site is more likely to ulcerate.

Many patients with diabetes will present with either "large" wounds (greater than 6 cm) or with

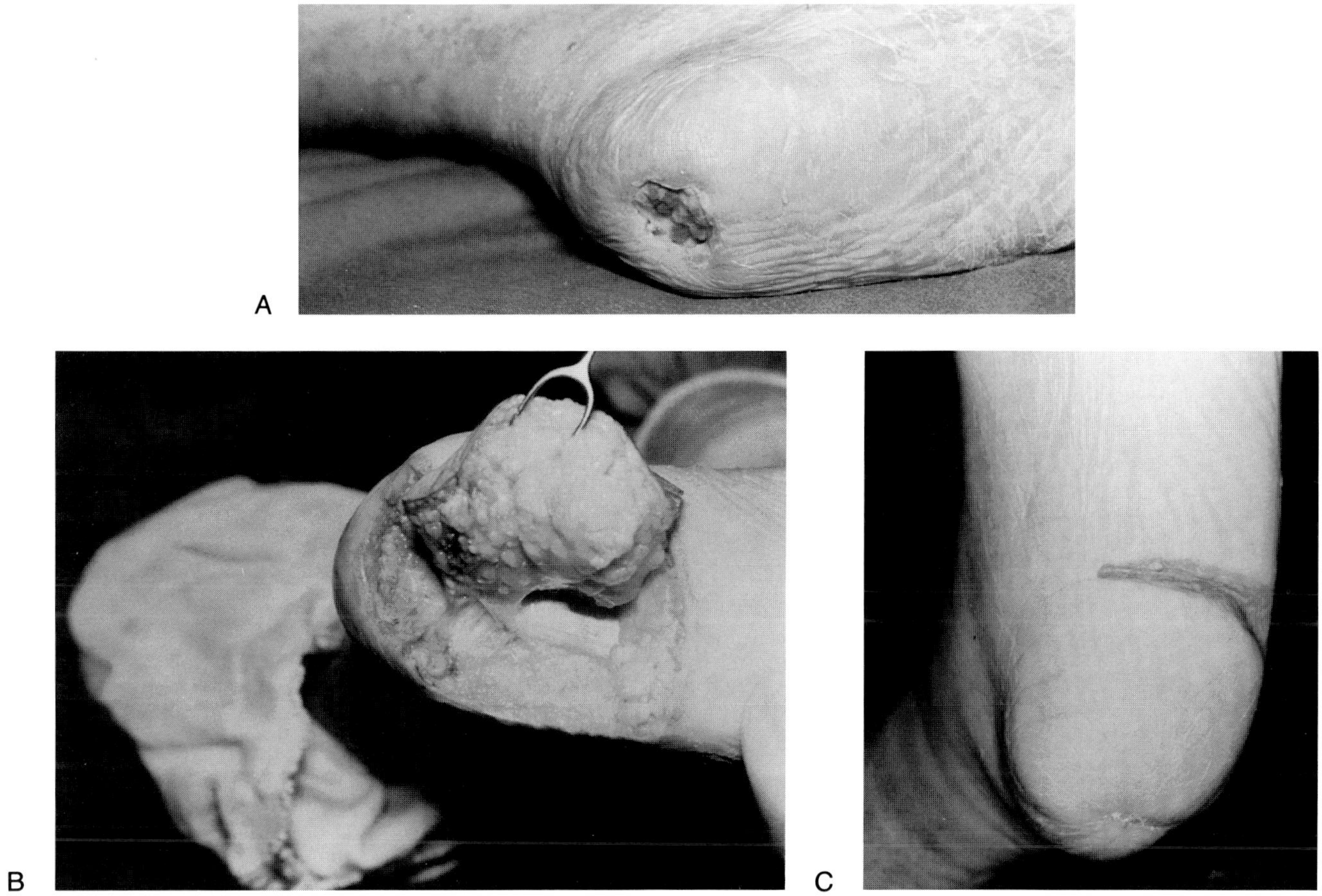

Fig. 19-11. (A) Small heel ulcer after aortofemoral bypass graft. (B) Heel pad elevated suprafascially, medially based. (C) Healed wound, skin-grafted donor site (non-weight-bearing).

significant peripheral vascular disease that would make using these flaps hazardous. Patients who have undergone distal vascular bypass surgery to the anterior tibial or peroneal vessels would benefit most from free-flap reconstruction. Free tissue transfer has therefore been our most common technique for the reconstruction of larger hindfoot (and midfoot) defects (Fig. 19-13). Flaps are generally harvested from the upper extremity or torso since the incidence of atherosclerosis in the donor pedicle is lessened. In patients who have undergone distal bypass vascular reconstruction, the arterial anastomoses may be performed directly to the in situ saphenous vein graft.[31]

ADJUNCTIVE TECHNIQUES

The importance of osseous manipulation cannot be overemphasized. Bone spurs, joint dislocations, and other causes of weight maldistribution must be addressed to help maintain a stable soft tissue envelope. Charcot deformity of the midfoot is often heralded by mild effusions, joint instability, crepitus, and soft tissue swelling before a fixed deformity is present. If these symptoms are identified early, casting may prevent permanent deformity.[23]

Recent evidence indicates that the "stocking/glove" distribution of peripheral neuropathy seen

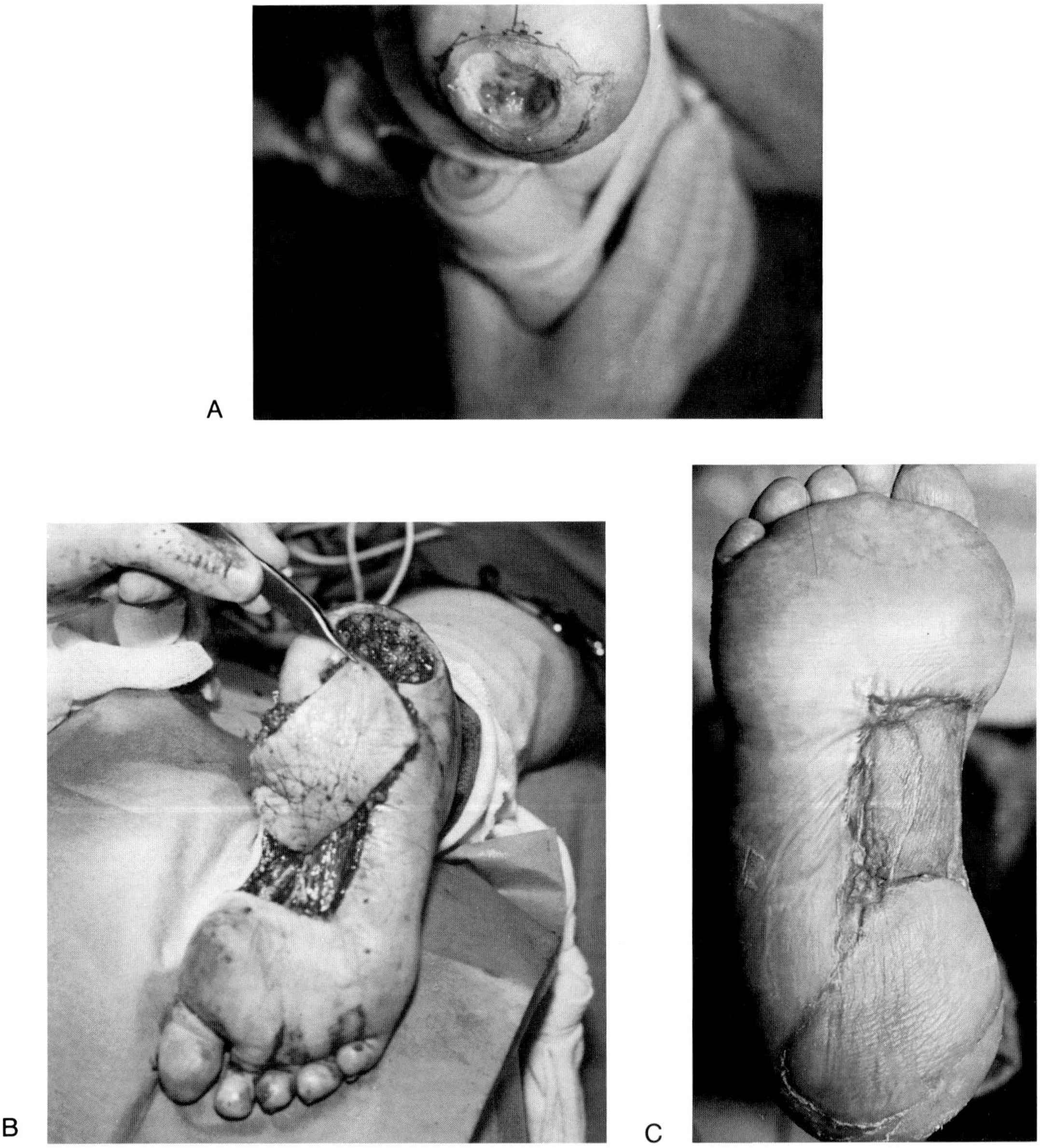

Fig. 19-12. (**A**) Heel ulcer. (**B**) Instep (medial plantar) fasciocutaneous flap elevated. (**C**) Closed wound with donor site skin grafted.

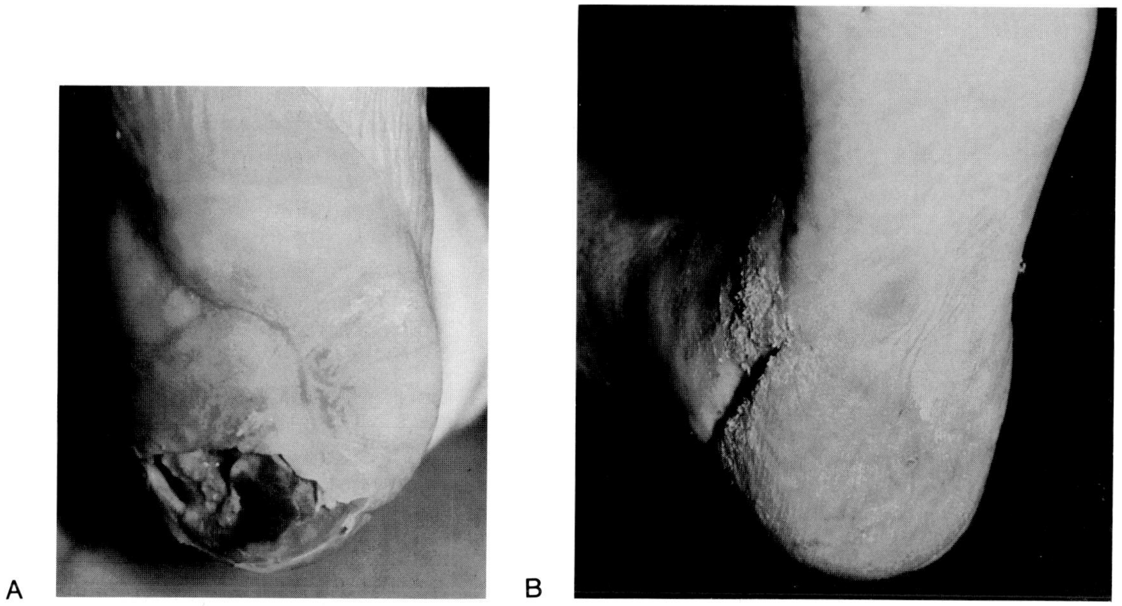

Fig. 19-13. (A) Recurrent heel ulceration and calcaneal osteomyelitis after numerous reconstructive procedures. (B) Stable soft tissue coverage and eradication of the bone infection with debridement, parenteral antibiotics, and staged closure using a serratus anterior free flap and skin graft.

in diabetes mellitus may be in part due to known sites of anatomic compression of the major peripheral nerves. It has been our experience and that of others that tarsal tunnel release performed at the time of definitive wound closure will significantly improve sensation to the plantar aspect of the foot.[16,18] Release is easily accomplished by dividing the flexor retinaculum as well as the origin of the abductor hallucis muscle. Epineurectomy and internal neurolysis may be performed as well, depending upon the findings at surgery (Fig. 19-14).

The importance of a multidisciplinary approach to the care of the diabetic patient with plantar ulceration cannot be overemphasized. The need for orthopaedic, vascular, and plastic surgical consultation is obvious. Routine prophylactic and therapeutic evaluation by the podiatric service is mandatory. Using this approach we have kept the below knee amputation rate at 3 percent over the past 6 years.[10]

FUTURE

Patient education, newer techniques of bone manipulation, improved weight-dispersion orthotics, and changes in both vascular and plastic surgical techniques will set the stage for significant advances in the care of the diabetic foot with plantar ulceration. Neuropathy continues to play the major role leading to the ulceration and its recurrence. The nonphysiologic dispersion of weight over insensate tissue is the major problem that remains to be resolved.

Effort should be directed toward the prevention and treatment of diabetic neuropathy, since a change in this part of the "diabetic foot syndrome" will have a major impact on the incidence of plantar ulceration in the future. The recent use of aldose reductase inhibitors has been promising in this regard. An increase of up to 54 percent in the hydra-

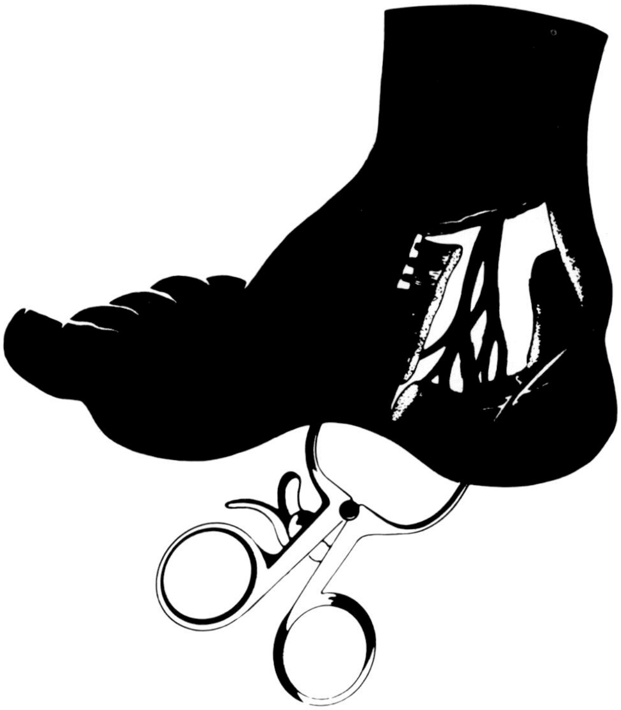

Fig. 19-14. Tarsal tunnel release performed through an incision posterior to the medial malleolus. The laciniate ligament (flexor retinaculum) and the origin of the abductor hallucis muscle divided.

tion of sural nerves of "untreated" type 1 diabetic patients with symptomatic polyneuropathy has been observed.[32] This is presumably due to an osmotically induced hydration secondary to the transformation of glucose to polyol through the aldose reductase pathway. Patients treated with aldose reductase inhibitors seem to have "normal" sural nerve hydration.[32] Resources spent in furthering this type of investigation may well be the key to the successful treatment and prevention of the peripheral neuropathy that plagues our patients with diabetes.

REFERENCES

1. Block P: The diabetic foot ulcer: a complex problem with a simple treatment approach. Milit Med 146:644, 1981
2. Warren R, Kihn RB: A survey of lower extremity amputations for ischemia. Surgery 63:107, 1968
3. A Report of the National Diabetes Advisory Board. p. 25. NIH Publications Number 81-2284, Bethesda, Maryland, November 1980
4. Goldner MG: The fate of the second leg in the diabetic amputee. Diabetes 9:100, 1960
5. Ecker ML, Jacobs BS: Lower extremity amputation in diabetic patients. Diabetes 19:189, 1970
6. Levin ME, O'Neal LW (eds): The Diabetic Foot. p. IX. 4th Ed. CV Mosby, St Louis, 1988
7. Rosenqvist U: An epidemiological survey of diabetic foot problems in the Stockholm County, 1982. Acta Med Scand, suppl. 687:55, 1984
8. Palumbo PJ, Melton LJ III: Peripheral vascular disease and diabetes. In Harris MI, Hamman RF (eds): Diabetes in America. Department of Health and Human Services, National Institute of Health, National Institute of Arthritis, Diabetes, and Digestive and Kidney Diseases, NIH Publications Number 85-1468, Bethesda, Maryland, 1985
9. The National Diabetes Data Group. Selected statistics on health and medical care of diabetes. p. A-3, 1980
10. Colen LB, Reus WR, Morain WD: Bipedal ambulation: the goal of diabetic foot management. Presented at the Annual Meeting of the American Association of Plastic Surgeons, Scottsdale, Arizona, May 1989
11. Schwartz RW, Logan NM, Johnson PJ et al: Pentoxifylline increases extremity blood flow in diabetic atherosclerotic patients. Arch Surg 124:434, 1989
12. Shults DW, Hunter GC, McIntyre KE et al: Value of radiographs and bone scans in determining the need for therapy in diabetic patients with foot ulcers. Am J Surg 158:525, 1989
13. Kristiansen B: Ankle and foot fractures in diabetics provoking neuropathic joint changes. Acta Orthop Scand 51:975, 1980
14. Johnson JTH: Neuropathic fractures and joint injuries. J Bone Joint Surg 49A:1, 1967
15. Lippmann HJ, Perotto A, Fanar R. The neuropathic foot of the diabetic. Bull NY Acad Med 52:1159, 1976
16. Dellon AL, Seiler WA, MacKinnon SE: Susceptibility of the diabetic nerve to chronic compression. Ann Plast Surg 20:117, 1988
17. Upton AR, McComas AJ: The double crush in nerve entrapment syndromes. Lancet 2:359, 1973
18. Dellon AL: A cause for optimism in diabetic neuropathy. Ann Plast Surg 20:103, 1988
19. Morain WD: Island toe flaps in neurotrophic ulcers of the foot and ankle. Ann Plast Surg 13:1, 1984
20. Buncke HJ, Colen LB: An island flap from the first webspace of the foot to cover plantar ulcers. Br J Plast Surg 33:242, 1980

21. Colen LB, Buncke HJ: Neurovascular island flaps from the plantar vessels and nerves for foot reconstruction. Ann Plast Surg 12:327, 1984
22. Colen LB, Replogle SL, Mathes SJ: The VY plantar flap for reconstruction of the forefoot. Plast Reconstr Surg 81:220, 1988
23. Cohn BT, Brahms MA: Diabetic arthropathy of the first metatarsal cuneiform joint. Introduction of a new surgical fusion technique. Orthop Rev 16:465, 1987
24. Heiple KG, Cammarn MR. Diabetic neurarthropathy with spontaneous peritalar fracture-dislocation. J Bone Joint Surg 48A:1177, 1966
25. McCraw JB, Arnold PG: McCraw and Arnold's Atlas of Muscle and Musculocutaneous Flaps. p. 597. Hampton Press, Norfolk, 1986
26. Grabb WC, Argenta LC: The lateral calcaneal artery skin flap (the lateral calcaneal artery, lesser saphenous vein, sural nerve skin flap). Plast Reconstr Surg 68:723, 1981
27. Haimovici H: Patterns of arteriosclerotic lesions of the lower extremity. Arch Surg 95:918, 1967
28. Hidalgo DA, Shaw WW: Anatomic basis of plantar flap design: clinical applications. Plast Reconstr Surg 78:637, 1986
29. Morrison WA, Crabb D, O'Brien B, Jenkins A: The instep of the foot as a fasciocutaneous island and as a free flap for heel defects. Plast Reconstr Surg 72:56, 1983
30. Baker GL, Newton ED, Franklin JD: Fasciocutaneous island flap based on the medial plantar artery: applications for leg, ankle and forefoot. Plast Reconstr Surg 85:1, 1990
31. Cronenwett JL, McDaniel MD, Zwolak RM et al. Limb salvage despite extensive tissue loss. Arch Surg 124:609, 1989
32. Griffey RH, Eaton P, Sibbitt RR, Sibbitt WL, Bicknell JM. Diabetic neuropathy: structural analysis of nerve hydration by magnetic resonance spectroscopy. J Am Med Assoc 260:2872, 1988

20

Antibiotic-Loaded Bone Cement in the Management of Diabetic Foot Infections

Allen M. Jacobs, D.P.M., F.A.C.F.S.
Ann M. Seifert, D.P.M.
Thomas J. Kirisits, D.P.M.
Hugh R. Protzel, D.P.M.

Soft tissue and bone infection frequently complicate the management of the diabetic foot. A variety of factors are known to increase the incidence of ulceration and infection in patients with diabetes mellitus. These factors include the presence of autonomic, motor, and sensory neuropathy. Not infrequently, impaired lymphocyte and leukocyte function, in the presence of poor long-term diabetic control, result in the persistence of trivial infections and their progression to involvement of deep soft tissue and osseous structures. The resolution of infectious disorders in the diabetic foot are further complicated by the presence of peripheral vascular disease in a large number of patients. The presence of such peripheral vascular occlusive disorders results in a diminished delivery of normal body immune defense mechanisms as well as antibiotics to the site of the necrosis and infection. The management of diabetic foot infection is frequently frustrating to both the patient as well as the treating physician. Under the best of circumstances, with ideal treatment, it is unfortunate that many such infectious disorders progress to a scenario of prolonged hospitalization, repeated surgical interventions with debridements, and, not infrequently, amputation. The subsequent disability, as well as social and financial burdens, frequently exceed the ability of the patient to tolerate such setbacks.

The use of antibiotic-loaded bone cement in the management of infections in the diabetic foot and ankle is an adjunctive measure, designed to decrease the incidence of recurrent infection as well as minimize hospitalization time for the patient. It must be emphasized that the use of antibiotic-loaded bone cement is not a substitute for standard techniques in the management of soft tissue and bone infections in the diabetic foot. The technique, it must be remembered, is used in conjunction with traditional methods in the management of infections to reduce the incidence of recurrent infection (Fig. 20-1). The use of antibiotic-loaded bone cement allows the clinician to obtain high levels of antibiotic in the area of contamination and infection. The levels of antibiotic thus obtained are not generally achievable by systemic administration of the same antibiotic without a concurrent high rate of complications such as impairment of hepatic or renal function. During the last 8 years, we have

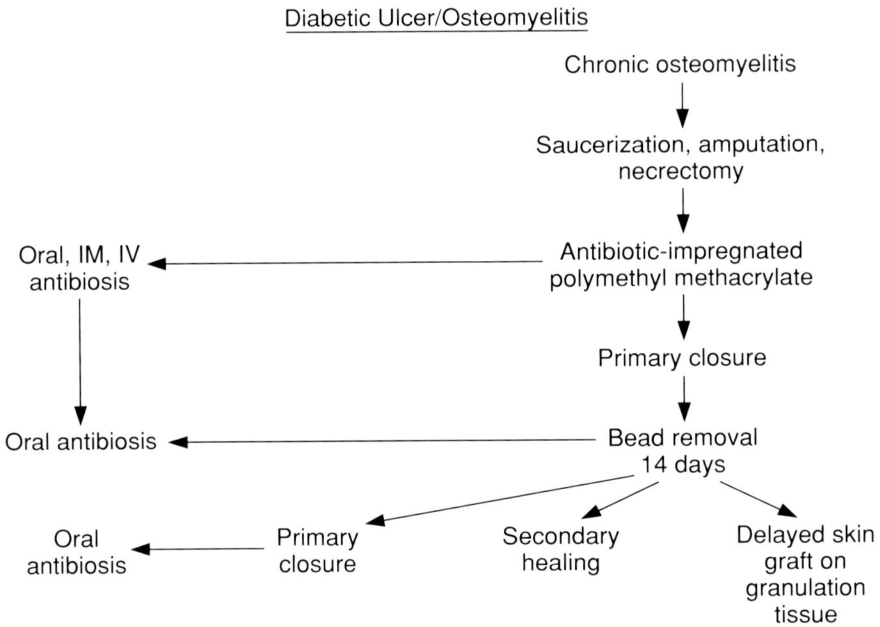

Fig. 20-1. Flowchart for the management of chronic osteomyelitis associated with diabetes mellitus.

used antibiotic-loaded bone cement in 200 clinical experiences. In this chapter, we review our technique for the employment of antibiotic-loaded bone cement in the management of bone and soft tissue infections in the diabetic patient. Our experience and conclusions are similar to those of others who have reported on their success using the same technique.[1–6]

GENERAL DISCUSSION

The successful resolution of soft tissue and bone infection in the foot and ankle of the patient with diabetes mellitus requires a combination of intense diagnostic, medical, and surgical intervention. The majority of cases require debridement and nettoyage of all necrotic tissue and foreign bodies, progressive local wound care based on daily observation, and the use of appropriate systemic antibiotics administered in such a manner as to achieve adequate tissue levels for the amelioration of the infectious process. Resolution of the initial infectious process together with the absence of recurrence of infection are the ultimate goal of management. Patients must be carefully observed for evidence of decreasing drainage, decreasing erythema, and resolution of edema and hyperthermia. Successful healing can only proceed in the absence of tissue necrosis or clinically obvious infection. Normalization of serum glucose levels, resolution of leukocytosis, decreasing erythrocyte sedimentation rate or C-reactive protein, or other measures of the acute inflammatory process should indicate response to therapy when such therapy is successful. Radiographically, a resolution of progressive destructive bone or soft tissue changes should be noted.

The management of diabetic infectious disorders is frequently complicated by the presence of bone and joint disease associated with diabetic neuropathy. The presence of neuropathic joint disease, particularly when associated with autonomic neuropathy, may result in a clinical and radiographic picture exaggerating the actual nature and extent of the infection. In the performance of debridement, as well as the all too frequent necessity for ablative procedures such as amputation, consideration must be given to the ultimate functional result that is to be obtained. In this regard, treatment of the initial infectious process may be followed by secondary surgical procedures in order to restore an anatomic configuration to the lower extremity that will maximize the ambulatory capacity and, therefore, the independence of the patient.

Not infrequently, an initial episode of soft tissue or bone infection in the diabetic foot may result in the recurrence of infection months or years following apparently successful obliteration of the initial infectious disorder. Historically, a variety of techniques have been employed with varying degrees of success in the management of initial osteomyelitis and in the prevention of recurrent or chronic osteomyelitis. These techniques have varied from the utilization of maggots for the debridement of infected soft tissue to the use of silver electrodes for the treatment of chronic osteomyelitis. Hyperbaric oxygen therapy, intraosseous antibiotic infusion pumps, and the use of various semi-closed and closed wound irrigation techniques represent other alternatives in the management of such disorders (Fig. 20-2).

The ultimate prognosis for the permanent resolution of infectious disease in the lower extremity of the diabetic patient is dependent on a variety of factors beyond the nature and extent of the foot infection itself. The presence of decreased peripheral vascular perfusion, relative or absolute nutritional deficiencies, the state of short- and long-term diabetic control, and concurrent disorders such as renal or cardiac pathology all influence the course of treatment for the infected diabetic lower extremity. In the assessment of such patients, all the medical circumstances that may influence the ability of the patient to heal must be considered in the determination of the most appropriate therapy.

Typically, osteomyelitis requires 6 weeks of antibiotic therapy administered at a bactericidal level. In certain circumstances, such as infectious disease

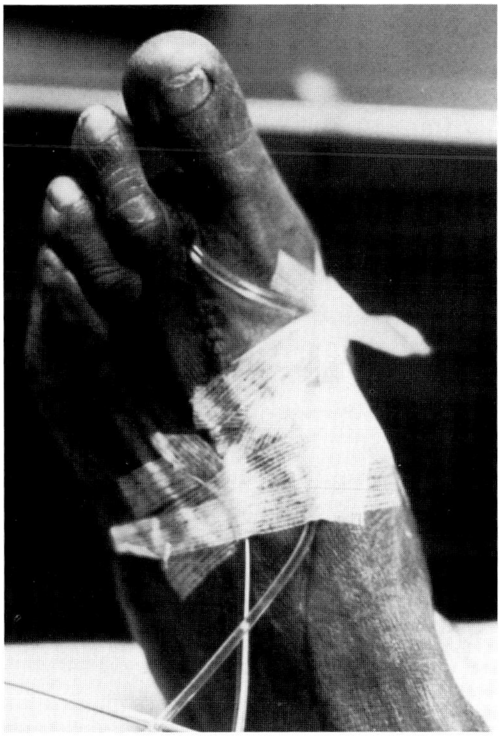

A

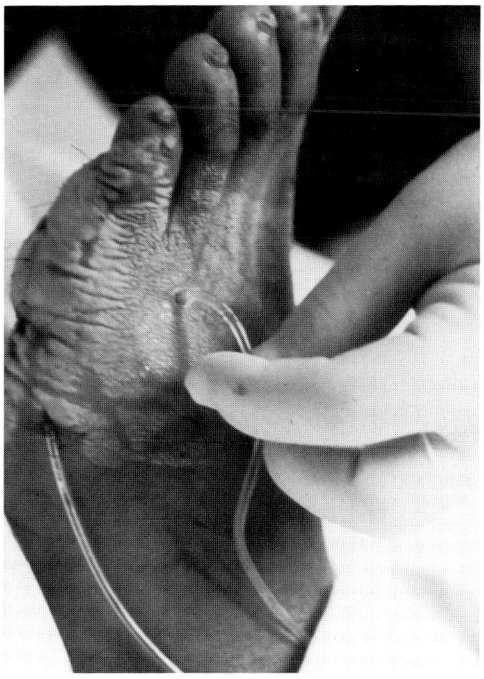

B

Fig. 20-2. (**A**) Continuous closed-suction irrigation represents an alternative technique to implantation of beads in achieving a high local concentration of antibiotic. (**B**) Complications of closed suction irrigation can occur when systems become occluded or overflow, resulting in maceration of the wound site and possible superinfection.

of the bones of the toe, amputation may remove the infected bone and soft tissue with a margin of safety. Under these circumstances, management of osteomyelitis may be varied from the traditional approach. Not infrequently, the concurrent use of continuous closed irrigation systems with or without antibiotics are employed in conjunction with local debridement or ablative surgery. The success rate for the resolution of soft tissue and bone infection in the management of the diabetic foot is extremely dependent not only on the nature of the local wound, but the variety of general medical factors listed previously. Techniques for the management of osteomyelitis that are appropriate in the young insulin-dependent diabetic patient with adequate peripheral vascular perfusion may very well fail to be appropriate in those patients with significant peripheral vascular disease or marked nutritional abnormality. Each patient must be individually considered as to the efficacy of a particular therapeutic approach for the resolution of bone and soft tissue infection associated with diabetes mellitus. In many circumstances, the successful resolution of initial soft tissue and bone infection, as well as the prevention of recurrent infection, may be achieved using antibiotic-loaded polymethyl methacrylate (PMMA) bone cement that has been impregnated with gentamicin sulfate. Reporting on a series of 583 patients, Buckholz used gentamicin-impregnated bone cement in the treatment of deep infections following total hip arthroplasty, with a 77 percent successful resolution rate.[2] In this study, clinical success was defined as the successful management of initial osteomyelitis with reimplantation of hip implant without recurrent infection. Muller, in a similar study of 146 patients with chronic osteomyelitis, reported only a 7 percent failure rate.[7]

Klemm first described premade gentamicin-impregnated PMMA (Septopal, E. Merck, FRG) and reported only eight recurrent infections at a 3-year postimplantation follow-up study.[8] Greiben reviewed 1,526 cases published in the orthopaedic literature using Septopal beads in the treatment of osteomyelitis and reported a success rate of 85 percent among all authors combined.[6] Jenny and Taglong reviewed their experience in the management of 200 cases of bone and soft tissue infections using antibiotic-loaded bone cement and reported a success rate of 75 percent. The successful resolution of osteomyelitis and soft tissue infection with the use of antibiotic-loaded bone cement has been similarly reported in a variety of studies, including those of Lidgren,[10] DeGroote et al.,[11] Harle,[12] Weise and Weller,[13] Walenkamp,[14] and Eberle.[15]

POLYMETHYL METHACRYLATE BEADS AND ANTIBIOTIC USE

In addition to the adequate removal of all necrotic bone and soft tissue, the successful management of osteomyelitis requires the attainment of a high local concentration of antibiotic for a prolonged time. Specifically, antibiotic levels must be maintained at a bactericidal level at the site of previous infection, particularly to decrease the incidence of recurrent infection. In the diabetic foot, the achievement of high wound concentrations of antibiotic at the site of previous necrosis and infection may be difficult to obtain owing to the presence of arterial disease. Antibiotic-loaded bone cement interdicts this problem by placing directly within the previously infected tissue high levels of antibiotics that are not dependent on the delivery of the antibiotic by circulatory means. A vehicle is necessary in order to allow the slow release of the antibiotic into surrounding tissues while not damaging either the soft tissue or bone or interfering with the desirable properties of the antibiotic. A variety of studies have demonstrated that thermostable antibiotics are eluted from PMMA in vitro in sufficient amounts to be bactericidal to organisms, thereby preventing, controlling, and curing infections. Water and similar molecules enter bone by diffusion, whereas antibiotics elute from bone cement because of diffusion concentration gradients that are significantly steeper than that of water between the antibiotic-loaded bone cement and surrounding soft tissue and bone.

In 1985, Buchholz presented the criteria that an ideal antibiotic should possess for incorporation in bone cement for local wound therapy.[1] These properties included (1) adequate elution quantitatively and temporally; (2) broad spectrum activity against both gram-positive and gram-negative organisms common in bone and soft tissue disease; (3)

a minimal bactericidal and minimal inhibitory concentration that are similar; (4) a low rate of resistance development by bacteria; (5) low protein bindings; (6) low sensitizing potential; (7) a high water solubility; (8) overall chemical stability (particularly against heat); and (9) a low potential for the induction of drug allergy.

Originally, Buchholz employed penicillin- and erythromycin-loaded bone cement.[3] Because of the potential for drug allergy as well as the development of resistant organisms, gentamicin was eventually used and became his antibiotic of choice. Gentamicin appears to act well in combination with PMMA because of its desirable bacteriologic as well as physiochemical properties. Gentamicin is a known broad spectrum antibiotic to which only few bacteria are resistant. This is of particular importance in the management of diabetic foot infections, where a polymicrobial flora is frequently encountered. The probability of the development of a bacteria resistant to gentamicin is known to be low when the gentamicin is administered at high levels. Additionally, gentamicin is well established as being associated with an extraordinarily low rate of allergy development. The polymerization process of PMMA is exothermic, thereby generating a significant amount of heat. Gentamicin is stable at high temperatures and therefore withstands the polymerization process without alteration in its biochemical or physiochemical properties. Gentamicin is hydrosoluble. Wahlig and Dingledein have demonstrated in vitro that gentamicin has the highest and most prolonged elution from PMMA of the common antibiotics that might be employed.[16] Following implantation at the site of debridement, gentamicin-impregnated bone cement continues to elute antibiotic into surrounding soft tissues for as long as 5 years following implantation. Local tissue levels of up to 110 mg/ml of gentamicin may be obtained when 500 mg of gentamicin is added to the standard 34 g of PMMA powder. These observations have been confirmed by Marks et al.[17] A variety of PMMA brands may be used together with gentamicin for the elution of the antibiotic into soft tissue and bone. Wahlig and Dingledein have demonstrated that of the available bone cements, Palacos brand bone cement allows the greatest elution of gentamicin into surrounding tissues.[16] This observation has been confirmed by other investigators, including Sattel and Nabert-Block,[18] as well as Marks.[17] The properties of Palacos bone cement that allow greater elution of gentamicin when compared to other bone cements is unknown. We have used Palacos bone cement in a limited number of cases, with the majority of our clinical experience associated with the use of Zimmer brand of PMMA. We have observed no apparent adverse sequellae in the clinical, laboratory, or radiographic evaluation of our patients using Zimmer bone cement when compared to those patients in whom Palacos bone cement was used.

Premade beads of gentamicin-impregnated PMMA were first designed by Klemm for the management of chronic osteomyelitis.[8] These beads are distributed under the trade name of Septopal. Each bead is 7 mm in diameter and contains 4.5 mg of gentamicin sulfate as well as 20 mg of zerconium dioxide as a radiographic contrast marker. Septopal beads are available in chains of 10, 30, or 60 beads on a monofilament wire. It is known that the amount of antibiotic that elutes from the bead into the surrounding soft tissue and bone is proportional to the surface area of the bone cement as well as the concentration of antibiotic within each bead. Because a spherical shape is associated with the greatest surface area per volume of bead, Septopal beads are provided in this form. Gentamicin-loaded bone cement is a special drug delivery system that allows high and prolonged bactericidal concentration of the antibiotic at the site of implantation without systemic effects. Wahlig implanted between 80 and 180 Septopal beads in canine femurs and demonstrated serum levels to never exceed 0.5 mc g/ml.[19] At the same time, wound concentrations of gentamicin were found to exceed 200 mc g/ml, a concentration at which gentamicin is bactericidal to almost all known bacteria.

The elution of gentamicin in vitro from Septopal beads has also been studied by Wahlig.[19] Initially, 400 to 600 mc g/ml of gentamicin is released per day. On the tenth day, 120 mc g/ml are detectable in the tissues surrounding implanted beads, while on the twentieth day following implantation, 50 mc g/ml are demonstrable. Eighty days following implantation, 10 mc g/ml of gentamicin continues to be eluted from beads and is deposited within surrounding tissue.

In vitro studies using rabbit kidney fibroblast have demonstrated no effect on cell viability or reproduction when exposed to high levels of gentamicin-impregnated PMMA when compared to conventional cell culture dishes. Rabbit kidney fibroblasts are used in such studies because of their known sensitivity to toxins, which may rapidly interfere with their growth and proliferation.

In vivo studies correlate with in vitro findings. Following the implantation of PMMA beads into the femoral canal of dogs, Wahlig found a concentration in osseous tissue between 5 and 24 mc g/g of tissue in cancellous bone, and between 2 and 20 mc g/g of tissue in cortical bone.[19] In the hematoma that develops following surgery and implantation of the beads, 100 to 200 mc g/g of tissue of gentamicin may be assayed. Correlated peak serum concentrations were noted to be only 0.3 mc g/ml whereas peak urine concentrations of 1.5 to 20 mc g/ml were observed immediately following implantation and rapidly declining thereafter. The minimal systemic absorption of gentamicin following its implantation within previously infected wounds is of significant importance in the diabetic patient. Frequently, the diabetic patient with foot sepsis has associated renal disease that may be accentuated by exposure to high levels of aminoglycoside antibiotics. Because of the minimal serum levels noted following local wound therapy with gentamicin-impregnated PMMA, nephrotoxicity from aminoglycosides should not represent a clinical concern in the management of diabetic foot sepsis.

In 62 humans in whom between 30 and 180 beads were implanted, studies of serum levels never exceeded 0.5 mc g/ml, while urine concentration of gentamicin never exceeded 10 mc g/ml. Studies of local wound exudate levels, however, demonstrated 50 to 80 mc g/ml of gentamicin. Between 30 and 70 days following implantation, soft tissue levels of 9.1 to 33.5 mc g/ml have been noted. Similarly, cancellous bone levels of gentamicin as far as 5 to 10 mm remote from the site of the implanted beads were noted to be 1.6 to as high as 4.3 mc g/g of tissue in cancellous bone, while cortical bone levels of gentamicin at the same distance averaged 3.0 mc g/g of cortical bone. In the diabetic patient, the intravenous administration of gentamicin results in a high serum level and elevated urine level of the antibiotic, although low tissue concentrations of the antibiotic may be present owing to associated arterial disease. The use of gentamicin-loaded bone cement results in high tissue concentrations without concurrent high serum or urine concentration. The application of gentamicin-impregnated bone cement therefore becomes attractive to patients with concurrent renal disease in whom nephrotoxic affects of antibiotics are of significance.

Antibiotic-loaded bone cement is only effective following the stabilization of the medical status of the diabetic patient as well as adequate debridement of necrotic and soft tissue. Harle and Ritzerfeld were able to demonstrate that gentamicin eluting from Septopal beads is able to penetrate 7 mm of dead bone.[20] The local wound concentration of gentamicin is between 10 and 100 times that which can be achieved by systemic administration. The local concentration of gentamicin that may be obtained by local implantation within PMMA is many times the minimal inhibitory concentration for most pathologic bacteria, a consideration of significant importance in the management of osteomyelitis, particularly in association with wounds of a polymicrobial nature, where it is desirable to achieve bactercidal levels. The concept of resistant organisms must be redefined in relation to local antibiotic therapy using antibiotic-loaded bone cement. It should be remembered that the typical culture and sensitivity report from which a determination is based as to the appropriateness of antibiotic selection is based on microbial sensitivities to antibiotics assuming a peak serum level achievable by parenteral administration. As a general rule, all bacteria with an antibiotic minimal inhibitory concentration greater than 4 mc ǵ/ml to gentamicin are regarded as not sensitive to the parenteral antibiotic. Harle, in his study of gentamicin released into wound secretions in vivo, concluded that there is no true entity of "total antibiotic resistance." [12] Specifically, Harle notes "the susceptible range of single germs to a given antibiotic is very broad; therefore, by increasing the local concentration of active substances, it is theoretically possible to eliminate all bacteria with a single bactericidal agent." [12]

Specifically, Vecsei, reviewed 102 cases of osteomyelitis treated with gentamicin-loaded bone cement.[21] *Staphylococcus aureus* was isolated in 40 percent of the cases, a single gram-negative organism in 33 percent of the cases, and mixed infections as the etiologic agent in the remaining cases. Only 15 of the cultured organisms were resistant to gentamicin. There was no evidence of clinical resistance of the microbial agents to gentamicin within the cases studied. Greiben reviewed 1,525 cases of gentamicin-impregnated PMMA beads.[6] Of pathogens, 1,126 were isolated using 1,106 culture and sensitivity tests. Ninety-two percent of the organisms were demonstrated as being sensitive to gentamicin using sensitivity discs with 10 mc g/ml of gentamicin. This study correlated well with the clinical results noted with an 85-percent success rate in clinical resolution of infection using antibiotic-loaded bone cement. In our personal experience, 56 percent of bacterial isolates for foot and ankle infections demonstrated a minimal inhibitory concentration (MIC) greater than 4 mc g/ml and would therefore be technically considered resistant to gentamicin. In fact, clinical resistance to the use of antibiotic-loaded bone cement containing gentamicin sulfate has not been observed in our patients. The achievement of high local wound concentrations of gentamicin sulfate achieved by elution from antibiotic-loaded bone cement is of significant clinical importance in the diabetic foot. In general, it may be assumed that most bacterial pathogens are killed, allowing the healing of wounds to progress in a noninfectious environment.

When a particular bacteria is gentamicin susceptible, it may be assumed that the use of antibiotic-loaded bone cement in the form of beads will be highly effective. When sensitivity testing indicates resistant bacterial strains, a broth dilution assay of the isolate may be performed. It may be assumed that bacterial strains inhibited by up to 50 mc g/ml of gentamicin are susceptible to local antibiotic treatment with gentamicin-impregnated PMMA beads. In our own experience, the highest minimum inhibitory concentration obtained has been 16 mc g/ml for one strain of *Staphylococcus aureus* and for *Streptococcus vicallous,* both cases of which went on to clinical cure.

INDICATIONS FOR USE

The successful employment of gentamicin-impregnated PMMA beads is dependent on radical debridement with removal of all necrotic soft tissue, bone, and foreign bodies (Fig. 20-3). Orthopaedic implants for the stabilization of dislocations and fractures may be allowed to remain if such fixation devices are stable within bone and the infectious process is not in direct contact with the orthopaedic material. Appropriate deep wound and bone culture and sensitivities should be obtained for aerobic and anaerobic, fungal and acid-fast organisms. Thorough lavage of the wound is essential. The peripheral vascular perfusion and nutritional status of the patient should also be consistent with the expectation of adequate wound healing.

In our experience, the primary use of antibiotic-loaded bone cement has been in the management of osteomyelitis in the diabetic foot. The beads are used adjunctively with traditional methods in the management of bone infection in order to decrease the incidence of recurrent infection. We avoid use of the terms "acute" or "chronic osteomyelitis." Not infrequently, the diabetic patient will present with clinical signs and symptoms suggestive of acute infectious disease with radiographs consistent with chronicity of bone infection. Similarly, recurrent or chronic osteomyelitis may be characterized with clinical signs and symptoms suggestive of acute inflammatory processes. We prefer to use the terms *initial* or *recurrent osteomyelitis* as appropriate to the particular situation encountered in each patient. The beads are implanted in order to gain a high wound concentration of antibiotic to create sterilization of previously infected bone and soft tissue cavities. When a chronic portal of entry for bacteria is present, such as a sinus tract or neuropathic ulcer, it is not uncommon for our service to resect such soft tissue defects concurrently with the resection of infected or devitalized bone. When the clinical, vascular, nutritional, and bacteriologic factors permit, these wounds are closed primarily over antibiotic loaded bone cement beads.

Gentamicin-impregnated PMMA beads may also be used as a prophylactic measure where signifi-

A

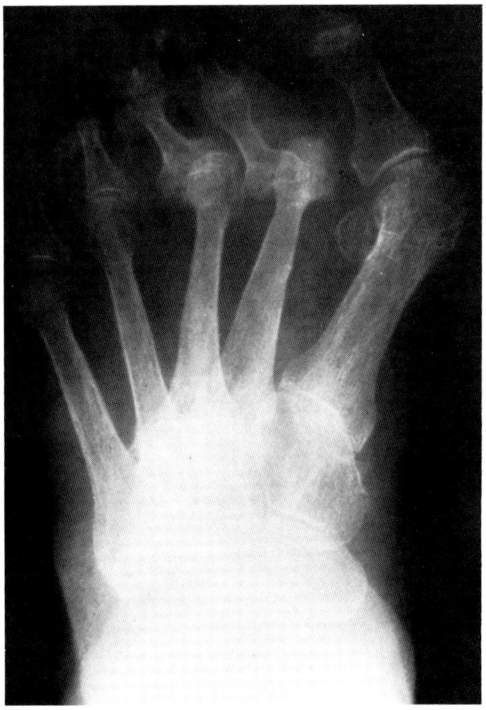

B

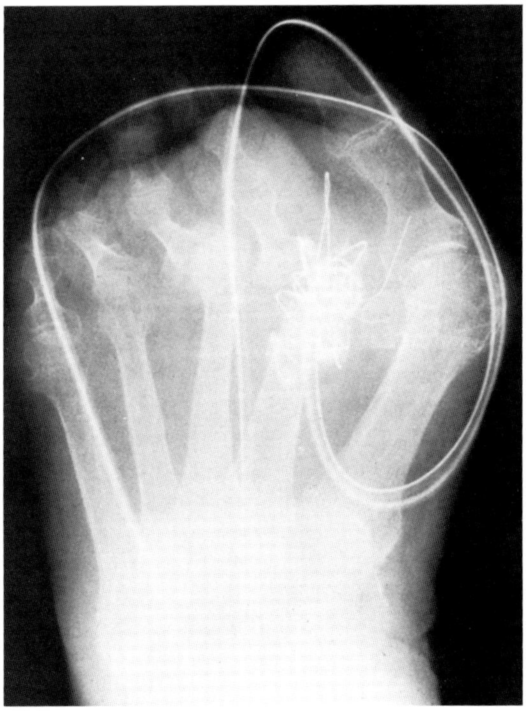

C

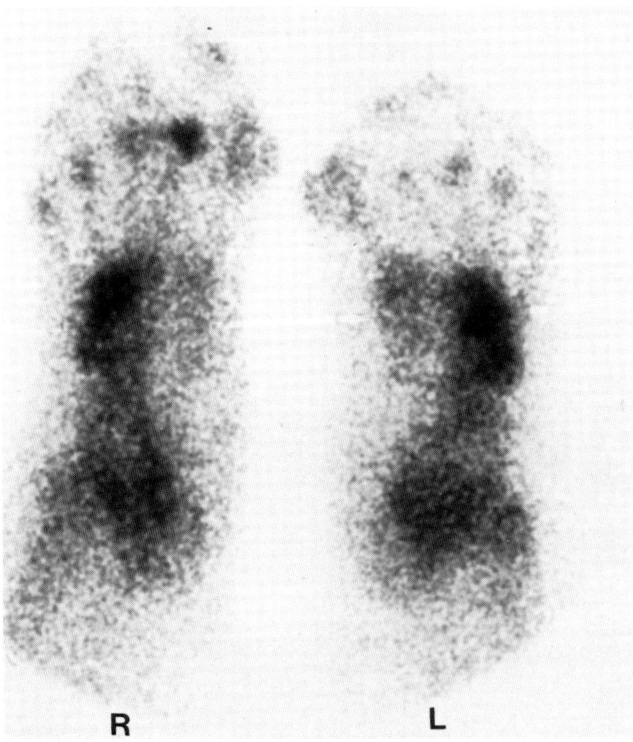

Fig. 20-3. (**A**) Early osteomyelitis of the second metatarsal. This patient had adult onset diabetes mellitus with an ulceration plantar to the second metatarsal head. Culture revealed coagulase positive *Staphylococcus aureus.* (**B**) The same patient following elliptical excision of the ulcer, resection of infected bone, and primary closure over antibiotic-loaded bone cement. The beads should be removed 2 weeks after implantation since the wound concentration of gentamicin will begin to fall below therapeutic levels at this time and the potential for resistant strains increases. (**C**) Bone scans can be used to determine the extent of bone resection required in each case.

cant concern exists for wound contamination or the spread of bacteria to previously noninfected sites. Common examples include the deployment of antibiotic-loaded bone cement beads at the site of amputation or bone revisional procedures where contiguous soft tissue or bone infection existed.

METHOD OF APPLICATION

Certain principles must be maintained in order to ensure the successful use of gentamicin beads in the treatment of both osteomyelitis and soft tissue

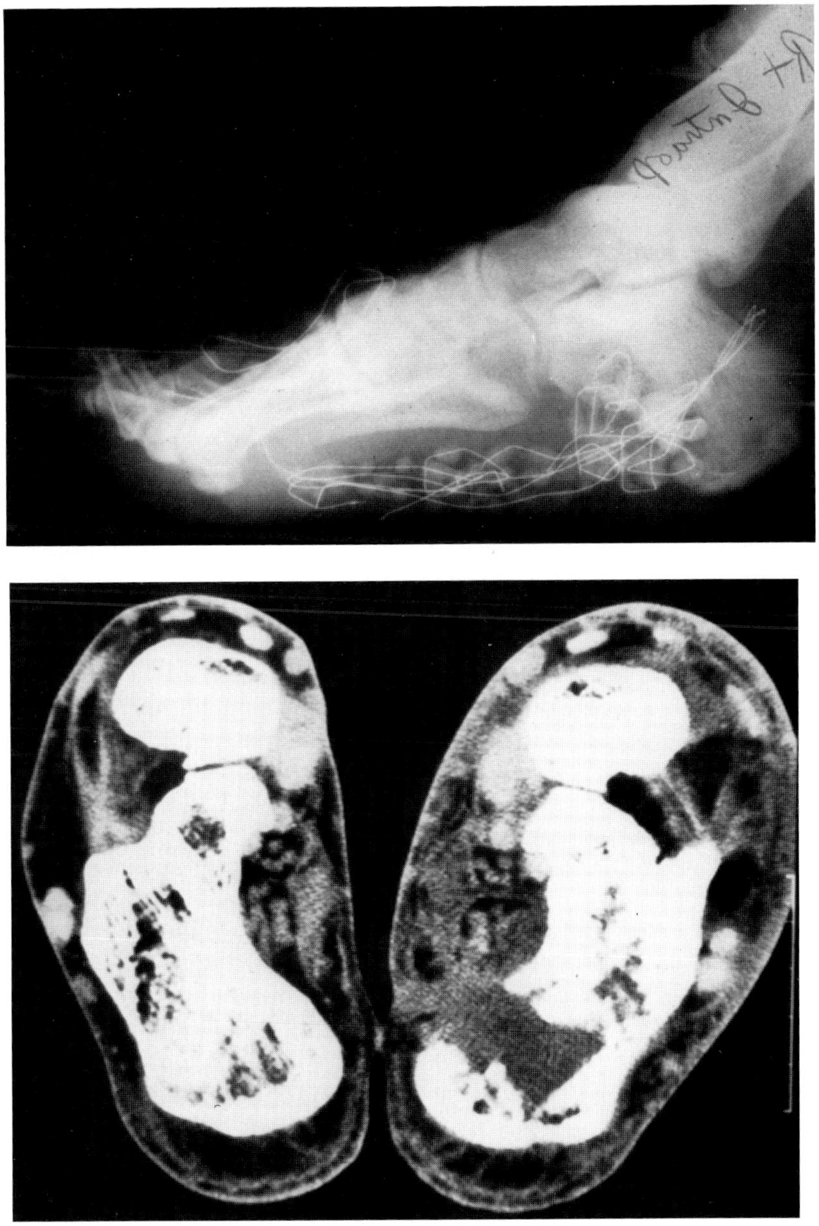

A

B

Fig. 20-4. (**A**) Postoperative radiograph demonstrates 113 beads in place in a patient with osteomyelitis of the fourth metatarsal and toe and calcaneus. (**B**) Postoperative computed tomograph (CT) scan. CT or magnetic resonance imaging scan may be needed of the foot in order to evaluate resolving infectious disease and bone healing.

infection. It must again be emphasized that radical debridement with removal of all necrotic soft tissue or bone must be completed. The wound should be copiously lavaged with either sterile saline or an antibiotic flush.

The gentamicin beads should be positioned as densely as possible within the wound and in as great a number within the cavity as possible (Fig. 20-4). The use of a large number of beads creates the highest possible concentration of active antibiotic for the achievement of a bactericidal affect. Klemm recommends that the last several beads be allowed to protrude through the incision to increase the ease with which they may be removed at a later date.[8] In the majority of our cases we allow several beads to protrude from the wound. Primary closure of the wound is essential in order to create a closed system in which the gentamicin may elute from the beads into a surrounding hematoma. The beads function best within a closed cavity so that high concentrations of gentamicin may be created by the diffusion process into the surrounding wound hematoma and seroma. In general, it appears advantageous not to allow a major flow of wound secretion for several days. In certain circumstances, it may be necessary, as determined by the surgeon, to concurrently use a closed-suction irrigation system. However, in each case the potential advantage in using such closed-suction irrigation systems must be weighed against the reduction in gentamicin-loaded hematoma as the result of its removal through the irrigation system. It must be remembered that the elution of gentamicin is possible only within a moist environment. The failure of fluid contact to be present adjacent to the beads results in minimal distribution of the gentamicin from within the beads to surrounding tissues. In the presence of open wounds, resistant organisms may develop due to the decreased concentration of gentamicin within the wound following implantation of beads that are not in contact with a moist environment. As a result, virulent organisms may colonize the wound secondarily or may not be killed, owing to the low concentration of gentamicin that is present. Within a closed wound, a high concentration of gentamicin may be expected to be present and may furthermore be expected to be bactericidal, thus allowing wound healing to occur in a sterile environment.

When primary wound closure without adequate coverage is not able to be obtained, secondary forms of closure such as the use of synthetic skin or other wound covering systems should be employed. Steri-strips, or loosely approximated sutures, are also acceptable alternatives. The objective is to maintain hematoma and seroma within the wound in order to achieve high levels of antibiotic within this site. At a later date, secondary closure or grafting may be achieved following removal of the antibiotic beads. If bone grafting is performed, a chain of beads should be placed in such a manner as to contact the top of the bone graft site. The use of synthetic skin may be employed when such bone grafts are performed in the presence of an open wound.

FABRICATION OF GENTAMICIN PMMA BEADS

Fabrication of antibiotic-loaded PMMA beads is carried out by adding 20 ml of the liquid monomer to 50 g of PMMA powder (Fig. 20-5). Mixing is continued until a homogenous paste is formed, which takes approximately 2 minutes. An evacuation system should be available in order to minimize the inhalation of toxic fumes generated by the polymerization process. Once a homogenous paste is formed, three-fourths of the paste is removed from the mixing bowl. Four-hundred-eighty mg of gentamicin sulfate powder or liquid is then added to the remaining one-fourth of the bone cement mixture that remains within the mixing bowl. The paste is then mixed until maximum incorporation of the gentamicin sulfate within the bone cement appears to have occurred. The paste is then spatulated up into a 6- or 10-cc syringe, and individual beads of gentamicin-impregnated PMMA are formed around two 2-0 monofilament wires, which have been previously twisted upon themselves in order to create a roughened surface. The beads are molded by hand into a size of approximately 7- to 10-mm diameter spheres. Every attempt should be made to make the beads as round as possible, in order to maximize the surface area per volume of bead and therefore maximize antibiotic elution.

A

B

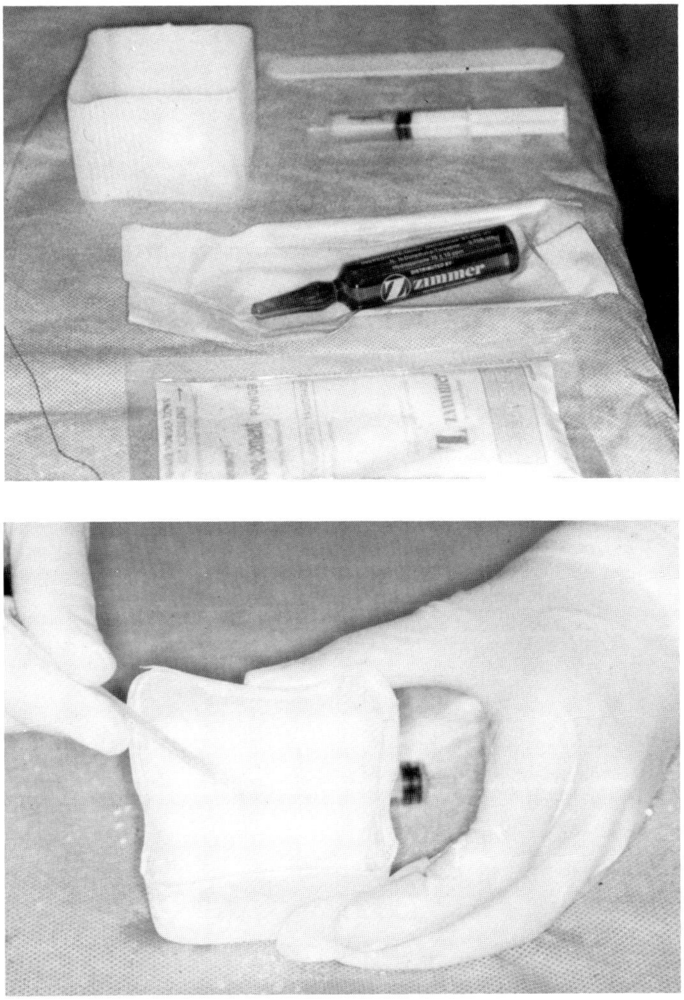

Fig. 20-5. (**A**) Bone cement and polymerizing agent. One should have everything ready at the time of mixing since only a few minutes will be available before the cement hardens. (**B**) Mixing of antibiotic-loaded bone cement (ALBC). After this is complete, three-fourths of the cement is discarded. Four-hundred-eighty mg of gentamicin powder or liquid is then folded into the remaining cement. *(Figure continues.)*

A variety of devices, generally resembling various forms of pressing machines, are available for the shaping and manufacturing of PMMA beads in the operating room. The adhesion of beads to the monofilament wires may be aided by holding the beads and wire out of contact with the operating room table or various towels. The ends of the wires are folded upon themselves and twisted. As many beads may be manufactured as are desired by the surgeon, depending on the size of the cul-de-sac to be filled in each case. The major limitation to the fabrication of the beads is that the cement hardens rather quickly and only 7 to 8 minutes of working time are actually available to the surgeon. It is best to work in an unheated portion of the operating room. The beads are allowed to harden for approximately 15 minutes in order to allow the exothermic reaction involved with the polymerization process to take its maximal effect outside of the surgical wound. To minimize operating time, it is generally recommended that the beads be manufactured before the initiation of the actual surgical debridement. It is most important to obtain deep cultures of bone and soft tissue before the implantation of

C

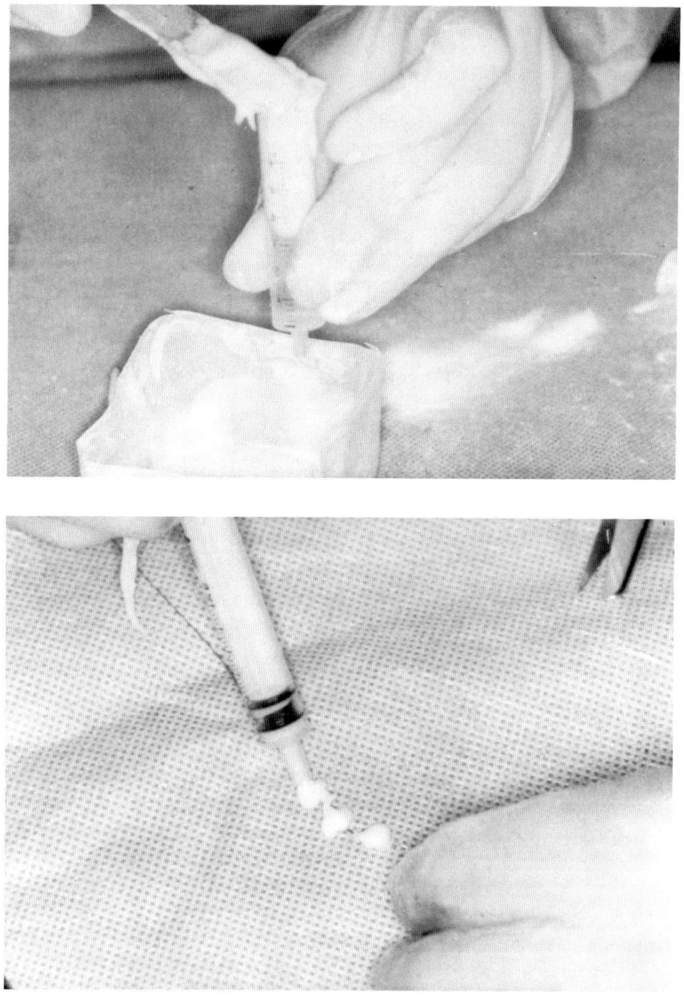

D

Fig. 20-5 *(Continued).* **(C)** The **ALBC** is then loaded into a 6- to 10-cc syringe. **(D)** The beads are then formed around two monofilament wires that have been twisted upon themselves. The beads should be as round as possible in order to ensure the greatest surface-to-volume ratio. *(Figure continues.)*

beads. All such cultures should be performed as mentioned earlier for fungal and acid-fast organisms as well as bacteria. Note should be taken of the number of beads implanted for reference at a later date when the beads are extirpated from the wound.

The wound is closed, allowing the end of the antibiotic-loaded bone cement chain to protrude with several beads outside the wound itself. The beads should be placed within the bone and soft tissue cavity in such a manner as to facilitate their later removal. In general, we do not recommend the simultaneous use of drains or a continuous closed-suction irrigation apparatus concurrently with the employment of gentamicin-impregnated bone cement. One bead that has been manufactured in the operating room is sent to the microbiology laboratory for a separate Kirby-Bauer plating with the organisms recovered from the deep wound. This technique allows reassurance that the bacteria that are present within the wound are in fact sensitive to the concentration of gentamicin obtained by the mixing of the beads in the operating room. Several such beads may be set aside for

E

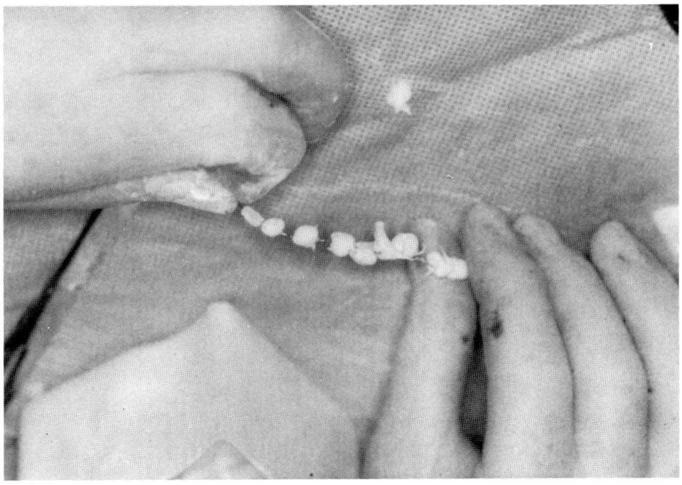

Fig. 20-5 *(Continued).* (E) Once the beads are counted and allowed to cool to hardness, they are ready to be implanted. One bead should be retained for laboratory analysis. The entire process should be performed in the operating room and under sterile conditions before setting up the back table.

use in this manner when polymicrobial infectious processes are present. Although a biochemical assay of the concentration of gentamicin per bead manufactured in this manner is difficult to perform in the usual hospital setting, it may be extrapolated that the addition of 480 mg of gentamicin sulfate added to 10 g of PMMA yields an average concentration of 9.6 mg of gentamicin for every 7-mm diameter bead. This compares favorably with premade Septopal beads, which demonstrate a concentration of 4.5 mg per bead.

USE OF ANTIBIOTIC-LOADED BONE CEMENT

It must again be stated that adequate surgical necrectomy consists of meticulous removal of all sinister appearing skin, soft tissue, and bone. Adequate debridement may at times necessitate partial amputation of healthy tissue in order to allow primary closure of the surgical wound over antibiotic-loaded bone cement beads. In general, anaerobic infections as well as severe necrotizing infections or streptococcal infections should not be treated in this manner. These wounds may be closed at an appropriate time over antibiotic-loaded bone cement; however, primary closure at the time of the initial debridement in such cases is generally not considered prudent.

Ideally the chains of beads are left in place for 10 to 14 days, the period during which maximal elution of the antibiotic occurs. The patient is then returned to the operating room where a small incision is performed and retrieval of the beads carried out without the disruption of the remaining wound tissues. A repeat Gram stain and culture should be obtained at the time of bead removal to determine if any remaining infection exists. If so, redebridement of the wound and reimplantation of a new chain of beads is performed. If at any time during the first 10 to 14 days following initial necrectomy and implantation of beads, clinical signs or symptoms of infection recur, re-exploration of the wound should be performed.

Typically a serous-appearing drainage occurs from the site of protrusion of the antibiotic beads. Not infrequently, we have found such drainage to be associated with the presence of noncandidal or candidal yeast organisms, which may be treated with appropriate antifungal therapy. Gram stains may be performed of the drainage, which in general demonstrate no organisms or may demonstrate *Staphylococcus epidermidis.* The presence of such drainage may be of concern to the uninitiated, but in the presence of decreasing wound pain, decreasing erythema, and decreasing signs of inflammatory disease the presence of such drainage should not be the cause of great concern by the clinician.

Drainage systems have been described for excess blood flow to guarantee a tension-free wound closure. This technique has recently been held in disfavor except in those cases where adequate hemostasis cannot be obtained. As noted, bead removal should be performed 10 to 14 days following implantation. At this time the beads will be found to have been firmly encapsulated within granulation tissue, often making bead removal difficult. Not uncommonly, the chain of beads will break off or several beads will slip from the wire. All that is required for removal is the removal of one or two sutures from either side of the wire exiting the wound and the application of gentle but persistent traction on the chain of antibiotic beads protruding from the wound. Alternately, the beads may be slowly removed on a daily basis, with removal of one to two beads per day beginning 2 days postoperatively, until all beads are removed.

The permanent filling of osteomyelitic cavities with beads has been advocated when insufficient development of connective tissue can be expected or when all possible sources of autologous cancellous bone have been exhausted. Jenny and Taglang reported on eight cases in which beads were implanted permanently, with one patient having the beads in place for 5 years without apparent adverse affect and without recurrence of infection.[9]

ADVANTAGES OF ANTIBIOTIC-LOADED BONE CEMENT

The advantages to the use of gentamicin-impregnated PMMA beads on chains are many, affecting patient, doctor, and hospital. The use of antibiotic beads creates a larger surface area to increase the release of antibiotic. The beads on a chain allow the use of an active substance to the actual site of infection and allow the use of a lower total amount of systemic antibiotic therapy, thereby reducing both cost and systemic side effects. The rapid decline in inflammation and quick control of infection and pain results in relief and comfort to the patient. Because there is no drainage or continuous irrigation system, there is decreased workload on the nursing staff, hospital hygiene is improved, and the possibility of secondary infection of a drainage system is avoided. Additionally, many soft tissue and bone infections become manageable on an outpatient basis, thereby reducing hospital cost.

The removal of beads is uncomplicated. Biomechanical properties of bone are not altered by the use of antibiotic-loaded bone cement. Secondary operations such as cancellous bone grafting may be executed with little risk. The rate of recurrence is decreased since there are few therapeutic failures. No cases of allergy or systemic toxicity have been reported with the use of gentamicin-impregnated PMMA in thousands of patients.

With the ability to provide high local concentrations of antibiotics, patients with peripheral vascular disease, which may otherwise impair parenteral antibiotics from reaching the area of infection, can be guaranteed therapeutic levels of the antibiotic within the wound. The technique, therefore, has been of significant value in the management of patients with diabetes mellitus as well as others with infection and concurrent diminished peripheral vascular perfusion.

DISADVANTAGES

Although the disadvantage to the use of gentamicin-loaded bone cement is relatively minimal, particularly when used correctly, several points must be reemphasized. Mixing antibiotics and bone cement creates a high risk of delayed allergic reaction due to long-term elution of the antibiotic from bone cement. This is more important in cases where the beads have been left in place for prolonged periods of time or have been permanently implanted. An increase in gentamicin-resistant organisms may theoretically occur since there is long-term exposure to the gentamicin, particularly with its chronic use and the exposure of bacteria to a lower dose of antibiotic later in the course of therapy. It is also important to note that anaerobic organisms are resistant to gentamicin, and they continue to be so even with significantly high levels of gentamicin present within wound concentrations. In such cases where closure may be considered, the use of clindamycin-impregnated beads or metronidazole-impregnated beads may be considered.

The most rational use of this technique is in those instances of known previous infection in which the organism and its sensitivities are known. The emergence of antibiotic-resistant bacteria is not likely. This is particularly so when the antibiotic beads are removed within 2 weeks.

The most common causes of failure in the use of antibiotic-loaded bone cement are related to the following factors: (1) marked sclerosis as the result of long-standing bone infections; (2) foreign material allowed to remain within the wound; (3) postoperative wound dehiscence and skin necrosis due to poor surgical technique or poor condition of the soft tissues; (4) inadequate length of chain of beads used to impregnate the surgical cavity; (5) severe peripheral vascular disease; (6) concurrent use of an irrigation or suction drainage system thereby reducing gentamicin concentration to less than optimal levels; (7) inability to obtain primary wound closure with the loss of gentamicin through the remaining wound orifice.

OTHER CONSIDERATIONS

Proper staging of the wound infection must be carried out before any surgical intervention except in those cases such as gas gangrene or necrotizing infections in which a surgical emergency is believed to exist. Although the diagnosis of osteomyelitis rests with recovery of micro-organisms from bone cultures, not infrequently the diagnosis can be inferred by the use of standard radiographs and the demonstration of progressive destructive osseous changes. Soft tissue swelling may represent the earliest sign of osteomyelitis. Radionuclide imaging using technetium methylene diphosphonate may be used to determine the extent of osteomyelitis and therefore determine the extent of bone resection if such tests are readily available and when the patient is not thought to be in an emergent situation. It must be remembered that radionuclide imaging with technetium methylene diphosphonate may overshoot or overestimate the extent of bone infection, with positive findings demonstrating bone that has become inflamed but not yet infected in the peri-infectious area. In our experience, we have found that the resection of bone on the basis of a bone scan provides for a wide margin of safety and allows for necrectomy to proceed through healthy noninfected bone. Because it is known that a variety of osseous problems in the diabetic foot may result in the development of a positive bone scan, we used either gallium citrate or indium 111-labeled leukocyte for further evaluation of bone and soft tissue when a nonemergent situation is present. When intense focal uptake is noted on all three phases of the technetium bone scan, an intense focal uptake is noted on either the gallium or indium scan, such imaging is considered consistent with osteomyelitis and our necrectomy proceeds in an appropriate manner.

USE OF ANTIBIOTIC-LOADED BLOOD CLOT

In certain circumstances, the use of antibiotic-loaded blood clot is appropriate for the management of osteomyelitis or soft tissue abscess associated with small defects where high levels of gentamicin are required for a short period of time. Such small defects may be inappropriate indications for the use of gentamicin-impregnated PMMA beads. In general, following use of a gentamicin-impregnated blood clot, high levels of antibiotic may be achieved at a bactericidal level for hours in local tissue, which may be sufficient to achieve clinical cure of soft tissue and bone infection. The use of this technique offers the availability of high levels of gentamicin within the wound without systemic absorption of gentamicin sulfate and its potential adverse effect on renal function.

The use of autologous antibiotic-loaded blood clot appears to have first been described by Winter in the management of recurrent osteomyelitis.[22] Ecke reported on 112 patients treated for recurrent osteomyelitis using antibiotic-loaded autologous blood clot.[4] The technique allows for the local management of osteomyelitis while simultaneously treating concurrent bone defects with cancellous grafting.

A significant advantage in this technique is that

by the use of a biologic carrier, later surgery for removal of antibiotic beads is not necessary. A variety of the antibiotics may be incorporated within blood clot, as they may with antibiotic-loaded bone cement. Gentamicin remains our antibiotic of choice. The use of gentamicin-impregnated blood clot is accompanied by the achievement of a bactericidal level of gentamicin within local wound tissues. Rapid infiltration of granulation tissue within the wound occurs into the hematoma. This is because the clot itself serves as a scaffold upon which soft tissue defects are rapidly filled. Primary wound closure is frequently possible with this technique.

MANAGEMENT OF THE NEUROPATHIC ULCER WITH LOCALIZED CHRONIC OSTEOMYELITIS OF THE ADJACENT BONE

Gentamicin-impregnated PMMA beads may be used adjunctively in the management of chronic neuropathic ulceration of the foot with associated contiguous resorptive bone pathology (Fig. 20-6). In such cases, initial resolution of cellulitis and acute soft tissue infection is of importance. The presence of inflammatory signs and symptoms due to autonomic neuropathy and masquerading as a cellulitic process should be considered in every case, as should the presence of diabetic osteolysis be considered as being responsible for bone pathology contiguous to an infected ulceration. Careful staging using standard radiographs, radiopharmaceutical studies as appropriate, or magnetic resonance imaging should be performed as appropriate in each case. The plantar ulcer is ellipsed for its full thickness. The incision should be of adequate length to ensure a tension-free closure on the plantar aspect of the foot. Appropriate cultures are taken. The wound margins are closed primarily. In the usual case, such as a submetatarsal ulcer, an incision is also made on the dorsum of the foot. The predetermined area of bone resection is then per-

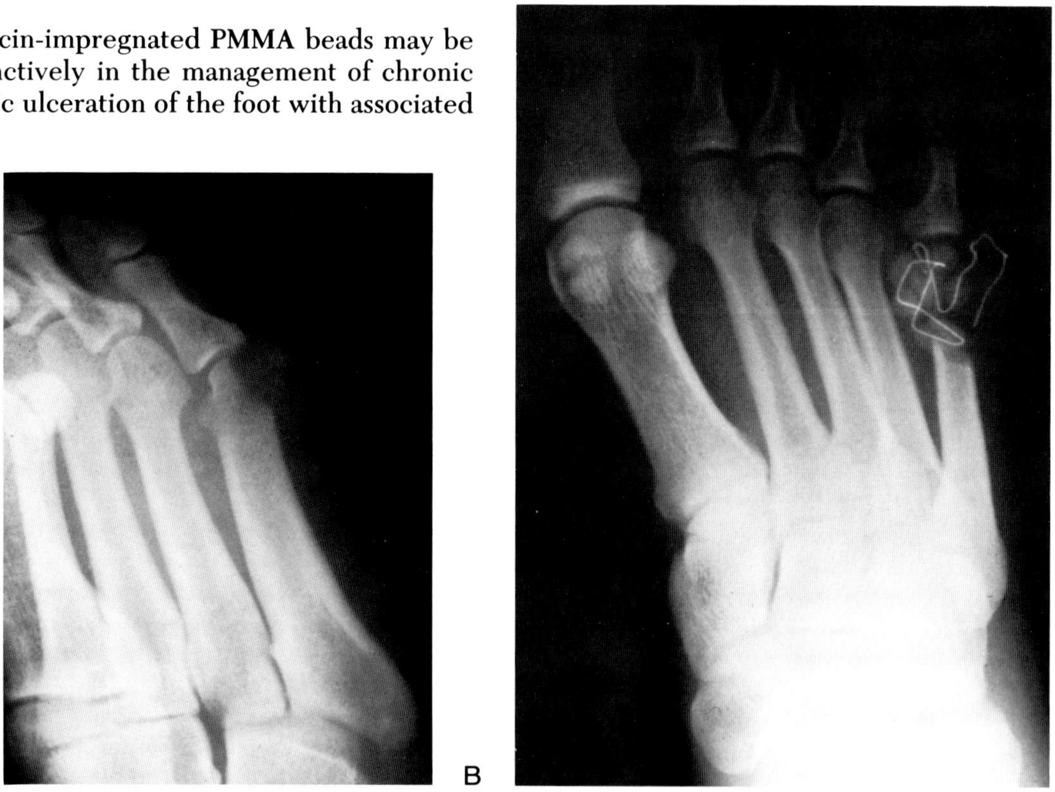

A B

Fig. 20-6. (**A**) Fifth metatarsal osteomyelitis following a puncture wound of the foot. Culture revealed *Staphylococcus aureus* and *Pseudomonas aeruginosa.* (**B**) Postoperative radiograph demonstrates resection of bone and soft tissue with implantation of antibiotic-loaded bone cement.

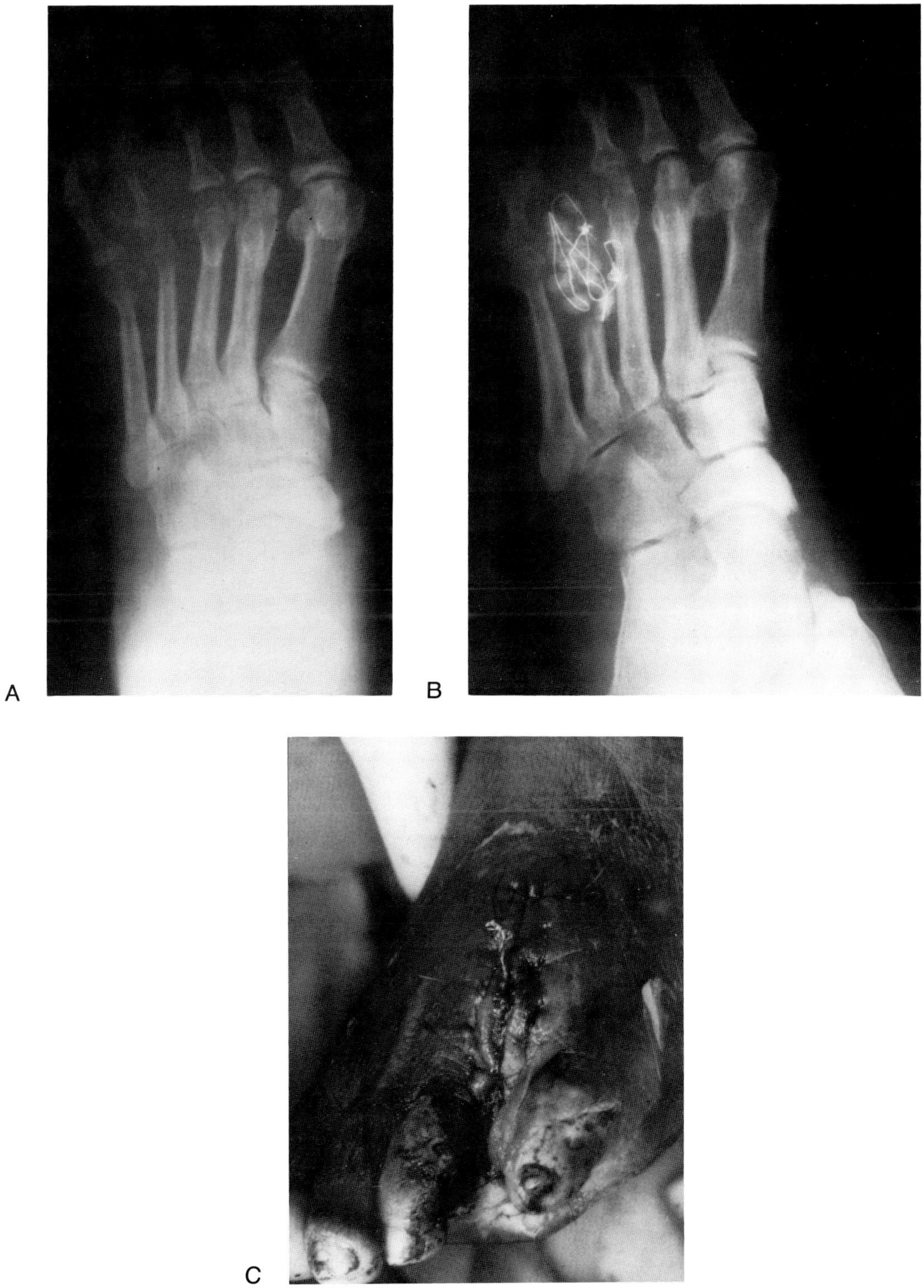

Fig. 20-7. (**A**) Osteomyelitis of a fourth metatarsal with extensive soft tissue necrosis of the toe. (**B**) Amputation of the fourth toe with implantation of antibiotic-loaded bone cement (ALBC). With amputations such as this, it may be preferable to include a one-stage procedure with primary closure over ALBC. In such cases, beads can be used to prevent recurrence of infection, although this type of amputation is best performed through clean tissue. (**C**) Clinical appearance after amputation and bead implantation. Bead wire exits the incision.

formed. The resection is carried out in such a manner as to remove all devitalized and infected osseous tissue. Antibiotic beads are then implanted within the wound cavity, and a primary closure is performed on the dorsal incision.

In the presence of acute inflammatory disease, we do not generally use antibiotic-loaded bone cement initially. When the management of the acute infectious process has been successful, as evidenced by decreasing signs and symptoms, secondary closure is performed with resection of infected bone and deep soft tissues with implantation of the beads and primary wound closure. In general, it is thought to be unwise to use this technique in association with severe necrotizing infections, anaerobic sepsis, severely dysvascular feet, or the presence of streptococcal disease.

Not infrequently, neuropathic ulcerations are complicated by recurrent infection and progressive necrosis. In many circumstances, it is prudent to perform a provisional or open amputation initially to minimize proximal extension of the infectious process. Antibiotic-loaded bone cement beads may be used at the time of amputation closure as a prophylactic measure to minimize the risk of septic contamination of the amputation stump (Fig. 20-7). We have found this technique useful when osteotomy, bone resection, or amputation are performed in an area contiguous to septic processes.

SUMMARY

Antibiotic-loaded bone cement and blood clot represent adjunctive measures in the management of soft tissue and bone infection in the diabetic foot. The technique allows the high concentration of antibiotic within previously infected tissue. The technique is performed in combination with radical debridement and excision of all necrotic-appearing bone and soft tissue. The levels of antibiotic obtained are bactericidal to the majority of pathogens encountered in clinical practice. The technique is of particular importance in the management of diabetic foot pathology, since such patients may not obtain adequate antibiotic wound levels by systemic administration of antibiotic owing to the presence of varying degrees of peripheral vascular disease. In addition, the broad spectrum activity of adequate levels of gentamicin sulfate are appropriate in the diabetic patient whose pedal infections are frequently polymicrobial in nature. When the volume of debrided bone and soft-tissue wounds does not permit the placement of antibiotic-loaded bone cement, the use of antibiotic-loaded autologous blood clot may be performed. Both techniques appear to speed the resolution of the initial infectious process while decreasing the incidence of recurrent infectious disease in the diabetic foot and ankle.

REFERENCES

1. Buchholz HW: Infection in total joint replacement: one stage exchange arthroplasty. In Uhthoff HK, Stahl E (eds): Current Concepts of Infection in Orthopedic Surgery. Springer-Verlag, Berlin, 1985
2. Buchholz HW, Elson RA, Engelbrecht E et al: Management of deep infection of total hip replacements. J Bone Joint Surg 63B:342, 1981
3. Buchholz HW, Engelbrecht E: Uber die Depotwirkung einiger Antibiotika bei Vermischung mit dem Kunstharz Palaces. Chirurg 41:511, 1970
4. Ecke H: Behandlung der chronischen Osteomyelitis mit plastischen operationsverfahren. Chirurg 33:123, 1962
5. Greiben A: Clinical results of Septopal in bone and soft tissue infection. A survey of clinical trials. In van Rens TJG, Kayser FH (eds): Local Antibiotic Treatment in Osteomyelitis and Soft Tissue Infections. Excerpta Medica, Amsterdam, 1981
6. Greiben A: Results of Septopal in more than 1500 cases of bone and soft tissue infections: a review of clinical trials. J Bone Joint Surg 62B:275, 1980
7. Muller KH: Experience with local antibiotic therapy in post-traumatic osteomyelitis by means of gentamycin polymethylmethacrylate. J Bone Joint Surg 62B:275, 1980
8. Klemm K: Septopal—a new way of local antibiotic therapy. In van Rens TJG, Kayser FH (eds): Local Antibiotic Treatment in Osteomyelitis and Soft Tissue Infections. Excerpta Medica, Amsterdam, 1981
9. Jenny G, Taglang G: Clinical experiences with the use of gentamycin-polymethylmethacrylate beads and chains in 200 cases of bone and soft tissue infections. In van Rens TJG, Kayser FH (eds): Local Anti-

biotic Treatment in Osteomyelitis and Soft Tissue Infections. Excerpta Medica, Amsterdam, 1981
10. Lidgren L: Basics in the treatment of orthopedic infections, with special reference to septopal. In van Rens TJG, Kayser FH (eds): Local Antibiotic Treatment in Osteomyelitis and Soft Tissue Infections. Excerpta Medica, Amsterdam, 1981
11. DeGroote W et al: The use of gentamycin polymethylmethacrylate beads in the treatment of osteomyelitis. In van Rens TJG, Kayser FH (eds): Local Antibiotic Treatment in Osteomyelitis and Soft Tissue Infections. Excerpta Medica, Amsterdam, 1981
12. Harle A: Surgical technique and results in the treatment of soft tissue infections with Septopal. In van Rens TJG, Kayser FH (eds): Local Antibiotic Treatment in Osteomyelitis and Soft Tissue Infections. Excerpta Medica, Amsterdam, 1981
13. Weise K, Weller S: Indication and use of Septopal in chronic osteitis. In van Rens TJG, Kayser FH (eds): Local Antibiotic Treatment in Osteomyelitis and Soft Tissue Infections. Excerpta Medica, Amsterdam, 1981
14. Walenkamp GHIM: Experiences in the treatment of osteomyelitis and infected endoprostheses with chains of gentamycin polymethylmethacrylate beads. In van Rens TJG, Kayser FH (eds): Local Antibiotic Treatment in Osteomyelitis and Soft Tissue Infections. Excerpta Medica, Amsterdam, 1981
15. Eberle H: Experiences in the treatment of post-traumatic osteomyelitis and soft tissue infection, especially in vascular surgery, with gentamycin polymethylmethacrylate chains. In van Rens TJG, Kayser FH (eds): Local Antibiotic Treatment in Osteomyelitis and Soft Tissue Infections. Excerpta Medica, Amsterdam, 1981
16. Wahlig H, Dingeldein E: Antibiotics and bone cements. Acta Orthop Scan 51:49, 1980
17. Marks KE, Nelson CC, Lauterschleger EP: Antibiotic impregnated acrylic bone cement. J Bone Joint Surg 58A:358, 1976
18. Sattel W, Nabert-Block G: Nachweis von Antibiotika aus Knochenzenmenten-Experimentelle und Klinlsche-Untersuchungen Wein, 94, 1973
19. Wahlig H: Gentamycin-polymethylmethacrylate beads, a drug delivery system; basic results. In van Rens TJG, Kayser FH (eds): Local Antibiotic Treatment in Osteomyelitis and Soft Tissue Infections. Excerpta Medica, Amsterdam, 1981
20. Harle A, Ritzerfeld W: The release of gentamycin into the wound secretions from polymethylmethacrylate beads. Arch Orthop Trauma Surgery 95:65, 1979
21. Vecsei V: Long term results in the treatment of septic bone and soft tissue diseases with gentamycin polymethylmethacrylate chains and beads. In van Rens TJG, Kayser FH (eds): Local Antibiotic Treatment in Osteomyelitis and Soft Tissue Infections. Excerpta Medica, Amsterdam, 1985
22. Winter L: Management of chronic osteitis and osteomyelitis with a coagulum of autogenous blood + penicillin + thrombin (on the basis of 56 case results). J Int Surg 1:510, 1951

SUGGESTED READINGS

Braun A, Gussbacher A, Wahlig H, Dingeldein E: Der Fibrin-Antibiotikum-Verbund als erganzende Lokalbehandlung der Osteomyelitis. p. 205. In Scheele J (ed): Fibrinklebung. Springer-Verlag, Berlin, 1984

Braun A, Schumacher G, Kratzat R et al: Der Fibrin-Antibiotikum-Verbund im Tierexperiment zur lokalen Therapie des staphylococceninfizierten Knochens. Vortrag 3. Deutsch-Osterisch-Schweizerische Unfalltagung. Vienna, 1979

Heine WD, Edinger D, Braun A: Wundheilung nach Fibrin-Klebung—Histopathologische Untersuchungen. p. 27. In Cotta H, Braun A (eds): Fibrinkleber in Orthopadie und Traumatologie. Thieme Verlag, Stuttgart, 1982

Heiss F, Ecke H, Sasse S, Bikfali A: Tierexperimentelle untersuchungen zum Wirkungsmechanismus der Eigenblut-Antibiotika-Plombe. Mschr Unfallheilk 66:262, 1963

Puhl W, Bohm E, Schimpf K, Braun A: Fibrin zur Blutstillung am spongiosen Knochen bei Hamophilie. p. 88. In Cotta H, Braun A: Fibrinkleber in Orthopadie und Traumatologie. Thieme Verlag, Stuttgart, 1982

21

Oxygen Therapy in the Diabetic Foot

Des F. Gorman, M.B., Ch.B., F.A.C.O.M., Ph.D.

The diabetic foot is often injured, and these injuries frequently do not heal because of a combination of hypoxia (secondary to ischemia) and infection.[1] Increasing local tissue oxygen tensions should be of considerable benefit. However, oxygen administration is still a potential rather than a proven therapy. This is in part because of ignorance about the effect on wound healing of varying oxygen dose,[2] the common but often unsuccessful practice of only applying oxygen topically,[3] and the anecdotal nature of most of the relevant clinical reports.[4]

Nevertheless, these anecdotal clinical data[4] and a single prospective controlled study[5] do suggest that oxygen therapy is useful in the overall treatment of foot wounds in diabetic patients. Consequently, this chapter will review both the mechanisms by which increased oxygen tensions can combat infection and accelerate wound healing and the supportive clinical data. Guidelines for patient selection will also be proposed along with possible modifications to conventional treatment regimens.

ADMINISTRATION AND MEASUREMENT OF OXYGEN

The fractional concentration of inspired oxygen ($F_{I}O_2$) varies from 0.21 to almost 1.0 in patients breathing oxygen at atmospheric pressure (1 atm) depending on the type of breathing circuit and delivery system being used. If $F_{I}O_2$ values are to approach 1.0, then a sealing mask such as an anesthetic mask and a gas reservoir, or high oxygen flow rates and a "demand" system are needed. Rebreathing systems (closed or semiclosed circuits), as compared to open-circuit "demand" systems, must be able to eliminate carbon dioxide (usually involving soda lime or lithium hydroxide), and unless the circuit is purged of all gas after the patient has been breathing on it for several minutes, the $F_{I}O_2$ will probably remain less than 0.85 because of nitrogen elimination from the patient.

Hyperbaric oxygen (HBO), that is, an inspired oxygen partial pressure ($P_{I}O_2$) of greater than normal atmospheric pressure (>1 atm), can only be delivered to patients in a pressure vessel. These are usually called *recompression chambers*, a relative misnomer and a reflection of the influence that diving medicine has had on the development of hyperbaric medicine in general. Recompression chambers vary considerably in both size and ancillary facilities.[6] The same need for adequate breathing circuits exists for HBO as for atmospheric pressure administration of oxygen, but in addition patients and their medical attendants are subject to hyperbaric pressures and hence are at risk of dysbaric illnesses such as barotrauma and decompression sickness. With care, the risk is very low.[7]

Oxygen diffuses slowly into tissues,[8] and for this reason topically administered oxygen usually fails to influence oxygen tensions in the base of wounds.[8,9] Many patients need a hyperbaric dose of oxygen to raise the tissue oxygen tension (the diffusion gradient is the difference between arterial and tissue oxygen partial pressures),[8] and any form of oxygen therapy will often fail to assist wound healing in hypovascular ischemic limbs.[10,11] Although some improvement of oxygen diffusion into tissues occurs with increased tissue temperature, oxygen transport and tissue oxygen consumption are primarily influenced by the arterial partial pressure of oxygen, which is itself virtually set by the PIO_2.[8]

Not only is there a wide range of potential oxygen doses that can be given, but also for even a given dose the changes in tissue oxygenation in and between individual patients is variable.[8] The bactericidal effect of oxygen increases with increasing oxygen tension,[12,13] but the beneficial effects of oxygen on wound healing appear confined to a narrow range of tissue oxygen tensions.[2] It follows that measurement of tissue oxygen tension is essential if the appropriate dose (PIO_2, duration, and frequency) is to be delivered. Oxygen concentrations or tensions can be measured by polarographic electrodes, mass spectrometers with radioactive tracers, and fiberoptic probes.[8] Of these, the transcutaneous polarographic electrode[14] is the most widely used for both patient selection and titration of dose. In this technique, the measured oxygen tension adjacent to the wound is often related to a normal reference area (e.g., the second left intercostal space) and may even be reduced to a simple percentage ratio. Changes in this relative value over time, such as after a course of oxygen therapy, are interpreted as changes in vascular density, as the actual arterial oxygen tension should be similar in the two regions.[15]

THE BIOLOGIC ACTIONS OF OXYGEN IN WOUND HEALING IN DIABETIC PATIENTS

Increased oxygen tensions may not have a direct effect on the diabetic disease process, although significantly reduced insulin needs have been reported after repeated HBO exposures.[16] In general, the beneficial actions of oxygen on the healing of diabetic foot wounds can be divided into antiseptic and wound-healing groups (Table 21-1).

Antisepsis

Increasing tissue oxygen tensions has a direct and toxic effect on obligate anaerobes.[17,18] Within the therapeutic range of PIO_2 that is not highly toxic to patients, oxygen has a direct toxicity only on those organisms that cannot synthetize the enzymes superoxide dismutase and catalase.[19-21] However, oxygen therapy can have significant indirect effects. The polymorphonuclear leukocyte killing of aerobic organisms such as *Staphylococcus aureus* is significantly impaired in hypoxic conditions.[12,13] Increasing tissue oxygen tensions substantially increases this killing capacity.[12,13] Hypoxia also will inhibit some antibiotic activity.[13] Vancomycin, sulfonamides, and aminoglycosides are known to be less effective under hypoxia,[13] and the effect of tobramycin on *Pseudomonas aeruginosa* is enhanced by oxygen administration both in vitro and in vivo.[22-24] In 1980, Keck et al.[25] showed that HBO also potentiated sulfonamides.

Perhaps because of these antibacterial effects, repeated HBO has been found to be a highly effective component of the treatment of refractory osteomyelitis.[26] Bone infection often underlies nonhealing foot wounds in diabetic patients,[4,27] and this may be another reason for the reported efficacy of oxygen therapy in diabetic foot injuries. In

Table 21-1. Beneficial Mechanisms of Oxygen in the Treatment of the Injured Diabetic Foot

Diabetic disease process
? Reduces insulin needs
Antisepsis
Toxic to anaerobes
Enhances neutrophils
Enhances aminoglycosides
Enhances sulfonamides
Enhances vancomycin
Wound healing
Stimulates angiogenesis
Improves microcirculation
Increases collagen
Enhances fibroblasts
?Enhances osteoclasts

addition to the antiseptic mechanisms listed above, relief of hypoxia may also enhance the scavenging activity of osteoclasts.

Wound Healing

Increasing the $P_{I}O_2$ can enhance tissue microcirculations by lowering interstitial fluid pressure and water content, most markedly with $P_{I}O_2$ of between 1 and 2 atm.[28,29] A raised $P_{I}O_2$ will also reduce the hematocrit (particularly with recurrent HBO application) and hence blood viscosity,[30] increase red blood cell elasticity,[30,31] and inhibit platelet aggregation.[32] Simultaneously, there will be an increase both in oxygen carriage by the blood and in the partial pressure diffusion gradient for oxygen into the tissues.[8] All of these processes can be expected to assist wound healing.

Conventionally it has been thought that the primary stimulus to wound repair was the release of growth and angiogenesis factors by hypoxic macrophages.[33] It is possible then that any oxygen therapy that produced normoxia or hyperoxia might inhibit the release of these factors, but this has not been demonstrated. The angiogenesis factor is also released by macrophages in response to lactate, and hyperoxia has little effect on wound lactate concentrations. Alternatively, growth and angiogenesis factor release may be more related to the oxygen gradient across the wound,[34,35] the greater the gradient the more stimulus to factor release. This gradient hypothesis could explain in part the nonhealing of wounds in hypovascular hypoxic tissues (no gradient) and the angiogenesis that has been found in these hypovascular tissues when HBO is administered.[15] The duration and frequency of oxygen administration is limited by oxygen's toxic effects on the patient's lungs and central nervous system.[36,37] If hypoxia is important to the stimulation of wound repair, then this will only be inhibited for the brief (1 to 2 hours per day) periods during which HBO can be given and for a short period afterward (0.5 to 4 hours) as tissue oxygen tensions return to normal.[8,38] It is even possible that maximal rates of wound healing are achieved when wounds are subject to alternating hypoxia and hyperoxia. Certainly, in experiments on animals, HBO administration has been clearly shown to stimulate both revascularization and re-epitheliazation of hypoxic wounds.[39] With the exception of premature neonates, breathing enriched oxygen mixtures or HBO has little or no effect on the vasculature in normal tissues.[15] Although it has been reported that the proliferative retinopathies in some juvenile-onset diabetic patients have apparently worsened when given HBO,[16] most (75 percent) diabetic patients given repeated HBO experience an increase in visual acuity without any macroscopic retinal changes.[16]

In addition to beneficial effects on the microcirculation and a possible stimulation of angiogenesis and growth factor release,[34,35] oxygen administration can also promote wound healing by stimulating fibroblast activity as well as collagen formation and cross-linking.[2] Indeed, hypoxia has been shown to inhibit the proline hydroxylation step in collagen synthesis,[2] fibroblast synthesis of collagen in general,[40,41] the tensile strength of collagen in healed skin wounds,[42] and the rate of epithelial proliferation in wounds.[39] Both the fibroblast proliferation and the hydroxylation of proline occur optimally at a slightly hyperoxic tissue oxygen tension of about 80 mmHg, (0.105 atm),[2] whereas a normal tissue oxygen tension is about 40 mmHg.[8] Above and below this 80 mmHg tension there is a progressive inhibition of both processes. Clearly, it is essential to titrate the oxygen dose to a tissue tension of about 80 mmHg, and to achieve this, the $P_{I}O_2$ required may be as low as 0.4 atm or may need to be hyperbaric. This also explains why fixed HBO regimens have such variable success,[4,27] and why the ideal oxygen dose to combat infection and that to promote wound healing will often be different. In addition, as wounds progressively revascularize,[15] the $P_{I}O_2$ needed to achieve a tissue oxygen tension of about 80 mmHg will decline. Adherence to the principles of a titrated dose using tissue oxygen measurement and effect will improve and widen the application of oxygen therapy to problem wounds.

Oxygen Toxicity

Oxygen is a toxic gas, and generally its toxicity in patients is manifested first in the lungs and the central nervous system.[36,37] This toxicity is essentially governed by the $P_{I}O_2$ and time, although it appears to be enhanced by anxiety, raised carbon dioxide tensions, work, fever, steroid and other drug administration, immersion in water, and changes in the type of inert gas being breathed as an oxygen diluent.[36,37,43] Nevertheless, a series of oxygen treatment regimens, usually HBO,[27] have evolved that avoid both overt and irreversible toxic changes. With these the permanent oxygen toxic morbidity rate in patients treated with oxygen is very low.

Doubts about using high oxygen tensions in treating nonhealing wounds have been raised because of concern that increased oxygen-radical formation may cause cell injury.[44] However, in vitro, modest hyperoxia has been shown to antagonize and not potentiate lipid peroxidation.[45] It is nevertheless possible that concurrent administration of oxygen-radical scavengers may enhance the beneficial effects of oxygen on wounds.

CLINICAL EXPERIENCE WITH OXYGEN TREATMENT OF INJURED DIABETIC FEET

Although the relative efficacy of systemic (inspired) and topical oxygen administration is difficult to determine as they are often administered simultaneously,[46,47] in general, topical oxygen administration alone does not significantly increase the oxygen tension at the base of wounds[8,9] and does not affect the outcome of wounds in diabetic patients.[3]

In contrast, the reported experience with systemic oxygen administration is generally favorable, although it is almost entirely limited to HBO. Indeed, the efficacy of breathing 100 percent oxygen at atmospheric pressure has not been determined.

Hart and Strauss[48] reported complete healing in 2 of 11 diabetic patients with previously nonhealing wounds when treated repeatedly with HBO at 2 atm. The remaining 9 had a "good response." Emhoff and Myers[49] reported a similarly favorable outcome in 10 patients, 8 of whom were shown at the outset to have hypoxic wounds by transcutaneous polarography. Perrins and Barr[11] achieved healing of wounds in 16 of 24 diabetic patients with HBO, and in 4 patients amputation was avoided. Pedesini et al.[50] achieved a good healing result in 23 of 26 diabetic patients. Kindwall and Goldmann[27] reported a much more variable success rate, except for the usual good control of any underlying osteomyelitis. The numbers in this latter series are not apparent. Davis et al.[4] presented a pictorial series of seven diabetic patients showing healing or successful grafting of ulcers and control of underlying osteomyelitis. Tufano and his coworkers[51] reported pain relief and a decrease in plasma ACTH and endorphin levels in 8 diabetic patients with vascular disease treated with HBO; while Cianci et al.[52] claimed an 89 percent successful salvage rate in 19 diabetic patients with lesions that threatened the viability of the involved limb.

Kindwall and Goldmann[27] reviewed a series of 62 diabetic patients with foot wounds and divided them into the following 3 groups on the basis of their outcomes and ankle perfusion pressures (measured using a Doppler blood pressure cuff): perfusion pressure greater than 90 mmHg, healing without assistance; perfusion pressure of 75 to 90 mmHg, healing probable with HBO; and perfusion pressure less than 75 mmHg, healing unlikely even with HBO.

None of these studies were adequately controlled. In the only prospective and controlled (but not randomized) study, Baroni and his co-workers[5] showed significantly improved healing and a reduced amputation rate in 18 diabetic patients with foot wounds treated with daily HBO in comparison to 10 diabetic patients with foot wounds treated without any oxygen breathing.

A randomized prospective controlled clinical study that includes a much wider range of oxygen doses and measurements of tissue oxygen tensions is obviously needed. In the interim, some conclusions can be made from the existing data. First, those diabetic patients who appear to respond in a cost effective fashion to HBO are those with only mild to moderate tissue hypoxia. Those with severe hypoxia do not heal, and those with very mild vascular disease heal well without any oxygen therapy. Second, the outcome for these patients is significantly improved by other ancillary measures such as regular and careful wound toilet, good metabolic control, and if antibiotic therapy of any osteomyelitis is indicated, by deep bone biopsy, with organism culture and assessment of sensitivities.[26]

SELECTION OF DIABETIC PATIENTS FOR OXYGEN THERAPY

The selection of diabetic patients with foot wounds for oxygen therapy should be based on assessments of peripheral vascular adequacy (i.e., a basis for angiogenesis) including palpation and Doppler evaluation of pedal pulses, ankle pressure determinations, angiography, and transcutaneous polarographic oxygen measurement (Table 21-2).[27]

In practice, the commonly used modalities are ankle perfusion pressure measurements, as described above, and transcutaneous polarography. The limitations of the latter are well described,[8] but the use of relative values, also as described above, has been successful. In my own experience a relative transcutaneous partial pressure of oxygen ($tcPO_2$) of greater than 0.85 indicates the wound will heal with conventional therapy, and a relative $tcPO_2$ of less than 0.2 indicates a poor prognosis regardless of oxygen therapy. The exception to this rule is if the $tcPO_2$ increases significantly above 0.2 when the patient is changed from breathing room air to 100 percent oxygen. These patients, and those with a relative $tcPO_2$ between 0.2 and 0.85, will probably heal if oxygen is administered adjuvant to appropriate wound care.[4]

Table 21-2. Selection Criteria for Oxygen Therapy for Injured Diabetic Feet

	Ankle Perfusion Pressure (mmHg)	*Relative $tcPO_2$*[a] (%)
Will heal without oxygen	>90	>85
Probable healing with oxygen	75–90	20–85
Unlikely to heal with or without oxygen	<75	<20[b]

[a] The $tcPO_2$ adjacent to the wound expressed as a relative value of that measured on the skin over the second left intercostal space.

[b] With the exception of those where the $tcPO_2$ increases by more than 50 percent within 15 minutes of the patient beginning to breathe 100 percent oxygen.

OXYGEN DOSE

The ideal oxygen dose (P_{IO_2}, duration and frequency) has not been determined, and from the preceding arguments it would appear that the P_{IO_2} should be titrated to achieve 80 mmHg wound oxygen tension on a daily basis. A trial of this approach is warranted, although careful attention to the method of oxygen tension assessment will be essential.

The only adequate human data exist for a P_{IO_2} of about 2 atm, administered daily for 1.5 to 2 hours, and continued until the wound heals or is successfully grafted.[4] The efficacy of 1 atm oxygen therapies cannot be determined from the available literature. Again, a trial of a much wider range of oxygen doses in conjunction with wound tension measurement is needed.

In summary, oxygen administration should be of benefit in selected diabetic patients with foot wounds. The mechanisms of action for oxygen in this context are well established and some supportive clinical data do exist. A change to an individually titrated dose of oxygen is strongly recommended.

REFERENCES

1. Kozak GP, Hoar CS, Jr, Rowbotham L et al: Management of diabetic foot problems. WB Saunders, Philadelphia, 1984
2. Mehm WJ, Pinsler M, Becker RL, Lissner CR: Effect of oxygen on in vitro fibroblast cell proliferation and collagen biosynthesis. J Hyper Med 3(4):227, 1988
3. Leslie CA, Sapico FL, Ginunas VJ, Adkins RH: Randomized controlled trial of topical hyperbaric oxygen for treatment of diabetic foot ulcers. Diabetes Care 11:111, 1988
4. Davis JC, Buckley CJ, Barr P-O: Compromised soft tissue wounds: correction of wound hypoxia. p. 141. In Davis JC, Hunt TK (eds): Problem Wounds. The Role of Oxygen. Elsevier, New York, 1988

5. Baroni G, Porro T, Faglia E et al: Hyperbaric oxygen in diabetic gangrene treatment. Diabetes Care 10:81, 1987
6. Davis JC, Hung TK (eds): Hyperbaric oxygen therapy. Undersea and Hyperbaric Medical Society, Bethesda, MD, 1977
7. Weathersby PK, Survanski SS, Hays JR, MacCallum ME: Statistically based decompression tables III: comparative risk using USN, British and Canadian standard air schedules. Naval Medical Research Institute, Bethesda, MD, 1986
8. Sheffield PJ: Tissue oxygen measurements. p. 17. In Davis JC, Hunt TK (eds): Problem Wounds. The Role of Oxygen. Elsevier, New York, 1988
9. Gruber RP, Heitkamp DH, Billy LJ et al: Skin permeability to oxygen and hyperbaric oxygen. Arch Surg 101:69, 1970
10. Jacobson JH: Effects of hyperbaric oxygen on peripheral vascular diseases. HBO Rev 2:227, 1981
11. Perrins JD, Barr P-O: Hyperbaric oxygenation and wound healing. p. 119. In Schmutz J (ed): Proceedings of the 1st Swiss Symposium on Hyperbaric Medicine. Foundation for Hyperbaric Medicine, Basel, 1986
12. Mader JT: Phagocytic killing and hyperbaric oxygen: antimicrobial mechanisms. HBO Rev 2(1):37, 1981
13. Mader JT, Adams KR, Sutton TE: Infectious diseases: pathophysiology and mechanisms of hyperbaric oxygen. J Hyper Med 2(3):133, 1987
14. Huch R, Lubbers DW, Huch A: Quantitative continuous measurement of partial oxygen pressure on the skin of adults and newborn babies. Pflugers Arch 337:185, 1972
15. Marx RE, Johnson RP: Problem wounds in oral and maxillofacial surgery: the role of hyperbaric oxygen. p. 65. In Davis JC, Hunt TK (eds): Problem Wounds. The Role of Oxygen. Elsevier, New York, 1988
16. Caamano JV, de lara Munoz Delgado A: Hyperbaric oxygen treatment of 525 cases of diabetic retinopathy. p. 169. In Desola Ala J (ed): Proceedings of the IX Congress of the European Undersea Biomedical Society. Barcelona, EUBS, 1984
17. Hill GB: Hyperbaric oxygen exposure for intrahepatic abscesses produced in mice by nonspore-forming anaerobic bacteria. Antimicrob Agents Chemother 9:312, 1976
18. Hill GB, Osterhout S: Experimental effects of hyperbaric oxygen on selected clostridial species. J Infect Dis 125:17, 1972
19. Brown GL, Thomson PD, Mader JT et al: Effects of hyperbaric oxygen upon *S. aureus, Ps. aeruginosa* and *C. albicans*. Aviat Space Environ Med 50:717, 1979
20. Gregory EM, Fridovich I: Induction of superoxide dismutase by molecular oxygen. J Bacteriol 114:543, 1973
21. McCord JM, Keele BB, Fridovich I: An enzyme-based theory of obligate anaerobiosis: the physiological function of superoxide dismutase. Proc Natl Acad Sci USA 68:1024, 1971
22. Adams KR, Mader JT: Aminoglycoside potentiation with adjunctive hyperbaric oxygen therapy in experimental Ps aeruginosa osteomyelitis. Undersea Biomed Res, suppl. 14(2):37, 1987
23. Adams KR, Sutton TE, Mader JT: In vitro potentiation of tobramycin under hyperoxic conditions. Undersea Biomed Res, suppl. 14(2):37, 1987
24. Norden CW, Kleti E: Experimental osteomyelitis caused by *Pseudomonas aeruginosa*. J Infect Dis 141:71, 1980
25. Keck PE, Gottlieb SF, Conley J: Interaction of increased pressures of oxygen and sulfonamides on the in vitro and in vivo growth of pathogenic bacteria. Undersea Biomed Res 7:95, 1980
26. Davis JC, Heckman JD: Refractory osteomyelitis. p. 125. In Davis JC, Hunt TK (eds): Problem Wounds. The Role of Oxygen. Elsevier, New York, 1988
27. Kindwall EP, Goldmann RW: Hyperbaric Medicine Procedures. St. Lukes Hospital, Milwaukee, 1984
28. Gu ZZ: Effect of oxygen at various pressures on intracranial pressure. Chung Hua Shen Ching Ching Shen Ko Tsa Chih 18:17, 1985
29. Isakov IV, Romasenko MV: Effect of hyperbaric oxygenation on total water content of brain tissue in experimental traumatic edema of the brain. Zh Vopr Neirokhir 50:25, 1986
30. Fischer B, Jain KK, Braun E, Lehrl S: Effect of hyperbaric oxygenation on disorders of the blood. p. 176. In Fischer B, Jain KK, Braun E, Lehrl S (eds): Handbook of Hyperbaric Oxygen Therapy. Springer-Verlag, Berlin, 1988
31. Mathieu D, Coget J, Vinchkier L et al: Red blood cell deformity and hyperbaric oxygenation. p. 27. In Proceedings of the 8th International Congress on Hyperbaric Medicine. Long Beach, CA, 1984
32. Hsu P, Zan-Shun W, Yong-Xing M: The effect of HBO on platelet aggregation, blood rheology, PaO_2 and cognitive function in the elderly. p. 19. In Proceedings of the 8th International Congress on Hyperbaric Medicine. Long Beach, CA 1984
33. Knighton DR, Oredsson S, Banda M et al: Regulation of repairs. Hypoxic control of macrophage mediated

angiogenesis. p. 41. In Hunt TK, Heppenstall RB, Pines E et al (eds): Soft and Hard Tissue Repair. Praeger Publishers, New York, 1984
34. Knighton DR, Hunt TK, Schencstuhl H et al: Oxygen tension regulates the expression of angiogenesis factor by macrophages. Science 221:1283, 1983
35. Knighton DR, Silver IA, Hunt TK: Regulation of wound healing angiogenesis: effect of oxygen gradients and inspired oxygen concentrations. Surgery 90:262, 1981
36. Donald KW: Oxygen poisoning in man. Part I. Br Med J 1:667, 1947
37. Donald KW: Oxygen poisoning in man. Part 2. Br Med J 1:712, 1947
38. Wells CH, Goodpasture JE, Horrigan DJ et al: Tissue gas measurements during hyperbaric oxygen exposure. p. 118. In Smith G (ed): Proceedings of the 6th International Congress on Hyperbaric Medicine. Aberdeen University Press, Aberdeen, Scotland, 1977
39. Miller TA, Korn HN: Epithelial burn injury and repair. p. 251. In Davis JC, Hunt TK (eds): Hyperbaric Oxygen Therapy. Undersea and Hyperbaric Medicine Society, Bethesda, MD, 1977
40. Gruber RP, Heitkamp DH, Amato JJ: Systemic absorption of topically applied hyperbaric oxygen. Tex Rep Biol Med 28:547, 1970
41. Niinikoski J, Henghan C, Hung TK: Oxygen and carbon dioxide tensions in experimental wounds. Surg Gynecol Obstet 133:1003, 1971
42. Kulonen E, Niinikoski J, Pentinen R: Effect of the supply of oxygen on the tensile strength of healing skin wound and granulation tissue. Acta Physiol Scand 70:112, 1967
43. Balentine JD: Pathology of Oxygen Toxicity. Academic Press, San Diego, 1982
44. Chance B, Boveris A: Hyperoxia and hydroperoxide metabolism. p. 185. In Robin EN (ed): Extrapulmonary Manifestations of Respiratory Disease, Vol. 8. DeKever, New York, 1978
45. Thom SR: Antagonism of lipid peroxidation by elevated partial pressures of oxygen. Undersea Biomed Res, suppl. 15:22, 1988
46. Heng MCY: Local hyperbaric oxygen administration for leg ulcers. Br J Dermatol 109:232, 1983
47. Heng MCY, Pilgrim JP, Beck FWJ: A simplified hyperbaric oxygen technique for leg ulcers. Clin Res 30:262A, 1982
48. Hart GB, Strauss MB: Responses of ischaemic ulcerative conditions to OHP. p. 312. In Smith G (ed): Hyperbaric Medicine. Aberdeen University Press, Aberdeen, Scotland, 1979
49. Emhoff TA, Myers RAM: Transcutaneous Oxygen Measurements and Wound Healing. MIEMSS, Baltimore, 1984
50. Pedesini G, Oriani G, Barini C et al: Hyperbaric oxygen therapy in the treatment of diabetic vasculopathies. p. 207. In Desola Ala J (ed): Proceedings of the IX Congress of the European Undersea Biomedical Society. Barcelona, EUBS, 1984
51. Tufano R, Del Gaudio A, De Gillis P: Hyperbaric oxygen effects on pain relief in patients with vascular disease. J Hyper Med 3(1):29, 1988
52. Cianci P, Petrone G, Drager S et al: Salvage of the problem wound and potential amputation with wound care and adjunctive hyperbaric oxygen therapy: an economic analysis. J Hyper Med 3(3):127, 1988

22

The Ambulatory Total Contact Cast

Stephen J. Kominsky, D.P.M., F.A.C.F.S., D.A.B.P.S.

HISTORICAL PERSPECTIVE

In Ceylon in the 1930s, an orthopaedic surgeon named Milroy Paul began treating plantar ulcers from Hansen's disease with a below knee walking cast. He had a moderate degree of success with this novel and controversial approach.[1] In 1939, Kahn, in India, used a plaster cast to treat similar conditions and had similar results.[2]

In India in the late 1950s at the trophic ulcer clinics of the Christian Medical College and Hospital in Vellore, Paul Brand and his colleagues were involved in treating trophic plantar ulcers on patients with Hansen's disease. They noted that many of these patients were able to be maintained with frequent dressing changes and local wound care for months and even years. The problems, however, became quite significant, since this type of treatment was not only costly in dollars and time, but in many cases it necessitated the patients' walking great distances to obtain the care. This, they found, increased the mechanical stresses, which in turn worsened the plantar wounds. Out of sheer necessity, it became imperative that these patients be treated in a manner that would allow ambulation without compromising healing. Thus, Brand and his co-workers adopted the early approach of Khan and began to immobilize these patients in plaster casts. They quickly found that the regularity and speed with which these ulcers healed was most impressive, and this supported the concept that the ulcer is directly related to mechanical stress. Support of this concept suggests that the ulcerations may be prevented and that recurrence of the ulcer may be avoided with the proper stress reduction technique (i.e., appropriate shoegear and accommodative insole).

After making some modifications to the basic cast, such as removing the padding, the total contact cast was born. This new approach to the treatment of foot ulcers and deformities came to the United States in the early 1960s.[1,2,3]

ULCER HEALING

In 1983, a study was completed demonstrating the efficacy of the ambulatory total contact cast for healing plantar ulcers.[4] In this protocol, a patient population with ulcerations was treated using this modality. The study investigated several factors affecting the rate of healing. The results of the study demonstrated that 72.7 percent of the population healed in 38.3 days using the casting technique. This is extremely rapid, since the majority of noncasted ulcers persist for a much longer period of time.

A patient with any condition that would benefit from cast immobilization should be considered for contact cast therapy. The ambulatory total contact cast, originally described by Brand et al., is a form of an occlusive dressing that immobilizes the foot sufficiently to allow various pedal pathologies to heal.

The most common conditions that develop on the foot of the diabetic patients are plantar ulcers and Charcot joint disease, also known as neuroarthropathy. These maladies are the direct result of biomechanical abnormalities, either in the shape of the foot, or in the weight-bearing pattern of the foot during gait.[2–5]

Several authors have identified the major cause of plantar ulcers in diabetic patients as being related to neuropathy, and unrelated to microvascular small vessel disease,[6] as has long been the theory. The contention of those researchers is that through the stresses of gait in a compromised foot (the insensate one), plantar keratosis develops and goes undetected (Fig. 22-1). If the pressure that has caused the lesions to develop continues, then through a process of enzymatic autolysis the soft tissue breaks down to form the plantar ulcer. Once this condition has developed, something has to be done to relieve the weight-bearing stress to allow the pressure lesion to resolve. This is the purpose of the total contact cast.

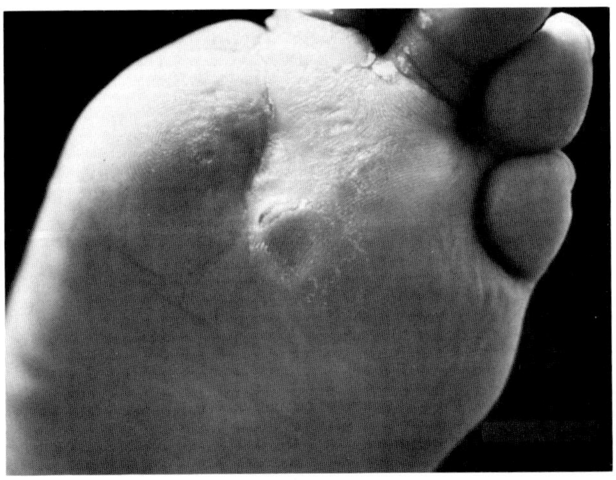

Fig. 22-1. One of the indications for the use of the total contact cast is a preulcerous lesion. In this case, note the blisterlike keratosis under the third metatarsal head. The first and second metatarsal heads were previously surgically removed. As a result, the remaining forces shifted to the third metatarsal head, whereby a keratosis developed. In this case, a partial thickness of the skin is evident. The lesion was debrided prior to the application of the cast. Lesions such as this respond quickly to cast therapy.

INDICATIONS FOR THE CAST

The total contact cast relieves the forces on the foot during gait in several different ways. First, it forces the wearer to shorten the stride length of each step. By doing so, the velocity of walking is decreased, which diminishes the vertical forces on the foot dramatically. Second, the cast eliminates motion at the ankle joint in the sagitttal plane. That in turn eliminates the propulsive phase of the gait cycle.[2,7] By accomplishing this, the forces on the forefoot are reduced considerably. It has been documented that the majority of plantar ulcers occur on the forefoot under the metatarsal heads.[4,5] These lesions are dynamic in nature, since they develop during the propulsive (dynamic) phase of the gait cycle. If forefoot propulsion is eliminated, the chances of healing the ulcer and preventing recurrence is very good.

The most direct effect that the total contact cast has on the foot is its ability to increase the plantar surface area. For example, a 150-pound person standing on a 1-inch-square block of wood, the force exerted on the bottom of the foot would equal 150 pounds per square inch. If, however, that same 150-pound person was standing on a 2-inch-square block, the forces on the foot would equal 75 pounds per square inch, or one-half the original amount.[1]

This becomes significant when there are bony prominences plantarly that are causing the pressure, and ultimately ulceration. As mentioned earlier, the vast majority of plantar ulcers are forefoot ulcers due to pressure from a metatarsal head prominence. Rocker bottom feet that have shifted bones plantarly from Charcot disease also fall into this category. Such cases are similar to the scenario of the man standing on the block of wood, only in these cases the prominence is smaller than 1 square inch, and so the force does not decrease, but increases instead.

An ischemic ulcer differs from a neuropathic ulcer not only in the etiology (dysvascularity versus vertical force) but also in the way that it responds to treatment. As previously mentioned, the neuropathic ulcer is related to a high amount of vertical force over a small surface area. Increasing the surface area decreases the vertical force, which allows healing. Little of this is relevant to cases involving ischemic ulcers. Generally these ulcers are not found on the plantar surface of the foot; more likely, they are located on the dorsum or adjacent to the malleoli. Therefore, since these are not weight-bearing lesions, use of the contact cast would not present any significant advantages.

Through the construction of the cast, which will be detailed later in this chapter, the surface area on the plantar surface of the foot is increased, which ultimately decreases the forces plantarly.[1,3,7] Another benefit of this cast is that it protects the foot from foreign objects. The makeup is such that it encloses the foot entirely, including the toes (Fig. 22-2). The major advantage of this is that while the person wearing it remains active, nothing will get into the cast. Since the foot is insensate, the feedback mechanism would not detect materials such as pebbles or twigs that could find their way into a cast with open toes.

Another feature that is beneficial as an adjunct with this cast is that it has the ability to control and reduce edema dramatically. Edema when present in a large amount has the potential to increase tissue hydrostatic pressure. As a result of this, enzymatic necrosis of tissue may occur. When this develops, ulceration occurs. In an already compromised patient, this could be catastrophic. Therefore, edema control becomes extremely important. The contact cast reduces edema so dramatically that it often becomes necessary to change the first cast after the initial 48 hours. Otherwise the cast will piston (slide) on the leg, which increases the shear force, potentially leading to soft tissue damage.

Thus far, the major focus of this chapter has been on the plantar ulcer. The person with Charcot joint involvement, or for that matter the diabetic patient who has a fractured bone, be it surgical or traumatic, would also progress very well with the total contact cast. As stated earlier, eliminating the propulsive phase of gait by fixing the ankle in the cast decreases the forces of walking dramatically. Therefore, either of these osseous conditions should be expected to heal without difficulty. One clarifying point with respect to the Charcot, however, is that it is dependent on the stage at which it is cast. If the pathology and deformity are far advanced, the cast may arrest further progression; however, it will not reverse deformity that is already present. The cast should, however, immobilize the foot sufficiently to allow whatever fractures are present to heal.

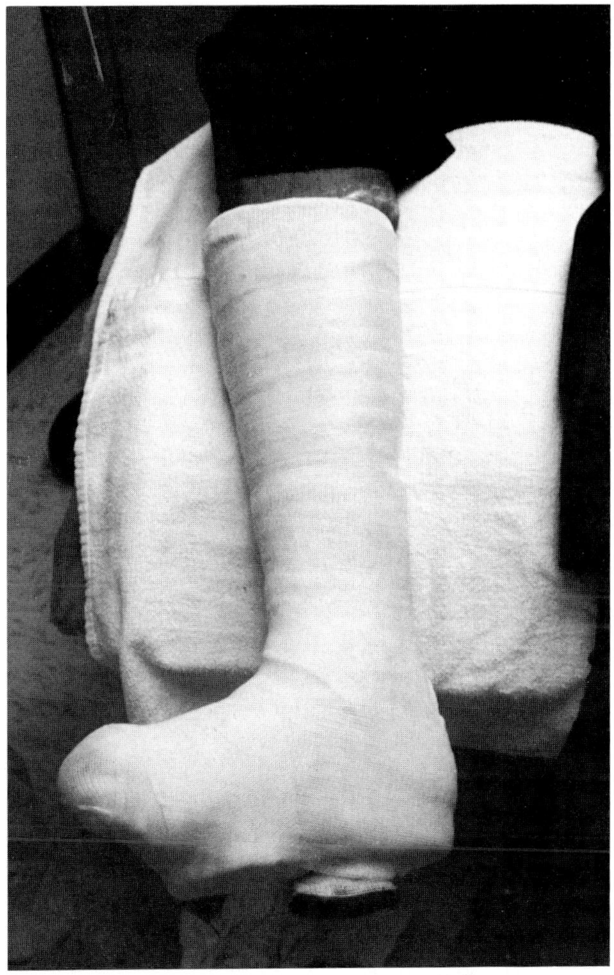

Fig. 22-2. An example of a total contact cast using synthetic material. Note that the toes are enclosed; this is for protection. The patient may ambulate on this cast 30 minutes after its application is completed (a major advantage to the synthetic material). Note the rubber walking heel and the platform on which it rests.

The ultimate goal in treating the Charcot joint is to allow consolidation of the involved joints to occur. The cast will immobilize the foot sufficiently

Table 22-1. Indications for the Use of the Ambulatory Total Contact Cast

1. To immobilize the foot in such a way as to diminish the forces of weight bearing on the limb
2. In the presence of a plantar ulcer or preulcerous lesion, to diminish the vertical forces of walking so as to allow the lesion to heal
3. In the presence of neuroarthropathy, to eliminate the stresses of weight bearing and allow the condition to consolidate
4. Postoperatively, to immobilize the surgical site to allow sufficient healing by minimizing the forces of weight bearing

so that the acute Charcot (that is, the one that presents with edema and increased skin temperatures) may be converted to the quiescent Charcot. This progress is monitored both radiographically, watching for joint consolidation, and with serial skin temperatures. The temperatures of the affected limb will eventually decrease and become symmetric with the contralateral limb. Once there is evidence of both of these things, then it is considered quiescent. Table 22-1 lists the various indications for the use of the total contact cast.

CONTRAINDICATIONS TO THE USE OF THE TOTAL CONTACT CAST

The previous sections have dealt with the indications for the use of the total contact cast. The contraindications to its use are equally important (Table 22-2). The major contraindication to the use of the total contact cast is the presence of an infected wound. Enclosing an infected ulcer could lead to catastrophic results. The cast provides a warm, dark, moist environment, one that bacteria would thrive in. Therefore, the first step when considering this type of therapy is to ensure that the wound is not infected.

Second, the ulcer must be wider at the surface than it is deep (Fig. 22-3). If this is not the case, the patient then runs the risk of epithelializing the surface of the wound before the depth has a chance to granulate and fill in. This would leave a cavity beneath the surface of the skin, which would potentially lead to the formation of an abscess. There-

Table 22-2. Contraindications for the Use of the Ambulatory Total Contact Cast

1. Noncompliant patients
2. Patients with claustrophobia
3. Patients with active dermatoses or with contact allergies to any components of the cast
4. Presence of active infection
5. Presence of an ulcer that is deeper than it is wide

A

B

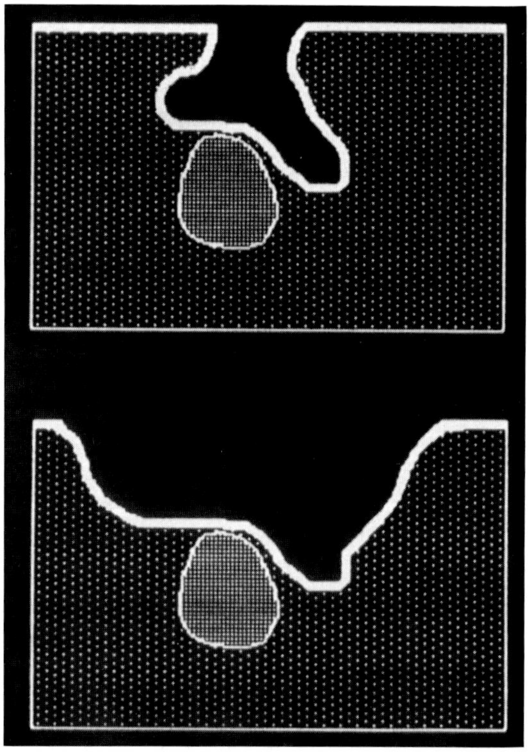

Fig. 22-3. One of the cardinal rules in contact cast therapy is that the wound must be wider at the surface than it is deep. **(A)** The thick white line in this figure represents skin, and the circle in the center represents bone. This figure demonstrates a wound that is deeper than the width of the surface opening. In order for this wound to be considered safe to cast, the surface opening must be debrided. In such cases the concern is that the surface will close before the depth has a chance to granulate in. **(B)** The wound after debridement. Note the difference in the width of the surface opening.

fore, it becomes necessary to sharply debride the surface wound, opening it sufficiently to accomplish this goal.

Patients who are claustrophobic do not tolerate being enclosed within a cast and often develop psychological complications as a result. Therefore, casts are not indicated for them.

Some people have skin sensitivities to one or several components of the cast. When this is the case, dermatologic considerations are important and often contraindicate the use of the cast.

Finally, patient compliance is a very important factor. The cast therapy requires a significant number of return or follow-up visits. This approach to treatment gives the patients a feeling that they have some control in their treatment. Some of them will respond positively to this, and some not. It is important that the doctor feel confident that the patient will alert him to problems if they arise. Based on that, compliance is an important aspect to this approach.

POTENTIAL COMPLICATIONS FROM CONTACT CAST THERAPY

As with any treatment modality, there exists the possibility of developing complications. It is of the utmost importance in contact cast therapy that every precaution be taken to minimize the chances of complications arising.

There are two categories of complications that may develop: those that are caused by using the cast on the "wrong patient," and those caused by the cast itself or its removal. With respect to the wrong patient concept, one would have to consider the list of contraindications to determine whether a given patient is suited for cast therapy.

In addition to the list of contraindications, there are several other factors that may lead to complications. For example, if the patient walks on the cast before the material has hardened, the plantar surface of the cast may collapse creating an area of high pressure under the foot (Fig. 22-4). This is a much greater risk when the entire cast is made of plaster. With the advent of synthetic materials, which cure in about 30 minutes, the risk of this problem has been reduced. If this problem does occur, it is usually detected before the patient leaves the office. If not, then on the first office visit when this is noted, the cast *must be changed*. Since this complication would cause a problem plantarly and, in the worst case scenario, cause an ulcer to develop, another cast should be applied to allow the patient to ambulate with diminished pressure.

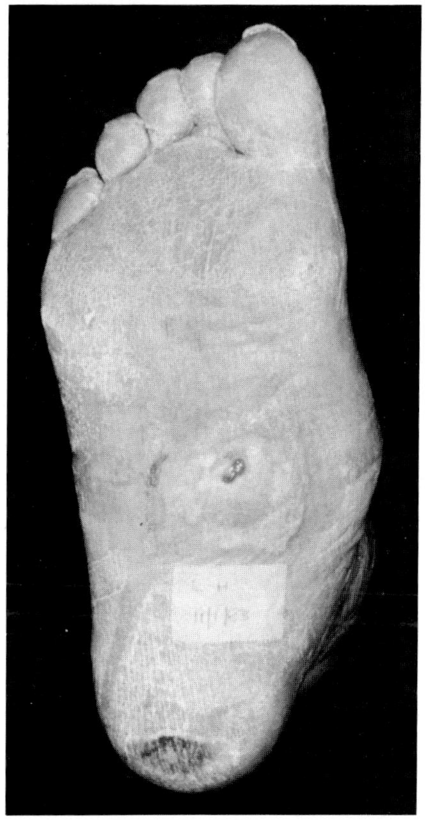

Fig. 22-4. A possible complication of walking on the contact cast before it hardens is the collapse of the plantar surface. If undetected, this may be a source of pressure, which would eventually lead to ulceration. The heel of this foot presents a hemorrhagic area consistent with a preulcerous lesion. When the cast was examined, it was noted to be indented in that spot. This patient was recasted to eliminate pressure from the heel as well as the midfoot.

Another problem that may arise is that caused by the overzealous use of the cast saw. If the person removing the cast bears down too hard with the saw, lacerations may ensue (Fig. 22-5). It is important to bear in mind that there is no cast padding in

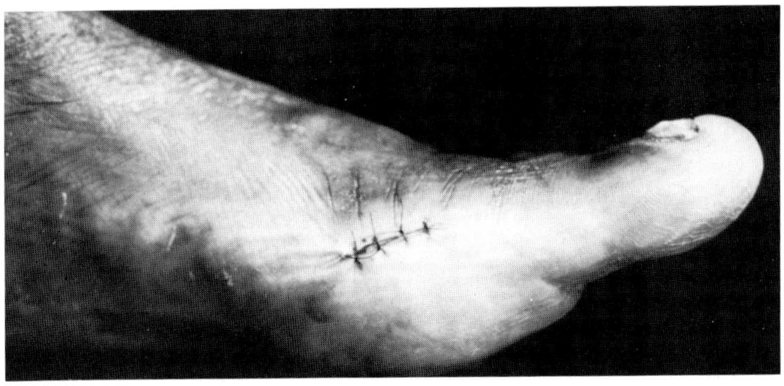

Fig. 22-5. Overzealous use of the cast saw or use of the saw in an unprotected place may lead to complications such as this. Special care must be taken when using the saw to remove the cast.

the total contact cast. Therefore, it is very important that the person responsible for removing the casts have some experience with the use of a cast saw before trying it on this type of cast (Fig. 22-6).

If the cast is applied either too low or too high on the leg, irritation at the edge of the cast may occur. Patients with large legs are especially prone to this problem. Ideally, the cast should stop at the tibial tuberosity.

APPLICATION OF THE TOTAL CONTACT CAST

Before the cast is applied, it is important to make sure that the toenails are debrided properly. This will prevent the risk of a nail gouging into an adjacent toe and potentially causing problems.

Once the ulcer has been properly measured, debrided, and dressed, the patient is placed in the prone position. Prone is the position of choice for several reasons. First, in this position the knee has to be flexed to position the foot. This allows the muscle mass of the gastronemius complex to "flow" proximally, which shifts it more proximally on the leg. This allows for a better fit of the cast distally. This point is more critical for the obese patient. Second, it is much easier to maintain the foot at a right angle to the leg with the patient prone. This will allow the person to walk with greater ease while in the cast.

The next step is to hydrate the skin. Generally, this is necessary for xerotic skin, which is a common

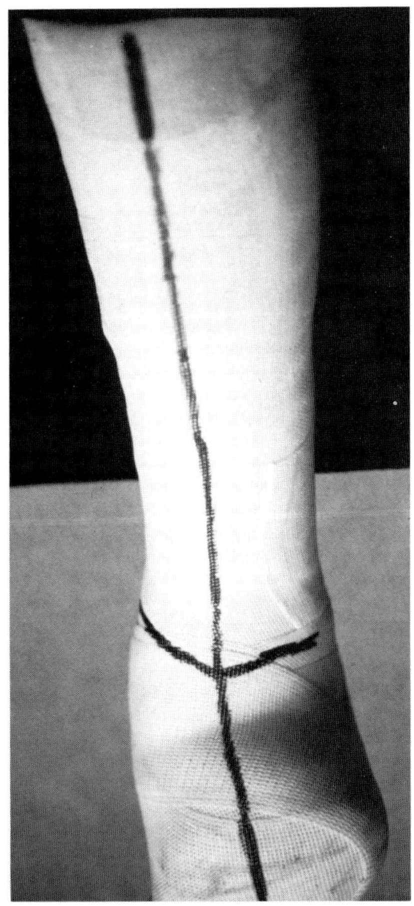

Fig. 22-6. The lines on the cast indicate the locations where the cast saw should be used to remove the cast safely. There is no padding in this cast; therefore, the saw must be introduced only in the areas that are protected by the adhesive felt, along the tibial crest and over the malleoli.

condition due to the autonomic component of the neuropathy. Hydration is accomplished two ways. First, a warm moist terrycloth towel is wrapped around the foot and leg for approximately 10 minutes. This is followed by the application of an emollient cream to the foot and leg. The brand of cream is left to the discretion of the doctor; there are many that work well. A small wisp of cotton should then be placed in each toe webspace to reduce maceration while in the cast. Lambswool should be avoided, as it might strangulate a toe or cut into the skin in the webspace.

At this stage, a section of cast stockinette is applied to the limb. The material should be snug enough to hug the leg, with no rolls or creases. It should not be so tight, however, that it restricts blood flow. The stockinette should go from the knee distally and extend several inches beyond the toes. The material should be folded loosely dorsally to cover the toes. Paper tape is applied to hold this fold in place.

A small cut should be made in the stockinette at the anterior ankle joint line, as this is a common location for the material to crease. Once the cut is made, a piece of paper tape is applied to hold the edges together.

Since there is no padding within this cast, provision has to be made for safe removal. This is accomplished by applying a 3-inch-wide strip of $\frac{1}{8}$-inch-thick adhesive felt along the crest of the tibia. This strip should extend from the tibial tuberosity to the dorsum of the toes. A circular button of the same material approximately 3 inches in diameter is also applied over the malleoli (Fig. 22-7). It is very important that all of the edges of this material be skived extremely thin so as to reduce the risk of edge pressure (shear stress). This can be accomplished with an ordinary skiving knife. Once these pieces are in place, they are secured with strips of paper tape.

A piece of sponge rubber, approximately 4 inches by 4 inches, is taped in place over the toes. It should extend from the toe sulcus plantarly to the dorsum of the toes. This, too, is anchored by using paper tape. The foot elongates with each step; therefore, the function of the rubber piece is to prevent the toes from jamming against the inside of the cast.

At no point should any of these pieces of tape encircle the leg or foot. The small strips merely need to anchor the materials in place.

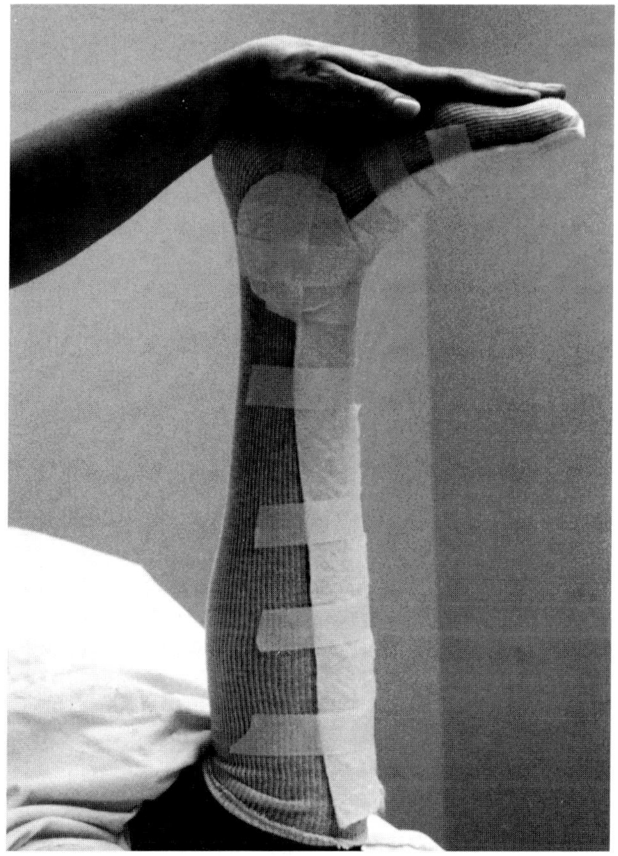

Fig. 22-7. The adhesive felt is skived along the edges and taped in place along the crest of the tibia. "Buttons" of felt cover the medial and lateral malleolus as well. The felt serves as protection against laceration from the cast saw. Note the perpendicular position of the foot relative to the leg. The toes are enclosed within the stockinette. There should not be any wrinkles or folds in the stockinette after it is applied.

Once the preliminary steps are complete, the first layer of plaster may be applied. Gypsona (Gypsona Plaster-Chaston, Inc., Melville, NY 11746) is a plaster material that is very creamy and extremely moldable. This property is critical for the interior layer of this type of cast. With the patient still in the prone position, the first layer is applied. A roll 4 inches wide by 5 yards long is applied from the toes to the tibial tuberosity. It is very important that this first layer be applied with no tucks, creases, or indentations in it (Fig. 22-8). If they do occur, the plaster should be removed and the cast started over. If left in place, the chances for complication due to increased pressure in those spots is dramatically increased. A second layer of Gypsona is applied to reinforce the first. Molding at this step is critical; the plaster should be molded carefully around the malleoli, the achilles tendon, into the medial arch, and around the anterior ankle joint line. The careful molding is what enables the cast to deliver the total contact (Fig. 22-9).

At this stage, the steps vary depending on whether one is applying a fiberglass or an all-plaster cast. Historically, the all-plaster cast has been described. There are advantages to both materials. The greatest advantage to the plaster cast is the cost factor. Plaster is far less expensive than the synthetic materials. Another advantage to the plaster is that it is easier to remove. The synthetics have the tendency to "snap back" after the cast spreader has been removed, making the spreading of the material more difficult.

Steps for a Plaster Cast

Two sets of 5-inch by 30-inch plaster splints are needed for this step. One group (five strips) is applied to the leg in a medial to lateral direction. The strips should extend from the medial side of the leg, go plantarly across the heel, and extend proximally up the lateral side of the leg. The second set of five splints should run in the direction of the plantar surface of the foot (starting at the toe sulcus) and extend proximally up the posterior surface of the

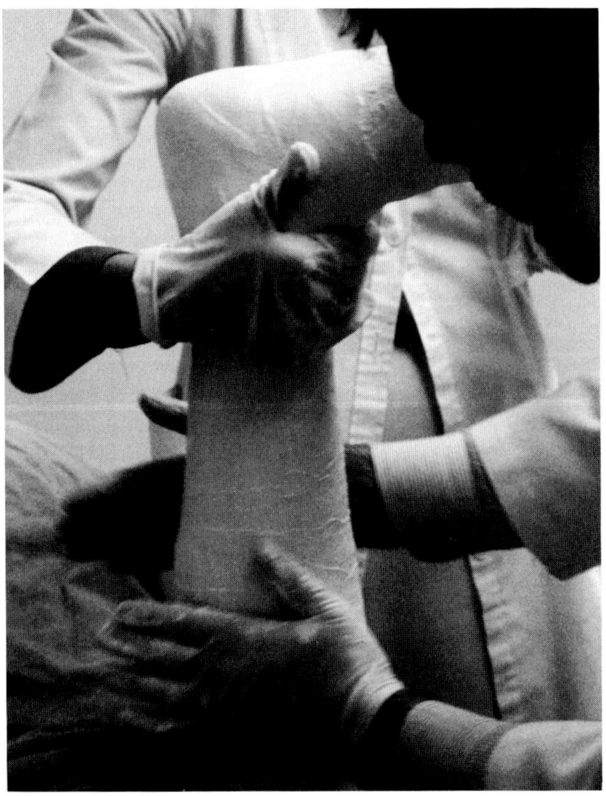

Fig. 22-8. Once the first layer of Gypsona is applied, the assistant must constantly maintain the foot and leg in position. The foot should be as perpendicular to the leg as possible. Note that the palms of the hand are used to mold the plaster, not the fingertips.

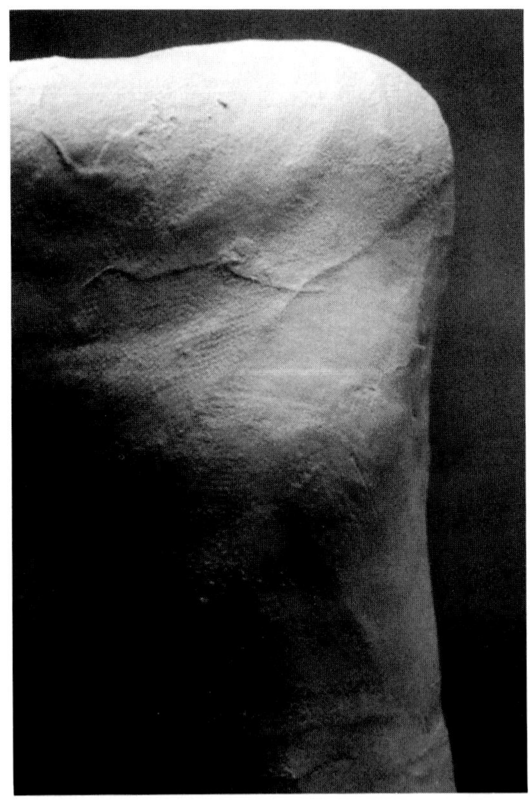

Fig. 22-9. There are no tucks, folds, or creases in the first layer of Gypsona. The textures should be like that of an eggshell. Note the degree of molding around the malleolus and the achilles tendon.

leg. The splints are molded well and locked in place with a 4-inch roll of plaster.

The next step is to address the plantar surface of the foot. A $\frac{1}{2}$-inch-thick piece of plywood cut into the shape of the foot is placed onto the bottom of the foot. The board should be arranged so that it is perpendicular with the longitudinal bisection of the leg. The spaces between the board and the bottom of the foot need to be filled in with small strips of plaster (Fig. 22-10). This is done so as to provide the board with a flat platform or surface on the bottom of the foot. A rubber walking peg is applied to the cast against the board as one would apply the peg to a regular cast.

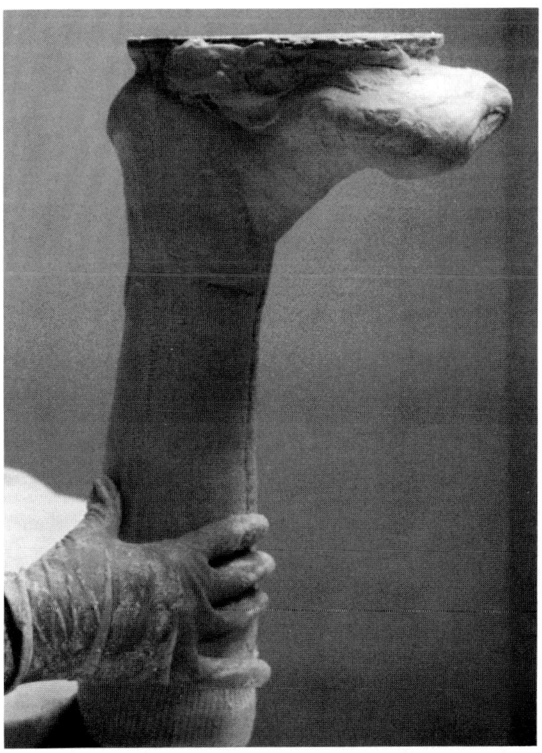

Fig. 22-10. Plaster strips are used to fill in the space between the foot and the board. This provides a stable flat surface for the walking heel. It also aids in distributing pressure evenly across the foot. The board should be perpendicular to the longitudinal bisection of the leg. The walking heel is fastened to the board as would be done on a regular fracture cast.

The final steps are to enclose the foot and cover the leg with two more rolls of 4-inch plaster. It is important to remember that plaster does not harden enough to support weight bearing for 48 hours. Therefore, the patient needs to provide some mechanism to remain non-weight bearing for that time period. Generally, crutches are the most effective and easiest way to accomplish this.

Advantages to the synthetic materials are that they are lighter in weight, they are more durable, and they "cure" faster, allowing the patient to bear full weight on them by the time they leave the office.

Steps for a Synthetic Cast

Once the initial Gypsona layer is applied, the next step is to support this layer with a roll of synthetic material. Generally, a roll of 4-inch cast tape is wrapped from the toes proximally to the top edge of the stockinette. This layer provides some strength to the Gypsona layer.

Following this, the plywood platform is applied in a way similar to the method used for the plaster cast. The only difference is that instead of filling in around the board with plaster strips, fiberglass material is used. Then the walking peg is applied in the way previously described. Finally, the entire cast is wrapped with a role of 4-inch fiberglass material to provide strength and support. This includes some wraps around and over the toes as well.

As mentioned earlier, the major advantage to the fiberglass as compared to the plaster is that the patient can bear weight on the cast in 30 minutes. This enables the patient to leave the office ambulating on the cast (Table 22-3).

The first cast should be changed after 48 hours. This is done for several reasons. The first has to do with the fit of the cast. This casting technique reduces pedal edema dramatically, and as a result, affects the fit of the cast. Therefore, to avoid a poorly fitting cast that may cause problems, the cast is changed early. Second, an early change of cast allows an early examination of the wound. Cast therapy has the potential to create anxiety in the treating physician because of all of the problems associated with casting the diabetic limb. Therefore, until the doctor has gained some confidence

Table 22-3. Fabrication of the Total Contact Cast

All steps should be done with the patient in a prone position.

I. Preparation of the foot
- A. *Ulcer*—Debride ulcer as necessary. Apply dressing, typically an antibiotic ointment, to ulcer with a 2-inch × 2-inch gauze sponge. This is held in place with paper tape. *No circlage dressing is applied,* as this would pose a risk of irritation to the skin or possible vascular compromise.
- B. *Charcot*—No specific wound care is necessary.
- C. Be sure that all toenails are debrided.
- D. Skin is well hydrated, using emollient of choice.
- E. Cotton may be placed between the toes to reduce maceration.

II. Cotton stockinette is applied to the foot and leg.
- A. Stockinette should be snug and form fitting.
- B. Fold stocking over the toes dorsally and tape it in place.
- C. Make a cut in the stockinette at anterior ankle and tape in place.

III. Apply a strip of ⅛-inch-thick, 2½-inch-wide adhesive felt along the tibial crest. This should extend from tuberosity of tibia to the dorsum of the toes. The edges of the felt should be skived thin.

IV. Cover each malleolus with a circular piece of felt also skived around the edge and tape in place.

V. Apply a 4-inch-square × 1-inch-thick piece of foam across the tips of the toes and tape it in place.

VI. Apply a 4-inch × 5-yard roll of Gypsona plaster extending from the toes proximally to the tibial tuberosity. It is very important that there be no tucks, bulges, or indentations in this layer of material.

VII. Apply a roll of fiberglass tape so as to cover the Gypsona.

VIII. Place a piece of ¼-inch plywood, cut into the shape of the foot, on the plantar surface. The board should be perpendicular to the long axis of the leg when viewed from the side. If it is not, it should be adjusted by placing strips of plaster under it to balance it until it is perpendicular.

IX. Place a conventional rubber walking heel on the board, proximal to the metatarsal heads, and affix using casting materials.

X. Wrap the cast from one end to the other (including the toes) with 1 to 2 more rolls of fiberglass.

XI. The patient must then remain non-weight bearing for ½ hour.

as well as experience with this therapy, the casts should be changed frequently. In addition, frequent changes allow close examination of the wound, with constant monitoring of the progress.

After a cast change visit, the patient is required to return to the office 48 hours later for a cast examination. During this visit the patient is questioned as to whether the patient perceived any problems with or within the cast. At the same time the cast is checked to make sure that it is still intact. If any cracks or breaks are noted or if the cast is soft in any areas, it must be removed and a new one applied.

Also during this visit the fit of the cast is checked. The examiner grabs ahold of the cast on the foot, then pushes and pulls on the cast. If the cast slides (pistons) up and down on the leg, the cast must be removed. If, on the other hand, the patient is practically being pulled off the seat with each tug on the cast, then there is a good fit and the cast is left in place.

Patients with plantar ulcers that are treated with this therapy should return to the office weekly for cast changes. The ulcer should be debrided as necessary. Once the ulcer is closed, the cast is an excellent means of protecting the foot from ulcer recurrence while the "definitive" shoe is being constructed. Once the shoes are ready, the patient may begin to wear the shoes, with partial weight bearing at first, to prevent stress fractures from occurring to bones that may have atrophied during the casting period.

Patients that are casted for Charcot disease generally endure the casting for a longer period of time. The average length of time from start to finish for a Charcot patient is 6 months. During that period, the cast is checked weekly, just as with the ulcer patients. Generally, however, if the fit is acceptable, each cast may remain in place longer since there is no open wound to be concerned about.

The cast is removed every 2 to 3 weeks, and radiographs are taken. In addition to radiographs, skin temperatures are also taken, as this is an excellent means to monitor the progress of the treatment. As previously mentioned, the goal of the cast therapy with the Charcot patient is to achieve consolidation of the involved bones and joints. Once this is achieved, the definitive therapy may be initiated at the doctors discretion. Once again, limited partial weight bearing should be initiated to allow the atrophied limb to strengthen.

Therapy with the total contact cast is but one part of a comprehensive approach to these most difficult patients. As any health care professional who has treated a diabetic patient with foot problems knows, the first steps in healing the immediate problem is in the recognition of the condition and in understanding the underlying pathology. Too many times, these conditions are written off as being associated with diabetic "microvascular disease," or poor healing potential because the underlying condition is diabetes. Instead of considering each case as one unto itself, they get pigeonholed into a class of "diabetic problems."

As mentioned earlier, there is more than one way to heal the diabetic plantar ulcer; however, the use of the ambulatory total contact cast provides some distinct advantages over other therapies. It does, however, come with some risks. In order to avoid the complications that may develop as a result of those risks, strict guidelines must be followed.

The diabetic patient is a "patient for life," and as such should be seen in the office frequently enough so as to provide the appropriate care needed to avoid the devastating complications. Treating these patients is extremely rewarding, but requires diligence and a thorough understanding of the pathologic process at work.

CASE STUDY

A 63-year-old man with a two-year history of a plantar ulceration presented to our office. This gentleman had diabetes mellitus for 18 years, and was insulin dependent.

On physical examination, he demonstrated bounding pulses at the dorsalis pedis and posterior tibial vessels bilaterally. Neurologic examination showed him to have a complete peripheral neuropathy, with total insensitivity from the midtibia distally. The right foot, which was the foot with the ulcer, presented with a rocker-bottom appearance as a result of a Charcot collapse of the midfoot.

The ulcer started as a callus directly under the prominence of the dislocated bone. The ulcer measured 2 cm in diameter and $\frac{3}{4}$ cm in depth. The base of the ulcer was clean (i.e., no fibrous tissue) and composed of healthy granulation tissue. There was no evidence of osteomyelitis or soft tissue infection noted (Fig. 22-11A).

For 2 years, this gentleman went to a plastic surgeon twice a week for debridements of the ulcer. According to the patient, no significant change in the size of the ulcer occurred over the 2-year period.

After it was ascertained that the etiology of the ulceration was the severe deformity of the foot and the extreme pressure associated with this deformity, it was decided that the patient would be placed into an ambulatory total contact cast. In this case, the purpose of the cast was to decrease and disperse more evenly the vertical forces of weight bearing.

The cast was applied following the appropriate guidelines and initial steps. Typically, the first case was changed after 48 hours due to the change in the fit of the cast. Most of the limbs that are casted are edematous, and this casting technique reduces the edema dramatically. Therefore, in order to maintain the total contact aspect of the cast, it must be replaced. This also allows for examination of the ulcer and foot.

As seen in Figure 22-11A, the borders and margins of the ulcer were discreet. Nineteen days after the first casting was initiated, significant improvement was noted (Fig. 22-11B). The base of the ulcer was shallower, and the diameter was reduced slightly.

At this point, the contact cast was changed approximately every 10 days. Exactly 4 months after the photograph in Figure 22-11A was taken, the ulcer was closed (Fig. 22-11C). The area was not quite healed, as there was still some keratosis present. This eventually disappeared due to further accommodation within the shoes.

This brief case represents one of the many successful results using the total contact cast as the primary treatment modality for the plantar ulceration. The rapid response in healing as evidenced by the photographs reinforces the premise that the

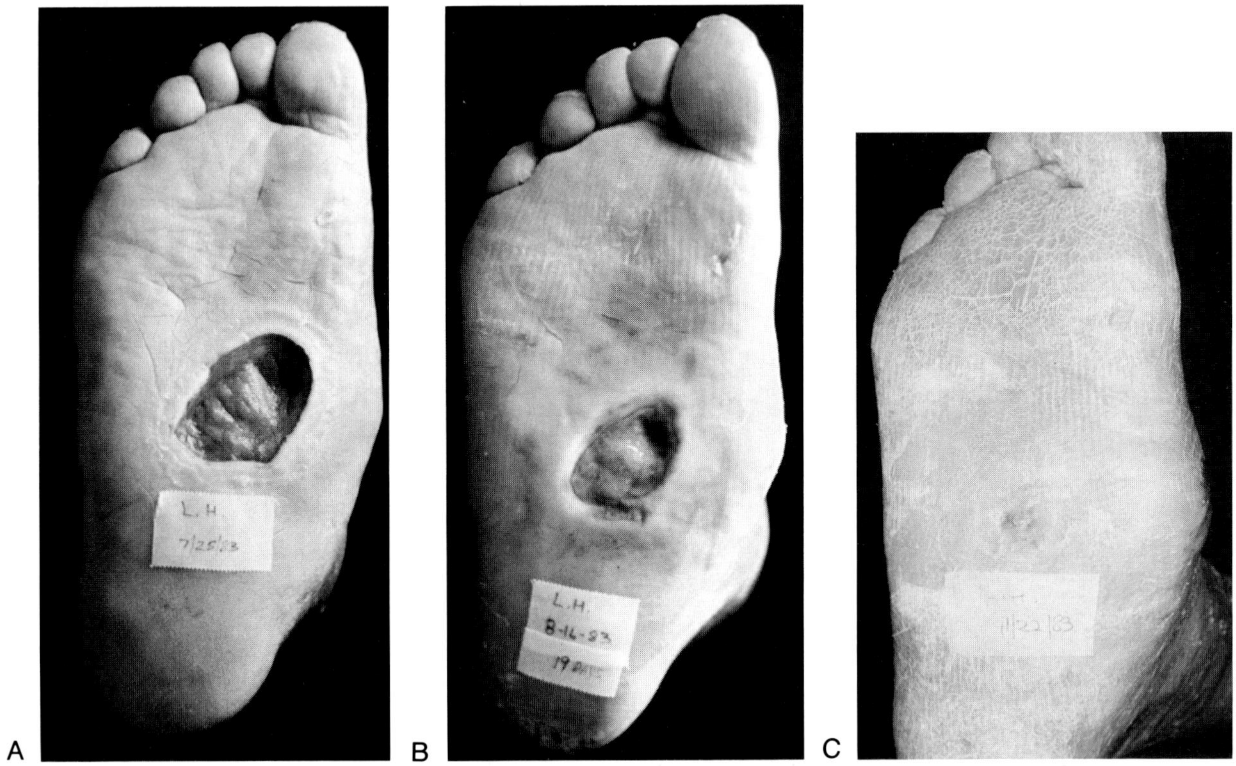

Fig. 22-11. (**A**) Ulcer on the right foot due to the extreme pressure associated with a Charcot collapse of the midfoot. (**B**) Appearance 19 days after the first casting. (**C**) Appearance 4 months after initial presentation.

plantar ulcers are caused by pressure and not small vessel disease.

REFERENCES

1. Bauman H, Girling JP, Brand PW: Plantar pressure and trophic ulceration. J Bone Joint Surg 45B:652, 1963
2. Coleman WC, Brand P, Birke J: The total contact cast: a therapy for plantar ulceration on insensitive feet. J Am Podiatr Med Assoc 11:548, 1987
3. Burnett O: The total contact cast. Clin Podiatr Med Surg 4:471, 1987
4. Boulton A, Hardisty C, Betts R et al: Dynamic foot pressure and other studies as diagnostic and management aids in diabetic neuropathy. Diabetes Care 6:26, 1983
5. Mueller M, Diamond J: Biomechanical treatment approach to diabetic plantar ulcers. Phys Therap 68:1917, 1988
6. LoGerfo F, Coffman J: Vascular and microvascular disease of the foot in diabetes. New Engl J Med 311:1615, 1984
7. Birke J, Sims DS, Buford WL: Walking casts: effect on plantar foot pressures. J Rehabil Res Dev 22:18, 1985

SUGGESTED READINGS

Ctercteko GC, Dhanendran M, Hutton W, Le Quesne P: Vertical forces acting on the feet of diabetic patients with neuropathic ulceration. Br J Surg 68:608, 1981

Gramuglia VJ, Palmarozzo PM, Rzonca E: Biomechanical concepts in the treatment of ulcers in the diabetic foot. Clin Podiatr Med Surg 5:613, 1988

Helm P, Walker S, Pulluim G: Total contact casting in

diabetic patients with neuropathic foot ulcerations. Arch Phys Med Rehabil 65:691

Hollander MR, Holton K, Mader D: Total contact providone-iodine perfusion cast for the treatment of neuropathic ulcers. J Foot Surg 25:484, 1986

Lippman HT, Perotto A, Farrar R: The neuropathic foot of the diabetic. Bull NY Acad Med 52:1159, 1976

Mooney V, Wagner WF: Neurocirculatory disorders of the foot. Clin Orthop 122:53, 1977

Pizur M, Smith D, Osterman H: Salvage of the infected or failed below-knee amputations with total contact casting and continued weight bearing. Orthopedics 11:437, 1988

Robson M, Edstrom L: The diabetic foot: an alternative approach to major amputation. Surg Clin North Am 57:1089, 1987

23

Prostheses and Orthoses for the Foot and Ankle

Gustav Rubin, M.D., F.A.C.S.
Ellen Cohen, D.P.M., Ph.D.
Edward C. Rzonca, D.P.M., F.A.C.F.O., D.A.B.P.O.

Diabetic neurovascular disease, with its accompanying arterial occlusion, loss of sensation, and loss of sensory feedback, is a potential antecedent of foot pathology. This includes ulceration secondary to shear and pressure trauma, flaccid paralysis of peripheral nerves, Charcot's disease of the foot or ankle, and even, ultimately, amputation. The aim of this chapter is to present current prosthetic and orthotic treatment modalities for problems such as these. The discussion that follows will be divided into separate prosthetic and orthotic sections as indicated below.

Mobility is often the key to survival. In less sophisticated societies, the individual may move about even on the stump of his partially amputated foot. Indeed, even in our present seemingly advanced state of knowledge about the biomechanics and treatment of the partial foot amputee, there are those who consider it unnecessary to provide the partial foot amputee with anything more than a shoe with a toe filler.[1]

It is important to consider the advantages of specific shoe corrections for the more distal levels of partial foot amputation as well as prosthetic devices and shoe corrections for the more proximal levels of amputation.

When the foot has been partially amputated, the foot lever has become shortened and less effective for push-off. Varying degrees of impairment of stability have occurred, and distal plantar push-off pressures have been introduced to areas that have either never been subjected to such forces, or, at best, have lost other supportive areas that would have allowed a broader distribution of push-off forces.

Shoe corrections should be introduced that would allow extension of the foot lever (long steel spring), substitution for the absent toe break (rocker bar), and, if ankle plantar flexion has been eliminated by the prosthetic or orthotic device, the solid ankle cushion heel (SACH) should be used to simulate plantar flexion and absorb impact.

The indications for appropriate prosthetic and orthotic devices and the applicable shoe corrections will be discussed below. Shoe inserts to cushion impact and protect localized areas of foot pathology may be applied over the prosthetic or orthotic device on the foot-device interface.

When the amputation is through the forefoot, as much length as possible should be preserved. When infection is present, a two-stage amputation may be necessary; that is, an open first stage and a definitive second stage after control of infection. Although it is possible to salvage a Chopart or a

Lisfranc amputation, these are generally undesirable amputation levels for adults (see below).

Most often the indication for amputation of the adult foot will be vascular insufficiency. Basic guidelines for amputation levels have undergone little change in recent years.[2] When only the distal phalanx of a toe manifests gangrene, the likelihood of complete healing after toe amputation is good. If one or more toes are gangrenous in their entirety, healing is more likely to be achieved if a transmetatarsal amputation is done. If the gangrene is more extensive and involves as much as a third of the foot, the most conservative amputation of the foot presents a potential for breakdown and should be avoided.

It is desirable to delay amputation, if the infection can be localized, until a line of demarcation develops.[3] The decision for delay must be carefully weighed against the general condition of the patient and the need to ward off rapid spread of infection. This is a surgical judgment.

Antibiotics will usually control infection, but if the patient is toxic, delay will probably not be possible, and a two-stage amputation may be indicated, the first stage to eliminate the infected area, and the second to amputate at a higher level to provide a definitive stump after control of infection.

When the amputation is nonemergent, a one-stage amputation should be done. Where the skin is thin and shiny and without hair growth, circulation will be poor. If the tissue above the area of gangrene is cyanotic and cyanosis persists during the elevation-depression test, this should be considered an additional manifestation of deficient circulation. Wagner describes the following[3]:

> Transcutaneous ultrasound has been coupled with the Doppler effect to provide an instrument that acts as a sensitive stethoscope or flow detector. . . . The ischemic index is calculated for each level by dividing the systolic pressure by the brachial artery pressure. . . . Study of a series of diabetic lower extremity amputations has shown over 93.3 percent successful healing when the ischemic index is over 0.45 at the level of amputation. Similar results were obtained in nondiabetics if the ischemic index is over 0.35.

BASIC SURGICAL PROCEDURES

Toe Amputation

It may not be feasible to use a long plantar flap; if it is not, then equal short flaps will be quite satisfactory. If the pathology is well localized to the toe tip, amputation through the proximal phalanx should be considered. If gangrene is more proximal, it may be necessary to amputate through the neck of the metatarsal, removing the toe and metatarsal head. This is least desirable in the case of the first and fifth toes. A preferred procedure would be toe disarticulation. The final decision will be dependent on the surgical judgment of the operator.

Transmetatarsal Amputation

If the diabetic gangrene is well demarcated, the infection controlled, and the gangrene does not extend into the web spaces, transmetatarsal amputation is feasible.[2,4] The incision should not be made through an area where there is absent sensation. The previously mentioned ischemic index guideline will be useful.

Ultimately, the final choice of the level of amputation will be decided at the operating table by the surgeon and will depend on the skin bleeding. Wagner states that "when the skin bleeds within three minutes after release of the (thigh) tourniquet there is an 80–85% successful healing."[3]

For transmetatarsal amputation, a transverse dorsal incision is made following the curve of the toes and extending down to bone. The metatarsals are sectioned and their edges smoothed. The tendons are placed under tension, severed, and not reattached. Closure is accomplished by bringing the longer plantar flap anteriorly. Kritter has used an irrigation tube placed though a stab wound on the dorsum of the foot and this is removed after 2 or 3 days.[3] Following removal of the tube, a cast is applied and the diabetic patient is allowed to ambulate in the cast after about 10 days.

Proximal Levels of Amputation

The prosthetist is not infrequently presented with the problem of fitting levels of amputation that may include the Lisfranc, Chopart, or hindfoot (Fig. 23-1) amputation, and occasionally even a Pirogoff or a Boyd procedure. These are not levels of amputation advisably selected for the adult vascularly impaired limb. They are usually the result of either an attempt to save all length of the traumatic amputation as a definitive procedure or as a planned first stage operation with a view to later revision. Not unusually, a patient will refuse the later revision, hoping to retain as much of the anatomy as possible. This is unfortunate and will present the prosthetist with a fitting problem.

The Boyd and Pirogoff procedures introduce the need to await bony union of the stump (residual limb) to the distal tibia. Such union is not easy to obtain, thereby extensively prolonging the rehabilitation process. Because of the excessively long stump, prosthetic fitting is a problem since there is not adequate room for a conventional prosthetic foot.

In the case of the adult, the Lisfranc amputation presents a borderline prosthetic fitting problem and can be successfully fitted if the equinus deformity is prevented by tendon transplant. The unmodified Chopart, in equinus, is to be condemned, although that level of amputation may be salvaged by the same method as with the Lisfranc or even by ankle fusion.[1] It is unfortunate that ankle fusion is not invariably successful and may require reoperation.

Amputations of the Child's Foot

Most amputations of the feet in children are post-traumatic. An occasional amputation may be

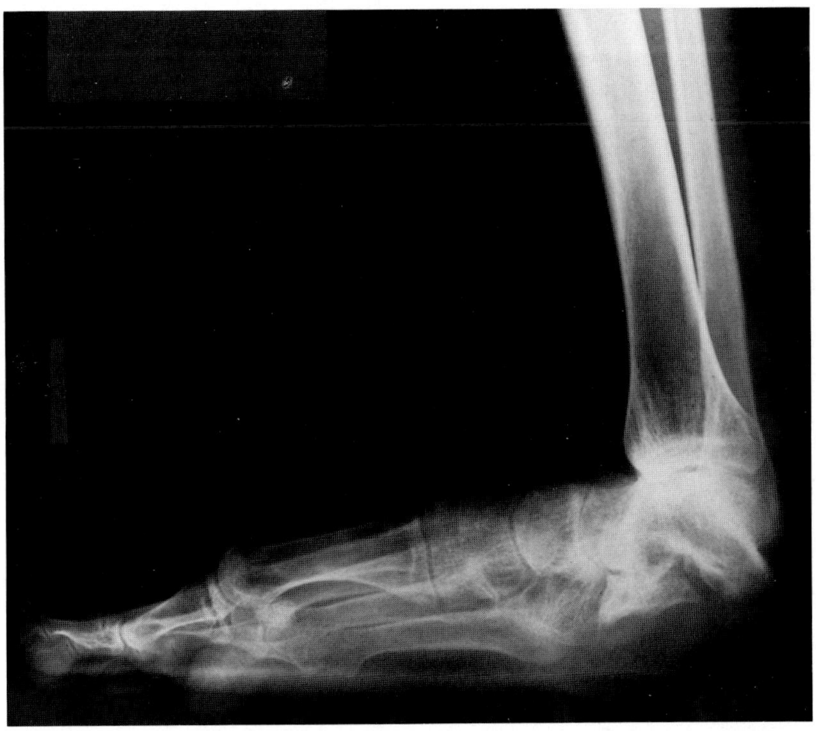

Fig. 23-1. War wound resulting in loss of bone elements of the hind foot. (From Rubin and Fischer,[55] with permission.)

secondary to a tumorous condition or a congenital abnormality, but trauma, such as a lawn mower accident, is the more frequent cause. Diabetic neurovascular disease is not a causative factor.

A review of children's partial foot amputation by Green et al.[5] concluded that the Lisfranc and Chopart were satisfactory procedures if the equinus contractures were prevented. When an equinus contracture was present, the Chopart provided the child amputee with a poorly functioning residual limb as compared with the Syme amputation, with respect to endurance, range of activity, and gait. In the latter instance, the child with the Chopart stump in equinus has the same problems as the adult with a similarly deformed Chopart.

Syme Amputation

The Syme amputation has been well documented and remains little changed since Dr. Syme first described it almost 150 years ago.[4] When indicated in situations such as trauma, tumors, and congenital deformities, the properly prepared Syme stump is an excellent amputation. Since detailed descriptions of the Syme amputation are readily available and are basically similar, the operation will not be described here.[3,4] If the heel pad is intact in the nonischemic limb, the one-stage Syme procedure can usually be done. When infection is present, it may be accomplished in two stages, initially an ankle disarticulation and secondarily a definitive procedure.

The two-stage procedure has been successful in a high percentage of diabetic patients when the previously described criterion for skin bleeding was employed, that is, incisional skin bleeding within 3 minutes after removal of a thigh tourniquet.

One of the problems with the two-stage procedure arises when the surgeon, inexperienced in prosthetic fitting, is able to obtain satisfactory secondary closure and accepts the ankle disarticulation as a definitive stump. It is a simple procedure to transect and remove the malleoli through small separate incisions.

PROSTHETIC MATERIALS

These may be classified into three broad groups: (1) shoe modification materials for the distal partial foot amputee, and the amputee requiring a solid ankle prosthesis; (2) materials employed to fabricate ankle-foot orthoses (AFOs) for the mid-foot amputee; and (3) materials employed to fabricate AFOs for the proximal and hind-foot amputees. The indications for the use of each of the materials referred to will be outlined in the section that follows.

The shoe may be modified by the addition of a flat long steel spring (16 or 18 gauge) placed in the sole from heel to toe, a rocker bar, and a SACH.[6] The SACH heel is compressible, absorbs impact at heel strike, and by virtue of its compressibility on heel strike simulates plantar flexion to a limited degree. The indications for the use of the materials mentioned in this section will be described below and will vary with the level of amputation and the device prescribed.

The AFOs for the midfoot amputee may be either the shoe attachment type or shoe insert type.[6,7] The shoe attachment type usually employed for the partial foot amputee consists of aluminum or steel double bar brace uprights, a solid ankle, or limited-motion ankle joint (5° in each direction, that is, plantar flexion and dorsiflexion) and stirrups attached to the shoe.

The aluminum uprights are lighter in weight, but less sturdy than the steel. The steel uprights are indicated for a heavy or very active individual.

The shoe insert AFO most commonly employed is fabricated of polypropylene, which is vacuum-formed over a cast of the limb and has a toe filler of Plastazote (Fig. 23-2). Polypropylene belongs to the olefin group of chemicals and is the most rigid of the olefins. Polyethylene, a member of the same family, not only has less rigidity but also has a poorer "memory," that is, after a period of flexion-extension use, it will not return to its original position, whereas polypropylene will do so. The shoe insert polypropylene's flexibility may be modified by the degree to which the posterior section of the upright is narrowed in the mediolateral direction

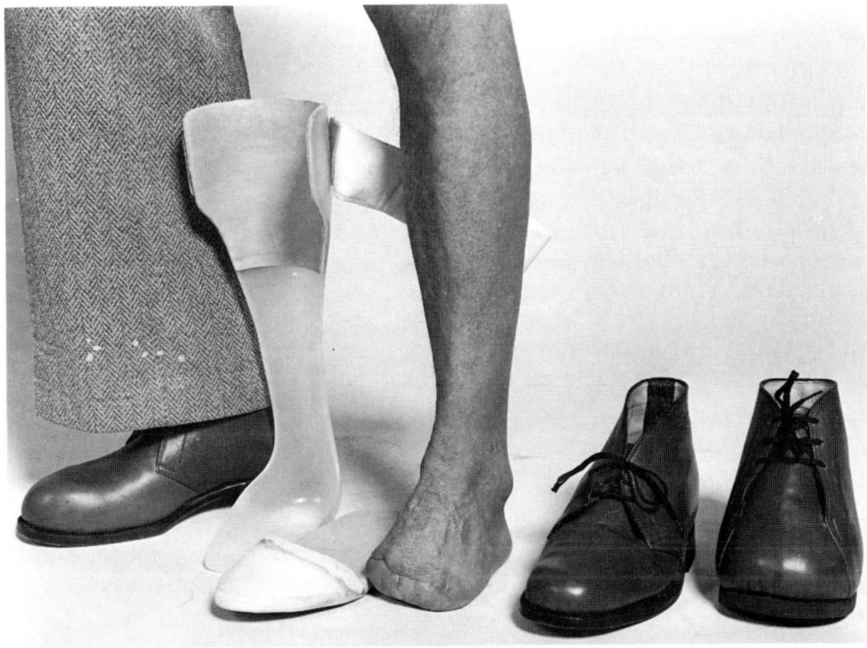

Fig. 23-2. Shoe insert ankle foot orthosis with toe filler for a transmetatarsal amputation. (From Rubin and Fischer,[55] with permission.)

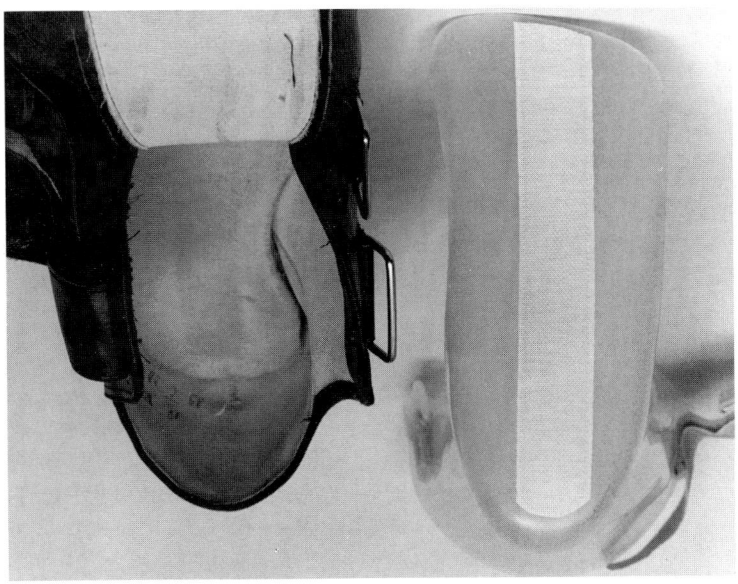

Fig. 23-3. Velcro stabilization of the partial foot polypropylene prosthesis.

posterior to the ankle (and graduating proximally) by the prosthetist. Both materials are vacuum formable.

Plastazote (Bakalite xylonite Ltd, U.K.) is a closed-cell polyethylene foam and is vacuum-formable if it has not been perforated. Pe-Lite (Bakalite xylonite Ltd, U.K.) is a similar material but somewhat more resistant to compression than Plastazote. Although both tend to "bottom-out," that is, not return to their original thickness after a time, they are useful for shoe inserts and are readily replaced if deformed. Soft inserts should be placed over the foot contact surface of the polypropylene shoe insert for sensitive, diabetic, or deformed feet.

On the inferior surface of the AFO and the opposing surface of the inner sole of the shoe it is advisable to attach matching Velcro strips (Fig. 23-3) to lock the AFO into place and thereby prevent slippage within the shoe.

AFOs for the proximal foot amputee, such as the Lisfranc or Chopart, must encompass the stump and leg entirely in order to transfer the forces generated during walking to the prosthesis.[4] A rigid device is therefore required (Fig. 23-4). As a first step in the preparation of the rigid prosthesis, the residual limb is wrapped with plaster of paris (calcium sulfate) and a negative mold prepared. The prosthetist will prepare a positive mold from this and the positive mold will be modified to provide relief for bone prominences and tender areas and to build up soft tissue areas that could more readily tolerate pressure.

A soft insert of a heat-moldable material such as Pe-Lite is drawn over a plaster mold and fitted to it. Nylon stockinette and Dacron felt are layered over the soft insert and a snugly fitted polyvinyl alcohol (PVA) sleeve is pulled over the positive mold, which is held upright in a clamp with the aid of a mandrel (an iron bar centrally placed within the cast) that had been positioned in the center of the positive plaster of paris mold before it hardened. The liquid polyester resin is mixed with a promoter and a catalyst. The combination is poured from above into the PVA sleeve and over the contained positive mold with its overlying stockinette and felt. As this is done the prosthetist blends the resin into the Dacron felt and nylon stockinette until they are thoroughly impregnated. After the resin has hardened, the mandrel and its plaster of paris positive are broken out of the mold and the prosthesis is trimmed.

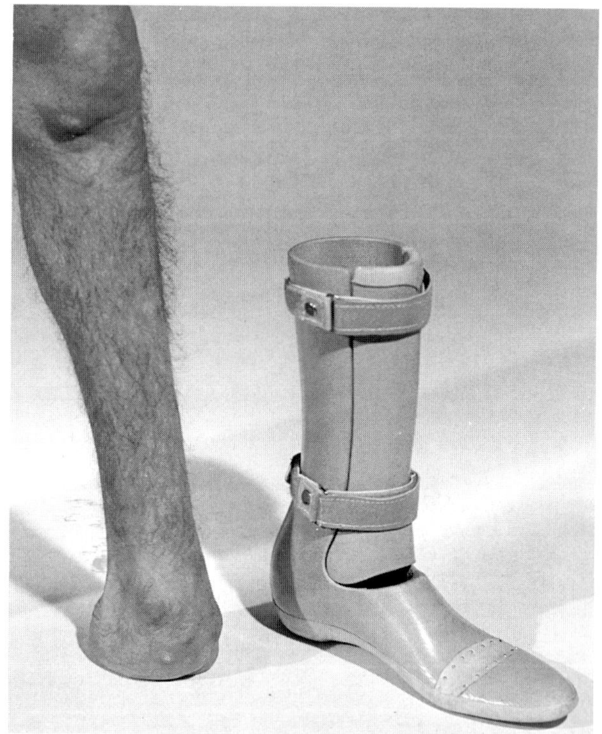

Fig. 23-4. Clamshell Chopart prosthesis. (From Rubin and Fischer,[55] with permission.)

Shoe Corrections and Prostheses for the Partial Foot Amputee

Absence of the first toe, multiple toes, an entire ray or rays adversely affects stability and push-off. A long steel spring (see above), 16 or 18 gauge, is inserted into the sole of the shoe.[5] This will extend the foot lever to restore length lost by the absence of anatomic elements, add spring to push-off, and increase stability. Deformity at the toe break of the shoe will be avoided as well. Since there will be a long steel spring stiffening the sole and an absent toe break, a rocker bar should be added to aid roll-over. This is usually $\frac{3}{16}$ to $\frac{1}{4}$ inch in height. When this

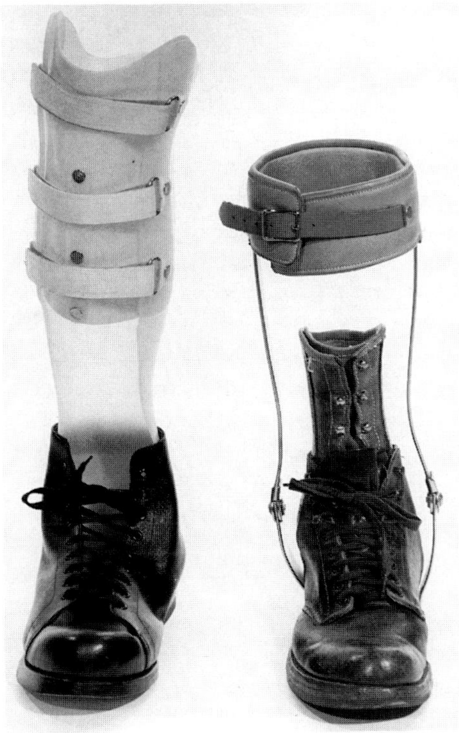

Fig. 23-5. A shoe insert type of PTB orthosis employed as a prosthesis for the hind-foot amputee is shown on the left. On the right is an old-style prosthesis.

is used, the heel of the involved shoe should be raised an equal amount but, to restore balance, it is important to remember to raise the heel of the other shoe.

These modifications are employed for major toe or ray amputations or distal transmetatarsal areas. For the more distal amputations in this group, which are uncomplicated, polypropylene shoe insert AFOs are modified by trimming of the posterior upright to allow plantar flexion on heel strike and dorsiflexion on push-off. A long steel spring and rocker bar correction are included in the shoe.

When the amputation is through the proximal metatarsals, the AFO is not trimmed posterior to the malleoli and remains rigid to fully stabilize the foot. The long steel spring and rocker bar are included, and, in addition, in view of the absence of ankle motion, a SACH heel is added. If there is mild edema, an elastic stocking may be used under a polypropylene shoe insert prosthesis. If there is significant edema or absent sensation, the shoe insert AFO is contraindicated and an external double bar shoe attachment AFO should be used.

If the Lisfranc procedure has been carried out and modified by tendon transplant to retain dorsiflexion, the above prosthesis and shoe corrections may be employed. If not, then the classic plastic laminated Chopart prosthesis is the most satisfactory functional approach, although this leaves much to be desired cosmetically.

The hindfoot (absent calcaneus) amputee requires the patellar tendon bearing (PTB) double bar device.[3] Because the socket resembles that of the socket for the below knee amputee, this device functions to partially unweight the heel area (Fig. 23-5).

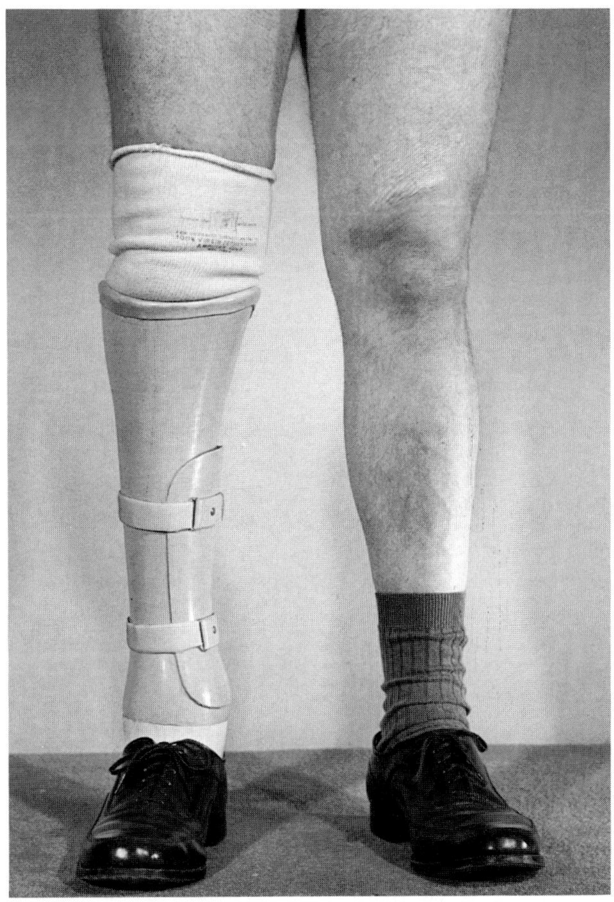

Fig. 23-6. The windowed Syme prosthesis.

Prosthesis for the Total Foot Amputee

The Syme amputation results in the removal of the entire foot. As a consequence, the prosthesis must incorporate an artificial foot. Although the Chopart prosthesis had to be fabricated in a clamshell design to allow the residual limb to enter it, the Syme residual limb, or stump, can enter the modern Syme prosthesis from above.[2,6] The modern designs are fabricated of plastic laminate using polyester (or acrylic) resin as previously described. The acrylic may be used if there is demonstrated sensitivity to polyester resin. Older Syme prostheses, prior to the plastic age, were of reinforced leather laced anteriorly, sometimes with a heavy, metal, movable ankle, the Berlin ankle. These components are no longer used. The foot is usually a Syme SACH or a somewhat more mobile Syme solid ankle flexible endoskeleton (SAFE) artificial foot as contrasted to the solid keel of the SACH.

There are two basic types of Syme prostheses: the windowed Syme, usually with the window placed medially (Fig. 23-6); and the closed Syme fabricated without the window.

The Syme stump has an hourglass shape with broadening across the malleoli distally. The stump enters the socket from above and the broad distal end is passed through the proximal part of the window, bypassing the narrow waist of the socket, and is then brought back through the distal end of the window. The window can be closed with Velcro. This closure over the narrow waist achieves very efficient suspension of the socket on the stump without piston motion of the stump within the socket on walking.

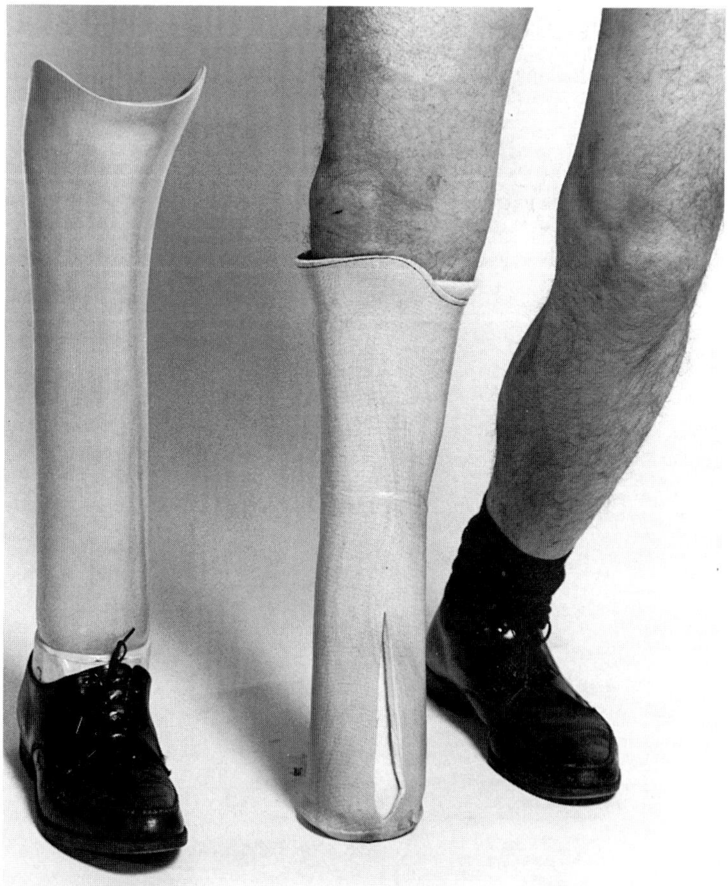

Fig. 23-7. The closed Syme prosthesis. Note the split insert.

The Syme prosthesis is fabricated without a window when the patient is overweight or very active, since the window weakens the prosthesis structurally. This type of prosthesis is tubular and chimney-shaped. The insert must be split to allow the stump to bypass the narrow area (Figs. 23-7 and 23-8). The outer configuration of the insert is similar to that of the socket so that it can enter the socket without difficulty. The inner configuration conforms to the residual limb.

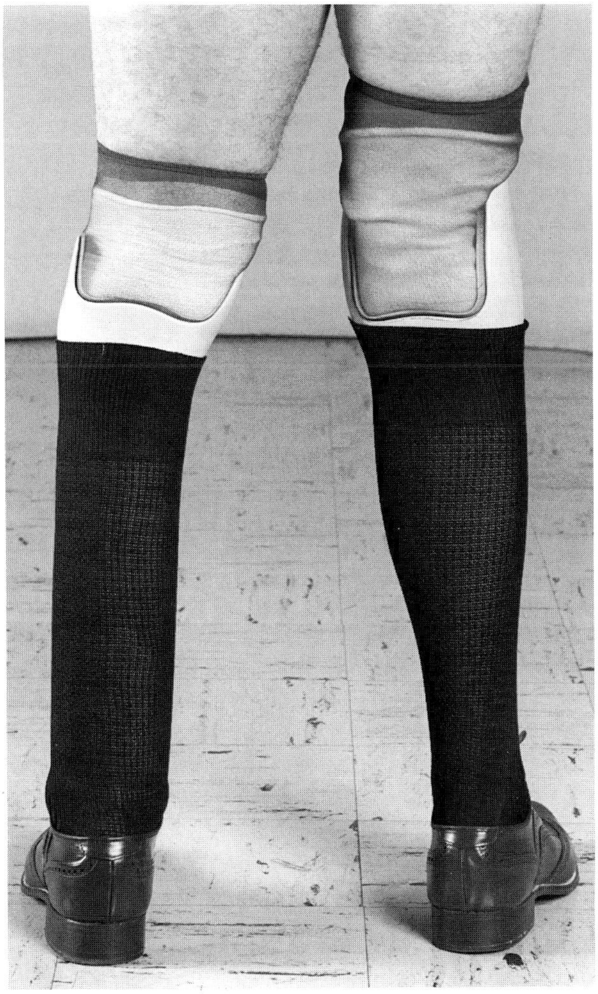

Fig. 23-8. Closed Syme prosthesis on the left and patellar tendon bearing prosthesis for below knee amputee on the right. Note the difference in cosmesis, that is, the tubular appearance of the closed Syme.

Amputation Problems

Unnecessary problems may be introduced when the surgeon applies extensive split thickness skin grafts to the distal end of a transmetatarsal amputation. This usually results in breakdown. A poorly stabilized Syme stump soft tissue pad will result in loss of the important end-bearing feature (Fig. 23-9). Syme amputations that are poorly planned and are not true Syme procedures will also result in stumps that cannot end-bear (Fig. 23-10).

In an attempt to save all length, retention of bone fragments may cause fitting problems for the prosthetist and difficulty in walking for the amputee. An egregious example of poor selection of components is illustrated in Figure 23-11. In this instance a Syme amputee was provided with an unstable high-top shoe and crutches. Good surgical judgment, meticulous surgery and aftercare, and appropriate selection of components and prosthetic fitting are all essential if the amputee is to be properly rehabilitated.

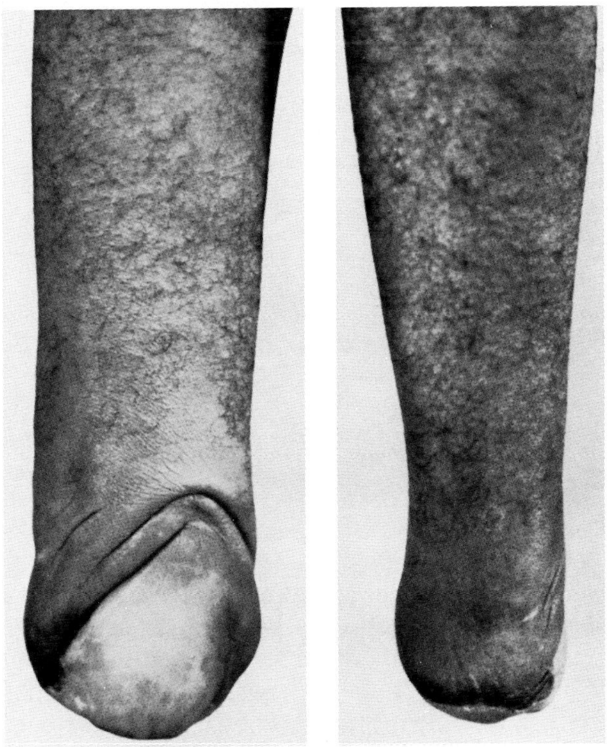

Fig. 23-9. A displaced Syme distal pad.

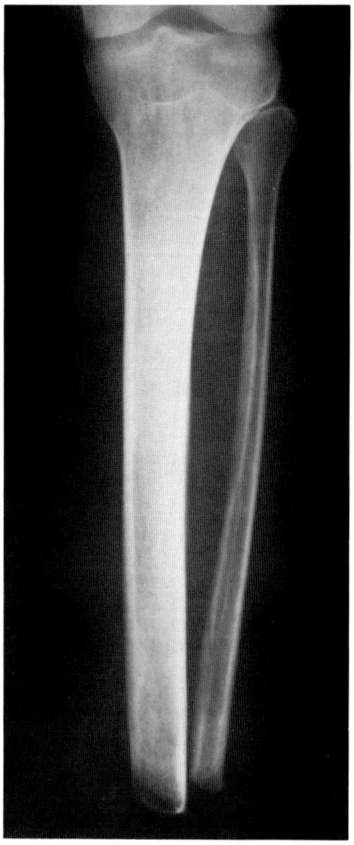

Fig. 23-10. Long amputation above the Syme level.

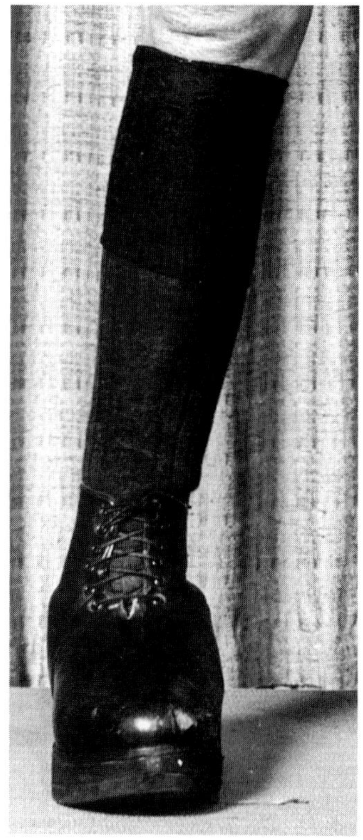

Fig. 23-11. A Syme amputee with a high-top shoe. (Modified Rubin et al.,[56] with permission.)

ANKLE-FOOT ORTHOSES

The use of the ankle-foot orthosis (AFO) for the diabetic foot is a subject that is frequently overlooked. There are numerous reports about the effectiveness of various insoles and orthotics[8–18] and special shoes to aid the diabetic patient.[19–22] However, diabetic patients have many problems both intrinsic to their diabetes and in addition to their diabetes that require the use of an AFO.

A large number of diabetic patients suffer with a peripheral neuropathy that results in a flaccid drop foot.[23] This group would benefit from an AFO. Many diabetic patients with Charcot feet need a patellar tendon bearing brace (PTB) to partially unweight the rear foot. Finally, many diabetic patients with upper motor neuron involvement including stokes, trauma, tumor, and multiple sclerosis require bracing.

There are certain differences that exist in bracing a diabetic patient with a stroke versus a nondiabetic patient with a similar condition. This section will deal with the use of the AFO with special elaboration of the diabetic individual.

The AFO is the most commonly used orthosis.[28] It is used in cases of paralysis and paresis from upper and lower motor neuron disease, weakness from motor pathology, and to prevent development of deformity.[29] The most common indication for the AFO is drop-foot gait.[30] The AFO is primarily a device for ambulatory patients who need help in walking. These patients can walk without the orthosis but they will tend to fall, stumble, and twist their ankles. The AFO is also used for the bedridden patient to prevent drop-foot contractures.

The specific purposes for prescribing AFOs are most commonly the following: (1) to provide toe pickup during swing phase to prevent dragging of the toe and tripping and falling; (2) to provide push-off stimulation during the latter part of stance phase; and (3) to provide medial-lateral stability at the ankle during stance to prevent inadvertent twisting of the ankle.[29] Table 23-1 summarizes some common uses of the AFO, exclusive of the PTB type of AFO, which will be discussed later.

There are a few basic generic types of AFOs. These include the traditional double upright steel or aluminum AFO, the polypropylene orthosis, Teufel (ortholene), spiral, shoe clasp, and patellar-tendon-bearing AFO. These will be discussed below.

Nomenclature

Type or class of orthosis is now designated by the joints or segments that it encompasses.[24] For example, what was previously referred to as a short leg brace is now known as an AFO because it encompasses the ankle joint. The former long leg brace is now classified as a knee-ankle-foot orthosis (KAFO) because it crosses both the knee and the ankle joint. The common "orthotic" that we use in podiatry is a foot orthosis (FO).

In the past orthoses were often prescribed on the basis of "disease bracing" with the automatic prescriptions for certain appliances to correspond to specific diseases. There is now an organized systematic approach to analysis of the patient for prescription on a biomechanical basis.[25]

McCollough lists five steps leading to the orthotic prescription. These include the biomechanical analysis, functional disability based on the biomechanical analysis, desired orthotic control, appropriate orthotic components, and the components combined into a prescription.[26] The orthosis controls joint motion in five general ways:

1. Free: allows free motion in any direction of the joint
2. Assist: application of external force for purposes of increasing range of motion
3. Resist: application of external force for purpose of decreasing velocity of force in desired motion
4. Stop: includes static unit to deter undesired motion
5. Hold: elimination of all motion in prescribed plane

A simplified example of how this system may be applied follows: A patient who on biomechanical analysis is found to have weak ankle dorsiflexors, a disability that causes loss of toe clearance during swing phase resulting in a drop-foot gait, is presented for evaluation. The orthotic control desired would be a dorsiflexion assist. The orthotic components considered most desirable for functional and cosmetic purposes would be a polypropylene AFO. The prescription selected would be a posterior leaf spring polypropylene AFO, which would provide a dorsiflexion assist.

Rubin lists eight steps leading to the prescription of an orthotic device.[27] These include (1) patient history, (2) job and life-style, (3) health, (4) gait, (5) functional requirements of components, (6) selection of components, (7) acceptance by patient, and (8) prescription. Of these he considers gait to be the most important single aspect of prescribing an orthosis. The gait abnormality is carefully analyzed and an orthotic device designed to correct that abnormality is selected.

Table 23-1. Common Conditions Requiring Ankle-Foot Orthoses

Malfunction	*Deficiency*	*Conditions*
Ankle dorsiflexors weak or absent	Loss of toe clear-swing-through	Drop-foot gait
Spasticity of posterior compartment	Plantar flexors tightly contracted	Equinus spastic gait
Absence of peroneal muscle function	Lateral instability of ankle joint also caused by torn ligaments or fixed deformity	Ankle sprain
Ankle plantar flexors weak or absent	Loss of push-off midstance to toe off	Apropulsive gait

Double Upright Ankle-Foot Orthosis

The double upright AFO was the standard brace used for drop-foot and various upper motor neuron lesions such as stroke, central nervous system (CNS) disorders, and lower motor neuron lesions such as poliomyelitis[31,32] (Fig. 23-12). It consists of two metal uprights whose proximal ends are connected to a metal or plastic calf band. The distal end of each upright is connected to a shoe stirrup through an intervening ankle-level orthotic joint. The stirrup is riveted directly to the sole of the shoe under the anterior section of the heel. The stirrup connects the shoe with the upright. The basic purpose of the device is to provide dorsiflexion assistance during swing and/or to stop or limit plantar flexion.

The variations in the double bar AFO functions are achieved by adjustments of the ankle joint.[33] The ankle joint can completely stop all motion for a patient with a very painful or arthritic joint. A plantar flexion stop may be employed to control spasticity. A dorsiflexion stop accommodates weak plantar flexors and avoids heel walking. A dorsiflexion assist is used for a drop foot to pick up the foot to clear the ground during swing phase of gait.

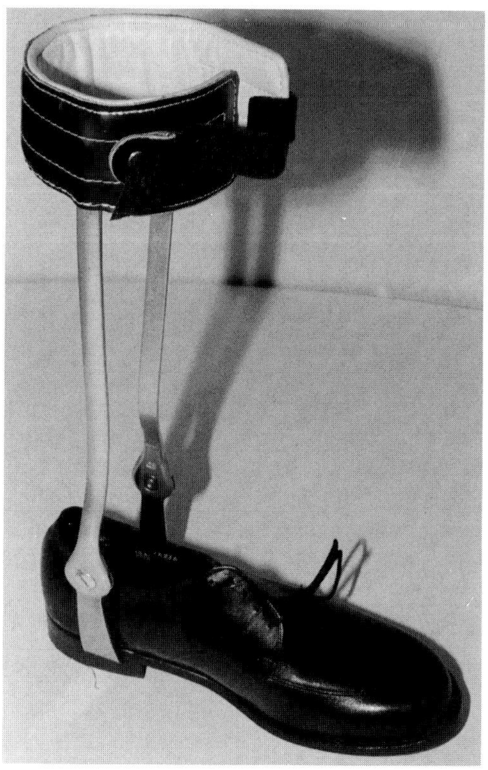

Fig. 23-12. Standard double upright metal orthosis. (From Rubin and Cohen,[57] with permission.)

A Blucher-type shoe with a leather sole, rubber heel, and strong shank is sufficient for a double-bar AFO with ankle joint motion. However, when the ankle joint motion is restricted by modification to a solid ankle or plantar flexion stop, a SACH is added to simulate plantar flexion on heel strike and cushion heel impact. A rocker bar aids rollover and dorsiflexion at heel off. A steel spring attached to the sole of the shoe aids push-off.[34] See Table 23-2 for summary of shoe corrections.

A varus T-strap, which is essentially a pull strap encompassing the lateral ankle with a fixation point on the medial bar of the orthosis, provides control of lateral ankle instability (Fig. 23-13).

The single-bar AFO has one metal upright on the lateral side. It has similar indications for use as the double bar, except that it may be fabricated to allow limited rotation of the orthotic joint. The round bar rotating single upright is accompanied by subtalar motion of the foot within the shoe.[35]

For ambulatory patients who need help walking due to various neuromuscular problems such as flaccidity, drop foot, or spasticity, the plastic AFOs have largely replaced the steel double-bar orthosis. The double-bar AFO is now used mainly in patients for whom a shoe insert may be contraindicated, such as those with leg edema or sensory deficit.[36]

In the diabetic patient a plastic shoe insert orthosis is often contraindicated due to both insensitivity and edema. It is desirable to keep the diabetic foot in contact with a soft shoe material rather than the hard plastic of a shoe insert type of AFO. Also, the foot plate and trimlines of the plastic orthosis may be too tight for the insensitive foot.

Polypropylene Ankle-Foot Orthosis

Plastic orthoses have now largely replaced the traditional steel double upright AFO. The most common materials are polypropylene, polyethylene, polycarbonate, and laminated plastics. The first plastic AFO was developed by Simons and Jebsen in 1967.[37] The polypropylene plastic AFO

Table 23-2. Purpose of Shoe Corrections

Shoe Modification	*Function*
SACH heel	Simulates plantar flexion at heel strike Absorbs shock on compression of heel
Rocker bar	Aids roll-over at heel off Provides dorsiflexion assistance
Steel spring	Provides assistance for push-off 1-inch wide, 16–18 gauge Stiffens sole of shoe Lengthens foot lever Prevents deformity of shoe at toe break

is composed of a thermoplastic material with a cuff and Velcro strap, and a shoe insert (Fig. 23-14).[33, 38]

When the calf shell is trimmed anterior to the malleoli, the orthosis will function as a solid ankle type (Fig. 23-15). When the orthosis is narrowed at the distal posterior ankle level of the calf shell, that is, trimmed posterior to the malleoli, it has been made flexible and becomes a posterior leaf spring variety depending on the narrowness of the posterior ankle shell (Fig. 23-16). The functional difference between the two is that the posterior leaf spring allows plantar flexion at heel strike, and following push-off returns the orthosis to neutral for the swing phase, providing toe pickup. The solid

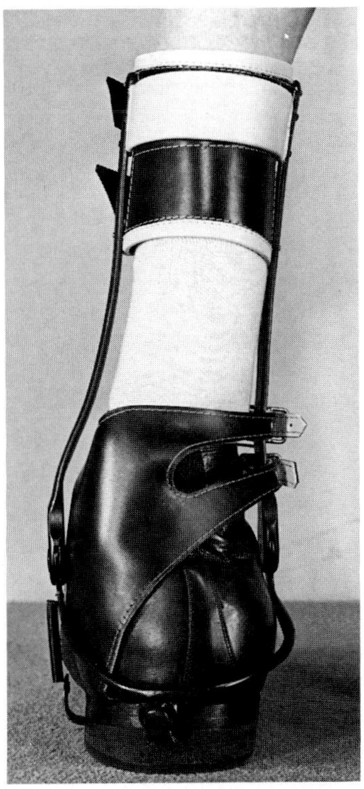

Fig. 23-13. Double upright orthosis with varus T-strap to correct ankle varus. (From Rubin and Cohen,[57] with permission.)

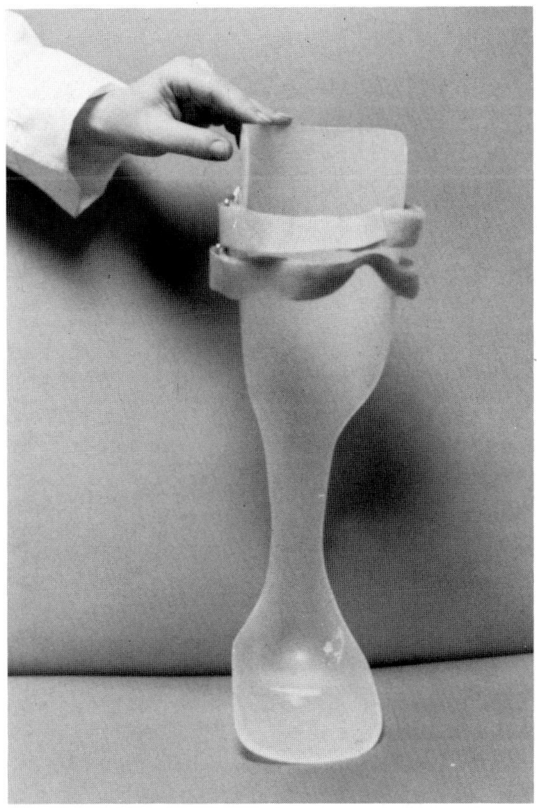

Fig. 23-14. Polypropylene plastic ankle-foot orthosis, posterior leaf spring variety. (From Rubin and Cohen,[57] with permission.)

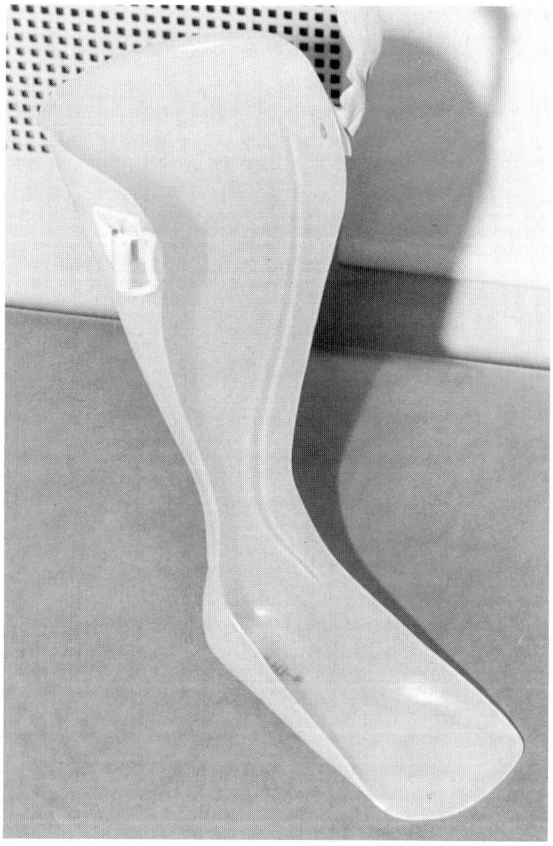

Fig. 23-15. Polypropylene plastic solid ankle-foot orthosis.

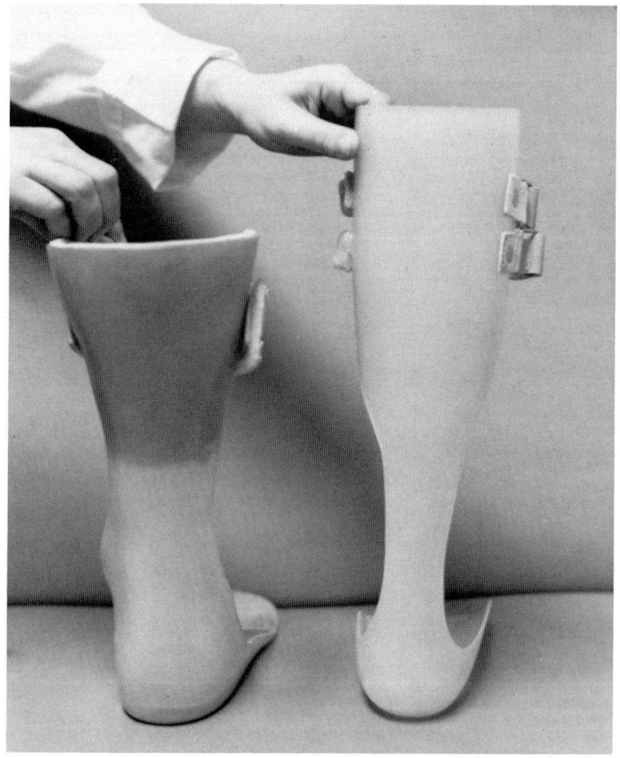

Fig. 23-16. Comparison of posterior leaf spring (right) and solid ankle polypropylene plastic ankle-foot orthosis (left). (From Rubin and Cohen,[57] with permission.)

ankle polypropylene orthosis does not allow plantar flexion at heel strike. It keeps the ankle rigidly immobilized.

The function of the polypropylene posterior leaf spring orthosis is to provide dorsiflexion assistance during swing phase. It is used mainly for a flaccid or mild spastic equinus deformity. The function of the solid ankle polypropylene orthosis is to restrict all motion at the ankle. It is indicated for traumatic arthritis of the ankle or other conditions in which ankle motion is significantly painful. It is also indicated for severe spasticity. Therefore, it is very useful in stroke and other upper motor neuron disease in which spasticity distorts foot placement.[39]

The only contraindication is edema pressure against rigid margins of the shoe insert, which creates irritation and an absence of sensation. The absence of sensation in the diabetic foot will remove a warning signal if irritations should occur. Since there is no ankle motion, the shoe modification must include a SACH-type heel, a long steel spring, and a rocker bar. The polypropylene AFO is used with a plantar flexion stop and free dorsiflexion for children with the spastic type of cerebral palsy. Figure 23-17 shows a polypropylene AFO with an ankle joint that has a 90° plantar flexion stop. This prevents the clonus of the spastic gait from occurring and allows dorsiflexion for a more normalized gait. It is of the shoe insert variety and can be placed in a shoe.

Generally, plastic shoe insert AFOs are not prescribed for diabetic patients with absent sensation. However, diabetic patients with neuropathy have been reported to use plastic AFOs worn in conjunction with extra-depth shoes.[40] The brace may be padded with a soft material such as Plastazote or

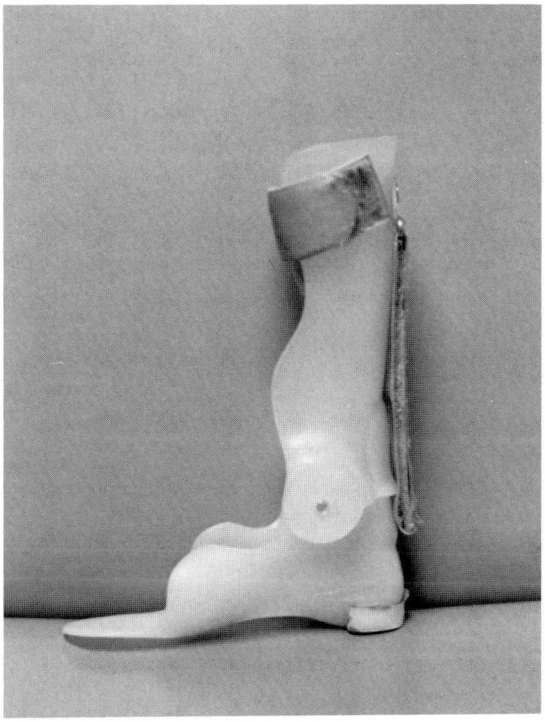

Fig. 23-17. Polypropylene plastic ankle-foot orthosis with 90° plantar flexion stop to be used for children with cerebral palsy. (From Rubin and Cohen,[57] with permission.)

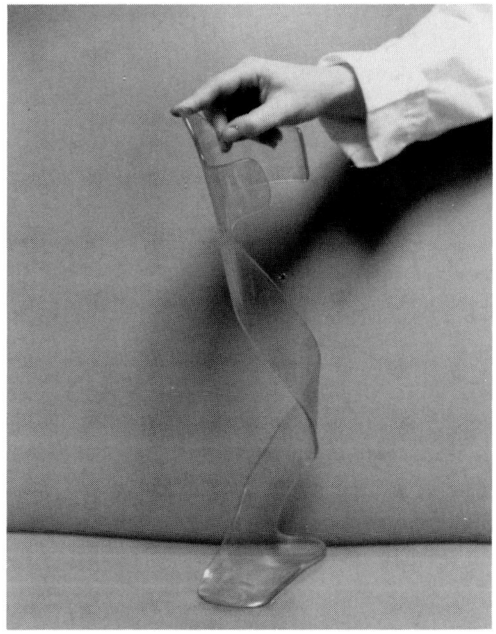

Fig. 23-18. Spiral orthosis. (From Rubin and Cohen,[57] with permission.)

Pe-Lite. The trim lines must be very carefully fit so as not to dig into the insensitive foot, and the foot plate must be checked to make sure there are no unusual pressure points. Patients must check their feet daily.

Spiral Orthosis

The spiral orthosis (Fig. 23-18) is a spiral configuration AFO, with a shoe insert segment connected to an upright at the medial side of the foot plate, spiraling around the leg posteriorly then across the anterior aspect, and terminating at the level of the tibial tubercle. A horizontal strap is attached to the spiral at the proximal level of the calf. It can be made from Plexidur, Nyloplex, or polypropylene.

The original concept of the design created by Lehneis in 1972 was to provide for controlled motion of the ankle-foot complex in all planes. It was indicated for patients who lack motor power in the entire foot-ankle complex.[41]

The mechanism of functioning in gait involves the unwinding of the spiral at heel strike to allow plantar flexion. From foot flat to midstance the forward motion of the tibia is assisted by the spiral as it returns to its unstressed position. From midstance to heel off, the orthosis is dorsiflexed as stored energy is released. At toe off the spiral assists in push-off, until it reaches its neutral position where the internal resistance of the orthosis acts to assist toe clearance during the swing phase of gait.[41–43]

Although the spiral orthosis offers the advantages of excellent cosmesis, light weight, and interchangeability of shoes, it tends to break at the ankle and is difficult to don. It is used infrequently for this reason.[36] Although designed to allow subtalar motion and concomitant tibial rotation, it does not do so, since subtalar motion is restricted by the foot plate attachment to the spiral upright component.

Patella Tendon Brace

The patella tendon bearing (PTB) brace is on the interface of the fields of prosthetics and orthotics. It was based on the concept of the below knee amputation prosthesis designed for below knee amputees to carry weight from the stump to the floor[44] (Fig. 23-19).

For the orthotics patient the PTB orthosis is used when it is necessary to unweight the limb below the knee. It reduces the biomechanical force on the ankle and foot by using primarily the patellar tendon, the flare of the medial condylar area of the tibia, and the posterior soft tissues of the calf for weight bearing. Therefore, it is indicated for many foot and ankle problems such as plantar heel lesions, hind-foot deformities interfering with weight bearing, ankle and foot disease, ankle arthritis, and the neuropathic hindfoot and ankle. It is also used in fracture repair and for delayed union of tibial fractures and surgical procedures that required unloading during healing.[39] It does not satisfactorily unweight the forefoot.

The structure of the PTB orthosis can effectively unload a very painful ankle particularly when the pain is related to direct weight bearing. Shoe modifications, arch supports, inserts, and AFOs are all ineffective for this purpose. Rubin and Dixon used the PTB orthosis to treat a rigid pes planus foot.[45] He states ". . . when the severely deformed pes planus foot is rigid, the deformity fixed and the arch totally dropped, to provide the patient with a conventionally molded arch support is an exercise in futility."

The PTB orthosis can be of the steel upright type or the plastic shoe insert type. The steel upright PTB orthosis is indicated for the diabetic patient with Charcot foot. It will unweight a painful rear foot. The plastic shoe insert type has a more limited range of adjustability.

A B
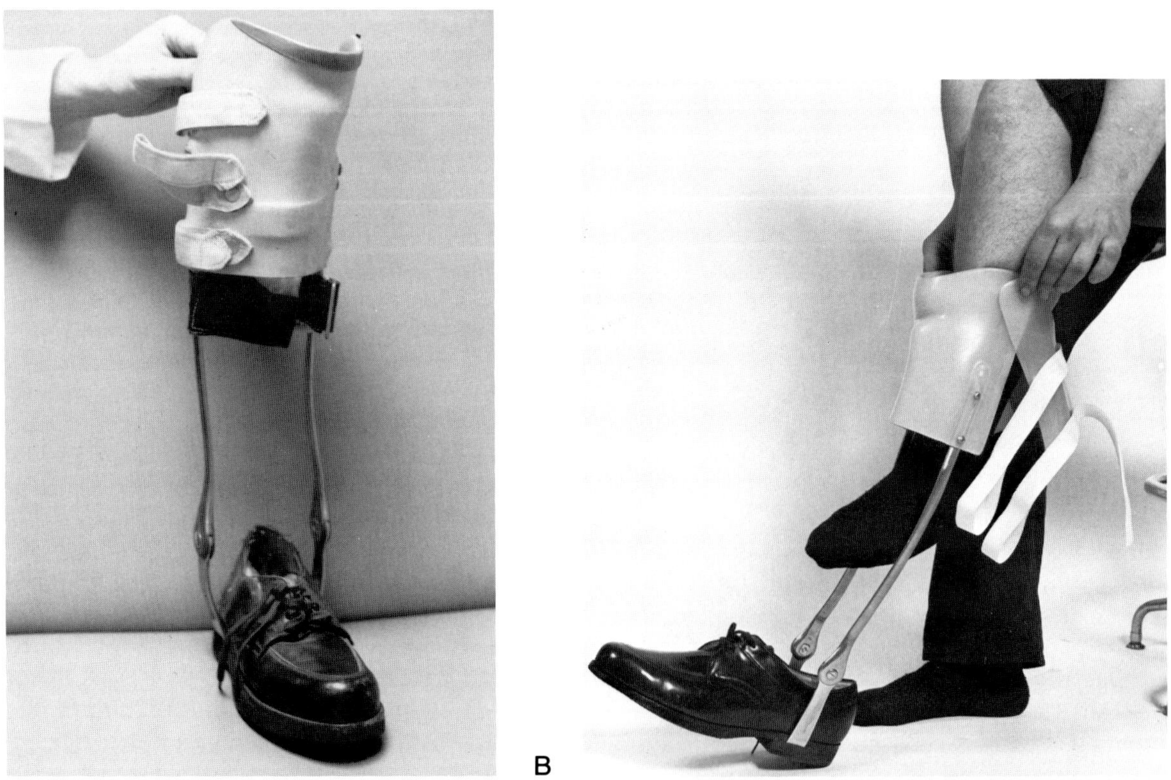

Fig. 23-19. (**A**) Patellar tendon bearing brace. (**B**) Donning the patellar tendon bearing brace. (From Rubin and Cohen,[57] with permission.)

Shoe-Clasp Orthosis

The shoe-clasp orthosis is a simple posterior leaf spring type device that attaches directly to the heel counter of the shoe (Fig. 23-20). It consists of a posterior flat bar made of epoxy fiberglass attached at the proximal end to a polyethylene slip-cuff. The distal end of the bar is attached to a clasp of stainless steel that clips directly on to the posterior heel counter of the shoe.

The posterior springlike component provides very efficient toe pickup. The ankle plantar-flexes on heel strike and is returned to the neutral position for swing-through by the posterior upright.

It is indicated for flaccid drop foot and mild spastic equinus. It provides dorsiflexion assistance during swing phase while providing slight lateral stability. Since the orthotic clasp attaches directly to the shoe counter, the type of shoe used becomes extremely important since the shoe is actually now functioning as an integral part of the orthosis. The shoe should be a Blucher type with leather sole, strong shank, stiff hard counter, and rubber heel.[34]

The orthosis offers the advantages of cosmesis, light weight, and interchangeability of shoes. Furthermore, the area of attachment of the shoe clasp to the counter is a source of continuous pressure if not adjusted properly by the orthotist. In addition the orthosis loses its efficiency if the counter breaks down.[27,46] It can be modified to attach directly to the posterior heel of the shoe via a flat caliper foot plate, instead of the counter. The modified shoe-clasp orthosis is especially good for the diabetic patient with peripheral neuropathy with a flaccid drop foot. It provides adequate toe pickup without direct foot contact, a great advantage for diabetics.

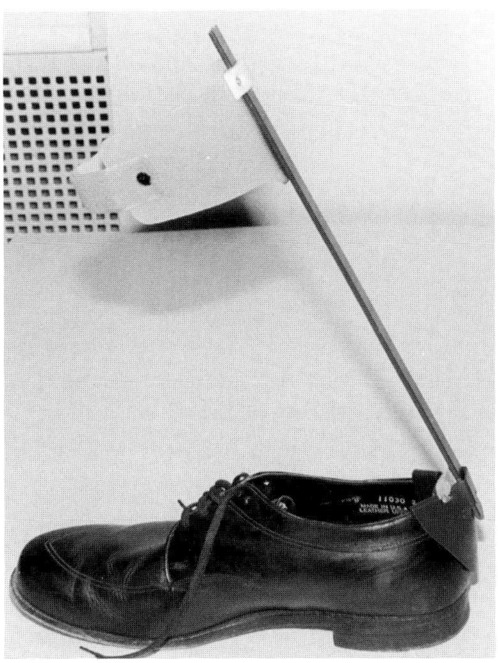

Fig. 23-20. The shoe clasp orthosis.

Teufel Orthosis

The Teufel orthosis is no longer being prescribed. However, one does encounter patients still wearing this device fabricated several years ago. The Teufel orthosis was replaced with the polypropylene orthosis. The Teufel orthosis is a shoe insert type of AFO that can be made either as a solid ankle AFO when the distal upright is trimmed anterior to the malleoli or as a posterior leaf spring type when the distal upright is trimmed posterior to the malleoli. The Teufel orthosis is made of the thermoplastic ortholene that was originally brought to the United States and Canada from Germany by Otto Bock.[37]

The posterior leaf spring Teufel AFO is basically a drop-foot brace. It is indicated for mild ankle instability with peroneal nerve lesion, flaccid drop foot, sciatic nerve lesions, and hemiplegics with mild to moderate spasticity. If the spasticity is moderate or severe and the Teufel orthosis as constructed above is unable to resist the strong plantar flexion forces, an AFO with a 90° plantar flexion stop is needed. This can be accomplished by appropriate trimming of the upright as was done in the case of the polypropylene (see above).

The Teufel posterior leaf spring orthosis functions by virtue of the flexibility and spring of the ortholene material. Plantar flexion occurs at heel strike due to the flexibility of the upright. Dorsiflexion returning the orthosis to neutral occurs as the foot passes into swing-through. The flexibility of the ortholene contributes to push-off.

The Teufel plastic posterior solid ankle AFO is indicated for complete flaccidity of the ankle dorsiflexors and plantar flexors.[30] Due to the relative thickness of the ortholene material it must be placed into an extra-depth shoe. It offers the advantages of simplicity, cosmesis, ease of application, and stability, and may be used for bilateral orthotic wearers. The main disadvantage is that of poor memory. The use of the AFO in the diabetic patient can be summarized as follows.

For the diabetic patient with peripheral neuropathy resulting in a flaccid drop foot, the posterior leaf spring shoe clasp orthoses should be tried. If in addition to the flaccid drop foot there is also peroneal nerve involvement resulting in an unstable ankle then a double-bar brace with a varus-valgus T-strap must be utilized.

For the diabetic patient with a stroke with vascular impairment and edema, the double upright steel AFO is required. In general the shoe insert plastic type should be avoided under such circumstances.

The diabetic with a Charcot foot can be helped by unweighting the rear foot with the PTB brace. If a shoe insert type is used, the shoe must have a SACH heel, a long steel spring, and a rocker bar.

FOOT ORTHOSES, INSOLES, AND DIGITAL SPLINTS

The diabetic patient with a peripheral decrease in sensation is biomechanically difficult to manage. Neuropathy accounts for over 40 percent of all diabetic foot lesions.[47] The foot cannot detect subtle or even gross changes in the surrounding environment of the shoe. The secondary breakdown of cutaneous and osseous structures are the direct result of a chronic insensitivity to pain and a faulty healing mechanism.[48–50] The following section will introduce types, indications, and contraindications for common foot orthoses, insoles, and digital splints used in the management of the diabetic.

Orthoses and Insoles

Orthosis in a generic sense refers to any material that supplements the function of a particular body part.[35,51] The scope of orthosis for the ensuing discussion will be limited to the foot orthosis as used in the diabetic individual for follow-up or preventative therapy.

Foot orthoses and insoles may be manufactured from an array of materials for the nondiabetic patient. However, the choices are fewer in number when considering management of the insensitive foot of the diabetic patient. The materials of the foot orthoses or insoles used should be consistent with the fragility of the soft tissue structures and the imminent chance of a future skin breakdown.[48] Therefore, the resultant choice of orthosis and insole is made primarily of the softer materials, e.g., leather, medium and firm polyethylene foams (Pe-Lite [Bakalite xylonite Ltd., U.K.], Plastazote [Bakalite xylonite Ltd., U.K.], Aliplast [Alimed, Dedham, MA], Spenco [Spenco Medical Corporation, Waco, TX], PPT [Langer Biomechanics Laboratory, Deer Park, NY], Lynco [Apex Foot Products, Hackensack, NJ], Sorbothane [Triad Research Inc., Strasburg, PA]).[51] Even with the most selective material chosen, there is no more than about a 20 to 30 percent reduction in pressure possible.[12]

The indications for the listed material and orthotic combinations would be to reduce friction and calluses that might result in possible ulcerations, and prevent subluxations as seen in the Charcot foot. Biomechanical deformities yielding potentially harmful calluses to the diabetic patient include, but are not limited to, hammer toes, claw toes, mallet toes, cavus and planus foot deformities, hallux valgus, and hallux limitus.

The goals for using foot orthoses in the diabetic patient are (1) control foot function, (2) decrease pain (if present), and (3) prevent further damage (e.g., joint subluxation or possible ulceration).[48] Patients with healed plantar ulcers with normal footwear face a 90 percent recurrence rate as compared to 19 percent recurrence rate for patients that wear modified shoes and orthoses.[52]

In preventing plantar ulcerations in the diabetic population, two types of foot orthoses are employed. One type of orthosis is a simple insole and the second type is the prescription foot orthosis. The insole is used primarily to redistribute the plantar weight forces acting on the metatarsal heads, distal tips of the digits, and other miscellaneous preulcerous sites plantarly.[10] If needed, it may be designed to add support to the longitudinal and transverse arches of the foot through the use of metatarsal and scaphoid type pads added to the underside of the insole.

Most commonly, the insole is a single layer of material measuring $\frac{1}{8}$ to $\frac{3}{8}$ inch in thickness (cut to the inside dimensions of the shoe). The thickness of the material chosen will initially depend upon the amount of available room inside the shoe with the patient's foot fitting comfortably from heel to toe. Thereafter, it is recommended that the patient purchase a pair of shoes to fit the required insole that would best accommodate the particular foot deformity. The choice of the insole material will be dependent upon the properties requested by the doctor in trying to manage the patient's pedal pathology. For example, shock absorption, plantar heat generation, degree of accommodation, and durability are properties of a material that help determine its usage. Polyurethane foams, viscoelastic materials and rubberized compounds (e.g., PPT, Sorbothane, and Spenco) are good for shock attenuation but not lesion accommodation, whereas, the polyethylene foams such as Pe-Lite and Plastazote are good for accommodation but not shock attenuation.[51] Rubberized products (e.g., Spenco and Lynco) tend to generate more heat than the polyethylene foams.[51] Often, a beneficial result is achieved through the use of an insole that is laminated with a shock-attenuative material on the bottom and an accommodative material on top.

Once the appropriate material is chosen, certain precautions must be taken to avoid causing lesions on other parts of the foot. The distal third of the insole is beveled along the underside of its border on a 45° angle to allow for adequate room for the digits. If the shoe already comes with an insole, it is best to remove it and replace it with the custom-made insole. After fabrication, the insole should be placed in the shoe to ensure a proper fit. It should be fitted flat and snug inside the shoe to prevent slippage. The edges should not be curled upward or bent over. The edges of the insole should contact the inner sides of the shoe. Otherwise, the digits, midfoot, or heel would come to rest on the edge of the insole material, thus producing an area for possible future irritation and ulceration.

The patient should be instructed to stand upon the insole inside the shoes after having been appropriately laced and tied. Care must be taken to evaluate the foot inside and outside the shoe for other areas of possible irritation. The shoe, with the insole inside, might put pressure on areas previously unaffected. The following checkpoints of concern should be observed: (1) distal tips of all the digits; (2) dorsal aspect of all the digits; (3) metatarsal heads, plantarly; (4) metatarsal heads, dorsally at the shoe crease; (5) lateral aspect of the fifth metatarsal head; (6) medial aspect of the first metatarsal head; (7) base of the fifth metatarsal, dorsal, plantar and lateral, (8) metatarsal cuneiform joint, dorsally; (9) cuneiform navicular joint, dorsally; (10) navicular, medially, (11) plantar arch; and (12) heel region, posterior, medial, lateral, and plantar.

For example, the dorsal aspect of all the digits should be palpated through the shoe, if possible. If there is dorsal distortion of the toe box, the digits are riding too high in the shoe. This could be alleviated by either a higher toe box, an extra-depth type of shoe, or thinning the distal plantar aspect of the insole. A similar evaluation can be performed for all the items on the list, both inside and outside of the shoe. Extra caution must be exercised in patients with decreased distal sensation, since they cannot experience the tightness or irritation caused by the shoe.

The last word of caution in preventing irritation and resultant breakdown would be to evaluate any apertures or dispersions applied to the insole for accommodation. Care must be exercised in assuring the dispersion does not have any rough edges, is wide and deep enough to allow for adequate accommodation, and is properly placed anatomically for the particular lesion.

A soft insole added to a shoe helps to spread the stresses of walking evenly across the foot. In one study, Sorbothane was used in neuropathic diabetic subjects both with and without a history of foot ulceration.[53] Dynamic foot pressure recordings were made over stress areas on all subjects and analysis performed first with the subjects barefoot and then with a 5-mm thick sheet of the viscoelastic polymer. The results showed a significant difference in peak pressures under the feet using the polymer insert; however, the reduction of peak pressure was greater in the subjects who had a history of ulcers than in those with no such history. Other studies have shown that walking on a sandal made of a deep soft material such as a soft microcell rubber or Plastazote will decrease abnormal pressures up to three times the original.[53]

The other type of orthosis used for the diabetic patient is the prescription foot support. This orthosis is custom-fabricated to a cast of a patient's foot. The advantage of the foot support over the insole is that it will allow for more biomechanical control of the complete foot. The prescription orthosis consists of a shell manufactured by using any one of the following materials: polyethylene thermoplastic, leather, Rohadur (Rohm Haas, Germany), carbon graphite, or polyethylene foam, that will retain its desired shape and control the foot biomechanically. The device may have a protective top cover made of any one of the aforementioned materials used for insoles.

The prescription orthosis is beneficial in preventing ulcerations by balancing not only the metatarsal heads (as insoles do) but also the shafts of the metatarsals. Orthoses can also provide support for the greater and lesser tarsus, which is imperative in diabetic patients that undergo Charcot joint changes. The diabetic patient may develop Charcot joints, which may present with varying degrees of difficulty depending upon the magnitude of destruction. In the early stage of the deformity, the joints are undergoing changes that can be attenuated by providing a more functional support when weight bearing is permitted or resumed. The support prevents abnormal ranges of motion from occurring, thereby retarding joint subluxations. This in turn will decrease the breakdown process. When it has reached the end stage of destruction, the foot can only be benefited by accommodative orthoses, insoles, or molded shoes that prevent the bony tarsus from bottoming out against the inside of the shoe. Prevention will consist of prudent forethought in evaluating patients with neurologic changes. The mainstay in the prevention of destructive osseous and soft tissue changes from Charcot joints is early recognition of subluxations and follow-up supportive therapy. The patient with diabetic neuropathic changes in the foot should be high on the suspect list for possible Charcot joint changes. The treatment is aimed at prevention of further trauma to the joints.[54] Orthotics can be effective toward meeting this goal by simultaneously balancing all three planes of the feet (Figs. 23-21 and 23-22).

For the diabetic patient, insoles and orthotics must undergo a break-in period before they may be used for a full working day. The usual break-in period would consist of wearing the orthotics or insoles for 1 hour the first day, 2 hours the second

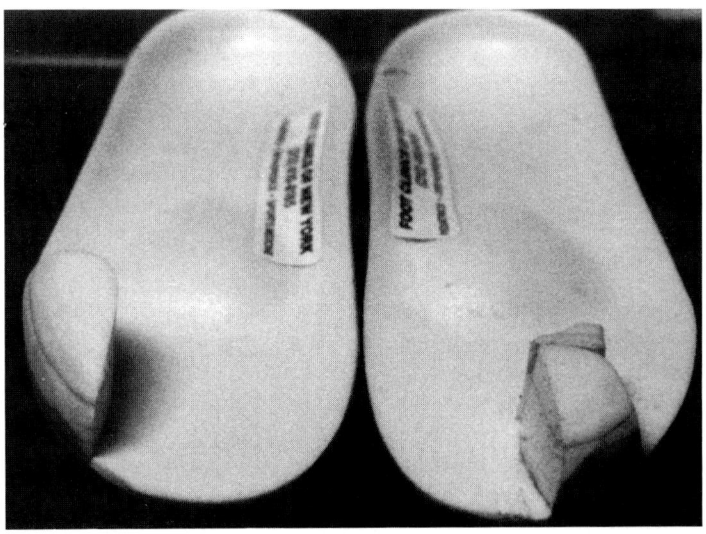

Fig. 23-21. The prescription orthotic fabricated from a plaster cast of the foot may be modified by adding a prosthetic toe filler. The toe filler prevents medial or lateral migration of the digits, which is a common problem after an amputation.

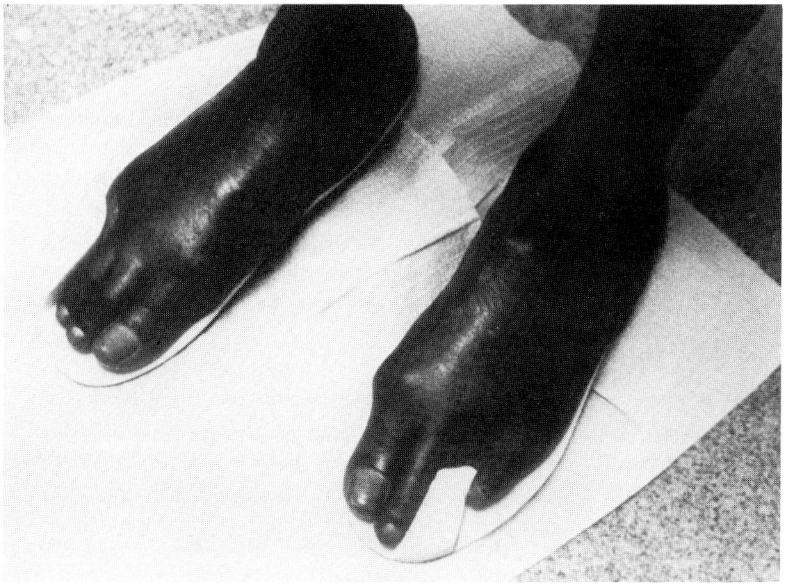

Fig. 23-22. While foot orthoses with prosthetic toe fillers may fit with stockings or sock off, another problem occurs with the application of hosiery. The prosthetic toe filler when made for digits two, three or four can be in the way and bothersome when donning shoes and stockings or socks.

day, 3 hours the third day, and so on until the patient is wearing them for a full 8-hour day. After that time the patient may wear them for the full working day. Caution must be given to diabetic patients who are starting to break in the orthoses. They must be reminded that their feet should be inspected for areas of irritation before and after each break-in period. These steps must be followed judiciously because diabetic patients with peripheral neuropathy will not have the appropriate feedback to discern pain in their feet.

Proper shoe inspection coupled with a thorough examination of the foot, as was performed for the insole, after the orthosis has been dispensed will minimize the risk of developing foot ulcers. Thus, the goals for using the foot orthoses will be accomplished: (1) control foot function, (2) decrease pain (if present), and (3) prevent further damage (e.g., joint subluxation or possible ulceration).

The contraindications for the aforementioned materials would be (1) known allergies to the component orthosis materials, (2) severely subluxed Charcot feet requiring molded shoe therapy, (3) use of orthoses with ill-fitting shoes, and (4) open or infected lesions.

Orthodigital Splints

Digital splinting in the diabetic patient is used extensively for the reduction of excessive pressures on the foot and digits and the prevention of ulceration. Digital splinting may be a reasonable conservative alternative where surgery is contraindicated. The most popular digital splints used on the diabetic patient are fabricated of either foam, silicone, or latex. The latex shield is the most durable product available for lasting results. For the latex shield, a negative plaster cast is made of the site of concern. The laboratory will then fabricate a latex splint around a plaster positive and disperse lesions as marked and instructed (Figs. 23-23 and 23-24).

Because of the impaired sensorium associated with so many diabetic patients, care must always be exercised when considering using a digital shield or splint that encircles an appendage. Inspection should be made to assess the circulatory status before and after the shield is applied.

The most common uses of digital splints would be to relieve excessive pressure or pain (if present) from bony prominences such as (1) the medial or dorsal eminence in hallux valgus or hallux limitus,

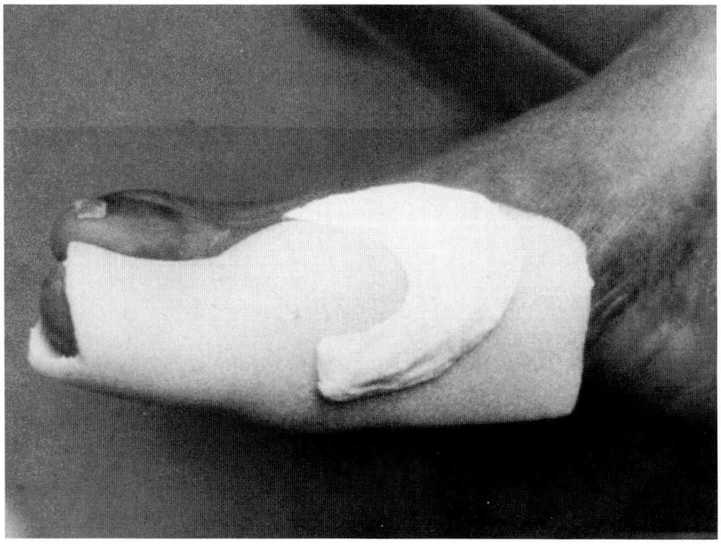

Fig. 23-23. A simple dispersion pad can be manufactured from foam sleeves and felt as a temporary aid in the relief of unwanted pressures over bony prominences.

respectively, (2) the distal digital tips as seen in claw or mallet toe deformities, (3) dorsal digital helloma durum, and (4) the tailor's bunion, dorsally or laterally.

The same cautions must be given to the patient as when dispensing any other orthopaedic device. Signs of irritation should be noted by the patient and doctor. Limited wearing time should be instituted when first dispensed.

Prevention and Management

The education of diabetic patients regarding the disease and how it affects their feet is a crucial facet in the total treatment plan. Proper advice to patients in preventing injuries and seeking early medical attention for all injuries are important measures. Patients should take an active role in the management of their disease by constantly moni-

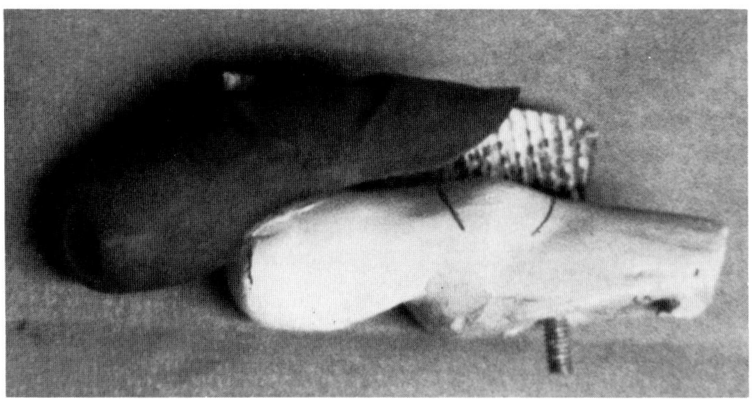

Fig. 23-24. A latex bunion shield can be fabricated to a plaster cast of the affected portion of the foot.

toring the status of their feet. The feet must be evaluated daily (preferably more often, especially after peak periods of activity) for areas of irritation either from the orthoses or shoes. Patients must be instructed to inspect inside their shoes daily for foreign objects, exposed nails, or areas of excessive wear of both orthoses and shoes. Instruction must be given to patients before the start of any new treatment for the precautions to be taken as well as any special recommendations to be followed. Occasional reinforcement of instructions should be made periodically during a treatment plan. The diabetic patient and the associated pedal abnormalities pose a particularly challenging problem for the doctor from both a management and prevention standpoint.

The biomechanical considerations that follow the primary management of the acute presentation of diabetic lesions are aimed at preventing further breakdown and lesion formation by minimizing the adverse effects of gait or ambulation. The use of insoles, orthoses, and orthodigital splints reduces the effects of increased pressures under the insensitive or subluxed foot.

ACKNOWLEDGMENTS

The authors would like to thank Jo-Ann Cooper for her assistance in the preparation of this manuscript and Les Mills for his expertise in medical photography.

REFERENCES

1. Christie J, Clowes CB, Lamb WE: Amputations through the middle part of the foot. J Bone Joint Surg 62B:473, 1980
2. Silbert S, Maimovici H: Criteria for the selection of the level of amputation for ischemic gangrene. JAMA 155:1554, 1954
3. American Academy of Orthopaedic Surgeons. Atlas of Limb Prosthetics. CV Mosby, St. Louis, 1981
4. Sarmiento A (ed): Symposium on amputation surgery and prosthetics. Orthop Clin North Am 3:1, 1972
5. Greene WB et al: Partial foot amputations in children. J Bone Joint Surg 64A:438, 1982
6. Rubin G: The partial foot amputations. J Am Podiatr Assoc 74:518, 1984
7. Rubin G: Indications for variants of the partial foot prosthesis. Orthop Rev 14:49, 1985
8. Hertzman, CA: Use of plastazote in foot disabilities. Am J Phys Med 52(6):289, 1973
9. Enna CD, Brand PW, Reed JK et al: The orthotic care of the denervated foot in Hansen's disease. Orthop Prosthet 30:33, 1976
10. Holstein P, Larsen K, Sager P: Decompression with the aid of insoles in the treatment of diabetic neuropathic ulcers. Acta Orthop Scand 47:463, 1976
11. Shipley, DE: Clinical evaluation and care of the insensitive foot. Phys Ther 59(1):13, 1979
12. Kalker AJ, Kolodny HD, Cavuto JW: The evaluation and treatment of diabetic foot ulcers. J Am Pod Med Assoc 72(10):491, 1982
13. Larsen K, Christiansen JS, Ebskov B: Prevention and treatment of ulcerations of the foot in unilaterally amputated diabetic patients. Acta Orthop Scand 53:481, 1982
14. Due TM, Jacobs RL: Molded foot orthosis after great toe or medial ray amputations in diabetic feet. Foot Ankle 6(3):150, 1985
15. Subbarao J, Gratzer M, Pinzur, MS et al: Diabetic neuro-osteoarthropathy rehabilitation of a patient with both ankle joints involved and associated skin problems. Orthop Rev 15(7):471, 1986
16. Larsen K, Holstein P: Abnormal extension of the big toe as a cause of ulceration in diabetic feet. Prosthet Orthop Inst 11:31, 1987
17. Brodsky JW, Kourosh S, Still M et al: Objective evaluation of insert material for diabetic and athletic footwear. Foot Ankle 9(3):111, 1988
18. Larsen K, Holstein P, Deckert T: Limb salvage in diabetics with foot ulcers. Prosthet Orthop Inst 13:100, 1989
19. Hampton GH: Therapeutic footwear for the insensitive foot. Phys Ther 59(1): 23, 1979
20. Lippmann HI, Farrar R: Prevention of amputation in diabetics. Angiology 30:649, 1979
21. Soulier SM: The use of running shoes in the prevention of plantar diabetic ulcers. J Am Pod Med Assoc 76(7):395, 1986
22. Coleman WC: Shoe gear in the insensitive foot. Clin Podiatr Med Surg 4:459, 1987
23. Ellenberg, M: Diabetic neuropathy. Diabetes 8(1): 21, 1982
24. McCollough NC: Lower extremity bracing. p. 124. In Introduction to Lower Extremity Orthotics. In-

structional Course Lectures. American Academy of Orthopaedic Surgeons, 1971
25. McCollough NC: Rationale for orthotic prescription in the lower extremity. Clin Orthop Rel Res 102:32, 1974
26. McCollough NC: Biomechanical analysis system. p. 169. In Atlas of Orthotics. American Academy of Orthopaedic Surgeons. CV Mosby, St. Louis, 1975
27. Rubin G, Dixon M, Danisi M: VAPC prescription procedures for knee orthoses and knee-ankle-foot orthoses. Orthop Prosthet 31:9, 1977
28. Halar E, Cardenas DD: Ankle-foot orthoses: clinical implications. Phys Med Rehabil 1(1):45, 1987
29. Lehmann JF: Lower extremity orthotics. p. 539. In Kotte FJ, Stillwell GK, Lehmann JF (eds): Krusen's Handbook of Physical Medicine and Rehabilitation. 3rd ed. WB Saunders, Philadelphia, 1982
30. Meyer PR: Lower limb orthotics. Clin Orthop Rel Res 102:58, 1974
31. Water R, Montgomery J: Lower extremity management of hemiparesis. Clin Orthop Rel Res, 102:133, 1974
32. Stills M: Lower-limb orthotics. Orthop Prosthet, 31(4):21, 1977
33. New York University: Post-Graduate Medical School Prosthetics and Orthotics. Lower-Limb Orthotics Revision. New York, 1981
34. Rubin G: The shoe as a component of the orthosis. Orthop Prosthet 30:13, 1976
35. Rose GR: Orthotics. p. 979. In Hassis NH (ed): Post Graduate Textbook of Clinical Orthopaedics. Wright PSG, Boston, 1983
36. Rubin G, Dixon M: The modern ankle-foot orthoses (AFO's). Bulletin of Prosthetics Research October 19, 1983, p. 20.
37. Lehmann JF: Biomechanics of ankle-foot orthosis: prescription and design. Arch Phys Med Rehabil 60:200, 1979
38. Rehabilitation Engineering Center: Lower-Limb Orthotics—A Manual. Massachusetts Rehabilitation Hospital, Philadelphia
39. Demopoulos JT: Orthotic and prosthetic management of foot disorders. p. 183. In Jahss (ed): Disorders of the Foot. WB Saunders, Philadelphia, 1982
40. Jacobs RL, Karmody AM: Management of the diabetic neurotrophic foot. p. 118. In American Association of Orthopaedic Surgeons. Instructional Course Lectures, 1982
41. Lehneis HR: Principles of orthotic alignment in the lower extremity. p. 131. American Academy of Orthopaedic Surgeons. Instructional Course Lectures, 1971
42. Lehneis HR: New concepts in lower extremity orthotics. Med Clin North Am 53:585, 1969
43. Lehneis HR: New developments in lower-limb orthotics through bioengineering. Arch Phys Med Rehabil 53:303, 1972
44. Rubin G: The patellar-tendon-bearing (PTB) orthosis. Bull Hosp Joint Dis. 33:155, 1972
45. Rubin G, Dixon M: The use of the AFO and PTB orthoses for severe pes planus. Clin Prosthet Orthop 10:24, 1986
46. LeBlanc MA: Clinical evaluation of a comprehensive approach to below-knee orthotics. Orthop Prosthet 26:27, 1972
47. Gibbons GW, Bothe A (eds): Diabetic Foot Management. Harvard Medical School, Cambridge, 1988
48. Gramuglia VJ, Palmarozzo PM, Rzonca EC: Biomechanical concepts in the treatment of ulcers in the diabetic foot. Clin Pod Med Surg 5:613, 1988
49. Boulton AJ: The diabetic foot. Med Clin North Am 72:1513, 1988
50. Habershaw G, Donovan J: Biomechanical considerations of the diabetic foot. p. 32. In Kozak GP et al: Management of Diabetic Foot Problems. WB Saunders, Philadelphia, 1984
51. Levitz SJ, Whiteside LS, Fitzgerald, TA: Biomechanical foot therapy. Clin Pod Med Surg 5:721, 1988
52. Dyck PJ, Thomas PK, Asbury AK et al (eds): Diabetic Neuropathy. WB Saunders, Philadelphia, 1987
53. Boulton AJM, Franks CI et al: Reduction of abnormal foot pressures in diabetic neuropathy using a new polymer insole material. Diabetes Care 7:42, 1984
54. Frykberg RG: Osteoarthopathy. Clin Pod Med Surg 4:351, 1987
55. Rubin G, Fischer E: Selection of components for lower limb amputation prostheses. Bull Hosp Jt Dis Orthop Inst 42:39, 1982
56. Rubin G, Dixon M, Fischer E: Avoidable amputation problems and responsibility of surgeon. Orthop Rev 14:73, 1985
57. Rubin G, Cohen E: Prostheses and orthoses for the foot and ankle. Clin Podiatr Med Surg 5:695, 1988

24

Footwear Considerations

William C. Coleman, D.P.M., D.A.B.P.O.

Proper footwear is the key factor in preventing injuries to insensate feet. Obtaining appropriate protective shoes and utilizing them in an effective injury prevention program is not a trivial task. However, it is rarely considered an essential component when diabetic foot services are being coordinated by medical professionals.

Footwear form and function should be a primary consideration whenever a diabetic patient is seen. Particularly during times when the foot may change or be more vulnerable to breakdown, such as prior to surgery or during rehabilitation from injury, footwear needs to be at the forefront of clinical decision making. Foot surgery is rarely planned on the basis of input from a shoe fitter. Successful healing of a surgical incision is often considered to be a satisfactory end point to this form of management. If footwear is considered at all by the foot surgeon, it often takes the form of a vague set of directions to a prescription shoe facility. Once this prescription is given to the patient few physicians schedule a follow-up evaluation of the completed footwear.

The cost of prescription footwear can often be the factor that determines the course of diabetic foot management. With third party payment for shoes still not available in most cases, the prescription is never written and patients without adequate financial resources must continue with unmodified footwear. Even after repeated episodes of injury the purchase of prescription shoes is beyond the financial means of many patients who require them.

When a prescription shoe fitter receives a prescription usually there is little information concerning the foot pathology to be addressed or the goals the physician wishes to achieve with footwear. It is not unusual, in the case of diabetic individuals that the shoe fitter be sent a patient with an open plantar ulcer. He is then expected to design footwear that will heal the wound or at least allow the patient to walk on the foot without making the injury worse. This attempt at foot management is conducted with little direct communication between shoe professional and medical professional. Neither is really sure of the expectations and techniques of the other. Until closer communication exists between physicians and those who fill shoe prescriptions, the diabetic population of the United States will continue to pay an unnecessarily high price in ulceration and amputation of their feet.

THE PHYSICIAN–SHOE FITTER RELATIONSHIP

A physician who plans to manage diabetic feet on a regular basis needs to become familiar with the basics of shoe fitting and design. Without this background knowledge the physician will be unable to evaluate the quality of the shoe fitter's product. The physician also needs to maintain a familiarity with current clinical footwear practices.

After becoming educated on the fundamental principles of footwear for diabetic patients, the physician will have a foundation upon which to contact a local shoe fitter and develop a close working relationship. The shoe fitter needs to become a critical part of decision making in the prevention of injury and rehabilitation of a previously injured foot. Whenever possible the shoe specialist should be present when the management plan for the patient is decided. The input of the shoe professional can then help determine the final plan.

The management of injury should not be the responsibility of the footwear specialist. Shoes are rarely indicated for the treatment of a damaged, insensitive foot. However, as the predominant means of injury prevention, footwear needs to take a more prominent role in patient management. For this reason, it is the responsibility of the medical professional who treats diabetic feet to become more conversant with proper prescription writing and shoe fitting protocols.

SHOE BASICS

Lasts are the solid forms over which shoes are constructed. Lasts determine the contours of shoes as materials are stretched, bonded, sewn, and nailed over them. It is the final shape, as determined by the last, that allows a shoe to fit or not to fit a particular foot. Lasts are the most precisely constructed component of shoemaking. The precision and range of last sizes is diminishing in the general commercial shoe market. Only the United States and Canada make precision lasts in the full range of widths. However, 80 percent of shoes purchased in the United States are imported from other countries.

The fit of footwear is not just determined by length or width. Many other factors need to be included to match a particular shoe with the foot. These include, but are not limited to, the distance from the back of the heel to the metatarsal heads on both sides, the adduction of the forefoot, the fit around the upper opening (top line), and the heel. To properly fit prescription footwear a professional shoe fitter needs to stock a variety of shoes built over a variety of last shapes in various lengths and widths.

Prescription footwear, in particular, should fit well over the dorsum of the midtarsal region. Currently, the preference for diabetic patients is footwear that laces up the front of the shoe in either a high-top or oxford style. The laces allow for the best adjustment of fit and control of the foot through the upper portions of the shoe. Adjustment can be more precise with a larger number of lacing eyelets (4 to 6 eyelets on each side of the shoe).

The heel counter is the stiffening that is built into most shoes around and behind the heel of the foot. A stiff heel counter is preferable in shoe design to help retain the shape of the upper material, to reinforce inserts, and to keep the heel of the foot from shifting side to side with each step.

The numbers and letters that constitute a shoe size can only be used as a general reference to begin fitting shoes. Due to the differences in last manufacturing and styles of lasts, identically numbered sizes can vary greatly in length and width. Patients with insensitive feet should never insist on only buying shoes of a specific numbered length or lettered width due to inconsistencies in fit between styles, manufacturers, and lasts. When a person does not have the sensations of touch or pain in his or her feet, an experienced, reliable, professional prescription shoe fitter should evaluate all shoes for proper fit.

In 1983 the Prescription Footwear Association surveyed 6,800 adults.[1] They found that 70 percent of men and women had one foot longer than the other. The longest foot could equally be the right or left. In three-fourths of these people the difference was one-half shoe size (about $\frac{1}{6}$ inch). The other fourth had a difference of one whole size or greater. The common practice in the United States is to fit the larger foot, and if the shoe on the smaller foot is noticeably loose the shoe fitter will place inserts to fill the space.[2]

For the best fit both feet should be measured. Laces should be tied and the fit should be evaluated with the person standing. The shoe should be $\frac{1}{2}$ to $\frac{5}{8}$ inch longer than the longest toe in this position. The metatarsal heads should match the angle and fit into the ball girth of the shoe. Footwear should not be too tight against the sides of the metatarsal heads and this should be the widest part of the shoe. This fit usually is determined by the shoe fitter pressing his thumb in against the leather at the metatarsal heads and, while maintaining the pressure, drawing his thumb across the dorsum of the shoe side to side (Fig. 24-1). The leather should have

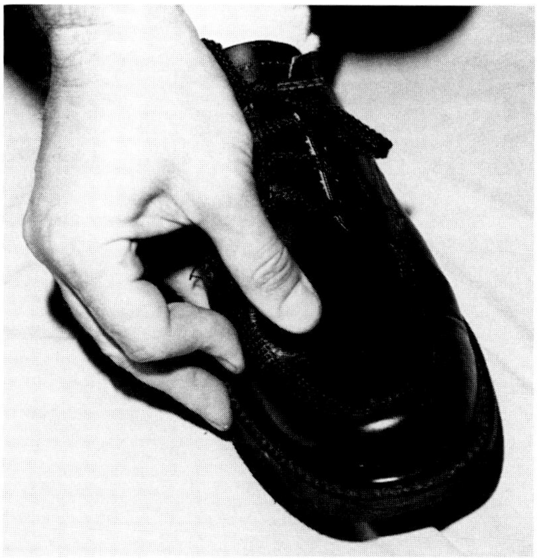

Fig. 24-1. The tightness of the shoe upper over the metatarsal heads can be evaluated by drawing the thumb over the dorsum of the shoe in this region side to side while pressing down. The leather should be slack enough for a low wrinkle to bulge up as this is done.

enough slack for a low wrinkle to form. The wrinkle should be too low to pinch between the thumb and index finger.

When a shoe is too tight across the front of the foot the lateral side of the fifth metatarsal head and the medial side of the first metatarsal head become very high risk locations for ulceration. These are the vulnerable areas of the foot because a tight shoe creates tension in the upper material of the shoe. This tension results in pressure when it is wrapped around the curved surfaces of the foot. When the tension in the leather curves around a small radius the highest pressures result (pressure is proportional to the tension divided by radius). Since the smallest radius of curvature is around the sides of the metatarsal heads, that is where the ulcers develop.

The direct pressures that result in the ischemic necrosis at the sides of the metatarsal heads are very low (1 to 5 pounds per square inch).[3] It is just enough pressure to block the flow of blood between the surface of the skin and metatarsal head. It is not the amount of pressure but the length of time the pressure remains in place without relief that results in the ulcers caused by tight shoes. If this pressure is applied for 5 or 6 hours the blood will not be kept from the tissues for a long enough period of time to cause ischemic damage. However, a person with insensate feet might keep a tight shoe on all day — 12 to 14 hours. To prevent this type of wound diabetic patients should not wear their shoes for longer than 5 or 6 hours. Once the shoes are removed blood will return to these tissues.

A shoe that is too loose will move excessively in relation to the foot and rub blisters on the skin. Ulcers from loose shoes usually develop around the heel or top line of the shoe.

The toe region of the shoe should not put pressure on the toes from the top or sides. The circumference of the shoe around the metatarsal heads is what determines the letter assigned to a given width of shoe. This is called the *ball girth.* As the letter designating width increases for a given size shoe, this circumference increases by $\frac{1}{4}$ inch. Many people have the misconception that they can make more room for the toes by buying a wider shoe, but it is the style and not the width that dictates the room for the toes. To make more room in the toe box a different style needs to be obtained.

Unless warranted by equinus or leg-length discrepancy, a diabetic patient should never wear a shoe with a relative heel height greater than $1\frac{1}{2}$ inches (Fig. 24-2). Heel heights greater than this result in an increase of pressure under the metatarsal heads.[4]

The upper parts of shoes should be made of leather. Unlike manmade materials, leather will gradually assume the shape of the foot and keep this shape between times when the shoes are worn. Leather can absorb foot perspiration and allow evaporation of moisture from the foot.[5] Leather can be stretched over areas of bony prominence to reduce pressure. The width of the shoe can also be increased with stretching, but stretching does not affect the length of shoes to any great degree.

Depth footwear is manufactured with additional vertical room within the shoe. The additional height is usually $\frac{1}{4}$ to $\frac{3}{8}$ inch. This additional volume can be used to accommodate thicker insoles or claw toe deformity. Due to motor neuropathy in the intrinsic muscles of the foot, claw toes are common among diabetic individuals. Claw toes can also be expected in patients who have had a tendon

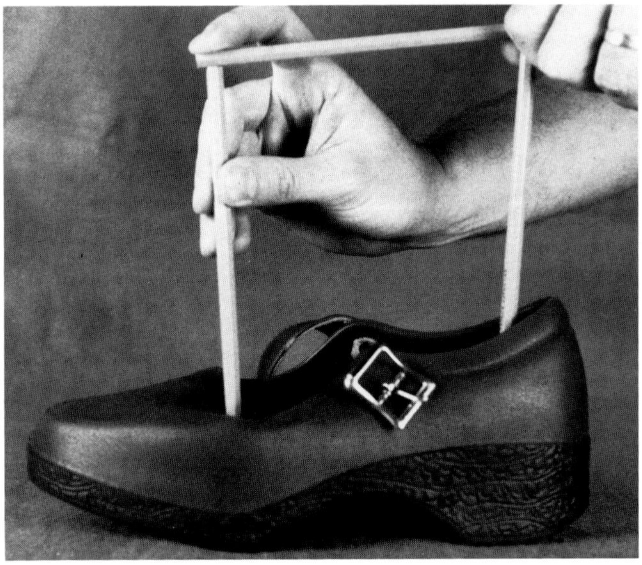

Fig. 24-2. Relative heel height can be easily determined by vertically placing the end of an unsharpened pencil inside the shoe at the location where the metatarsal heads would be and another pencil of equal length vertically at the center of the heel (about where the tubercles of the calcaneus would press). The difference in height of the top of the pencils will reflect the relative heel height.

transfer for drop-foot correction. Without additional room in the toe box of the footwear the claw toes will lead to high pressures at the end of the toes, over the proximal interphalangeal joints, and under the metatarsal heads (Fig. 24-3). It is not unusual to find depth footwear with insoles so thick as to eliminate the benefits of additional vertical room. Both the medical professional and shoe fitter need to ensure that the shoe does leave the necessary room for toe deformity and not assume that the depth shoe is doing all that is needed.

INTERIM FOOTWEAR

A fundamental principle in the management of insensate feet is to educate patients never to walk without protection between their feet and the walking surface. It is the sole of the footwear that should take the penetration of a thumb tack or piece of glass, not the bottom of an insensitive foot.

During the course of protecting insensitive feet from injury, definitive long-term footwear will not always be available for the patient to wear. Prescription shoes may need repair or may not have arrived from the factory. Some form of protective footwear must be worn at these times.

There can be some advantage in using trial footwear to evaluate different protective techniques

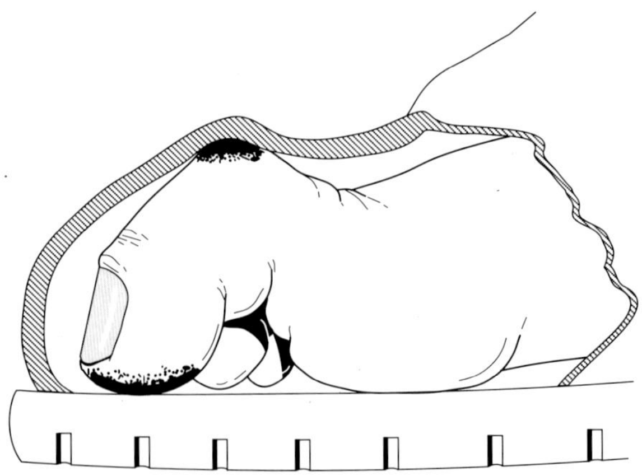

Fig. 24-3. Without the additional vertical room in depth footwear claw toes will result in increased stress under the metatarsal heads, over the proximal joint in the toe, and at the end of the toe.

before ordering the final shoe. Sometimes, a physician may require a much bulkier form of footwear postoperatively or during rehabilitation from injury. These are some of the reasons why foot care providers need to develop a form of footwear that can be quickly assembled for short-term use by the patient. Eventually, after the prescription shoes are being worn, many of the forms of temporary footwear can be used as house shoes. The patient should be aware that many commercial house slippers have soles too thin to provide adequate protection from stepping on sharp objects.

At the present time, Plastazote is the material most frequently used in the construction of molded foot beds for interim footwear. It is a light, closed-cell polyethylene foam that can be molded directly to the bottom of the foot without burning the skin. A thick foam rubber block can be used to improve the molding (Fig. 24-4). For over twenty years, the Hansen's Disease Center at Carville, Louisiana, has used sandals constructed from Plastazote for interim use.[6] For clinics without shoemakers the foot bed can still be constructed quickly and placed in a commercial form of footwear such as a Darco shoe (Fig. 24-5).

THE FOOT AT RISK

Persons with sensory loss in the feet will rarely seek foot care on their own before an injury has occurred. To become effectively involved in their own injury prevention, all diabetic patients need education on footwear selection and injury prevention. Prevention needs to begin when the diagnosis of diabetes is made. Shoes are best used as a defense against injury rather than a means of managing active wounds. However, not all diabetic patients need the same degree of protection. By classifying patients according to their degree of risk of injury, prevention can become more effective by concentrating attention to those who need it most

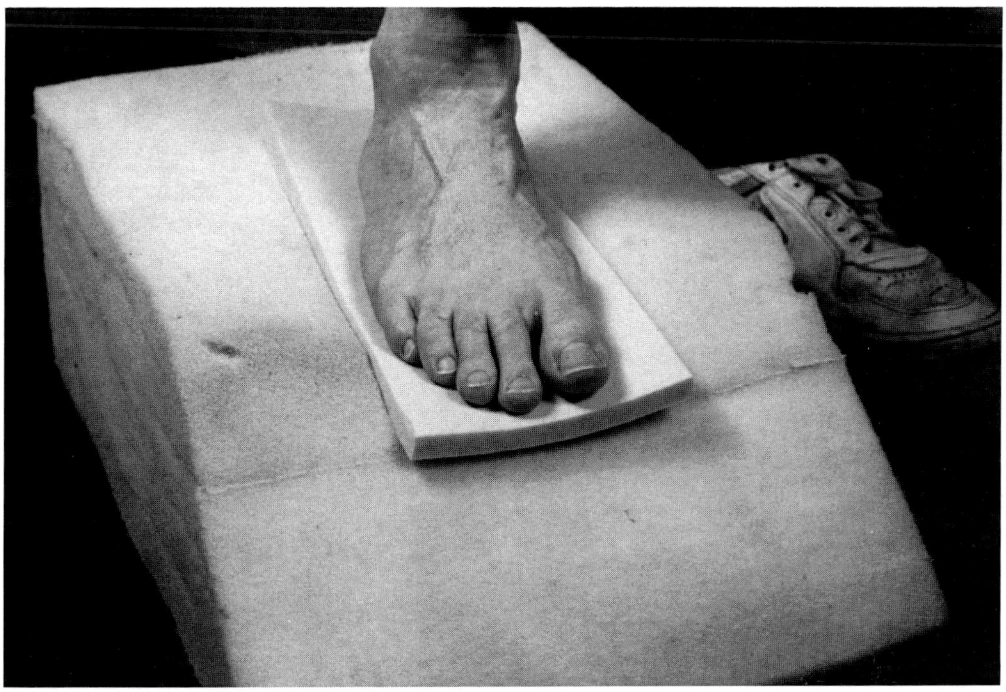

Fig. 24-4. A foam rubber block can be used to mold Plastazote foot beds for interim use. This block is angled at the front so as not to create a ridge in the material anterior to the toes. Such a ridge could lead to toe ulceration.

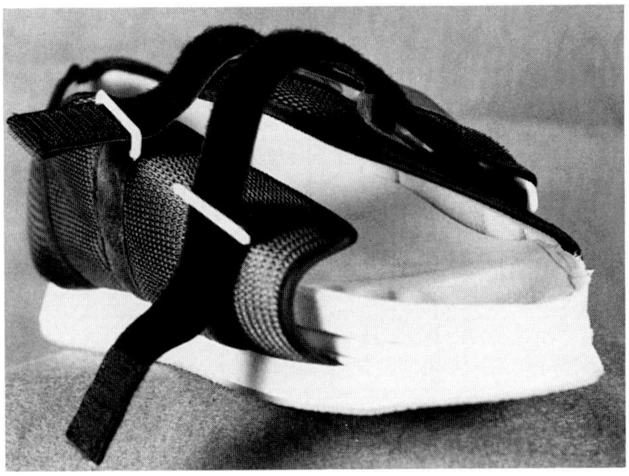

Fig. 24-5. Shoes such as the Darco shoe can be used to contain the foot and a molded polyethylene foot bed can be used as interim footwear.

while still protecting those at less risk. One means of categorization can be found in Table 24-1.

In this table category 0 includes all patients with diabetes who have not lost sensation and have adequate circulation to their feet. Even these patients should begin adapting their purchases of footwear to styles that will pose the least risk to their feet. It is not unusual for the sensory loss to be detected clinically after the first ulcer is already present.

Category 1 patients are those who do not have foot deformity or a history of plantar foot ulcers, but who have lost protective levels of sensation in their feet. More than anything else in diabetes, it is the loss of protective sensation that leads to foot injuries. Once sensation is lost the person is at much higher risk of injury. Such people need a high level of professional assistance and prevention. All of their shoes that are regularly worn should be evaluated for fit and style. Thin cushioned inserts such as Spenco or PPT can be used to reduce stress against the bottom of the foot.[7] Recent studies indicate that socks with plantar padding can also reduce pressures under the foot as compared to using conventional hosiery.[8]

Patients in category 2 not only have lost sensation but also have a foot deformity. Deformity often results in an increase of pressure to tissues over the deformity. If surgery is not used to eliminate the deformity, then the footwear needs to be modified or constructed to accommodate the shape. Once proper shoes are obtained it is essential that the physician and shoe fitter work closely together to ensure the shoe continues to function properly and the foot is not becoming injured. The patient

Table 24-1. Risk and Management Categories for Diabetic Feet Without Ulceration

Risk Category	Management Category
Risk Category 0[a] Has protective sensation Has not had a plantar ulcer May have foot deformity Has a disease that could lead to insensitivity	**Management Category 0**[a] Foot clinic visit once a year Patient education, to include footwear selection that may require style changes
Risk Category 1 Does not have protective sensation Has not had a plantar ulcer Does not have a foot deformity	**Management Category 1** Footwear style changes Soft insoles—Spenco, nylon-covered PPT Foot clinic visit every 6 months
Risk Category 2 Does not have protective sensation Has not had a plantar ulcer Does have foot deformity	**Management Category 2** Foot clinic visit every 3 to 4 months Custom-molded orthotic device Prescription footwear
Risk Category 3 Does not have protective sensation Has history of foot ulceration and/or vascular laboratory findings indicate significant vascular disease	**Management Category 3** Foot clinic visit every 1 to 2 months Custom orthotic devices Prescription shoes

[a]Protective threshold of sensation is lost if the patient cannot feel Semmes-Weinstein monofilament 5.07 (10 grams).[18] Diabetic patients who have foot deformity but have not yet lost protective sensation should have a sensory examination every 4 months.

should be scheduled more frequently for these inspections.

The most common site of ulceration on insensate feet is a part that was ulcerated before.[9] Category 3 patients with a history of foot ulcers should be seen even more often than category 1 or 2 patients for footwear inspection and foot evaluation. It is not unusual to see these patients once a month to ensure an ulcer is not emerging or the shoe is not wearing down. During these frequent visits the shoe fitter or physician should try to encourage the patients' own vigilance and reinforce their education on foot care. All professionals contributing to the management of a diabetic patient should reinforce the need for the patient to continue to wear proper footwear at all times.

SHOE MODIFICATIONS

The most common cause of plantar ulceration on insensate feet is the repetitive stress of walking.[3] Unlike persons with normal sensation, those with sensory loss never alter the way the foot meets the ground when excessive stress begins to cause tissue injury. Although the initial injury consists of microtrauma that would be a slight discomfort to the person with sensation, in the insensitive foot continued walking leads to continuous inflammation. The area becomes more and more inflamed with additional walking that is only occurring because no pain is restricting the patient's activity. Due to the inflammatory process the number of white cells is continually increasing. It is this white blood cell density that eventually leads to the autolysis of the tissues and ulceration.[3] If the first small trauma had led to discomfort the whole process would have stopped there. When sensation has been lost the principle of stopping the progression of injury remains valid. The stress has to be reduced to stop the inflammation. Proper footwear design can decrease the mechanical stress of walking to safe levels.

When inflammation is present in the foot the surface of the skin will become warmer in that region. If the increase of surface temperature is detected soon enough the shoe can be modified before an ulcer emerges. The more frequent clinic visits for patients at higher risk enables the foot care professional to look for these focal areas of inflammation.

The most common locations for plantar ulcers to occur are under the metatarsal heads and first toe.[10,11,12] Therefore, the primary focus of prevention for diabetic patients whose feet have never been ulcerated should be toward minimizing the repetitive pressure that occurs under the forefoot of such patients while walking.

There are three general means of relieving stress between the foot and ground: softness, molding, and rocking.

Softness

Soft materials cushion the shock of the foot meeting the ground by conforming to its plantar surface as they are compressed and by slowing the rate of deceleration as the foot comes against the walking surface. Running shoes have greatly improved shoe sole cushioning. A preliminary study in 1986 indicated that running shoes can be used as a means of relieving pressure and reducing the size of plantar callus formation.[13] The techniques of design and use of materials that has evolved through the natural selection of the purchases and endorsements of long distance runners are gradually being incorporated into a wider range of footwear, particularly walking shoes.

Molding

Pressure is defined as force divided by area ($P = F/A$). Force is generated by the body weight. Area is the amount of the foot meeting the walking surface at any given time. By increasing the surface of the foot through which the force passes, the pressure on any part of the foot can be reduced. Properly molded firm insoles are more efficient at spreading stress than unmolded soft materials. The viscoelastic properties of human soft tissues are the best cushion under the foot. Firm materials are also better at maintaining these structures under the foot.

Rocking

By making the sole of a shoe rigid and by changing the shape of the bottom of the sole (Fig. 24-6) the vectors of force can be redirected as the leg passes over the foot during weight-bearing phases of gait.

Shear stress, which is stress applied parallel to the surface, often leads to tearing of the tissue or blistering. Shear can be reduced by making the shoe sole rigid from the heel to the toe.[14] If a shoe sole was made rigid from the heel to the toe without any other sole modification, the patient would pull the heel of the foot out of the shoe during each toe-off phase of gait.

With a rocker contour added to the bottom of the shoe sole, as the patient tries to apply force to the forefoot when the heel is lifted in gait, the shoe will roll forward like a wheel. The shoe sole must be made rigid from heel to toe for the rocking mechanism to best relieve plantar forefoot pressure. Rather than letting the patient lift heel in gait onto the metatarsal heads, the rocker sole, by rolling, will transfer the pressure from under the shoe sole forward as the heel is lifted from the ground.[15] These designs can be particularly effective at reducing forefoot stress.

The most effective form of rocker sole design begins to curve up away from the floor in the middle of the total shoe length as viewed from the side.[16] This may begin the rocker too far posterior for some patients. They may feel unstable while standing. When this occurs the rocker can be moved forward. However, the rocker should never begin curving anterior to the vertical alignment with the first metatarsal head. The heel of the foot is lifted from the shoe during gait when such rockers are used.

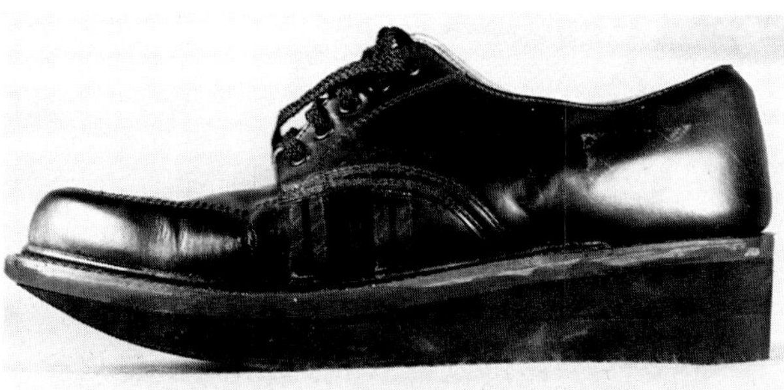

Fig. 24-6. This rocker sole design was constructed by increasing the toe spring of the shoe by 20° on a sole rigid from heel to toe. Metal strips were used to make the sole rigid. These strips were glued in place between laminations of the soling material. A curvature was then built onto the bottom of the sole. This curve begins from a point 50 percent of the shoe length and curves on a perpendicular radius of 60 percent of the shoe length. This rocker design reduced pressure under the third metatarsal head by over 20 percent.[17]

As a general guideline, rocker soles are more effective at minimizing plantar pressure when the radius of shoe sole curvature is decreased.[17] Smaller radii require the sole to be thicker at the midfoot. A compromise must be made between the curvature and sole thickness for each individual patient.

Other Footwear Considerations

Many of the most commonly used additions to the outer sole, such as metatarsal bars, Denver heels, Mayo crescents, and Hauser bars, are not advisable for use with diabetic patients. These modifications are means of molding the inside of a shoe by applying pressure from under the outer sole. These techniques are usually imprecise and in the past have led to diabetic foot ulceration.

Stability and reinforcement can be added to the shoe by attaching extensions, sometimes referred to as flares or outriggers, to the sides of the shoe sole (Fig. 24-7). Lateral sole extensions greatly enhance a person's lateral stability and can be angled out to the side. Medial sole extensions can also add to stability by providing a broader base of support in the sole. On the medial side, extensions must not be angled out toward the other foot. If the sole extension angled away from the shoe on the medial side, during swing phase of gait the flare would hit the medial malleolus of the opposite foot.

For people who have a three-part stance phase of gait (heel contact, midstance, and toe-off), the sole should not be extended posteriorly. Posterior extensions will create a rapid plantar flexion of the ankle joint at heel contact. This rapid plantar flexion is sometimes referred to as foot slap, a description of the end of the plantar flexion.

Some people do not walk with a three-part

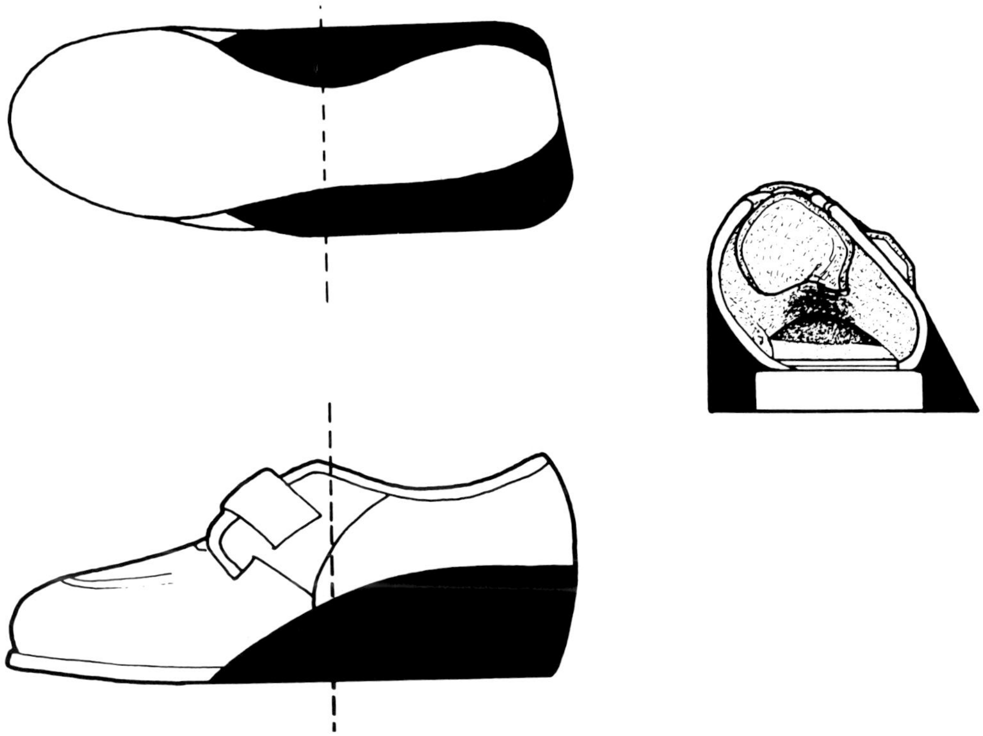

Fig. 24-7. Extensions to the sole can be added to the sides of the shoe sole to provide additional stability to the patient as he walks. The extensions can come higher on the shoe to reinforce the heel counter and inserts, particularly under the medial arch of the shoe.

weight-bearing phase, but rather shuffle when they walk. For these persons a posterior extension can be used to provide posterior stability, since many of them shuffle because they feel unstable.

Sometimes shoe inserts press out against the sides of the shoe and distort the shoe conformity. Most shoe uppers curve in just above where they attach to the sole. This can be filled in with the sole extension, and even brought up the sides of the shoe to reinforce the upper (Fig. 24-7).

Sole extensions would rarely provide any benefit if placed anterior to the neck of the metatarsals. This metatarsal-toe area should already be the widest part of the shoe. The shoe sole is usually thinner in this area and this would minimize the benefit of a lateral extension.

The goal of prescription footwear for diabetic patients is to provide an extra level of protection from the mechanical stress of walking for patients who have lost or may loose the ability to perceive for themselves excessive mechanical stress in their feet. A combination of principles described above can be tailored to the needs of the individual patient. Molding, softness, and rocker soles can be combined to provide plantar pressure relief in a properly fitted shoe. The sole can also be extended to the sides when additional stability is required.

GENERAL FOOTWEAR RECOMMENDATIONS FOR DIABETIC PATIENTS

1. Patients with pedal neuropathy must never walk barefoot. Footwear should be appropriate to the needs of each patient in the environments where he or she will be walking.
2. Patients with ulcerated or fractured foot should have footwear in preparation for immediate use during rehabilitation, and definitive footwear should be ready when rehabilitation from injury is completed.

3. Prior to putting footwear on, the patient should inspect the inside for foreign objects, torn lining or insoles, or signs of excessive wear.
4. New shoes should always be broken in gradually. Initially shoes should be worn for only 1 or 2 hours at a time for the first 2 weeks. Even after the break-in period, shoes should be removed at midday and in the evening to relieve low pressure stresses from the sides of the metatarsal heads and toes.[3]
5. Prescription footwear does not last forever. Frequent assessment for needed repairs needs to be performed by patients, medical personnel, and the shoe provider.
6. The best prescription shoe is no good if it is not worn. Some compromise and bargaining may be necessary to find something the patient will wear at least most of the time they walk. The best compromises would be in color and decorative patterns rather than toe box heighth or width. One study in England has shown an 83 percent recurrence of foot ulcers when patients stopped using prescription shoes. Only 26 percent had recurrence when they followed prescription shoe recommendations.[16]
7. Persons with insensitive feet need to be vigilant at all times to protect their feet. A higher level of awareness should come whenever they may be exposed to possible threats such as excessive heat or cold. Steam pipes, hot floors, exposure to the cold, and corrosive chemicals should be avoided; if such potential hazards are a part of the person's occupation, special footwear considerations should be made.

REFERENCES

1. Rossi WA: The high incidence of mismated feet in the population. Foot Ankle 4:105, 1983
2. Rossi WA: The futile search for perfect fit. J Test Eval 16:393, 1988
3. Brand PW: The diabetic foot. p. 829. In Ellenberg M, Rifkin H (eds): Diabetes Mellitus, Theory and Practice. 3rd Ed. Medical Examination Publishing, New Hyde Park, NY, 1983
4. Schwartz RP, Heath AL: Preliminary findings from roentgenographic study of the influence of heel height and empirical shank curvature on osteo-articular relationships in the normal female foot. J Bone Jt Surg 41A:1065, 1959
5. Rossi WA, Tennant R: Professional Shoe Fitting. National Shoe Retailers Association, New York, 1984
6. Coleman WC, Plaia A: Soft molded sandals for insensitive foot care. Clin Pros Orthot 12:67, 1988
7. Smith L, Plehwe W, Yue DK, Turtle JR: Electrodynogram in objective assessment of bearing pressures in the feet of diabetic patients. Diab Res Clin Pract 5:S312, 1988
8. Veves A, Masson EA, Fernando DJS, Boulton AJM: Use of experimental padded hosiery to reduce abnormal foot pressures in diabetic neuropathy. Diab Care 12:653, 1989
9. Brand PW: Insensitive Feet: A Practical Handbook for Foot Problems in Leprosy. The Leprosy Mission, London, 1981
10. Barrett JP, Mooney V: Neuropathy and diabetic pressure lesions. Orthop Clin North Amer 4:43, 1973
11. Ctercteko GC, Dhanendran M, Hutton WC et al: Vertical forces acting on the foot of diabetic patients with neuropathic ulceration. Br J Surg 68:608, 1981
12. Duckworth T, Boulton AJM, Betts RP et al: Plantar pressure measurements and prevention of ulceration in the diabetic foot. J Bone Jt Surg 67(B):79, 1985
13. Soulier SM: The use of running shoes in the prevention of plantar diabetic ulcers. J Am Podiatr Med Assoc 76:395, 1986
14. Price EW: Studies on plantar ulceration in leprosy; IV; the management of plantar ulcers. Lep Rev 31:159, 1960
15. Coleman WC: The relief of forefoot pressures using outer shoe sole modifications. Proceedings of the International Congress on Biomechanics and Kinesiology of the Hand and Foot. Madras, India, 1985
16. Edmonds ME, Blundell MP, Morris HE et al: Improved survival of the diabetic foot: the role of the specialized foot clinic. Q J Med 60:763, 1986
17. Nawoczenski DA, Birke JA, Coleman WC: Effect of rocker sole design on plantar forefoot pressures. J Am Podiatr Med Assoc 78:455, 1988
18. Birke JA, Sims DS: Plantar sensory threshold in the ulcerative foot. Lep Rev 57:261, 1986

25

Rehabilitation of the Diabetic Patient

James Allen Birke, M.S., P.T.

Rehabilitation is the restoration to and maintenance of an optimal level of physical, occupational, psychological, and social function. This chapter presents specific areas to consider when rehabilitating the diabetic patient with a high risk foot. These guidelines are based on treatment approaches developed at the Gillis W. Long Hansen's Disease Center in Carville, Louisiana.

Implicit in the rehabilitation process is the involvement of a multidisciplinary team approach. Experience has shown that no single medical discipline can adequately care for the total needs of the diabetic patient with high risk feet. The various disciplines should be brought together on a regular basis in order to interact and develop treatment strategies. At this facility, patients can be presented at weekly "foot clinics." The core team (consisting of a podiatrist, a physical therapist, and a shoemaker) offers treatment alternatives and can be assisted during these sessions by team members (orthopaedic surgeon, physiatrist, vascular surgeon, nurse, social worker, orthotist, prosthetist). Edmonds et al. presented a British model for a diabetic foot clinic which consists of a chiropodist, a nurse, a surgeon, and a physician. A significant decrease in amputations was reported with the inception of the clinic.[1]

The opinions or assertions contained herein are the private views of the author and are not to be construed as official or as reflecting the views of the Public Health Service.

Within any diabetic foot program, rehabilitation should include the following important elements:

1. Exercise programs
2. Restoration of functional activity
3. Prevention and care of foot problems
4. Management of the residual limb (postamputation)

EXERCISE PROGRAMS

General Conditioning

Prescribed exercise programs incorporating moderate aerobic exercise may have specific benefits for the type 2 diabetic patient. These positive effects of exercise include the following[2–4]:

1. Decreased blood lipids, including triglycerides and very low and low density lipoprotein cholesterol
2. Decreased blood glucose levels
3. Increased insulin sensitivity and increased insulin receptor binding
4. Decreased platelet adhesiveness (reducing the danger of thrombotic phenomenon)
5. Increased cardiovascular endurance
6. Assistance in control of obesity

Response to exercise by the type 1 patient is variable and is dependent on insulin availability. During periods of insulin deficiency, exercise may cause poor uptake of glucose, plasma hyperglycemia, and the rapid development of ketosis. This is in contrast to the more common situation in which insulin availability is increased by exercise-induced insulin sensitivity with resultant hypoglycemia. Injection of insulin into the exercising skeletal muscle further aggravates the problem in the type 1 diabetic patient by increasing insulin availability.

The problems associated with hypo- or hyperglycemia in the type 1 patient during exercise may be minimized by the following [2-4]:

1. Progressing exercise slowly and adjusting insulin and food intake via self-monitoring and documentation of the glycemic response
2. Avoiding the exercising extremities as insulin injection sites prior to exercise
3. Consuming meals 1 to 3 hours prior to exercise

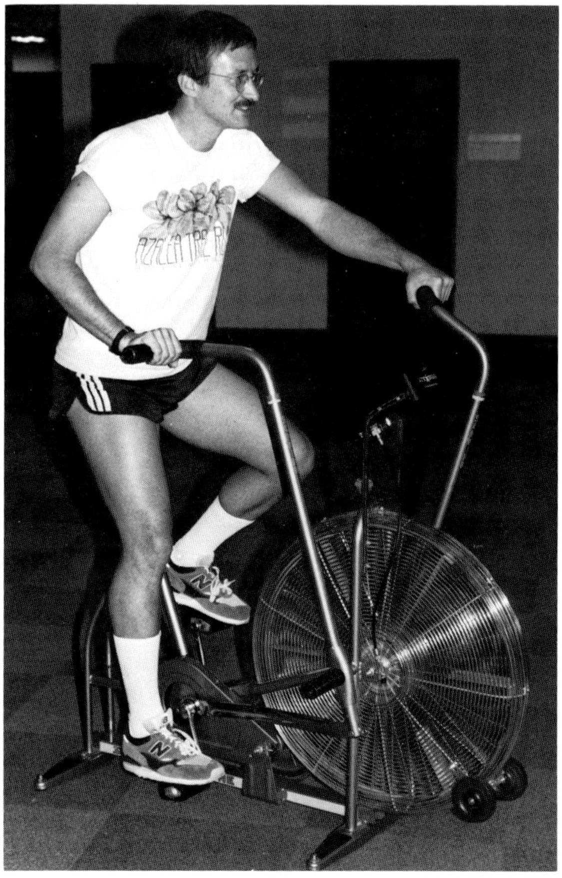

Fig. 25-1. Stationary bicycle with arm resistance exercise (Air-Dyne, Schwinn Sales South, Atlanta, GA).

The exercise prescriptions must be uniquely designed for each individual. The patient's age, sex, level of fitness, degree of diabetic control, and level of risk for foot injuries should be considered.[3,5] In addition, the medical history should be reviewed for conditions that may be aggravated by vigorous activity. These conditions include proliferative retinopathy, cardiovascular disease, nephropathy, and neuropathy.

In general, the following guidelines can be suggested. Exercise intensity should be moderate and result in a heart rate increase of 55 to 75 percent of maximum. Each session should last 15 to 60 minutes and should be performed 3 to 5 days per week. The exercises should involve the larger muscles, ideally both the arms and legs (Fig. 25-1). Activities most often selected are walking, jogging, cycling, swimming, and racquet games.[4,5] However, ambulatory limitations may restrict the exercise to the upper extremities and trunk.[6] Individuals with problematic feet should select activities such as swimming, cycling, and rowing, which minimize the impact on the feet. New exercise modes, which optimize cardiovascular fitness but minimize foot stresses, need to be developed in response to the recent awareness of diabetic foot problems.

Range of Motion Exercises

Exercises may also be designed to increase or maintain joint range of motion. Evidence indicates that diabetic patients are more likely to develop joint limitations as compared to nondiabetic individuals.[8] Heel cord tightness, subtalar joint hypomobility, hallux limitus, and clawing of the lesser toes is seen with greater frequency among diabetic patients.[8] Collagen accumulates in the lower dermis and may cause periarticular stiffness. The neuropathy also contributes to development of joint limitation by creating muscular imbalances around a joint secondary to weakness. Limitation of joint motion may result in abnormal pressure distributions on the plantar surface of the foot and lead to plantar ulceration.[9,10] Gentle passive stretching, active range of motion exercises, and joint mobilization techniques specifically designed to improve and maintain ankle, foot, and toe mobility may be indicated (Fig. 25-2). Studies are

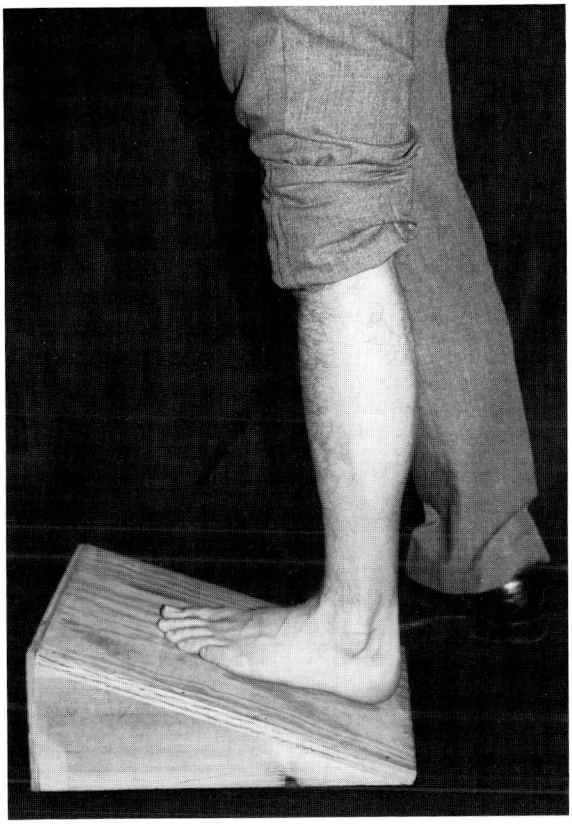

Fig. 25-2. Stretching exercise for heelcord tightness using an incline board.

needed to evaluate the value of range of motion exercises in the prevention of foot lesions. Additionally, exercises can be prescribed for dysfunctions of the spine and other peripheral joints.

Strengthening Exercises

Diabetic polyneuropathy in the lower extremity commonly involves the peroneal and tibial nerves. This results in weakness in the foot and ankle due to involvement of the intrinsic muscles and ankle dorsiflexors-evertors, and to a lesser extent ankle plantar flexor-invertors. In the upper extremity the ulnar and median innervated muscles of the hand are often involved, resulting in loss of grip strength and fine motor control. In the chronic neuropathic process onset is insidious and significant motor improvement is unlikely. However, physical therapy is indicated for the prevention or slowing of motor wasting.[4]

Mononeuropathies secondary to entrapment syndromes or ischemic infarction of the vasa nervorum arterial capillaries may be present in a cranial, spinal, or peripheral distribution. Diabetic amyotrophy is a disorder characterized by a unilateral weakness, pain, and wasting of the muscles of the pelvic girdle and thigh; improvement usually occurs within two years.[4] In both cases, physical therapy may be beneficial.

RESTORATION OF FUNCTIONAL ACTIVITY

Functional independence can be severely impaired by the neuropathic, metabolic, cardiovascular, cerebrovascular, renal, and retinal complications of diabetes. These are compounded by the debilitating effects of prolonged inactivity and bedrest. Restoration of the activities of daily living can only begin after a thorough assessment of such factors as strength, balance, sensation, and vision (Fig. 25-3). The numerous techniques for improving functional deficits are beyond the scope of this text.

FOOT PROBLEMS

Prevention

Since there are approximately 12 million diabetic patients in the United States, preventative foot programs must direct their resources to the patients with greatest need.[11] The identification of the patient at highest risk of developing plantar ulceration then becomes a critical component of a preventative program.

There are several mechanisms responsible for ulceration of the foot. Diminished sensation and abnormal stresses are considered the major factors in the development of plantar ulcers. In addition, ischemic lesions, often painful, are initiated by trauma or abnormal stress, and are slow to heal due to poor circulation. Conversely, ischemic lesions

FUNCTIONAL EXAMINATION

Name: ______________________ **Date:** __________
Patient Complaints: ______________________
Medical History: ______________________
Social History: ______________________
Living Environment: ______________________
Orientation: ______________________
Vision/hearing: ______________________
Balance: ______________________
Sensation: ______________________
Skin Condition: ______________________

Activities:

	Indep	Assistance Min	Mod	Max	Comments
supine > sit					
bed > chair					
sit > stand					
toilet					
car transfers					
wheelchair mobility					
ambulation					
stairs					

(note cane, quad cane, walker, special footwear, prosthesis)
distance __________

Strength/ROM:

Left ROM	Left Strength		Right ROM	Right Strength
		shoulder flexion		
		elbow flexion		
		elbow extension		
		wrist flexion		
		wrist extension		
		hip flexion		
		hip extension		
		knee flexion		
		knee extension		
		ankle dorsi flexion		
		ankle plantar flexion		

KEY

5 - Full resistance against gravity
4 - Some resistance against gravity
3 - Full range of motion against gravity
2 - Full range of motion gravity eliminated
1 - Muscle contraction; no joint motion
0 - No muscle contraction

Assessment: ______________________

Fig. 25-3. Functional evaluation form.

DIABETIC FOOT SCREEN

Date:

Patient's Name(Last, First, Middle)____________________

ID No:

Fill in the following blanks with an **R**, **L**, or **B** to indicate positive findings on the right, left or both feet.

Has there been a change in the foot since last evaluation?	Yes__	No__	N/A__
Is there a foot ulcer now or history of foot ulcer?	Yes__	No__	
Does the foot have an abnormal shape?	Yes__	No__	
Is there weakness in the ankle or foot?	Yes__	No__	
Are the nails thick, too long or ingrown?	Yes__	No__	

Label: Sensory Level with a "+" in the circled areas of the foot if the patient can feel the 10 gram (5.07 Semmes-Weinstein) nylon filament and "–" if he/she can not feel the 10 gram filament.

RIGHT

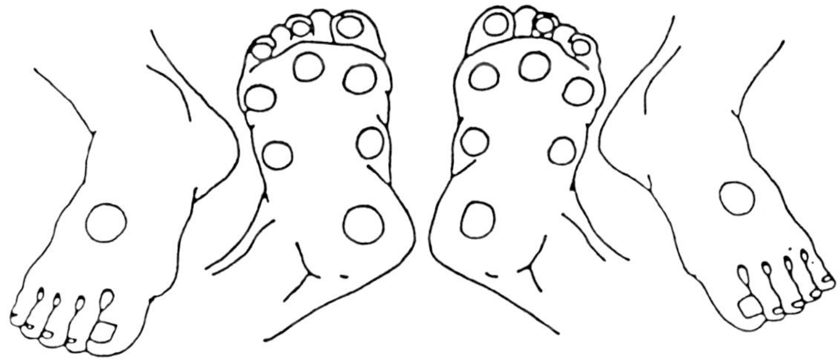

LEFT

Draw in and Label: Callus ▨ , Pre-ulcer ▩ , Ulcer ■ (Note width/depth in cm.)
Skin Condition with **R** - Redness, **S** - Swelling, **W** - Warmth, **D** - Dryness, **M** - Maceration

Vascular:

Brachial Systolic Pressure	R__	L__
Ankle Systolic Pressure	R__	L__
Ischemic Index	R__	L__

Does the patient use footwear appropriate for his/her category? Yes__ No__

RISK CATEGORY:

__ 0 No loss of protective sensation.

__ 1 Loss of protective sensation (no weakness, deformity, callus, pre-ulcer or Hx. ulceration.)

__ 2 Loss of protective sensation with weakness, deformity, pre-ulcer or callus but no Hx. ulceration.

__ 3 History of plantar ulceration or Ischemic Index < 0.45.

Fig. 25-4. Foot screening form.

can be painless and attributed to prolonged pressure on an insensitive foot. Charcot fractures occur in a neuropathic foot as a result of abnormal stress or trauma and are exacerbated by the resultant hyperemia and continued painless ambulation.[12]

Foot Screen

A foot screen should be a brief examination designed to determine the present status of the patient and identify factors which place the foot at potential risk for problems (Fig. 25-4). Two clinical tests have been recommended for identifying loss of protective sensation: vibrometry and nylon monofilaments.[13–16] At our facility the vibrometer failed to identify risk in some patients with known history of ulceration. The filaments are preferred due to their relative ease of application.

Abnormal stresses on the foot are often the result of observable foot deformities. Deformities include muscle weakness, claw toes, hallux limitus, plantar flexed first ray, rear and forefoot varus, equinus, Charcot foot, and forefoot amputations. With sensation loss or ischemia these deformities result in abnormal pressure distributions and focal lesions. The skin is inspected for callus formation, redness, or preulcerative lesions. Previous ulceration and the resultant scar formation place a patient at high risk of future ulceration. A Harris mat pressure test may also be used to screen the foot for local areas of high pressure.[17]

The Doppler probe for calculation of the ischemic index is the most popular method for screening circulatory dysfunction in the foot.[18–20] A limitation of the test occurs when blood flow cannot be occluded due to calcific arteries. The simplicity of the technique, however, makes it an excellent screening tool. The identification of patients with potential vascular risk would indicate a need for further vascular evaluation.

Risk Categories

Once the screen is completed, the patient can be assigned to a risk category which provides a basis for prescribing preventative treatment measures.[21] Those patients at risk of developing foot complications may benefit from a prevention program including patient education, protective footwear, callus and skin care, exercise, and surgical correction of deformities.[21,22] These aspects are discussed elsewhere in this text. Risk categories also serve as a basis for scheduled follow-up. For example, patients in risk category 3 usually need routine follow-up monthly for callus and nail care and to make adjustments to or replace footwear. Risk category 0 patients only require screens annually.

Foot Injury Management

Whirlpool and debridement have been part of traditional treatment regimes for foot ulcerations. This treatment approach alone is often ineffective because it does not focus on the mechanical factors of ulceration.[23] Without resting the foot, plantar ulcerations are extremely difficult to heal. Rest minimizes joint movement and weight-bearing stresses on the foot. Bed rest is often inadequate because patients continue to weight bear during short trips to the bathroom and hospital appointments. Furthermore, the debilitative effects of bed rest can be detrimental to the patient's medical status. For these reasons rest appliances have been devised.

Rest Appliances

Several studies have shown the effectiveness of walking casts in healing plantar ulcers, with average healing rates of about 6 weeks.[24–28] Walking casts have also been shown to be more effective than traditional methods in promoting ulcer healing.[29] When casts have not been advisable, other rest appliances such as walking splints (Fig. 25-5) or cutout sandals have been used successfully. Each of these devices has been designed to relieve stresses at the ulcer site.[21]

The insensitive or ischemic foot is also at risk of non-weight-bearing lesions on the bony areas of the foot, ankle, posterior heel, and lower leg. A custom-molded Plastazote boot designed with ulcer reliefs and protective shields has proven to be an excellent device for eliminating harmful contact stresses and direct trauma (Fig. 25-6). The device should be worn continuously during the day and may even be worn in bed.

The interim period between wound closure and full healing is critical.[21,22] A newly closed plantar ulcer is likely to reulcerate unless the foot is carefully protected and monitored. Often, prescribed

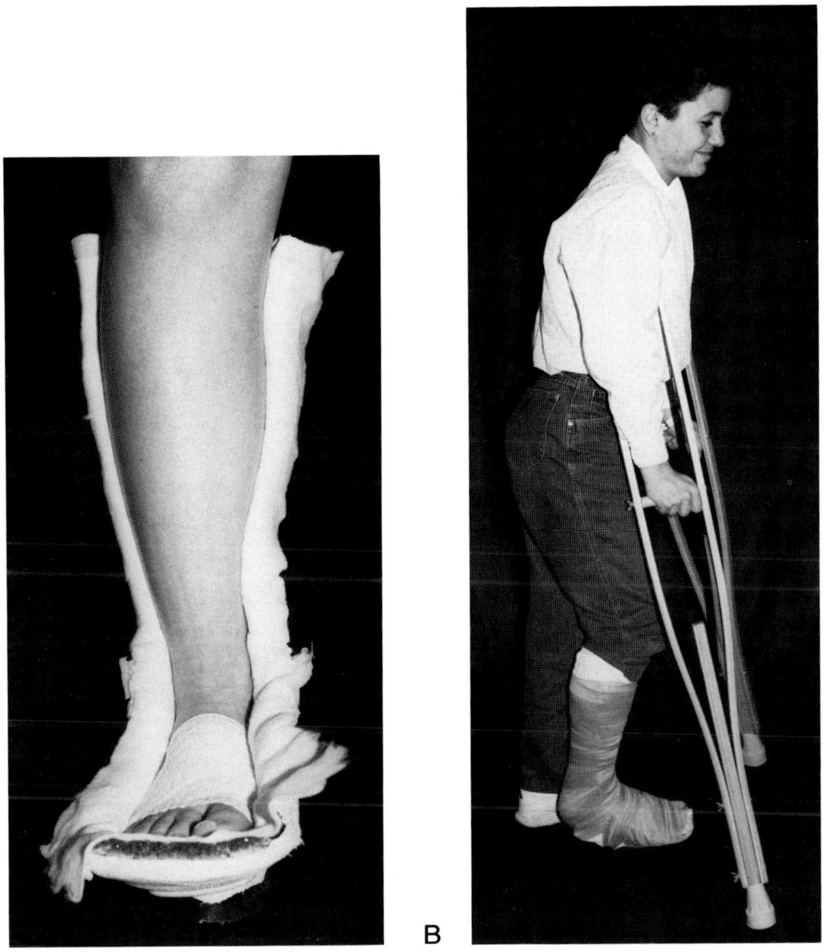

Fig. 25-5. (**A**) Walking splint. (**B**) An elastic bandage attaches the splint to the foot. Partial weight-bearing with crutches provides additional reduction of stress to the lesion area.

footwear takes days or weeks to obtain or fabricate. When the rest appliance is no longer needed, the foot should be fit immediately with temporary protective footwear before the patient resumes ambulation. Healing shoes or sandals with molded Plastazote footbeds are convenient and easy to fabricate. Patients should also remain partially weight-bearing with careful monitoring until the lesion appears fully healed. Temperatures provide a means of evaluating healing progress and soft tissue stress. Normal temperatures usually vary within 1 °C when compared to the same area on the contralateral side.[22,30] When skin temperature is greater than 1 °C difference when compared to the contralateral side, the rehabilitation progression of the patient should be modified. Several good skin thermometers and radiometers are available to detect elevated skin temperatures (Fig. 25-7).

Modified Footwear

When the foot is fully healed, definitive footwear is provided. Creativity is essential to adapt the shoe to the patient's foot and to his environment. The footwear should fit the shape of the foot and provide adequate depth for custom-molded orthoses. Orthotic devices incorporate elements of molding, softness, pressure relief, and control of abnormal foot motion. Forefoot lesions may benefit from a rocker sole modification. Cupped heel orthoses and cushioned heels are used after ulceration of the

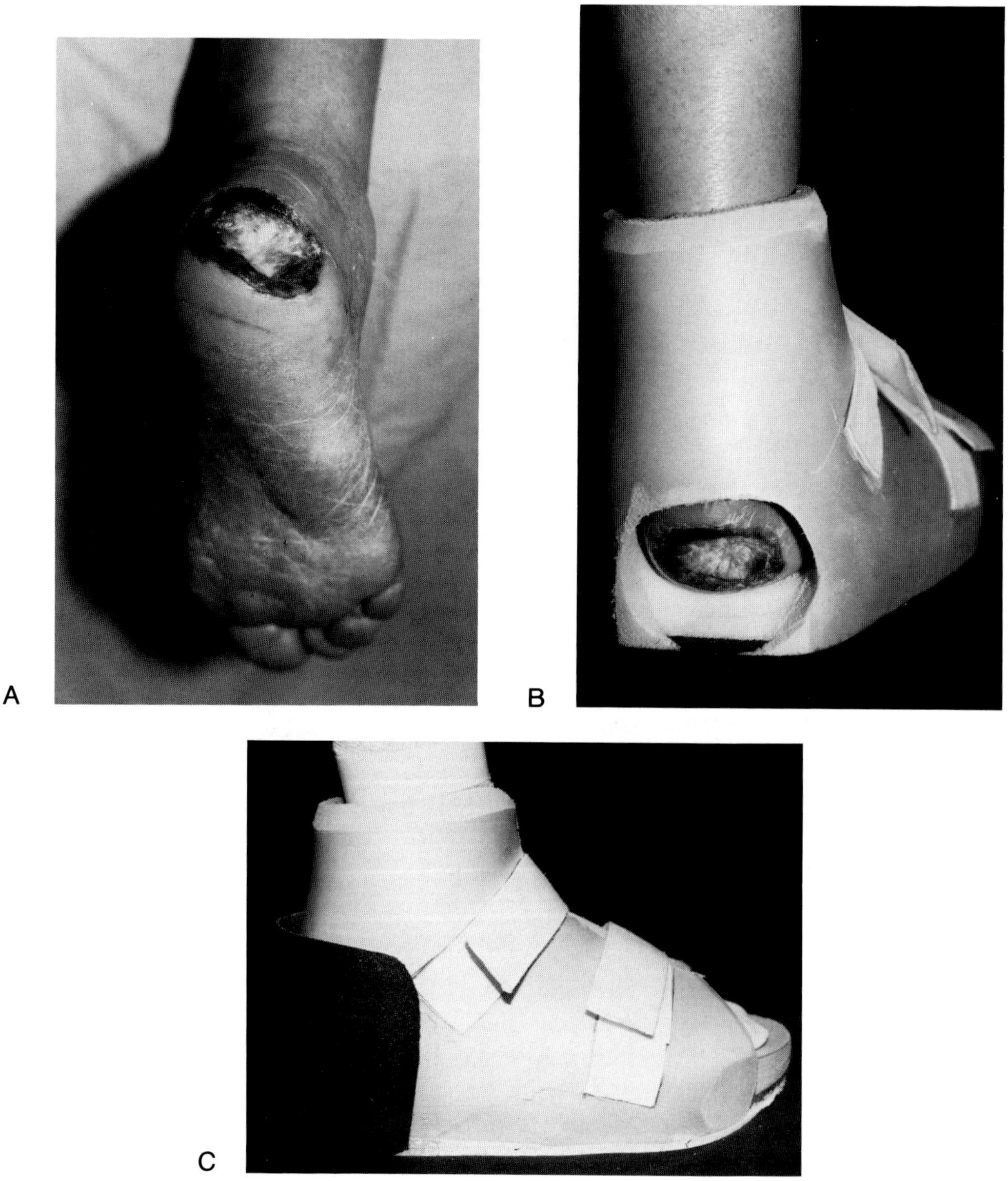

Fig. 25-6. Custom-molded Plastazote boot. (**A**) Posterior heel ulceration in a diabetic patient. (**B**) Cutout in boot to relieve stresses at the lesion site. (**C**) An additional piece of rigid plastazote provides protection from external pressure.

heel. All footwear should be carefully checked on the patient and specific instructions should be given on footwear break-in. New footwear should generally not be worn for longer than 1 hour per day the first week, then increase gradually over time. The foot should be carefully inspected after shoe removal and each morning and evening.[21]

Charcot Foot

Acute neuropathic fractures may be treated with prolonged immobilization, surgery followed by immobilization, or amputation (in cases of severe hypomobility or deformity).[31,32] Following periods of immobilization ambulation is resumed with careful monitoring (Table 25-1). The rate of ambulation

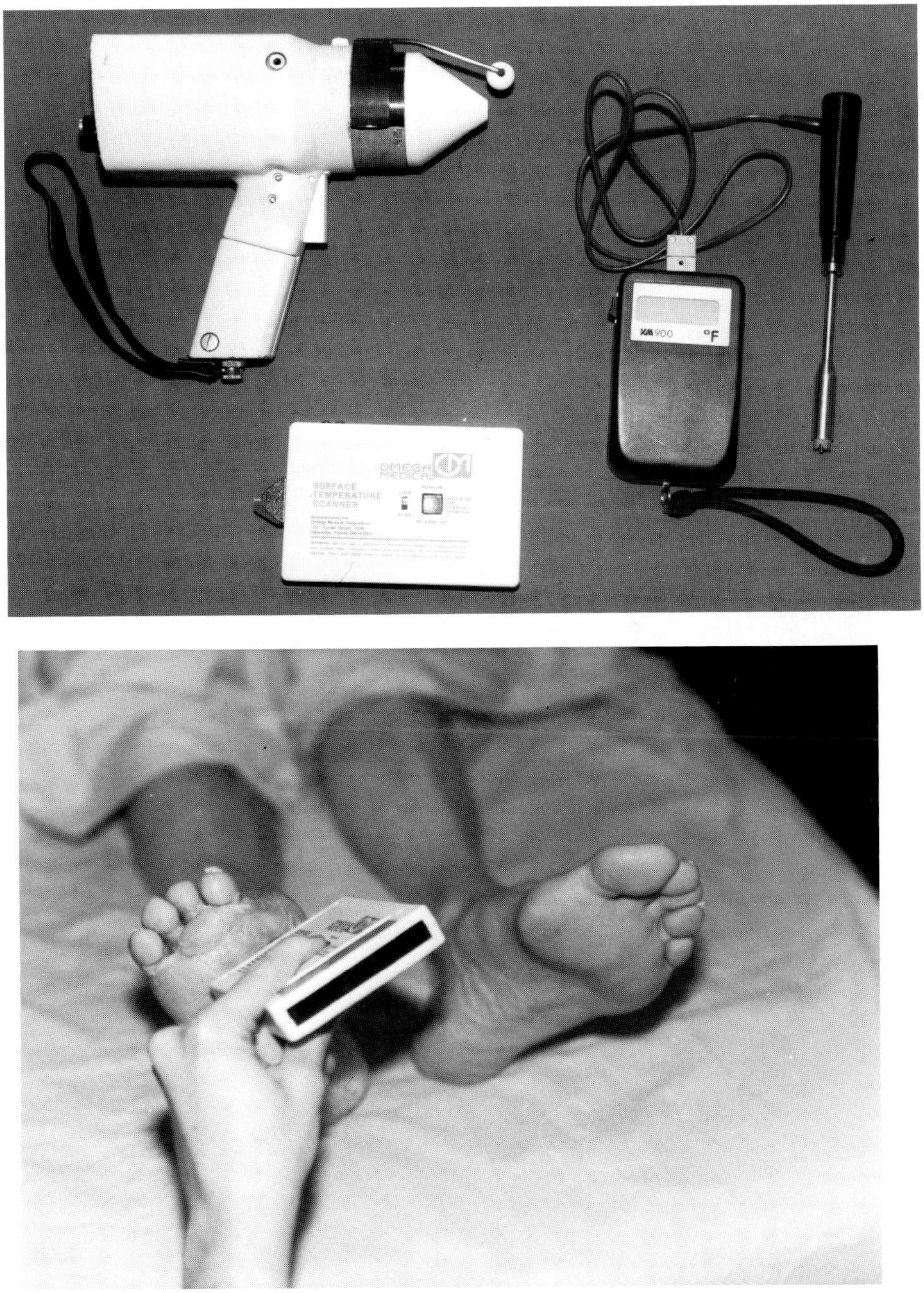

A

B

Fig. 25-7. (**A**) Left, portable digital infrared thermometer (Mikron Instrument Co., Wyckoff, NJ); center, surface temperature scanner (Omega Medical Corp., Clearwater, FL); right, electronic thermometer and probe (Kane May Instruments, Measurements Inc., New Orleans, LA). (**B**) Comparison of skin temperature with the contralateral foot.

Table 25-1. Ambulation Progressions for the Charcot Foot

Walking cast
Orthopaedic walker
Orthopaedic walker and break-in of custom footwear PWB
Custom-molded footwear PWB
PWB for long distances
Full weight-bearing

Abbreviation: PWB, partial weight-bearing (use of crutches or walker).

progression is based on the comparison of skin temperature with the contralateral side. Orthopedic walkers (Fig. 25-8) have been useful as a means of progression from cast immobilization.[33] Patients with a Charcot foot may eventually progress to custom footwear. These shoes are constructed from plaster foot models and will accommodate abnormal foot shape. Custom boots with rocker soles provide support above the ankle and control movement at the foot and ankle.

MANAGEMENT OF THE RESIDUAL LIMB

Presurgical Care

The treatment goals of the patient prior to amputation are to prepare the patient psychologically, instruct in strengthening and range of motion exercises, and instruct in ambulation with assistive devices. Well-informed patients with realistic expectations are better prepared for rehabilitation.

A B

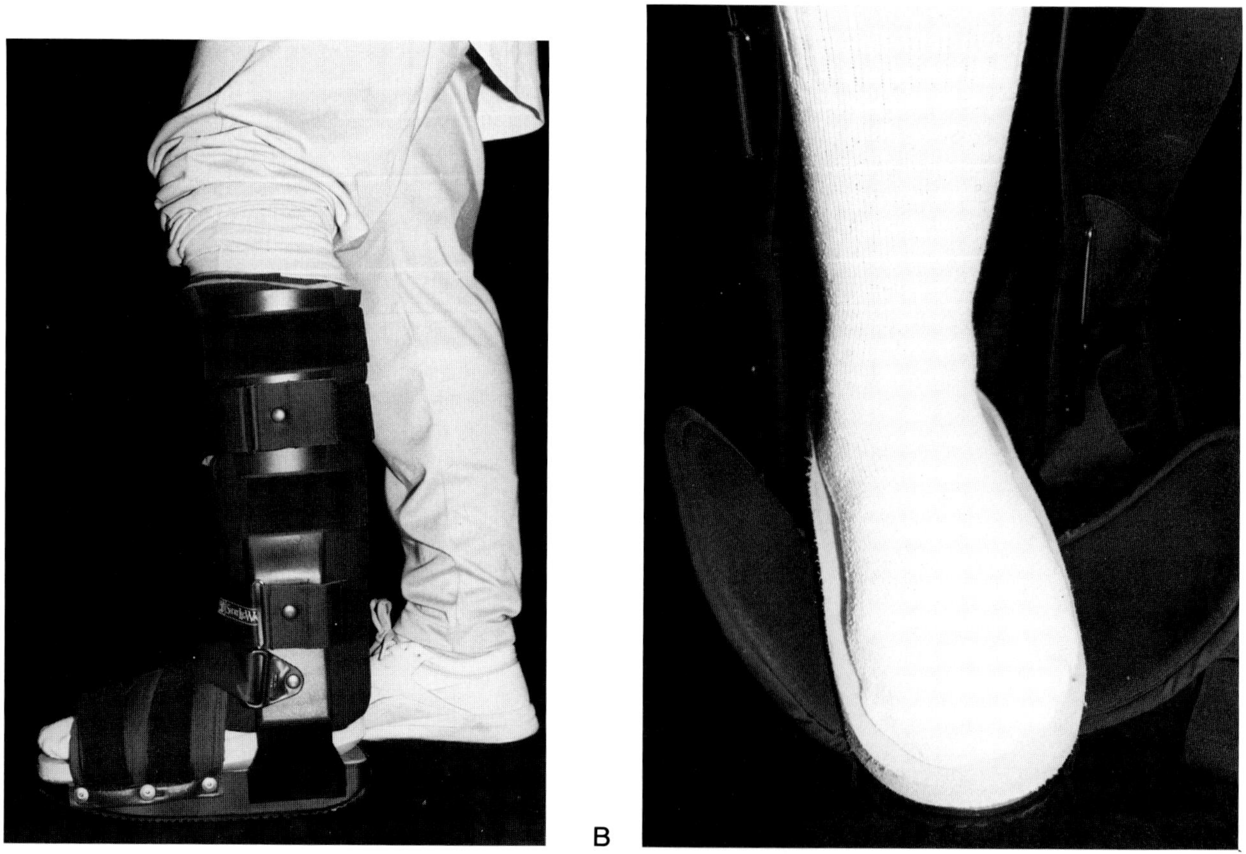

Fig. 25-8. **(A)** Short leg walker (3D Orthopedic, Inc., Dallas, TX). **(B)** Short leg walker modified with a molded Plastazote footbed.

Exercises are more easily taught before than after surgery and are important in preventing weakness and joint limitation. After surgery, the development of knee and hip flexion contractures is the most common cause of failure in prosthetic rehabilitation.

Considerations for Level of Amputation

When salvage of the foot is not possible, amputation and subsequent prosthetic fitting offer the diabetic an opportunity to return to normal functional activities. In general, as the length of the residual limb is increased, function is improved and energy cost is reduced.[34] For this reason, above knee amputations should be considered as a last resort.

Syme Amputation

A Syme procedure may be recommended for unmanageable neuropathic fractures and ulcerations. Also, unsalvageable ischemic foot lesions may be candidates for a Syme amputation after adequate circulation has been restored through vascular reconstruction.[35] The advantage of the Syme procedure is the long residual lever arm and the ability for distal end weight-bearing. The amputation is not appropriate when the heel pad has been destroyed or if circulation to the ankle is compromised. Arguments against this procedure include inadequacy of blood supply and the difficulty in constructing a satisfactory prosthetic device. The conventional medial window and expandable Syme prostheses are proven as acceptable designs; their disadvantage is poor cosmesis because of a wide ankle girth.

Below Knee Amputation

The below knee (BK) level is the most common site for amputation in the diabetic patient. Unilateral and even bilateral BK amputees are capable of normal functional activities but at a lower level of performance. Care must be taken to ensure adequate length of the BK stump. Short stumps result in an inadequate lever arm, encourage flexion deformities, and provide a limited surface area for weight-bearing stresses. The traditional range for acceptable stump length is $3\frac{1}{2}$ to $5\frac{1}{2}$ inches below the tibial plateau.[36] However, this range does not provide for variations in body size. Lengths to the calf tendinous junction or 40 percent of the length of the lower leg have been considered ideal.

Preprosthetic Care

Following surgery, the goals of preprosthetic rehabilitation care are maintenance of strength and range of motion, promotion of stump healing, shrinkage and shaping, progressive ambulation, and the fitting and assessment of temporary prostheses.

Rigid Dressing

The application of a plaster cast, or rigid dressing, at the time of surgical amputation has been shown to be an effective method to prevent edema, decrease pain, and promote healing.[37,38] A sterile heavy cotton stump sock is placed over the stump and extends above the knee. A reticular foam pad is placed over the incisional area to provide pressure relief and absorb drainage. A drain tube is easily removed when placed at the medial side of the cast sock. The knee should be maintained in full extension during plaster application. Elastic plaster is carefully wrapped around the stump and a gentle posterior to anterior pull is provided across the distal stump (in the direction of the anterior stump flap). Additional layers of standard extra-fast-drying plaster are applied for strength. The plaster should extend at least 5 inches above the knee, and before fully set, pressure is applied above the medial and lateral condyles to create suspension contours. An elastic waist strap provides additional suspension.

The initial rigid dressing is usually removed after 1 week to inspect the wound and a second cast is applied for 2 weeks (Fig. 25-9). If the incision is fully closed, sutures may be removed at 3 weeks. Early removal of sutures may result in wound dehiscence. Additional casts are applied until the incision line is fully healed. Rigid dressings are often described in conjuction with immediate prosthetic fitting and ambulation. In the diabetic patient immediate prosthetic fitting is not recommended.

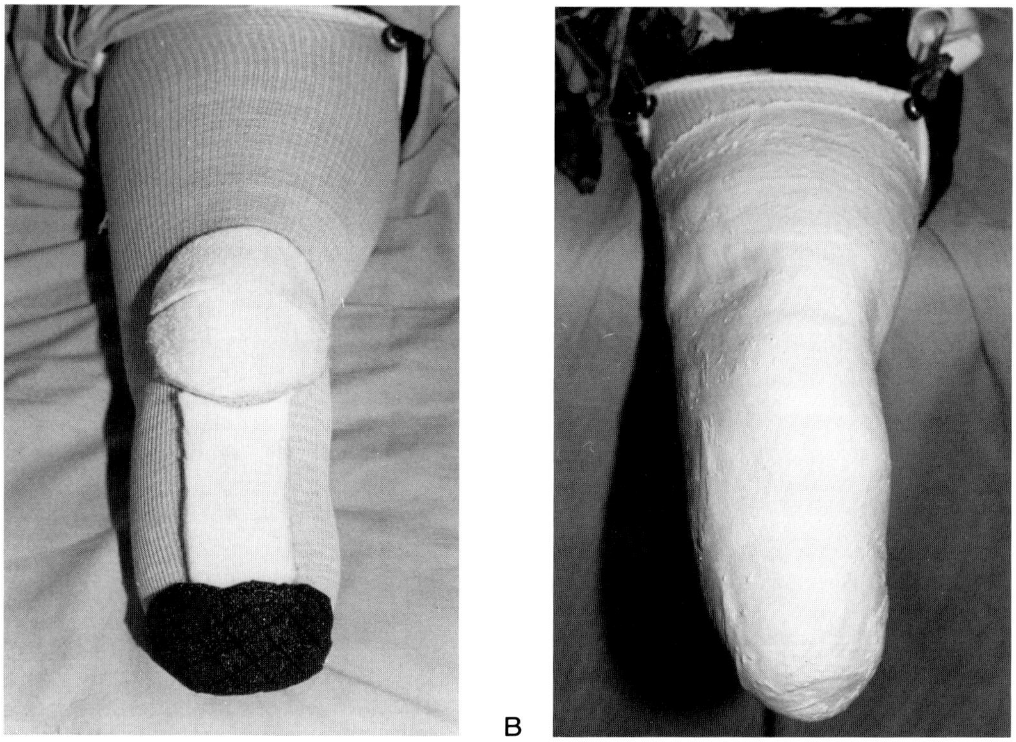

Fig. 25-9. Rigid dressing. (**A**) Padding over the incisional area, tibial crest, and patella. Not shown, several layers of cotton cast padding applied around and below the knee to pad other pressure sensitive areas. (**B**) Finished rigid dressing. Note that the plaster has been molded above the femoral condyles to aid in suspension.

If rigid dressings are not applied at surgery, postoperative swelling is a problem. Elastic bandages should be applied carefully to prevent uneven pressures on the stump and resultant skin breakdown. A removable rigid dressing has been reported to be effective in controlling edema and promoting wound healing while providing ease in wound inspection.[39–41] Other alternative devices include Unna's boots, shrinker socks, and air splints.[42–44]

Within the first 48 hours after surgery, correct bed positioning should be reviewed with the patient, family, and nursing staff. The knee should be maintained in full extension, and hip flexion and external rotation should be minimized. Gentle range of motion and quadriceps strengthening exercises are begun. Periods of prone lying should be encouraged as soon as tolerated, and the knee should be supported in full extension when sitting or in a wheelchair.

Prosthetic Fit

The patient may be fit with a definitive prosthesis when the stump is fully healed and there is no postoperative edema. Since the stump continues to shrink significantly during the initial months of full-time prosthetic use, the patient will often need a second prosthesis within 1 year. To minimize the cost of prosthetic refitting, a temporary prosthesis is often prescribed as an initial device. The temporary prosthesis may be made with a plastic, fiberglass, or plaster socket attached to an adjustable aluminum pylon and standard prosthetic foot[42] (Fig. 25-10). Temporary prostheses are also valu-

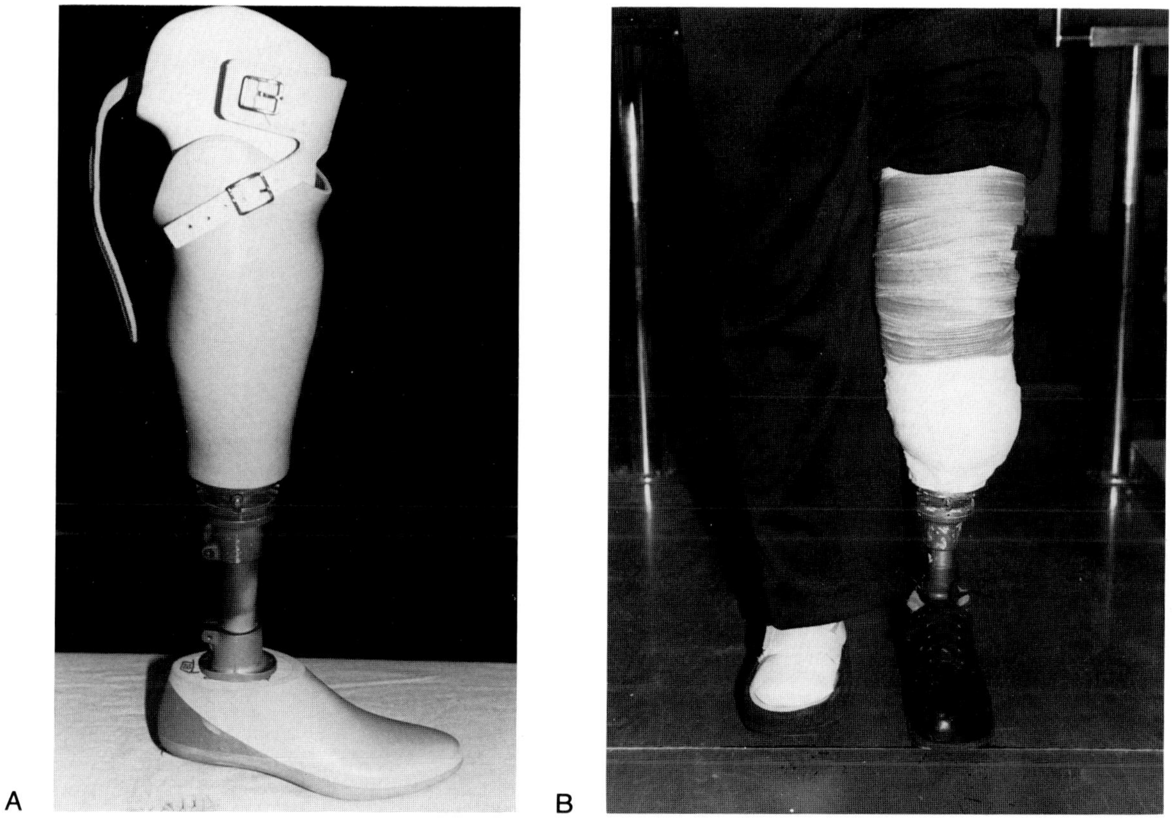

Fig. 25-10. Temporary below knee prostheses. (**A**) Plastic patella tendon bearing socket, soft liner, adjustable pylon and solid ankle cushion heel (SACH) foot. (**B**) Patient ambulating 4 weeks post amputation with a temporary prosthesis made of a plaster socket lined with plastazote and reinforced with fiberglass taping. This type limb is suitable for supervised walking only. The opposite foot is protected with a molded Plastazote sandal.

able for fitting patients that are considered marginal candidates for prosthetic use.

Prostheses

The standard BK prosthesis with a patella tendon bearing socket design, cuff, or supracondylar suspension and SACH (solid ankle cushion heel) foot are still the most popular. Recently developed energy-storing prosthetic feet, the Seattle Foot, Flex-Foot, and Carbon Copy II, are designed to conserve energy during activity and sports[46,47] (Fig. 25-11). Further studies are needed to evaluate their applicability within a diabetic population.

Contralateral Foot

Amputation places additional weight-bearing stresses on the uninvolved limb. Studies have shown that these stresses often result in a second amputation within a few years of the initial procedure.[45] Preventative measures should be initiated, including protective footwear, patient education, and routine monitoring (Fig. 25-10B).

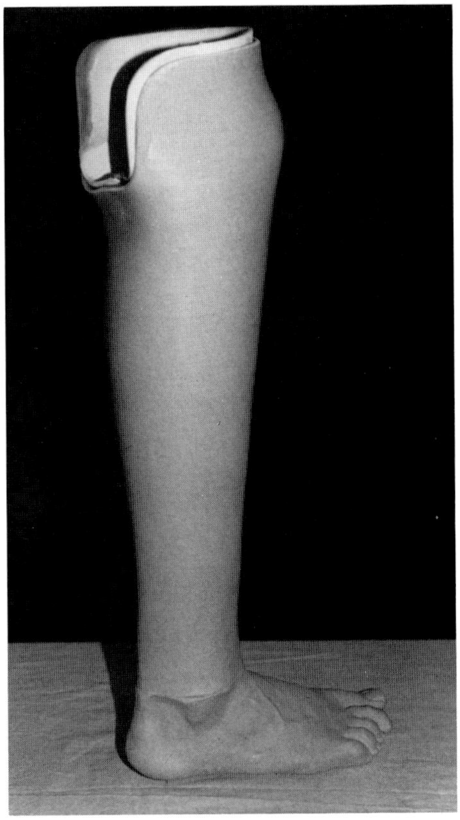

Fig. 25-11. Below knee prosthesis. Patella tendon bearing socket with supracondylar suspension, soft liner and Seattle foot.

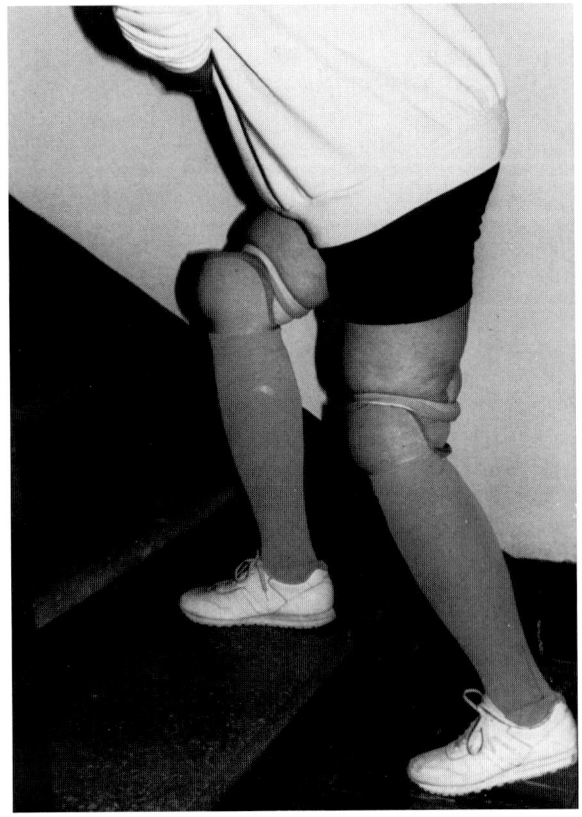

Fig. 25-12. Bilateral below knee amputee demonstrates normal function in stair climbing.

Prosthetic Checkout and Training

Definitive prostheses should be evaluated for proper fit and workmanship. Analysis of the patient's gait may reveal problems in fit or alignment. Training and progressive ambulation should be carefully monitored by the clinician as well as by the patient and family. As with footwear break-in, stump soft tissue tolerance improves over time. Areas of high stress should be immediately brought to the attention of the prosthetist to avoid skin breakdown.

Patients need specific instruction in donning the device, correctly adjusting the number of prosthetic socks, using assistive devices, getting up from the floor, and ambulation on inclines, declines, uneven surfaces, and stairs[42] (Fig. 25-12). Extensive training may be needed in the above knee or bilateral amputee.

REFERENCES

1. Edmonds ME, Blundell MP, Morris ME, et al: Improved survival of the diabetic foot: the role of a specialised foot clinic. Q J Med, new series, 60:763, 1986
2. Zinman B, Vranic M: Diabetes and exercise. Med Clin North Am 69:145, 1985
3. Horton ES: Exercise and diabetes mellitus. Med Clin North Am 72:1301, 1988
4. Olson CO: Diagnosis and Management of Diabetes Mellitus. Raven Press, New York, 1987

5. American College of Sports Medicine, Guidelines for Exercise Testing and Prescription. 3rd Ed. Lea & Febiger, Philadelphia, 1986
6. Doucete MM, Hohkanan B, Mianulli M, Roehr C: Non-ambulatory cardiovascular conditioning for individuals with diabetes mellitus, abstracted. Arch Phys Med Rehabil 68:663, 1987
7. Shinabarger NI: Limited joint mobility in adults with diabetes mellitus. Phys Ther 67:215, 1987
8. Mueller MJ, Diamond JE, Delitto A, Sinacore DR: Insensitivity, limited joint mobility and plantar ulcers in patients with diabetes mellitus. Phys Ther 69:453, 1989
9. Delbridge L, Perry P, Marr S, et al: Limited joint mobility in the diabetic foot: relationship to neuropathic ulceration. Diabetes Management 5:333, 1988
10. Birke JA, Cornwall MW, Jackson M: Relationship between hallux limitus and ulceration of the great toe. J Orthop Sports Phys Ther 10:172, 1988
11. Scarlet JJ, Blais MR: Statistics on the diabetic foot. J Am Pod Med Assoc 79:306, 1989
12. Levin ME: The diabetic foot: pathophysiology, evaluation and treatment. p. 1. In Levin ME, O'Neil LW (eds): The Diabetic Foot. CV Mosby, St Louis, 1988
13. Birke JA, Sims DS: Plantar sensory threshold in the ulcerative foot. Lepr Rev 57:261, 1986
14. Boulton AJ, Hardesty CW, Betts RP et al: Dynamic foot pressure and other studies as diagnostic and management aids in diabetic neuropathy. Diabetes Care 6:26, 1983
15. Holewski JJ, Stess RM, Graf PM, Grunfeld C: Aethesiometric quantification of cutaneous pressure sensation in diabetic peripheral neuropathy. J Rehabil Res Dev 25:1, 1988
16. Hammond CJ, Klinerman P: Protective sensation in the foot in leprosy. Lepr Rev 59:347, 1988
17. Shipley DE: Clinical evaluation and care of the insensitive foot. Phys Ther 59:13, 1979
18. Barnes RW, Shanik GD, Slaymaker EE: A index of healing in below-knee amputation: leg blood pressure by doppler ultrasound. Surgery 79:13, 1976
19. Boone GE and Pomajzl JM: Toe blood pressure by photoplethysmography: an index of healing in forefoot amputation. Surgery 89:569, 1981
20. Ramsey DE, Manke DA, Sumner DS: Toe blood pressure: a valuable adjunct to ankle pressure measurement for assessing peripheral arterial disease. J Cardiovasc Surg 24:43, 1983
21. Hampton GH, Birke JA: Treatment of wounds caused by pressure and insensitivity. p. 196. In McCullough J (ed): Contemporary Perspectives in Rehabilitation: Wound Healing. FA Davis, Philadelphia, 1990
22. Birke JA, Sims DS: The insensitive foot. p. 133. In Hunt GC (ed): Physical Therapy of the Foot Ankle. Churchill Livingstone, New York, 1988
23. Levin ME: To soak or not to soak. Clin Diabetes 4:44, 1986
24. Coleman WC, Brand PW, Birke JA: The total contact cast. J Am Pod Med Assoc 74:548, 1984
25. Mooney V, Wagner FW: Neurocirculatory disorders of the foot. Clin Orthop Rel Res 122:53, 1977
26. Pollard JP, Le Quesne LP, Tappin JW: Forces under the foot. J Biomed Eng 5:37, 1983
27. Birke JA, Sims DS, Buford WL: Walking casts: effect on plantar foot pressures. J Rehabil Res Dev 22:18, 1985
28. Sinacore DR, Mueller MJ, Diamond JE et al: Diabetic plantar ulcers treated by total contact casting. Phys Ther 67:1543, 1987
29. Mueller MJ, Diamond JE, Sinacore DR, et al: Total contact casting in treatment of diabetic plantar ulcers. Diabetes Care 12:384, 1989
30. Bergtholdt HT: Temperature assessment of the insensitive foot. Phys Ther 59:18, 1979
31. Warren AG: Tarsal bone disintegration in leprosy. J Bone Joint Surg (Br) 53:688, 1971
32. Goldman F: Identification, treatment, and prognosis of Charcot joint in diabetes mellitus. J Am Pod Med Assoc 72:485, 1982
33. Nawoczenski DA, Birke JA, Graham SL, Koziatek E: The neuropathic foot: a management scheme. Phys Ther 69:287, 1989
34. Waters RL, Perry J, Antonelli D, Hislop H: Energy cost of walking of amputees: the influence of level of amputation. J Bone Joint Surg 58A:42, 1976
35. Bowker JH: Partial foot and Symes amputation: an overview. Clin Prosth Orthot 12:10, 1987/8
36. Murdoch G: Levels of amputation and limiting factors. p. 41. Lower Limb Prosthetics. New York University, Post Graduate Medical School, 1980
37. Burgess EM, Raub JE, Wilson AB: Immediate post-surgical prosthesis in the management of lower extremity amputees. TR10-5, Veterans Administration, Washington DC, 1967
38. Mooney V, Harve JP, McBride W, Snelson R: Comparison of postoperative stump management: plaster vs. soft dressing. J Bone Joint Surg 53A:241, 1971
39. Wu Y, Krick H: Removable rigid dressing for below-knee amputees. Clin Orthot Prosth 11:33, 1987
40. Richter KJ, Hurvitz EA, Girardot K: Rigid remov-

able dressing in a case of poor wound healing. Arch Phys Med Rehabil 69:128, 1988

41. Mueller MJ: Comparison of removable rigid dressings and elastic bandages in preprosthetic management of patients with below-knee amputations. Phys Ther 62:1438, 1982
42. McCollough NC, Harris AR, Hampton FR: Below-knee amputation. p. 341. In American Academy of Orthopedic Surgeons: Atlas of Limb Prosthetics. CV Mosby, St Louis, 1981
43. Manella KJ: Comparing the effectiveness of elastic bandages and shrinker socks for lower extremity amputees. Phys Ther 61:334, 1981
44. Rausch RW, Khalili AA: Air splint in preprosthetic rehabilitation of lower extremity amputated limbs. Phys Ther 65:912, 1985
45. Thornhill HL, Jones GD, Brodzka W, VanBockstaele P: Bilateral below-knee amputations: experience with 80 patients. Arch Phys Med Rehabil 67:159, 1986
46. Michael J: Energy storing feet: a clinical comparison. Clin Orthot Prosth 11:154, 1987
47. Edelstein JE: Prosthetic feet: state of the art. Phys Ther 68:1874, 1988

26

Prophylactic Surgery in the Diabetic Foot

Bonnie Johng Nicklas, D.P.M., F.A.C.F.S., D.A.B.P.S.

THE NEED FOR PROPHYLACTIC SURGERY

In the most basic terms, prophylactic or preventive surgery in the diabetic foot focuses on reduction of pressure areas (i.e., prevention of callus formation, cell death, hemorrhage, and ultimate ulceration). The hazard of a diabetic patient developing an infection once an ulcer has formed is dangerously high. A diabetic individual is much more likely to develop gangrene than a nondiabetic person; in fact, approximately 45 percent of all nontraumatic leg and foot amputations in the United States are caused by diabetes.[1] It has been estimated that 30 percent of patients with unilateral limb amputations will revisit the surgical arena for treatment of the contralateral limb within 3 years.[2] The 5-year survival rate for patients with unilateral amputations has been predicted to be as low as 30 percent, making it vital to exhaust all attempts at preserving the limb. Preservation of a limb not only allows the patient to ambulate more easily, but also helps to minimize the psychological disturbances burdening the diabetic patient.[3]

Probably one of the earliest descriptions of diabetic gangrene in part states, "In the 39th year of his reign King Asa became affected with gangrene of his feet; he rested with his forefathers in the 41st year of his reign."[4] Historically, surgeons were called in to treat a case of diabetes because conservative prophylactic measures taken to avoid serious foot problems had failed. In the past, this usually translated to amputation at some level, either in the infected neuropathic foot or in the ischemic foot with or without infection. In 1975, Moschella wrote, "The function and importance of physically intact hands and feet are often taken for granted until impaired by disease."[5] This often translates into ulceration, infection, and gangrene. In 1979, Dormandy wrote, "Lacking the glamour of a classic surgical set piece, the treatment of these patients is too often considered an unwelcome cross that surgeons have to bear."[6] Frequently this treatment was nothing more than salvage surgery, with the primary variable being the level of amputation. The focus now, however, is changing toward preventive, or prophylactic, surgery, with the emphasis being to look intelligently into the future needs of these patients. Choosing appropriate surgical procedures that prevent these catastrophic and devastating effects of diabetes before they occur is the goal of prophylactic surgery in the diabetic foot. This is accomplished by altering the structure and function of the foot.

GOALS OF PROPHYLACTIC SURGERY

The primary goal of prophylactic surgery in the diabetic patient is to reduce and/or minimize pressure areas. Because of neuropathy, patients with a diabetic foot may lack the normal protective mechanism of pain. As stated by Brand, "Pain is the most valuable sensation we have."[7] The measurable pressure capable of causing pressure necrosis is very low. One pound per square inch, or 50 mmHg, will block capillary blood flow.[7] After several hours of continuous pressure it may take only 3 lb/in^2 to cause a pressure ulcer.[8] All persons with normal sensation experience pressure in excess of this every time they stand or sit still. Unlike the patient with an insensitive limb, however, they shift their weight and move about, often subconsciously, in response to pain. They will protect the foot by limping (i.e., changing their gait), which will change the distribution of force so that the same area does not endure repetitive stress beyond the inflammatory stage. Patients lacking this protection as a result of neuropathy will continue to stand or walk in the face of inflammation. Continuous pressure on focal, inflamed areas results in necrosis from local ischemia. Diabetes is not a rare disease, in fact it is quite prevalent. Studies from the American Diabetes Association (ADA) report that more than 11 million people in the United States have diabetes, and each year over 150,000 die as a result of its complications. Since health care and related costs for treatment of the diabetic patient run to $20.4 billion annually, more emphasis should be placed on preventive surgical care. The total economic costs of diabetes were estimated at $14 billion in 1984.[9] Clearly the costs are increasing.

HISTORY OF PROPHYLACTIC SURGERY

Historically, diabetic "prophylaxis" was synonymous with "conservative care." Consisting of proper hygiene, protective foot gear, and observation, it was considered to be of paramount importance, and failure of this conservative care program generally meant amputation. There was little consideration for the middle ground, that is, prophylactic surgical care. Many authors have written on preventive or prophylactic surgery in the diabetic patient.[10–13] The common theme remains consistent: to reduce pressure on discrete areas, particularly over bony prominences. These areas can change in the diabetic foot. This is primarily because of the neuropathy and its effects on the intrinsic musculature. Neuropathy involving motor innervation of the intrinsic muscles results in atrophy of the muscles, which leads to instability and malalignment of the forefoot (Fig. 26-1). This is why hammer toes and hallux abducto valgus deformities are so common in the diabetic foot.

With changes in the configuration of the foot, the gait is altered and new pressure points are created, often resulting in ulceration at these sites.[14] Ulceration often leads to infection, which may lead to amputation. Reestablishing and maintaining optimal pressure distribution in the diabetic patient with two lower limbs is challenging, and even more so in the patient who has had unilateral amputation, since the prognosis for the remaining limb is extremely poor.[15–17] The altered pressure distribution results in callus formation. Blood and serum, extravasated from capillaries, accumulate under

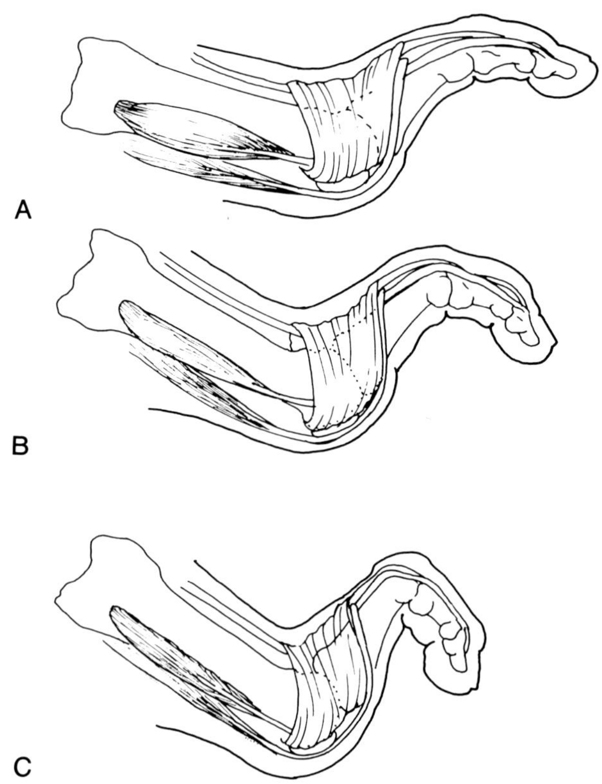

Fig. 26-1. (**A**) Normal intrinsic musculature. (**B**) Mild intrinsic muscle wasting. (**C**) Severe intrinsic muscle wasting.

the callus as subcutaneous tissue is bruised and capillary damage occurs. The capillary damage results in ischemia. The collected fluids provide a culture medium for bacteria as an abscess forms. The hard, callused tissue is often impenetrable by the underlying infection, and the infection can therefore more easily invade the underlying soft tissue and joint capsule than penetrate the callus itself. Deeper penetration into the subcutaneous layer may result in spread along fascial planes, tendon sheaths, and naturally occurring anatomic spaces, and eventually into the periosteum and bone. This process can occur at any pressure point, such as on the plantar aspect of the foot under the metatarsal heads, medially or laterally over the bony prominences of hallux valgus and tailor's bunion deformities, or on the dorsal or distal surfaces of contracted digits. Vesignie coined the term *plantaire mal perforant* for these ulcers, owing to their tendency to perforate through tissue layers, beginning at skin level and eventually penetrating bone.[18] A study by Classen in 1963 reported that in a series of 45 patients with perforating ulcers, 40 had diabetes.[19] In the past 23 years since that study, little has changed. The appearance of ulcer is classic. It was described as early as 1818 by Mott,[20] who commented on the thick, hard cuticle surrounding the ulcer, known today as the "halo." Brand described the four pathomechanical entities leading to development of ulceration in the insensitive foot as follows[21]:

1. Low pressure plus time (ischemic necrosis)
2. High pressure (mechanical destruction)
3. Moderate pressure and repetition (inflammation)
4. Moderate pressure and infection (spreading sepsis)

Many authors recommend orthotic devices and molded shoes as a means of redistributing pressure points.[22–24] For many patients, however, orthotic devices or molded shoes are not acceptable options. Various social activities, employment, or other life-style constraints often make this type of footwear either impractical or impossible. For these patients, reconstructive surgery of the foot, to realign the internal osseous architecture and reestablish balance of the periarticular structures, should be considered. Prophylactic surgery is indicated in the well-vascularized diabetic patient with recalcitrant ulcers, those resistant to all conservative therapy for longer than 3 months, and those with gross osseous deformities.[25] Specific deformities will now be described, along with recommended surgical procedures, postoperative management, and the rationale for selecting a treatment plan.

THE SURGICAL CANDIDATE

Prior to the selection of a particular surgical procedure, one must establish that the patient is a good surgical candidate; elective surgery should be performed only on patients who are well controlled. Poor blood-sugar control may lead to impaired circulation.[26]

The diabetic neuropathic foot is generally amenable to surgical reconstruction. It typically presents as a healthy foot that is warm to touch and well vascularized, as evidenced by its capillary filling time and palpable pulses. It demonstrates some level of neuropathy, which is partly sensory and partly motor. The diabetic ischemic foot, on the contrary, presents as a very unhealthy foot. It is cool to the touch, often painful to palpation, and pulseless. Lack of hair growth, dystrophic skin and nails, and often areas of necrosis or gangrene accompany an already threatened clinical situation. This type of foot must be identified and addressed immediately, either by careful and frequent monitoring and protective conservative care, or by surgical revascularization or amputation when necessary. This type of foot must be identified as that which is not amenable to elective surgery; in fact, it would probably not heal following surgery distal to the ankle.

After it is established that the foot has the capacity to heal, the nutritional status of the patient should be considered. Basic nutrient requirements of the diabetic patient are generally in accordance with those of any healthy individual.[27] The three primary nutrients to consider are carbohydrates, proteins, and fat. High-carbohydrate, low-fat diets have been shown to have beneficial effects in diabetes management. Higher percentages of calories from complex CH_2O sources appear to result in a decrease in the plasma glucose concentration and a favorable reduction in serum cholesterol.[28] Accelerated nutrient needs associated with biosynthetic activities such as wound repair must also be considered when planning diets for these individuals.[29] Particular attention must be paid to the diet of the diabetic patient, since the inefficient usage of nutrients associated with diabetes is frequently accompanied by suboptimal healing of wounds and ulcers.[30]

Vitamins

Vitamin C

Unlike most animal species, humans cannot synthesize ascorbic acid, owing to lack of the enzyme needed to convert L-gulonic acid to ascorbic acid. It was noted in the sixteenth century that scurvy, caused by vitamin C deficiency, results in poor wound healing. Since then, many studies have focused on this issue, but the pioneering work of Wolbach and Howe 50 years ago provided the basis for studies that have now largely defined the clinical and biochemical roles of ascorbic acid in wound repair.[31]

A lack of of ascorbic acid leads to increased capillary permeability, fragility, rupture, and hemorrhage of these vessels, and to a failure to form new capillaries in the healing wound.[32] Fibroblast function is impaired in the presence of vitamin C deficiency. The final result may be reflected in an inability to synthesize an adequate amount of basement-membrane collagen.

Vitamin B Complex

Since B vitamins serve as cofactors in a variety of enzyme systems, serious deficits in some of them may hamper healing. Few clinical studies have been performed on wound healing and the B vitamins. Bosse and Axelrod, experimenting with riboflavin and pyridoxine deficiency, reported markedly delayed healing in open skin wounds.[33]

Vitamin A

Frank vitamin A deficit is rare in the United States. In underdeveloped countries it is associated with widespread retarded wound healing. Experimentally induced deficiencies of the vitamin retard epithelialization, wound closure, and collagen synthesis rates, prolong hydroxylase activity of healing tissue, and may prolong the crosslinking of new collagen.[34]

Vitamin D and Ca^{2+}

Vitamin D has an important role in Ca^{2+} homeostasis. For vitamin D to act, adequate dietary protein must be supplied and gut function must permit synthesis of the necessary transport protein and absorption of nutrients. Vitamin D deficit is not commonly encountered in surgical patients unless there is a malabsorption syndrome present.[35]

Additional Factors Affecting Healing

Healing tissue requires adequate vascularization for delivery of oxygen. Anything that diminishes oxygenation of tissues is therefore detrimental to the healing process, and should be discontinued prior to surgical intervention. A major example of this phenomenon occurs with cigarette smoking in diabetic patients, which must be stopped or significantly decreased prior to surgery.[36] Cigarette smoking has been associated with an increased incidence of foot lesions in diabetic patients.[37] Clinical experience strongly confirms that patients who smoke and have chronic occlusive arterial disease affecting the extremities do not do well.[38] The physiologic effects of smoking on blood flow were shown many years ago by the study of Allison and Roth.[39] This study demonstrated that smoking causes a decreased blood flow to the extremities and subsequently a decreased temperature of the digits. A single cigarette can cause narrowing of the arteries and a reduction in blood flow that may last for one hour or more.[38]

Smoking has also been shown to increase platelet aggregation,[40] decrease blood flow to the skin in experimental animals,[41] and increase the entry of cholesterol into endothelial cells.[42] The series of Beach and Strandness[43] on arteriosclerosis obliterans and associated risk factors in diabetic patients showed a high correlation between smoking and atherosclerosis. Because of the likelihood of vascular disease in the diabetic foot, any additional threat to essential tissue perfusion could be disastrous, particularly in situations of increased need, such as the healing surgical wound.

DEFORMITIES

Hyperkeratotic lesions are no more frequent in the diabetic than in the nondiabetic individual, but in the neuropathic foot these lesions are potential sources of trouble because of possible ulceration in the absence of the normal protective response to friction and pain.[44]

Musculoskeletal disorders primarily involve the forefoot. Hammer toes, bunions, and "metatarsalgia" are by far the most frequent musculoskeletal findings in any patient population regardless of foot type.[44] Various foot deformities may be found in patients with neurologic disease and insensitivity.[45]

Tissue will break down at those areas of high pressure that receive repetitive stress (Fig. 26-2).[46] Intense pressure of short duration and low pressure applied for extended periods are equally detrimental.[8] Reconstructive podiatric surgery should be done in patients who are predisposed to ulcer formation because of external pressures on underlying bony deformities. Musculoskeletal malalignment may have a structural or biomechanical/functional etiology.

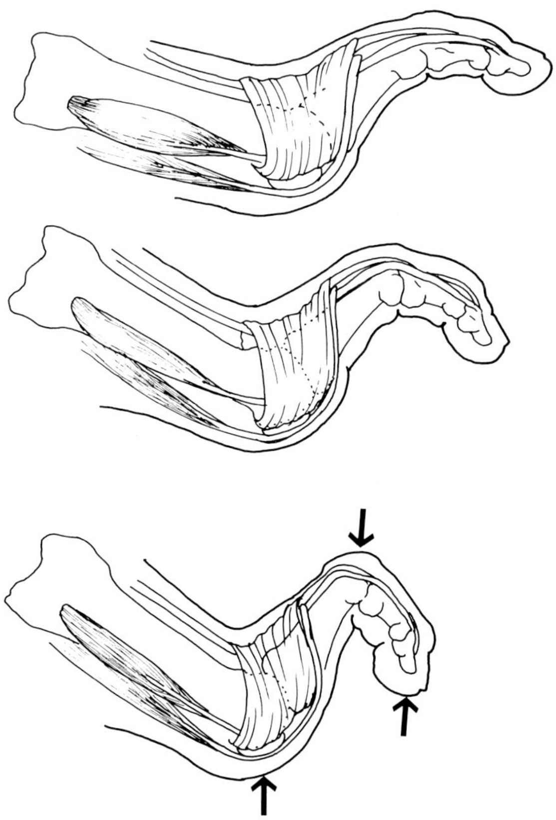

Fig. 26-2. Areas of increased pressure.

Preoperative Management

It is important to properly determine the etiology of a deformity in order to maximize the potential for future function and alignment of the foot. The surgical patient must have adequate vascular perfusion for healing, and have a blood glucose level that is under good medical control. General anesthesia is accompanied by a higher incidence of complications than is local anesthesia, and therefore local anesthesia should be used whenever possible.

Postoperative Management

It is important to control postoperative edema in the diabetic patient. Edema interferes with delivery of neutrophils into the area by creating an increased distance from the capillary to the cell and a decrease in the rate of diffusion that is proportional to the distance.[47] Additionally, the removal of metabolites and cell debris is impaired in the presence of edema.[48–50] Whenever possible, the potential for healing the surgical wound in the diabetic patient should be maximized, in order to minimize the burden on the immune system. Immune deficiency in the diabetic patient has been reported by various authors.[51–57] The polymorphonuclear leukocyte (PMN) seems to be the cell in which the malfunction occurs. The impaired humoral and cell-mediated immunity that accompany malnutrition decrease a patient's ability to fight infection.[47]

Depression of cell-mediated immunity (T-cell function) has also been reported; this defect in leukocyte function may be partly responsible for defects in wound healing that occur in the diabetic patient even in the absence of infection.[58]

A discussion of the most commonly encountered

forefoot deformities amenable to surgical correction follows, beginning with the type of deformity, the procedure of choice, technique, and postoperative management. Finally, a rationale for the chosen procedure is presented.

NAIL SURGERY ON THE DIABETIC FOOT

Pathologic nail conditions amenable to surgical correction include onychocryptosis, onychogryphosis, paronychia, subungual exostosis, and subungual neoplasms. Although these conditions are not generally of a serious nature by themselves, in the diabetic patient a simple ingrown nail border can become infected, resulting in gangrene and potentially in the loss of a digit or limb. In fact, deep-space infections can result from local infection anywhere on the toe. Toes with pathologic nail conditions are subjected to various forms of trauma, ranging from pressure phenomena to self-inflicted injuries consequent to "bathroom surgery." Suspicious subungual lesions or neoplasms should be appropriately excised and evaluated histologically by a pathologist.

When performing permanent removal of a nail or one of its borders in the diabetic patient, it is generally recommended that a cold-steel procedure rather than a chemical matrixectomy be performed, in order to maximize the healing potential and minimize complications secondary to a chemical burn. In the healing surgical wound, particular consideration must be given to the process of neovascularization. Neovascularization is a constant feature of repair, at least in part because the needs of inflammation and repair overwhelm the injured nutritional supply.[59] By the third or fourth postoperative day, evidence of granulation tissue begins to appear where the first new vessels are forming. The vascular and nutritional demands for healing tissue are greater than those required for mere survival, and the vascular demands are greater for the burn wound than for the scalpel-surgical wound.

Technically speaking, a chemical matrixectomy may be classified as a deep or third-degree burn (i.e., one that extends below the level of the dermis, damages blood vessels, and leaves no viable epithelial cells at the point of chemical contact). Applying a chemical cauterizing substance such as phenol or NaOH creates an immediate chemical burn resulting in necrosis at the site of contact. The severity of tissue necrosis is determined by vascular factors as the local hemodynamics stabilize. Necrotic tissue is easily infected. Infection tends to further compromise local vessels, and a second deepening of the wound may result.

While scalpel wounds begin neovascularization within a few days, burn injuries do not show significant neovascularization for well over a week.[60] The inflammatory reaction and neovascularization are both delayed, even in tiny deep burn wounds.[60] It would not, therefore, seem advisable to utilize a chemical burning agent in the diabetic foot, which almost invariably has some degree of vascular disease, may ultimately lack the healing capacity necessary to recover.

Chemical matrixectomies in the diabetic foot pose another problem to the patient. Because the chemical creates a burn, the wound will drain fluid as a normal response. Local destruction of capillaries results in capillary oozing, increased capillary permeability, and liquefaction necrosis of the destroyed cells. In most cases, these patients are instructed to soak the foot within the guidelines established by the practitioner until the capillaries are repaired and all necrotic fluids and tissue are removed. But in the diabetic patient, foot soaks are controversial at best, and in fact they should not be part of the care of this select patient population for several reasons. Because of neuropathy, discrimination between tepid and hot water may be impossible, and the result may be a serious burn. Also, soaking the feet in warm or hot water requires a significant increase in blood flow to the skin to dissipate the heat. Patients with circulatory problems are unable to increase this arterial blood flow, and skin injury and ulceration often result.[61]

The normal skin temperature of the foot is variable, depending on factors such as outside temperature, room temperature, and the emotional state of the individual.[62] The body's thermal symmetry allows a comparison of the temperatures of various body parts. Meaningful information from skin temperature measurements can be obtained by comparing the temperature of an inflamed area to that of the contralateral side and measuring the difference (ΔT). A ΔT greater than 1°C has been considered significant.[63] Differences of up to 6°C are often seen in the feet when an injury or inflammation is present.[62] Thus, immersion and soaking of the diabetic foot could produce inflammation and ensuing complications.

In addition, soaking the feet often leads to tissue maceration, fissuring, and cracking of the skin. When the integrity of the skin is broken, avenues are established for invading organisms including bacteria, fungi, and viruses. With breaks in the skin, the risk of infection becomes very high.

Performing "cold steel" or surgical matrixectomies allows the permanent nail procedure to be performed without the hazards and increased risk involved in postoperative soaking. The procedure should be done in the operating room under usual sterile conditions. Epinephrine should not be used in the digit; instead, a digital tourniquet can be applied until the matrix is removed, and can then be released prior to skin closure. A fluffy sterile dressing is applied postoperatively, and a follow-up plan is established, as in any surgical procedure.

Problem: Paronychia of the Nail Border

Procedure of Choice: Temporary Partial Nail Avulsion

Technique

1. Perform a digital block with local anesthesia.
2. Using a Freer elevator, separate the lateral nail skinfold from the nail plate while firmly grasping the digit, keeping the thumb over the nail plate.
3. Using a nail nipper or English anvil, split the nail plate distally at the appropriate level.
4. Using a #61 or #62 blade, continue to split the nail proximally, taking care to avoid laceration of the nail bed. Raise the back of the handle up when the blade is at the level of the eponychium, continuing to move the blade proximally. Complete the incision through the proximal edge of the nail plate, and incise the matrix.
5. Insert the Freer elevator between the nail plate and nail bed at the distal tip of the toe, taking care not to gouge the nail bed.
6. Insert one side of a straight hemostat under the nail plate, below the eponychium, and clamp.
7. Using a rotating motion, grasp the jaws of the hemostat and pull, rotating as the hemostat is pulled out.
8. Irrigate the surgical site with sterile saline. Carefully inspect the wound for debris, callused tissue, or nail fragments.
9. Fabricate a "wick" using sterile gauze or cotton, and place it into the surgical site, gently tucking it under the margin of the eponychium.
10. Apply a sterile dressing, taking care to check capillary refilling to ensure that the dressing is not too constrictive.

Postoperative Management

1. Two days postoperatively: Dressing change. Apply a new sterile dressing.
2. One week postoperatively: Dressing change. Apply light dressing.
3. Two weekly visits. Begin using a small bandage.
4. Follow-up visits 1 month and 3 months later.

Rationale and Discussion

Temporary removal of a nail or nail margin is necessary when the surrounding tissue has become inflamed, and particularly when the surrounding tissue is infected. In the presence of infection, local anesthesia may be less effective, owing to the pH changes in local tissues, and a more proximal block may be indicated. A tourniquet is not needed so long as the nail bed is protected and not lacerated, since there will be very little bleeding until the incision extends into the matrix. Carefully placed sterile wicks, povidone-iodine (Betadine) wet-to-dry dressings, and frequent dressing changes are required to monitor the resolution of the infection. Antibiotics should be considered, as well as hospitalization, if the infection is not localized to the nail border or if cellulitis or lymphangitis are evident. Infection anywhere in the toe may reach the plantar space by local spreading until the flexor tendon sheath is involved by suppurative tenosynovitis.[64] Therefore, infections in and around the nail apparatus must be addressed immediately and aggressively.

Problem: Onychocryptosis

Procedure: Frost[65]

Technique

1. Split the nail at the point where the "arc" of the nail begins. Continue proximally through the eponychium.
2. Place the blade in this groove and make a vertical incision down to but not into the phalanx at the level of the eponychium. (Fig. 26-3A).
3. Make a second incision at the proximal end of the first incision, at a 90° angulation, going through the skin only (Fig. 26-3B).
4. Create an epidermal flap by underscoring at the reticular dermis.
5. Make a third incision beneath the flap, parallel to the first incision, but curving distally to converge with the first incision.
6. Dissect out the nail, matrix, and partial nail bed.
7. Place one 5-0 nonabsorbable suture in the flap, avoiding the apex (Fig. 26-3C).
8. Apply povidone/iodine (Betadine) paint, a fluffy dressing, and a surgical shoe.

Postoperative Management

1. Three days postoperatively: Dressing change. Apply a new sterile dressing.
2. Ten days postoperatively: Suture removal and dressing change.
3. Follow up with two weekly visits. Twenty-four days postoperatively discontinue dressing.
4. Follow up 2 weeks later with a checkup.
5. Follow up visits 1 month and 3 months later.

Rationale and Discussion

The Frost technique is an effective means for excising one or both nail borders. When reported in the Journal of the National Association of Chiropodists in 1950, mention was made of sloughing of the skin flap, which was attributed to the use of a skin suture. It was more likely due to the fact that procaine hydrochloride (Novocain) with epinephrine at a concentration of 1:25,000 was used in conjunction with a digital tourniquet. If placed properly, a single suture should not cause vascular impairment of the flap resulting in necrosis and sloughing. There should be no tension on the skin, and if possible the apex of the flap should be avoided either by using an apical stitch or a single suture in the longitudinally placed incision. When performed properly, the Frost technique allows for adequate visualization of the nail matrix, and in general heals uneventfully with a good permanent surgical result.

Problem: Onychocryptosis/Granuloma

Procedure: Winograd[66]

Technique

1. Split the nail along the striation.
2. Following the split, incise the nail bed and matrix down to but not into the phalanx for the entire length of the nail (Fig. 26-4A).

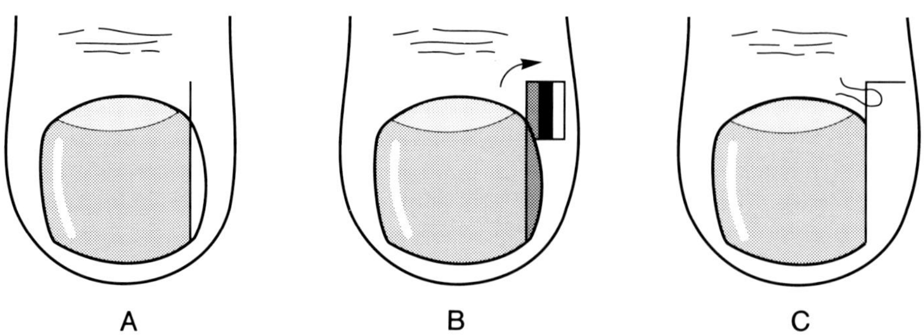

Fig. 26-3. Frost procedure. (**A**) Nail plate incision. (**B**) Proximal incision, 90° to first incision. (**C**) Single skin suture.

3. Make a second semi-elliptical incision converging with the first incision at its proximal and distal aspects (Fig. 26-4B).
4. Dissect out the nail, matrix, and soft tissue granuloma formation, as well as the nail bed and partial nail skinfold.
5. Coapt the soft tissue (lateral nailfold) to the nail with 5-0 nonabsorbable suture material (Fig. 26-4C).
6. Apply povidone/iodine (Betadine) solution and a fluffy sterile dressing.
7. Apply a surgical shoe.

Postoperative Management
Same as in the Frost procedure.

Rationale and Discussion
The Winograd procedure is a very effective way to permanently remove the nail border and the hypertrophied lateral nailfold, as well as any granulomatous tissue in the same region. The incision allows for adequate visualization of the nail matrix and complete excision of pathologic tissue adjacent to the nail. Particular care must be taken to ensure that all pathologic soft tissue has been removed, since inadvertently leaving a portion of the callused skin or any superficial tissues inside the wound and closing skin over it will result in a rapid foreign-body reaction and probable infection. Skin closure, as always, should be carefully performed, with no clamping of skin edges, no tension on skin edges, and no overlap of skin edges. Since its publication in 1929,[66] the Winograd procedure has without question stood the test of time, and is one of the most successful and commonly performed surgical nail procedures.

Problem: Deformed Nail Over the Entire Plate

Procedure: Zadik[67]

Technique

1. Avulse the entire nail plate.
2. Incise the eponychium at its proximal corners at 45° angles (Fig. 26-5A).
3. Create a skin flap by underscoring the reticular dermis to release it from the matrix (Fig. 26-5B).
4. Reflect the skin flap proximally to expose the matrix.
5. Make transverse incision at the proximal margin of the matrix.
6. Make a transverse incision at the distal margin of the matrix (lunula).
7. Connect the two incisions at the fibular and tibial borders.
8. Dissect out the matrix, partial nail bed, and soft tissues.
9. Coapt the skin flaps and eponychial margin with 5-0 nonabsorbable suture material (Fig. 26-5C).
10. Apply povidone/iodine (Betadine) paint, a fluffy dressing, and a surgical shoe.

Postoperative Management
Same as in the Frost procedure.

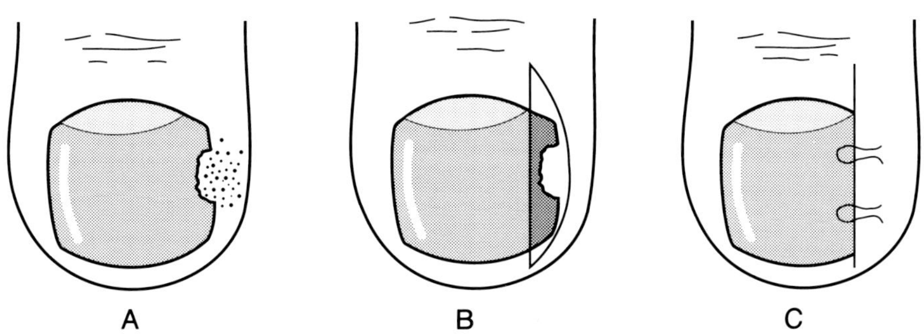

Fig. 26-4. Winograd procedure. (**A**) Nail and skin incision. (**B**) Second incision: Semielliptical. (**C**) Closure: Skin to nail plate.

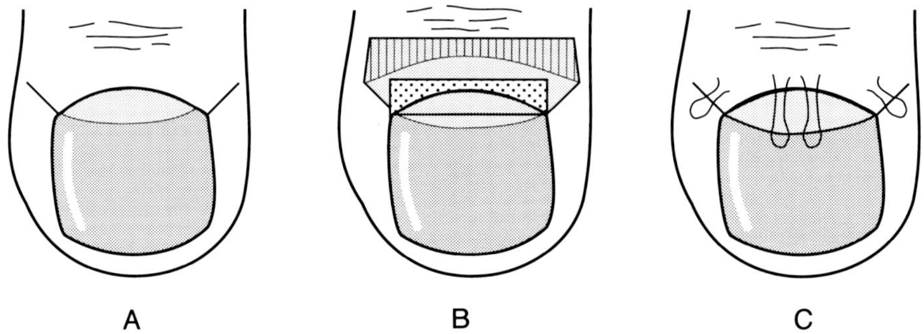

Fig. 26-5. Zadik procedure. (A) Skin incisions at 45° to nail margins. (B) Create skin flap. (C) Skin closure.

Rationale and Discussion

The Zadik procedure described in 1950,[67] was originally designed to permanently remove the nail plate and matrix in an attempt to avoid the complications of procedures that were in vogue at the time, and which specifically involved shortening of the digit subsequent to the distal Syme amputation, which was very popular. The Zadik procedure allows for adequate visualization of the entire nail matrix, without tension on or excessive retraction of the skin flap. As always, particular care must be taken to avoid trauma to the skin flap, either by clamping, retraction, heat and dessication, or suture damage. The sutures should be placed in such a way that there is minimal if any tension on the skin edges and no overlap of edges; most importantly, the needle should not pass through the apices of the skin flaps. The Zadik procedure was important in changing the philosophy of nail surgery and remains a very valuable and commonly used technique.

DIGITAL SURGERY IN THE DIABETIC FOOT

Digital deformities[20] are very common in the diabetic foot. Prior to surgical intervention, the etiology of the deformity must be carefully identified. The etiology may be mechanical or biomechanical, static or dynamic, a single deformity or the result of multiple deformities. Ellenberg, in 1968, attributed hammering and contracture of digits in the diabetic foot with neuropathy to weakness and imbalances of intrinsic muscles of the foot.[68] Stokes found a reduction of the load on the toes that was significant in the diabetic patient even without evidence of ulceration.[69,70] Significant numbers of hammer toe deformities with accompanying limitation of dorsiflexion were observed in the San Francisco VA cross-sectional study.[71] Articular malalignment secondary to contracture causes joint damage over time, and the digit progressively loses flexibility and often forms a rigid deformity. Extrinsic shoe pressure and friction create helomata dura over bony prominences, which may ulcerate (Fig. 26-6). Mal perforans ulcers occur mainly on weight-bearing surfaces, but may also occur on the dorsal surfaces of digits in hammer toes and claw toes, and on the distal tips of digits exhibiting the typical mallet toe deformity (Fig. 26-7). The digital deformity should therefore be addressed surgically to reduce the contracture, eliminate excessive and abnormal pressure and friction points, and stabilize the digit at the metatarsophalangeal joint when necessary. Levin refers to this type of deformity as the "tip-top-toe ulcer syndrome," and states that patients who have this type of foot deformity should be considered for prophylactic surgery long before ulceration occurs and when the circulation of the foot is still adequate.[38] Once the etiology has been identified, appropriate surgical procedures are selected and executed. A successful surgical outcome begins with a proper skin incision, performing those procedures necessary to completely address the deformity, and ends with careful postoperative management. One of the most important

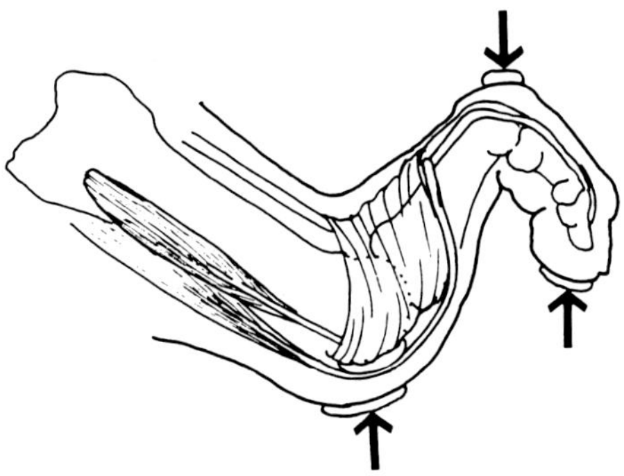

Fig. 26-6. Helomata dura over bony prominences.

points to observe is to control the bleeding of the digit during surgery, through careful tissue handling, anatomic dissection, and vessel ligation. Control of the bleeding will in most cases control postoperative edema. The integrity of the skin must be preserved. Avoid clamping, thermal damage, retraction trauma, and irrigation trauma. Any trauma to the skin and underlying soft tissues will contribute to postoperative edema and prolong rehabilitation.

Tissue handling is extremely important in digits, because available space to allow for swelling is very limited. Minimal swelling will cause significant discomfort and may persist for weeks or months. Damage to the skin edges will result in necrosis of skin cells, sloughing of skin, and possible dehiscence and infection. Postoperative dressing techniques are designed to stabilize the digit(s) during the healing process and provide gentle compression to control swelling. Postoperative splints may be used when sterile bandages are discontinued, to further stabilize the digit and control swelling as the patient's activity level increases. When surgery is done on multiple digits, or when an isolated digital operation with a significant dynamic component is performed at the metatarsophalangeal joint, the digit should be stabilized using a 0.045 Kirschner wire in retrograde fashion. To do this, the stump of the proximal phalanx is first stabilized and the central canal of the bone is located with manual pressure using a 0.035 Kirschner wire. This is easily done after complete or partial head resection. Once the canal is established, the 0.045 wire is power driven through the middle phalanx and out the end of the digit. The wire driver is then relocated to the distal end of the wire, and the wire is power driven proximally, taking care to place the proximal end of the wire into the canal that has

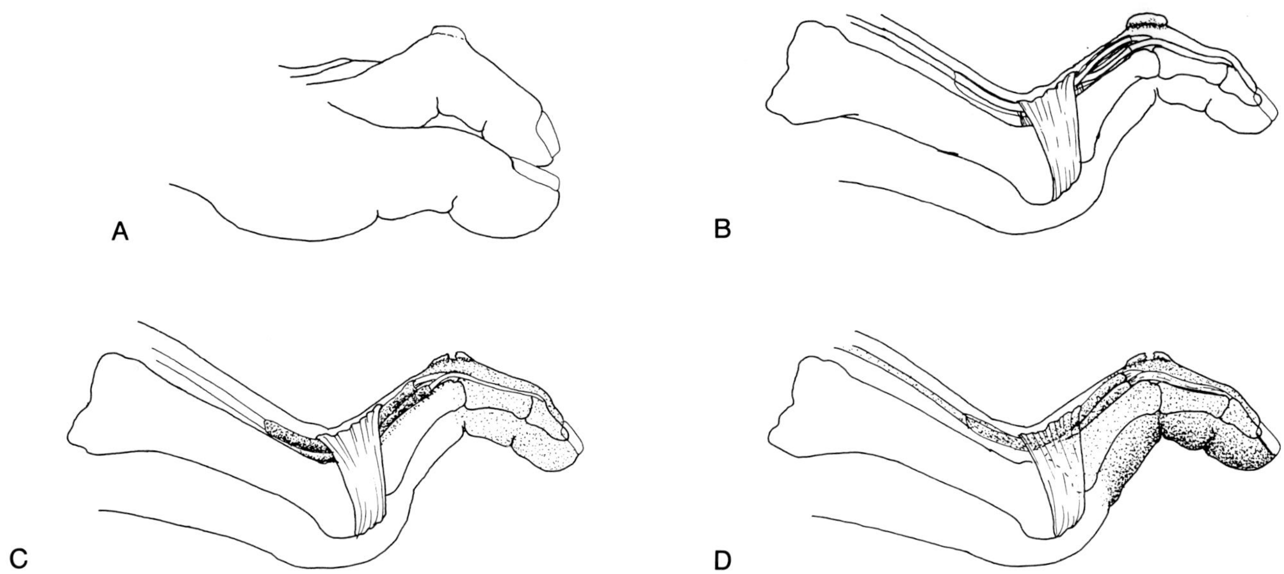

Fig. 26-7. (A) Dorsal callus formation. (B) Subcutaneous bruising, capillary damage. (C) Invasion of tendon sheath, joint capsule, and deep fascia; localized infection. (D) Cell death, ischemic changes in digit due to vascular occlusion, edema of digit, proximal extension of infection.

been established with the 0.035 wire. The wire is driven to the base of the digit, the wire driver removed, and the distal end of the wire bent, cut, and covered by a pin cap. If needed, the wire can be driven through the base of the proximal phalanx, across the metatarsophalangeal joint, and into the metatarsal head with one clean pass. In this case the surgical shoe must be modified to reduce bending forces across the metatarsophalangeal joint to avoid pin fracture.[72] To protect the pins from trauma, the surgical shoe should have a toe guard attached, which should extend distally and dorsally to allow for adequate protection.

Problem: Subungual Exostosis (Fig. 26-8A)

Procedure of Choice: Exostectomy

Technique

1. Perform an appropriate digital block with local anesthesia.
2. Make a transverse stab incision at the tip of the toe, about 2 mm inferior to the nail bed (Fig. 26-8B). The stab incision is carried to the level of the distal phalanx, and the periosteum is carefully incised.
3. Insert a Freer elevator into the incision and bluntly separate the periosteum from the bone, elevating all soft tissue attachments from the exostosis.
4. A thin power burr is inserted into the surgical site and the exostosis is carefully removed (Fig. 26-8C). Final recontouring of the dorsal surface is done with a hand rasp.
5. The surgical site is aggressively irrigated with normal sterile saline injected with a large syringe.
6. The surgical incision is coapted with a single, simple interrupted suture of 5-0 nylon or 5-0 polypropylene on a plastic surgery needle. The surgical site may be painted with povidone/iodine (Betadine) solution.
7. A dry sterile fluff dressing is applied, taking particular care not to cause compression at the distal tip of the toe.

Postoperative Management

1. Three days postoperatively: Dressing change. Apply a new sterile dressing.
2. Ten days postoperatively: Suture removal and application of an adhesive bandage.
3. Follow up with two weekly visits. Discontinue dressing.
4. Follow-up visits 1 month and 3 months later.

Rationale and Discussion

Although small and relatively harmless, the subungual extosis is extremely painful, and in the significantly neuropathic foot can cause pressure-induced nail bed ulceration and subsequent infection. The surgery is relatively simple, with minimal if any rehabilitation inconvenience, and is very gratifying to both the practitioner and the patient. A postoperative lateral radiograph with the hallux elevated should be taken immediately after removal of the exostosis, and repeated 3 and 6

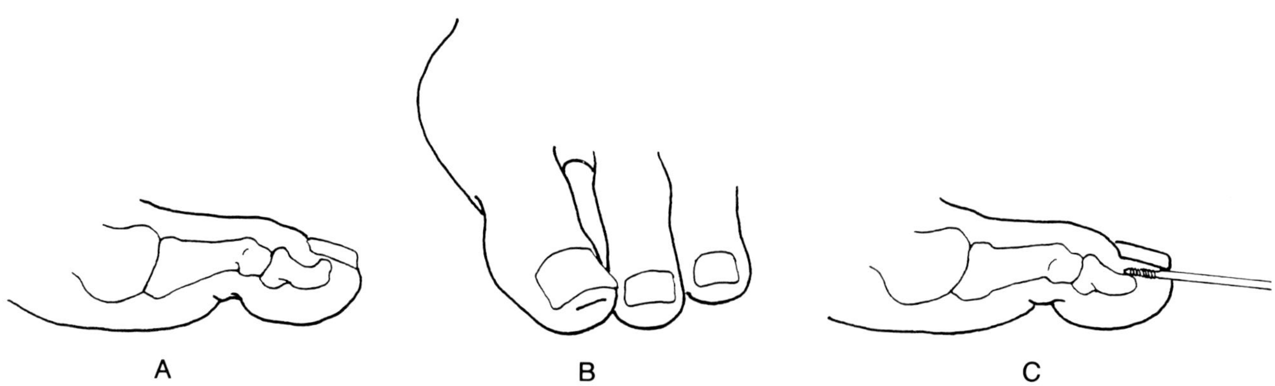

Fig. 26-8. (A) Subungual exostosis. (B) Skin incision. (C) Small power burr.

months later to monitor possible recurrence. Caution must be taken during the procedure to remove all bone fragments and debris from the wound by inserting a rasp upside down (teeth dorsally and rasping the soft tissues).[44] The digit is then carefully squeezed to remove this debris through the operative site.

Problem: Isolated Hammer Toe Deformity (Fig. 26-9A)

Procedure of Choice: Proximal Interphalangeal Joint Arthroplasty

Technique

1. Make a dorsal linear skin incision centered over the digit and crossing the proximal interphalangeal joint (PIPJ) (Fig. 26-9B).
2. Dissect down through the subcutaneous tissue to the level of the deep fascia.
3. Plantar-flex the digit and transect the extensor digitorum longus tendon at the level of the PIPJ. Release the collateral ligaments and deliver the head of the proximal phalanx through the operative site.
4. Using an oscillating saw, resect the head of the proximal phalanx cleanly and smoothly, perpendicular to the long axis (Fig. 26-9C).
5. Using a power burr, remodel the edges of the remaining stump to remove any sharp borders.
6. Irrigate the surgical site with normal sterile saline.
7. Reapproximate the tendon ends with 3-0 absorbable suture material, the subcutaneous tissue with 4-0 absorbable suture material, and the skin closure with 5-0 nylon or polypropylene on a plastic-surgery needle.
8. Paint the digit with povidone/iodine (Betadine) solution and apply a dry sterile dressing.

Postoperative Management

1. Three days postoperatively: Dressing change. Apply a new sterile dressing.
2. See in 1 week (10 days postoperatively). Remove sutures. Apply a sterile dressing with mild compression.
3. See in 1 week. Discontinue dressings and begin splinting materials.
4. Follow up thrice at 2-week intervals.
5. At 6 weeks, discontinue the surgical shoe and apply an athletic shoe.
6. Postoperative radiographs: Immediately after surgery and at 6 weeks and 3 months to evaluate for alignment or osseous regrowth.

Rationale and Discussion

Arthroplasty of the PIPJ for the isolated hammer toe deformity is very successful in reducing dorsal prominences, over which hyperkeratotic tissue forms, which may lead to ulceration. The procedure may also be performed at the level of the distal interphalangeal joint, removing the head of the middle phalanx, for a mallet toe deformity. These simple procedures are performed for static deformities as opposed to the dynamic deformities, which would require stabilization of the PIPJ via arthrodesis, and external Kirschner wire stabili-

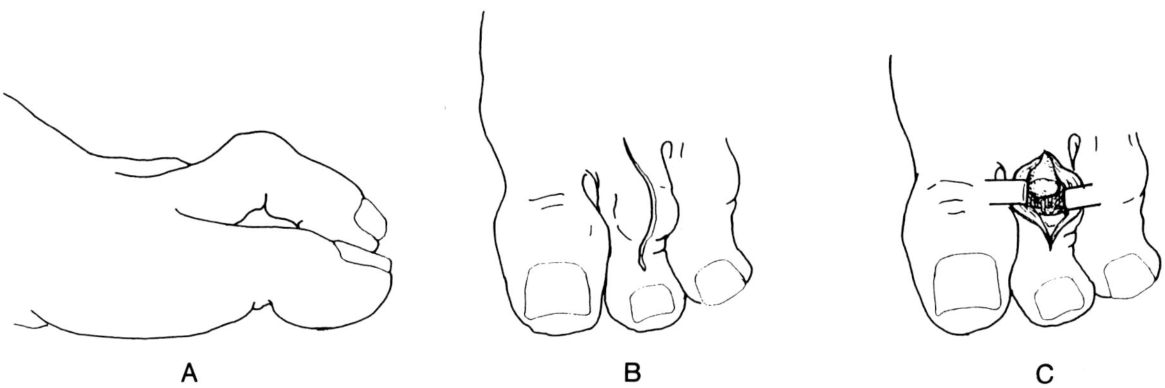

Fig. 26-9. (A) Isolated hammer toe deformity. (B) Skin incision. (C) Proximal phalangeal head resection.

zation. The longitudinal linear incision allows for excellent exposure and avoidance of vital neurovascular structures through careful anatomic dissection.

Problem: Multiple Hammer Toe or Claw Toe Deformities with Dislocation at the Metatarsophalangeal Joint (Fig. 26-10)

Procedure of Choice: Sequential Reduction of Digits with Stabilization

Technique

1. Make a dorsal linear skin incision that curves gently over the metatarsophalangeal joint (MPJ) (Fig. 26-11A). Lightly brush through the subcutaneous layer with a #15 blade to the level of the deep fascia and long extensor tendon.
2. Perform a Z-plasty technique on the long extensor tendon, reflecting one end proximally and the other distally, exposing the PIPJ of the involved digit (Fig. 26-11B). (The tendon may be severed at the level of the PIPJ as an alternative procedure, depending on the severity of the contracture at the MPJ).
3. If an arthroplasty is being performed, the head resection is done at this point* (Fig. 26-11C).

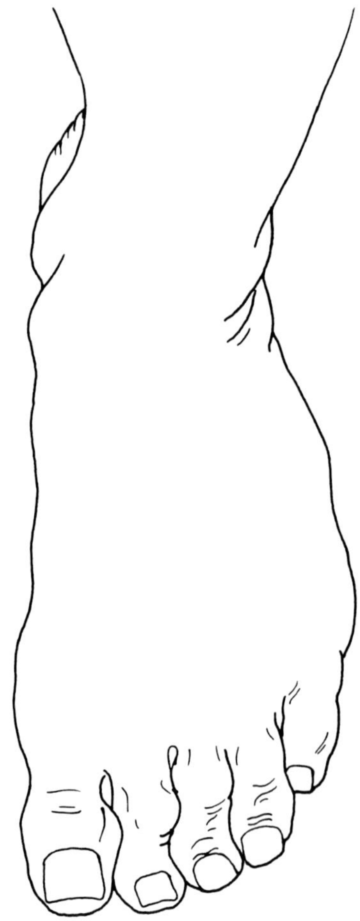

Fig. 26-10. Multiple hammer toe/claw toe deformities with metatarsophalangeal joint dislocation.

4. After the bone is resected, the "push-up" test as described by Kelikian[73] is performed by putting upward pressure on the metatarsal heads. If the digit remains elevated, the next step in the sequence is performed.
5. The extensor hood recession is now performed over the level of the MPJ and proximally, using a #15 blade (Fig. 26-11D). The tendon is grasped with a pair of pick-ups, and the fibers of the hood apparatus are released in a sweeping-type motion under the tendon. Particular care is taken to avoid the tendon or its delicate covering, as well as the periosteum, which is left intact throughout the procedure.
6. The Kelikian push-up-test is again performed,

* If an end-to-end arthrodesis is being performed, it is done at this point, first by delivering the head of the proximal phalanx and then manually resecting the cartilaginous surface of the proximal phalangeal head and middle phalangeal base. If a peg-in-hole arthrodesis is being performed, it is also done at this point. The head of the proximal phalanx is partially removed transversely with a power oscillating saw. Next the medial, lateral, and plantar cortical surfaces of the stump are removed. The dorsal cortex is left intact for strength. A hole is then fashioned in the middle phalanx, using a thin side-cutting burr first, followed by a series of ball burrs of increasing size. The peg is inserted into the hole and additional remodeling is performed as needed.

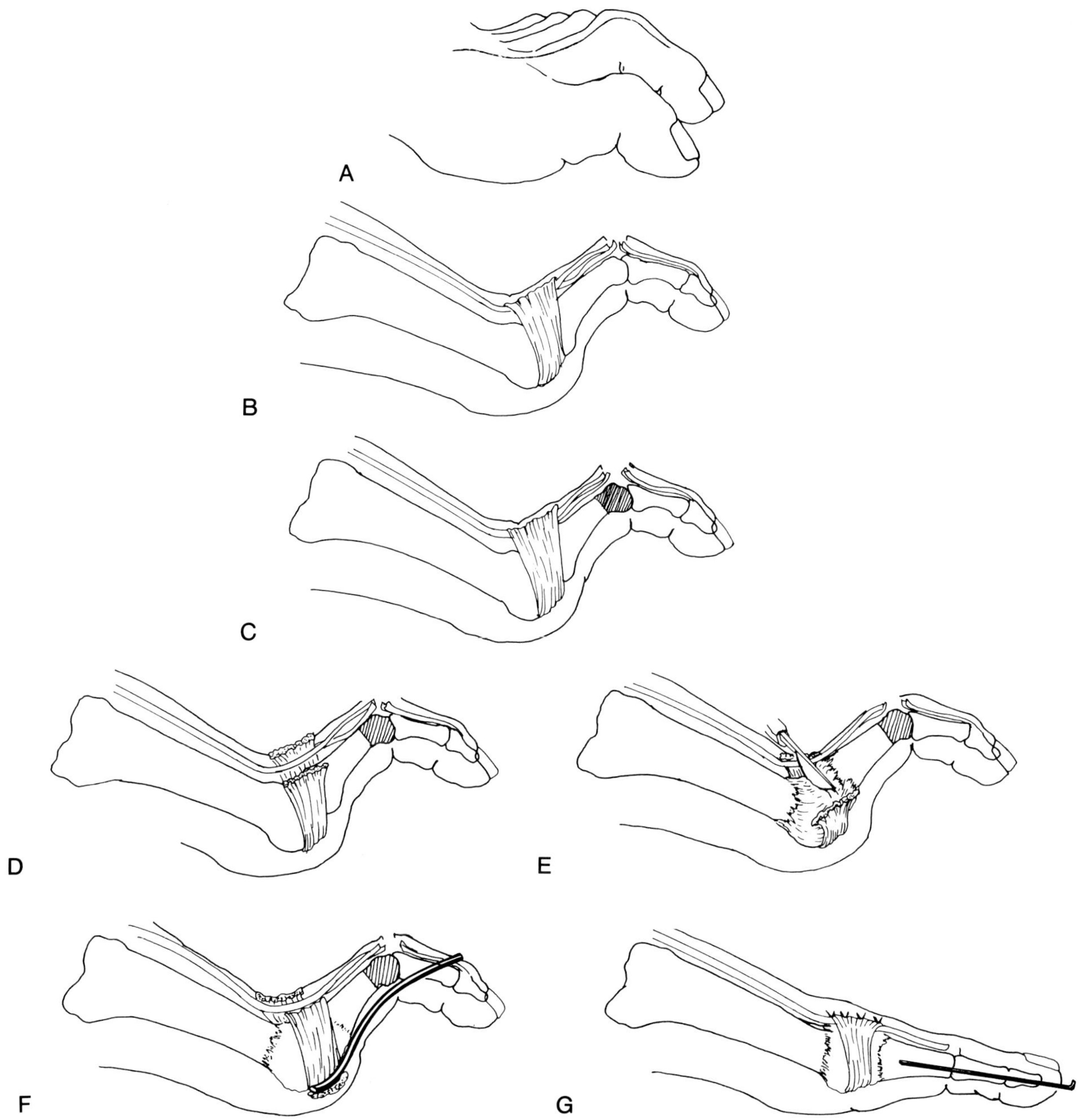

Fig. 26-11. (**A**) Dorsal linear skin incision. (**B**) Z-plasty lengthening extensor digitorum longus tendon. (**C**) Head resection (partial or total) proximal phalanx. (**D**) Extensor hood recession. (**E**) Metatarsophalangeal joint capsulotomy. (**F**) Flexor plate release. (**G**) Kirschner wire stabilization.

and if the digit remains elevated, the next step in the sequence is performed.

7. The MPJ capsule is now incised on the dorsal, medial, and lateral sides using a #64 blade (Fig. 26-11E).
8. The Kelikian push-up-test is again repeated, and if the digit remains elevated, the next step in the sequence is performed.
9. The flexor plate is now released using a metatarsal elevator, by gently but firmly inserting

the elevator under the metatarsal head and advancing it proximally (Fig. 26-11F). The flexor plate will be released, and the sequential reduction is completed.

10. The digits are stabilized using 0.045 Kirschner wires in retrograde fashion as previously described, usually to the base of the proximal phalanges (Fig. 26-11G). If the digit exhibits residual elevation, the pins are placed across the MPJ.

Postoperative Management

The postoperative plan is basically the same as for the other digital procedures. The Kirschner wires are left intact for a period of 6 weeks, at which time they are easily removed with a pair of pliers. On weekly visits, the exit sites of the pins are carefully inspected for blanching, inflammation, or drainage. They are cleaned at each visit, and a new layer of povidone/iodine (Betadine) ointment is applied at the site. Radiographs should be taken immediately after surgery, at 3 weeks, and at 6 weeks, particularly in the arthrodesis procedures, to monitor osseous healing. Light compression splints are utilized to avoid swelling of the digits as the patient's activity level increases, or when the sutures or pins are removed. In some patients, removal of sutures and/or pins may cause some mild temporary swelling.

Rationale and Discussion

Multiple claw toe deformities are a frequent finding in the diabetic patient, owing to the neuropathy and atrophy of the intrinsic musculature. Contracted digits are subjected to excessive extrinsic pressures, creating inflammation, callus formation, and often ulceration (Fig. 26-12). In addition to obvious digital deformities, the contraction and dislocation at the MPJ cause secondary plantarflexion of the metatarsal heads (Fig. 26-13). The result, as it is anywhere on the diabetic foot, is often inflammation, callus formation, ulceration, and ultimate infection. Often, metatarsal lesions can and should be corrected by relocating the dislocated digits at the MPJ. In this situation, the submetatarsal lesion is secondary and the digital dislocation is primary. It is clearly demonstrated that the etiology of the deformity must be accurately ascertained prior to attempting surgical correction. When lesser-metatarsal osteotomies are performed on the patient with severe digital contractures and normal metatarsal declination, the surgery is doomed to failure. The arthroplasty is generally performed on those digits where flexibility at the PIPJ is needed (Fig. 26-14). The end-to-end arthrodesis is generally performed in those digits that are mildly contracted, have some dynamic component, and are of normal length (Fig. 26-15). The peg-in-hole procedure is generally performed on those digits that are severely contracted, have a significant dynamic component, and are excessively long (Fig. 26-16). The peg-in-hole procedure provides tremendous shortening capabilities through its design. The sequential reduction and Kirschner-wire stabilization will allow for healing in the proper position.

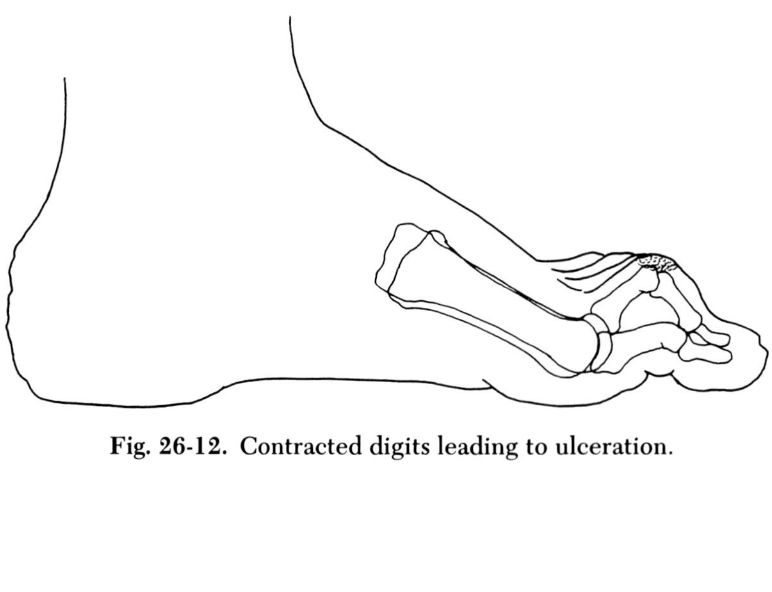

Fig. 26-12. Contracted digits leading to ulceration.

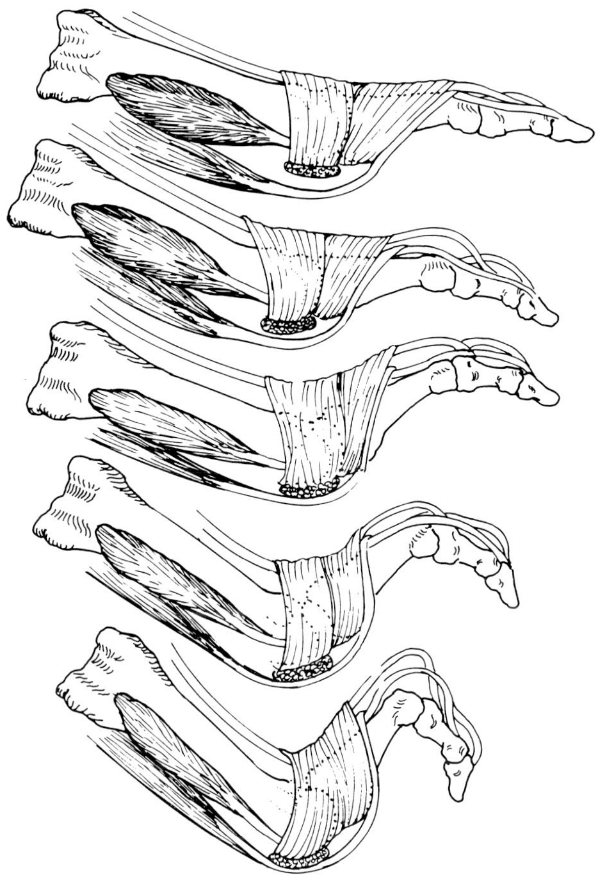

Fig. 26-13. Contraction of digits leading to plantar flexion of metatarsal heads.

Because of loss of function of the intrinsic musculature, the proximal phalanges of the digits are not stabilized against the ground during gait, and instead undergo buckling at the MPJ. Stabilizing the digits through this complex repair restores some of the stability that has been lost, allowing better function of the digits, better propulsion in gait, and improved alignment of the metatarsal heads in the transverse plane. When all of the lesser toes are addressed in this manner, the second and third toes are generally arthrodesed, while the fourth and fifth toes undergo arthroplasty procedures. The fifth toe is never arthrodesed.

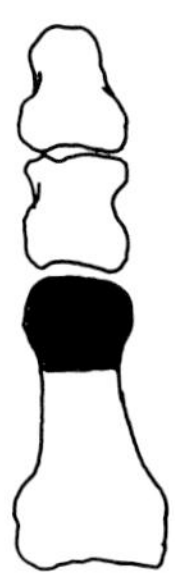

Fig. 26-14. Arthroplasty-proximal phalangeal head resection.

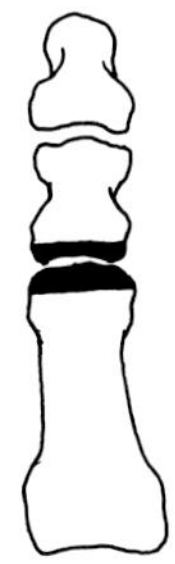

Fig. 26-15. End-to-end arthrodesis.

The sequential reduction of complex claw toe and hammer toe deformities, described by Jimenez, McGlamry, and Greene,[72] is an excellent method for reducing severe digital contractures, and often eliminates accompanying metatarsalgia secondary to digital dislocation.

Problem: Adductovarus Deformity — Fifth Toe (Fig. 26-17A)

Procedure of Choice: Derotational Arthroplasty

Technique

1. Debride hyperkeratotic tissue (heloma durum) prior to surgery (Fig. 26-17B).
2. Using a sterile skin scribe, mark the two semiel-

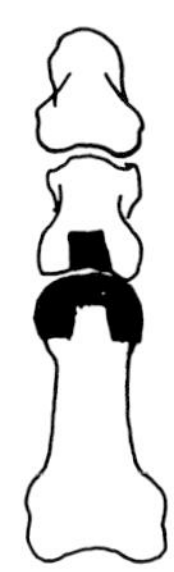

Fig. 26-16. Peg-in-hole arthrodesis.

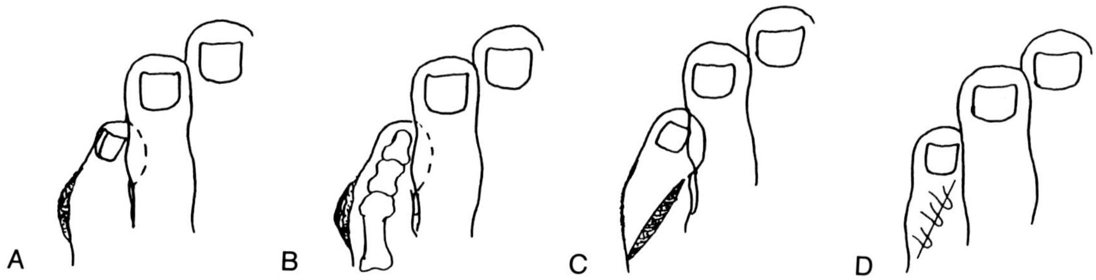

Fig. 26-17. (A) Adductovarus deformity, fifth toe. (B) Heloma durum over proximal interphalangeal joint. (C) Incision: Two semi-elliptical oblique incisions. (D) Skin closure with digit derotated.

liptical skin incisions, going in a proximal-lateral to distal-medial direction (Fig. 26-17C). The skin ellipse should maintain a 3 : 1 ratio of length to width.

3. Using a #15 blade, make the two incisions, taking care to converge the incisions proximally and distally. Grasping the skin with a pickup, gently remove it from the digit using a #15 blade at the dermal-subcutaneous junction. Only epidermis and dermis are removed, leaving all subcutaneous tissues intact in the digit.
4. Perform a head resection of the proximal phalanx as previously described.
5. Upon closure of the skin, the digit should derotate and sit in an upright position, its alignment restored. Apply povidone/iodine (Betadine) splint (Fig. 26-17D).

Postoperative Management
The treatment is the same as that described for the simple arthroplasty.

Rationale and Discussion
The adductovarus deformity of the fifth toe is a very common occurrence. Because of its position, extrinsic shoe pressure frequently leads to hyperkeratotic tissue formation in the form of heloma durum, over the dorsal or dorsolateral aspect of the digit. The fifth toe is particularly subject to trauma because of its location and size. Peripheral neuropathy in the diabetic foot may render the lesion relatively painless, leading to continued trauma and eventual ulceration. The derotational arthroplasty is an excellent way to achieve precise realignment of the digit and removal of underlying bony prominences, which often develop pathologic changes, beginning with a callus and ending with an ulcer that may become infected.

Problem: Congenitally Overlapping Fifth Toe

Procedure of Choice: Relocation of Digit

Technique

1. Perform a V-Y skin plasty technique over the MPJ (metatarsophalangeal joint) in line with the contracture (Fig. 26-18A).
2. Create a flap, dissect down through the subcutaneous tissue to the level of the deep fascia, and locate the extensor digitorum longus tendon to the fifth toe.
3. Perform a Z-plasty lengthening of the fifth extensor digitorum longus tendon (Fig. 26-18B). Reflect the tendon ends, one distally and one proximally.
4. Locate the fifth MPJ. Using a #64 blade perform a medial, dorsal, and lateral fifth MPJ capsulotomy (Fig. 26-18C).
5. Make a dorsal linear incision, either separately or by extending the arm of the "V" to "Y" (short Y to long Y), centered over the fifth digit. In the fashion previously described, perform an arthroplasty technique via proximal phalangeal head resection (Fig. 26-18D).
6. Irrigate the surgical site with normal sterile saline, and retrograde a 0.045 Kirschner wire through the digit, extending it across the MPJ (Fig. 26-18E).

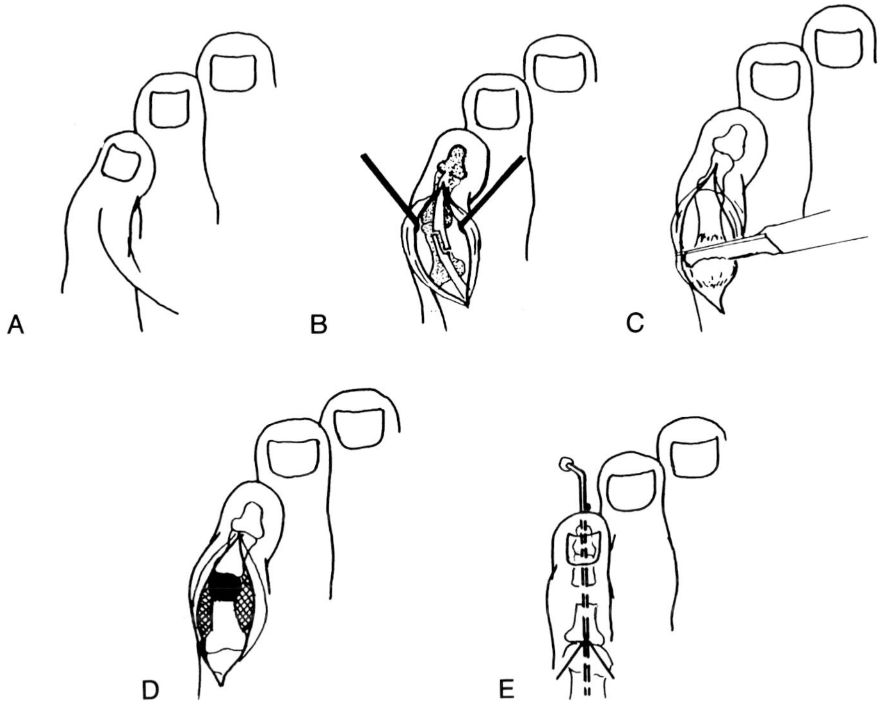

Fig. 26-18. (**A**) Skin incision: "Y." (**B**) Z-plasty lengthening of extensor digitorum longus tendon. (**C**) Capsulotomy-metatarsophalangeal joint. (**D**) Head resection, proximal phalanx.

7. Reapproximate the tendon ends at physiologic length using 3-0 absorbable suture, and the subcutaneous tissue with a 4-0 absorbable suture. The apex of the flap should be closed with an "apical stitch," taking particular care not to pass the needle through the tip of the flap. Skin closure is accomplished with 5-0 nonabsorbable suture material.
8. Apply povidone/iodine (Betadine) splint dressing and a surgical shoe with a toe guard.

Postoperative Management

1. Three days postoperatively: Dressing change. Apply a new dressing.
2. See in 1 week (10 days postoperatively). Remove sutures. Apply a light sterile dressing with mild compression. Apply povidone/iodine (Betadine) ointment at the pin exit site at each visit.
3. Follow up weekly until 4 weeks postoperatively. At 4 weeks, back the pin out across the MPJ and shorten and rebend the pin, leaving it in the digit only for another 2 weeks. See the patient in 2 more weeks, remove the pin, and apply a digital splint.

Rationale and Discussion

Because of significant malalignment, the overlapping fifth toe is particularly prone to injury and trauma, callus formation, and eventual ulceration. It should therefore be relocated whenever possible. Historically, many procedures have failed to correct this deformity, most likely because one of the four components of the deformity was not addressed. The shortened dorsal skin must be lengthened, the contracted extensor tendon and the MPJ capsule must be lengthened, and some bone must be removed in order to relocate the digit without putting significant stretch on the surrounding neurovascular structures.

Problem: Severe Recurrent Helomata Molle: Fourth Web Space (Fig. 26-19A)

Procedure of Choice: Syndactylization

Technique

1. Debride hyperkeratotic tissue; inspect for sinuses, ulceration, infection, and necrotic tissue.
2. Using a sterile skin scribe, mark the area of skin removal on one of the digits. With the ink still wet, gently touch the two inner surfaces of the digits together, creating a mirror image on the opposite side.
3. Using a #15 blade, circumscribe the area indicated by the ink, being careful not to skive the edges (Fig. 26-19B).
4. Remove the entire flap of skin, taking care to remove only epidermis and dermis, and leave all subcutaneous tissues intact in the digits. From within the wound, locate the proximal phalanx of the fifth digit. Free up surrounding soft tissues, and deliver the head through the surgical site. Resect appropriate portions of bone (Fig. 26-19C), remodel the stump, irrigate the site, and bury the stump in the surrounding soft tissues.
5. Attach suture material across the incision site, but let the material lay in place, with the incision open. Repeat this process for the entire length of the incision, and with all pieces in place, begin to close the incision by carefully hand-tying the ends of the material until all are used and the ends are reapproximated (Fig. 26-19D).
6. Apply povidone/iodine (Betadine) split-sterile dressing, and a surgical shoe.

Postoperative Management

The postoperative management is the same as that described for simple arthroplasty.

Rationale and Discussion

Although it may appear harmless and unimportant to the patient, a heloma molle in any web space can quickly become infected, and particularly in the diabetic foot, may undergo rapid progression into the deep plantar spaces of the foot, depending on location. The heloma molle should therefore always be sought by the physician, and if it does not respond to conservative treatment, consideration should be given to syndactylization. Important points to remember in performing the procedure are to map out the skin incision carefully, and when the skin flap is removed, to leave all subcutaneous tissues intact for vascular supply. Placing the sutures across the site, leaving them open, and later tying them all by hand avoids the sometimes difficult closure that is often encountered when closing one suture at a time with the needle, owing to the limited space within which the surgeon must work. An assistant should gently stabilize and align the digit while the surgeon performs the closure.

Syndactylization is an excellent procedure for severe, recurrent helomata molle or those that have been previously infected. Particular care should be taken to remove adequate portions of bone to avoid irritation of adjacent osseous segments.

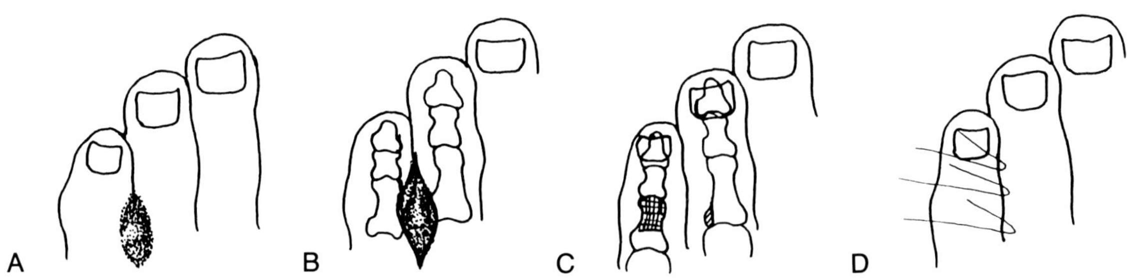

Fig. 26-19. (**A**) Recurrent heloma molle, fourth web space. (**B**) Incision of circumscribed area. (**C**) Appropriate bone resection. (**D**) Skin closure.

LESSER METATARSAL SURGERY IN THE DIABETIC FOOT

The diabetic foot often exhibits submetatarsal lesions, often callus formations, which sometimes lead to ulcers. As stated previously, when these lesions are attributed to digital dislocation at the metatarsophalangeal joints, reduction of the digits is usually necessary. There are situations, however, when the etiology of the lesion stems from the metatarsal itself, and in those situations the focus of surgery is on the metatarsal.

It has been shown by sonographic examination that patients with diabetes who exhibit significant neuropathy have atrophic plantar fat pads.[74] In these patients, any accentuated plantar-flexion of a metatarsal head results in an excessive focal weight load, causing inflammation, callus, and possible ulceration. Although it is a rare occurrence, a patient with a truly rigid plantar-flexed metatarsal head may be a candidate for elevation of that metatarsal, either at the head or at the base. After a thorough physical examination and gait analysis, preoperative evaluation should consist of weight-bearing ink impressions, dorsal-plantar standard radiographs with the foot in angle and base-of-gait positions and a marker on the lesion, a forefoot axial radiograph with a lesion marker, and a lateral radiograph with a lesion marker.

When it has been thoroughly established that a rigid plantar-flexory deformity exists, a surgical procedure is selected and executed. The osteotomy at the metatarsal head traditionally has been performed and allowed to "float." It is now recommended that some type of fixation be used across the osteotomy to ensure stability across the osteotomy and aid in primary bone healing.

Problem: Rigid Plantarflexed Metatarsal Head, Normal Width

Procedure of Choice: Distal V-Osteotomy with K-wire Fixation

Technique

1. Make a dorsal linear skin incision centered over the distal third of the metatarsal to the level of the joint.
2. Brush down gently through the subcutaneous tissues with a #15 blade to the level of the deep fascia/long extensor tendon. Retract the extensor tendon to one side or the other. Release of the proximal extensor hood fibers may be necessary to mobilize the tendon.
3. The metatarsal head and neck are located by palpation. Make a linear incision through the deep tissues to the level of bone, centered over the metatarsal, taking care not to let the scalpel blade slip off laterally or medially.
4. Using a Freer elevator, reflect the periosteum off the bone, exposing the metatarsal neck at the metaphyseal flare (Fig. 26-20A).

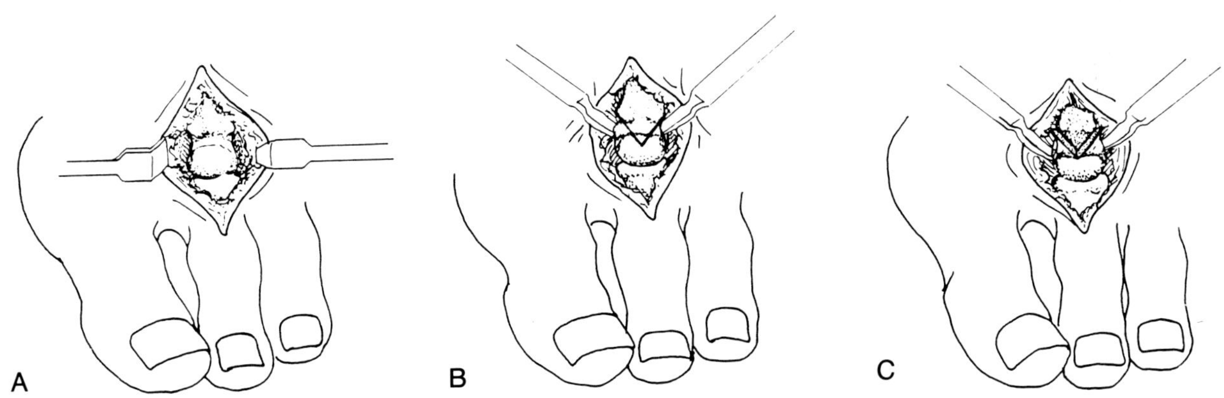

Fig. 26-20. (A) Exposure of metatarsal head. (B) V-osteotomy at metaphyseal neck. (C) Distal capital fragment is repositioned/realigned for improved weight distribution.

5. Using a 1.5-mm drill bit, create a pilot hole in the metaphyseal region, taking care to tilt the drill bit slightly distally (approximately 15°) to avoid violating the plantar condyles. For a guide, a 0.045 Kirschner wire may be inserted, shortened, and used to keep the saw blade in proper line.
6. The V-osteotomy is performed with the apex distal (Fig. 26-20B). This is a through-and-through cut, and when it is completed, the distal capital fragment is repositioned and realigned for equal weight distribution (Fig. 26-20C).
7. When satisfactory alignment is achieved, the correction is maintained with a single .045 Kirschner wire. The wire may be placed across the osteotomy percutaneously and left exiting the skin, or may be bent, cut, and buried under the periosteum, subcutaneous tissue, and skin.
8. Periosteum and deep fascia are closed with 3-0 absorbable sutures, subcutaneous tissue with 4-0 absorbable sutures, and skin closure is accomplished with 5-0 absorbable material in intradermal fashion.

Postoperative Management

1. The first dressing change is performed 3 days postoperatively. If the osteotomy fixation is stable, the patient may be ambulatory in a rigid surgical shoe. Four weekly visits should ensue, followed by visits every 2 weeks. The patient should wear a surgical shoe for 6 weeks, and at that time convert to normal shoe gear if radiographs demonstrate osseous healing.

Rationale and Discussion

Although not technically difficult to perform, the long-term outcome for the lesser metatarsal osteotomies is difficult to predict. Placement of the distal capital fragment is critical prior to pinning, and much of this decision is based on palpation of the metatarsal heads plantarly. This procedure, more so than procedures that are more easily quantifiable and measurable, demonstrates the art rather than the science of surgical medicine.

Regarding the fixation, it is always preferable to bury the wire rather than have it exiting the skin. The buried wire is not prone to damage, as is the wire that exits the skin. The scar left by the external wire is also unsightly, and may develop in a thicker, irritated manner if there is tension on the skin. Not only does the buried wire allow the patient to bathe the foot sooner, but the likelihood of infection is greater in the accidently immersed foot with a Kirschner wire exiting the skin than in one in which all of the skin is closed. Whether internal or external, the Kirschner wire should be placed in a dorsal-proximal to plantar-distal direction, parallel with the metatarsal (i.e., without obliquity of the pin). An oblique pin will probably not be as effective in preventing the distal capital fragment from rotating.

With regard to the procedure, it is quite effective in dorsiflexing the distal segment of the metatarsal. If additional shortening of the metatarsal is needed, the surgeon can simply perform the two additional cuts, making the procedure the "Chevron."

FIFTH RAY SURGERY ON THE DIABETIC FOOT

Problem: Tailor's Bunion Deformity

Procedure: Reverse Austin (Fig. 26-21)

Technique

1. Make a dorsal-linear skin incision centered over the fifth metatarsal to the level of the MPJ (Fig. 26-21A).
2. Brush down gently through the subcutaneous tissues to the level of the deep fascia/long extensor tendon. Retract the extensor tendon medially and locate the MPJ by palpation.
3. Make a linear incision through the deep fascia and periosteum to the bone. Using a Freer elevator, reflect the periosteum cleanly off the bone, exposing the metatarsal neck. A #15 blade is required to completely reflect the deep tissues from the lateral aspect of the head, due to Sharpy's fibers.
4. Visualizing the head as a circle, make a dot in the center and insert a 0.045 Kirschner wire as a guide from lateral to medial.

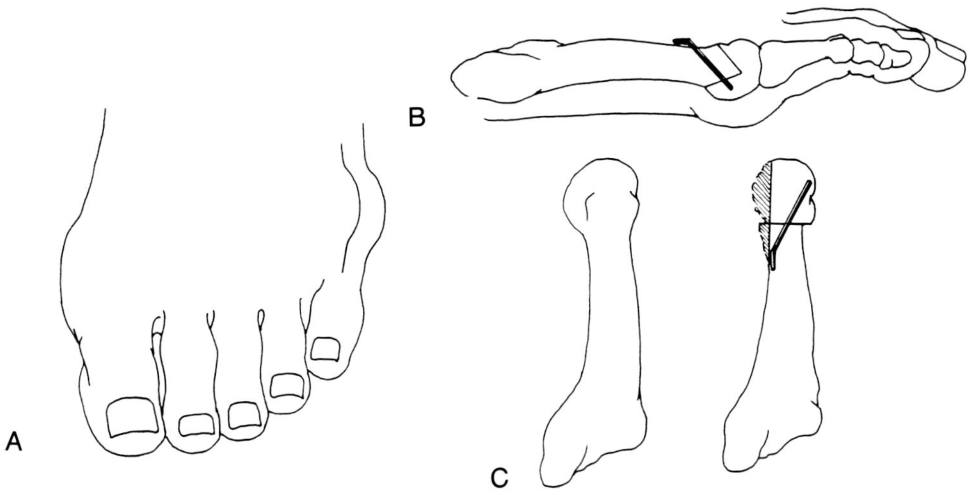

Fig. 26-21. (A) Dorsal linear skin incision over deformity. (B) Osteotomies cut through and through. (C) Distal capital fragment is repositioned medially and fixated with 0.045 Kirschner wire.

5. Perform two through-and-through osteotomies in the metatarsal head, with the apex at the pin, angulated at 60° to one another (Fig. 26-21B).
6. Displace the capital fragment medially to the desired position (Fig. 26-21C).
7. Fixate using one 0.045 Kirschner wire from dorsal-proximal-lateral to plantar-distal-medial. Bend, cut, and bury the Kirschner wire. Irrigate.
8. The periosteal tissues are reapproximated over the wire using 3-0 absorbable suture material, the subcutaneous tissues are reapproximated with 4-0 absorbable suture material, and skin closure is accomplished with 5-0 absorbable suture material in an intradermal fashion.

Postoperative Management

The postoperative management is the same as for the lesser metatarsal osteotomy.

Rationale and Discussion

Because of the lateral prominence caused by the tailor's bunion deformity, callus can form, followed by ulceration extending into the periarticular structures, joint, and bone. Should such an ulceration go unchecked and become infected, it can lead to loss of the fifth ray and a subsequent balance problem. It is therefore important to surgically reposition the fifth metatarsal while it is in a healthy, uninfected state. If the entire metatarsal is splayed, a wedge-type osteotomy may have to be performed at the base. If the metatarsal is not splayed but an enlarged head exists, the lateral condylectomy may suffice. The traditional "slide" osteotomy done transversely and without fixation is very unstable and should not be performed in these patients.

Prolonged bone healing at the cellular level has been described in the diabetic foot, from the effects of insulin and diabetes on bone and mineral metabolism.[47] Because of the already increased risk of delayed bone healing in the diabetic foot, bone fixation is recommended to maximize healing capability.

FIRST-RAY SURGERY IN THE DIABETIC FOOT

Criteria for the surgical correction of a hallux abducto valgus deformity are basically the same for diabetic and nondiabetic feet. Forefoot pathology is very common in the diabetic foot, including digital, lesser metatarsal, and first-ray involvement. As noted previously, neuropathy of intrinsic musculature causes digital instability, lesser metatarsal malalignment, and abnormal distribution of weight. This instability and malalignment may have a direct effect on the load bearing of the first ray. Ctercteko found significantly greater forces acting on the first ray area in diabetic patients both with and without ulceration.[75]

As a result of underlying osseous malalignment, the foot displays the typical medial eminence formation. Friction and pressure from normal footgear cause inflammation and irritation at the first metatarsophalangeal joint. Since the involved area is fairly distal, it frequently has some degree of neuropathy in the diabetic foot. Consequently, pain sensation is diminished or absent, and the patient continues to wear footgear beyond the early signs of inflammation. Blister, callus, and ulcer formation often result. Penetration at this level may invade through the skin and subcutaneous tissues to the level of the joint capsule, which may be eroded. Septic arthritis and osteomyelitis may then result, causing massive destruction of articular surfaces. Infected ulcerations over the plantar-medial aspect of the first metatarsal head may allow access to the medial plantar space of the foot, which contains the abductor hallucis and flexor hallucis brevis. In order to avoid the potentially devastating consequences of spreading infection in the medial column of the foot, bony prominences should be reduced when they are prone to blister, callus, and ulcer formation. Standard criteria are followed to determine the particular procedure to be utilized. One exception to this general rule is with implant arthroplasty. Silastic joint-replacement implants are not recommented for diabetic patients because of their increased potential for reactivity.[47] When a joint-destructive procedure is warranted, it should be performed as a traditional Keller, with no insertion of foreign materials such as an implant. Fixation of the osteotomies should be done to aid in primary bone healing, as previously described in the section on lesser metatarsal surgery.

In summary, it is important to realize that the healthy neuropathic diabetic foot has the capability of healing after surgical reconstruction, and should be considered for prophylactic surgery under appropriate circumstances, in order to avoid the devastating and catastrophic events that may occur in the foot that has significant structural malalignment.

Problem: Hallux Abducto Valgus Deformity

Procedure: Modified McBride Bunionectomy with Distal Osteotomy

Technique

1. Make a dorsal linear incision centered over the first metatarsal and extending across the first MPJ (Fig. 26-22).
2. Gently brush down through the subcutaneous tissues to the level of the deep fascia. Reflect subcutaneous fat off the deep fascia with a wet sponge. Locate the deep fascia "pocket" at the base of the proximal phalanx, on its medial aspect. Insert the back of the scalpel handle into the pocket and extend it proximally, continuing to separate the tissue layers.

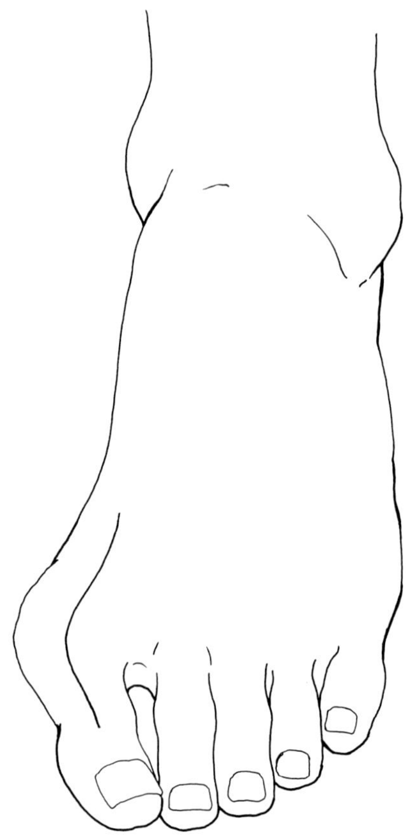

Fig. 26-22. Dorsal linear skin incision over bunion deformity.

3. To perform the interspace dissection, separate subcutaneous tissue off the deep fascia extending into the interspace. Insert a Whietlander retractor and dissect down with Metzenbaum scissors. Locate the deep transverse intermetatarsal ligament, suspend it with the Metzenbaum scissors, and transect. Make a stab incision into the MPJ, release the adductor tendon proximally, and remove a portion. Locate, isolate, and release the fibular sesamoidal ligament. Examine relocation of the sesamoid apparatus and if necessary remove fibular sesamoid at this time.
4. Return to the first metatarsal and make a linear "press cut"-type of incision, bisecting the first metatarsal through the deep fascia, capsule, and periosteum. Make a vertical incision just distal to the medial epicondyle. Reflect all soft tissues from the medial eminence, exposing the medial eminence. Disarticulate the MPJ. Examine the first metatarsal head. Perform appropriate osteotomy as needed.
5. *Austin osteotomy*: Place a 0.045 Kirschner wire into the metatarsal head centrally, on the medial aspect. Using the pin as a guide, perform two through-and-through osteotomies from medial to lateral, angulated at 60° to one another. Displace the capital fragment laterally. Fixate using 0.062 Kirschner wire from a dorsal-proximal medial position to a plantar-distal-lateral position (Fig. 26-23).
   Reverdin osteotomy: Using an oscillating saw, perform two osteotomies in the metatarsal head, making the proximal cut perpendicular to the longitudinal bisection of the metatarsal and the distal cut parallel with the articular cartilage of the metatarsal head. Preserve a lateral cortical hinge. Remove the wedge of bone. Close the osteotomy site. Fixate with a scaphoid staple device across the osteotomy (Fig. 26-24).
   Keller arthroplasty: Using an oscillating saw, perform an osteotomy at the base of the proximal phalanx of the hallux, just distal to the flare. Caution should be taken to protect the flexor hallucis longus tendon from the saw blade. Sharply dissect out the segment of bone, taking care not to sever the tendon. Stabilize the proximal phalanx to the flexor hallucis longus tendon by suturing the plantar aspect of the proximal phalanx to the tendon through a small drill hole (Fig. 26-25).
6. Medial capsulorrhaphy is performed with 2-0 polyester suture material. The periosteum, capsule, and deep tissues are reapproximated with 3-0 absorbable suture material, the subcutaneous tissues with 4-0 absorbable suture material, and skin closure is accomplished with 5-0 absorbable material in an intradermal fashion.

Postoperative Management

The first dressing change is performed 3 days postoperatively. If the osteotomy fixation is stable, the patient may be ambulatory in a rigid surgical shoe. Four weekly visits should be followed by visits

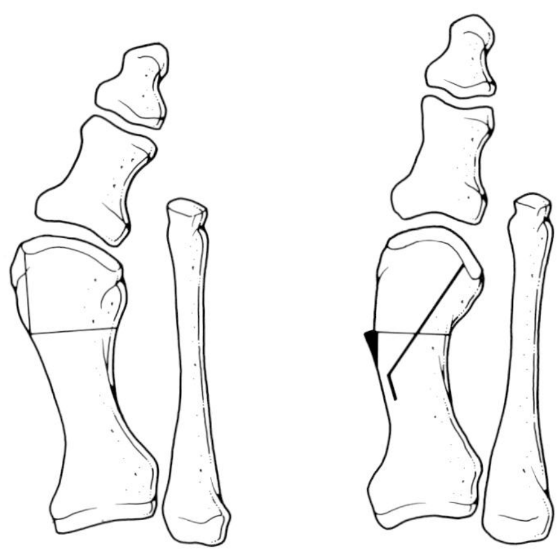

Fig. 26-23. Austin procedure.

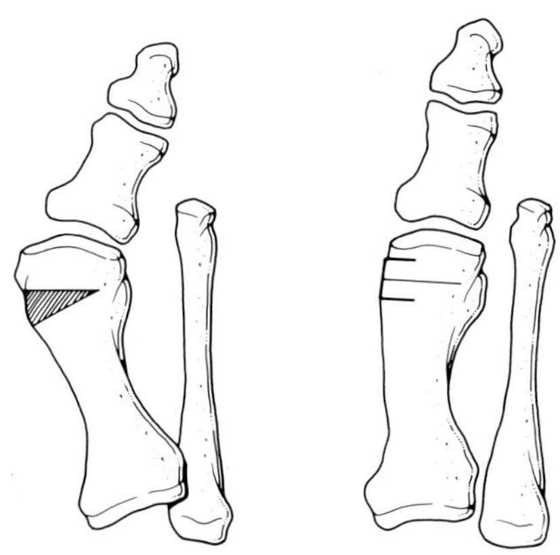

Fig. 26-24. Reverdin procedure.

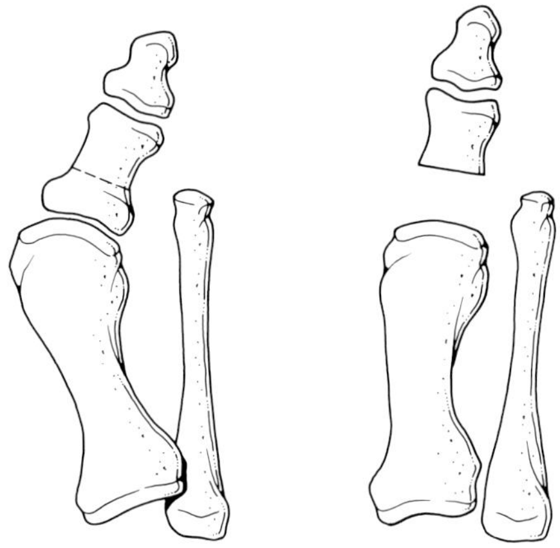

Fig. 26-25. Keller procedure.

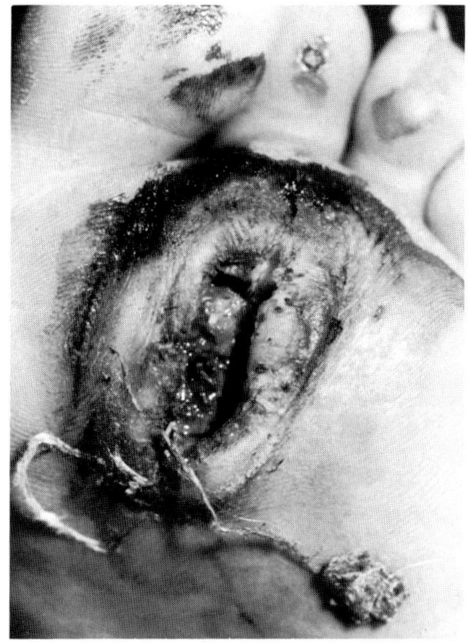

Fig. 26-27. Callus under plantar-flexed metatarsal leading to severe mal perforans ulceration.

every 2 weeks. The patient should wear the surgical shoe for 6 weeks, and at that time convert to normal shoe gear if radiographs demonstrate osseus healing. Bunion splints may be used to maintain the correction after dressings have been discontinued.

Rationale and Discussion

Diabetic patients generally do quite well following bunion surgery provided they have adequate circulation and perioperative management is followed carefully. When performing distal osteotomy procedures on the metatarsal, the complete anatomic dissection, as previously described, is performed. If a Keller arthroplasty procedure is to be performed, the surgery will differ in that the lateral interspace dissection will not be performed. Particular care should be taken in all procedures to avoid applying dressings that may be too constrictive, causing circulatory compromise and possible pressure blisters or pressure necrosis. Always remember that the patient with neuropathy may not realize that a bandage is too tight or is irritative to the skin. A good rule of thumb is to always have dressings well padded with many sterile 4- × 4-inch gauze pads wrapped with conforming gauze bandages.

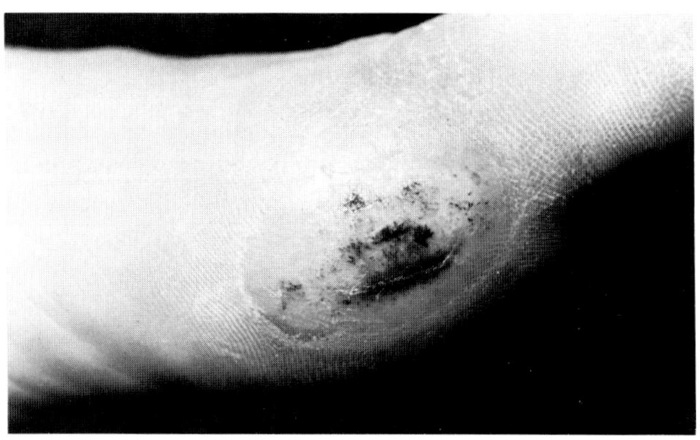

Fig. 26-26. Pressure over bunion leading to callus formation with subcutaneous bleeding.

Postoperative radiographs should be taken immediately after surgery and at six weeks, 3 months, 6 months, and 1 year for long-term follow up. The patient is generally maintained in a rigid-soled surgical shoe for the first 4 weeks postoperatively, then moved to a more flexible surgical shoe for 2 weeks, and then to athletic shoes (running or walking shoes) at 6 weeks for a period of 2 weeks. At 8 weeks, the patient may generally return to any type of conventional footgear.

As stated previously, forefoot pathology in the diabetic foot is very common, and may lead to callus formation, ulceration, and infection. Pres-

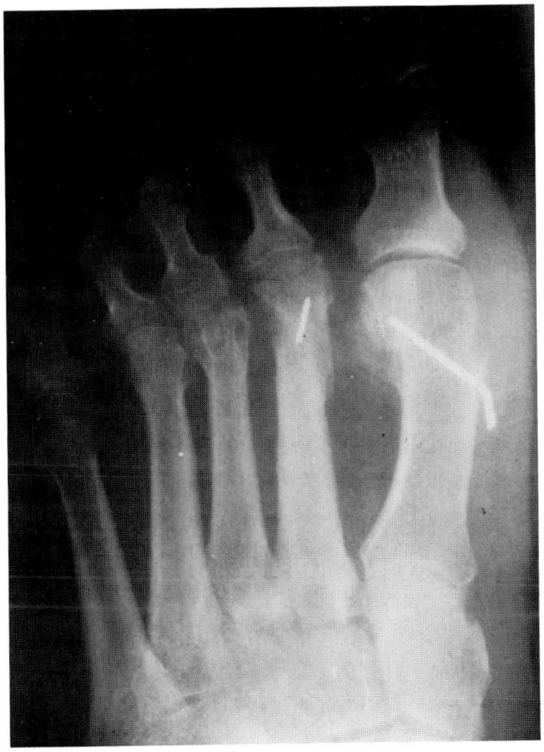

Fig. 26-28. Status post Austin bunionectomy and V-osteotomy of the second metatarsal with internal fixation devices.

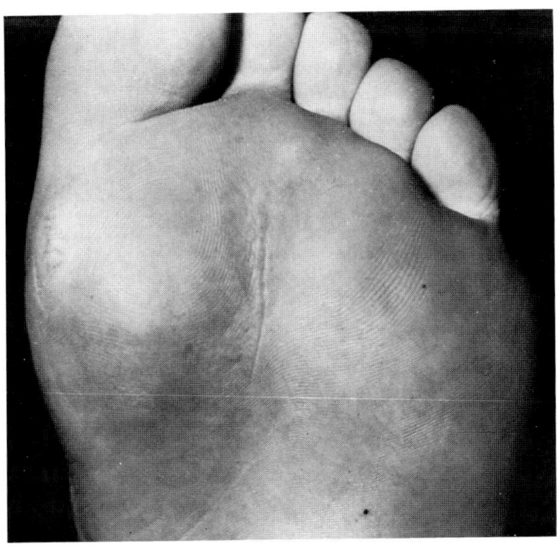

Fig. 26-29. Complete resolution of calluses/ulcerations.

sure over a bunion formation may lead to callus with subcutaneous bleeding (Fig. 26-26). If left untreated, a callus under a plantar-flexed lesser metatarsal may lead to severe mal perforans ulceration (Fig. 26-27). Addressed surgically, lesser metatarsals and first metatarsals may be repositioned for improved weight distribution and held in place by internal fixation devices (Fig. 26-28), leading to resolution of the deformity and avoidance of the devastating results of massive diabetic infection (Fig. 26-29).

REFERENCES

1. American Diabetes Association Newsletter. January 1989
2. Kalish SR: Limb salvage procedures in the diabetic. p. 131. In Brenner MA (ed): Management of the Diabetic Foot. Williams & Wilkins, Baltimore, 1987
3. Most RS, Sinnock P.: The epidemiology of lower extremity amputations in diabetic individuals. Diabetes Care 6:87, 1983
4. Chronicles XVI, 12–14
5. Moschella SL: Hypersensitive and insensitive extremities. Br J Dermatol 93:151, 1975
6. Dormandy JA: Management of the diabetic foot. Ann R Coll Surg Engl 61:305, 1979
7. Brand PW: Management of the insensitive limb. Ch. 2. In: The Insensitive Limb. American Physical Therapy Association, Feb. 1979
8. Kosiak M: Etiology and pathology of ischemic ulcers: Arch Phys Med Rehab 40:62, 1959
9. Entmacher PS, Sinnock P, Bostic E et al: Economic Impact of Diabetes in America. U.S. Government Printing Office, U.S. Department of Health and Human Services, Washington D.C., August, 1985
10. Ger R: Prevention of major amputations in the diabetic patient. Arch Surg 120:1317, 1985
11. Kozak GP, Koar CS, Rowbotham JL et al: Management of Diabetic Foot Problems. WB Saunders, Philadelphia, 1984
12. Gudas C: Prophylactic surgery in the diabetic foot. Clin Podiatr Med Surg 4:445, 1987
13. Towne JE: Management of foot lesions in the diabetic patient. Vasc Surg Nov. 1985
14. Larsen K, Christiansen J, Sandahl, Ebskor B: Prevention and treatment of ulcerations of the foot in unilaterally amputated diabetic patients. Acta Orthop Scand 53:481, 1982

15. Smith AG, Casingal EL: Management of diabetic patients with foot lesions. Surg Gynecol Obstet 128:85, 1969
16. Viskum B: Prognosis of conservatively treated diabetic gangrene. Acta Med Scand 185:319, 1969
17. Ebskor B, Josephenson P: Incidence of reamputation and death after gangrene of the lower extremity. Prosthet Orthot Int 4:77, 1980
18. Vesignie S: Sur une affection singulière des os de pied. Gaz Hôp Paris, 25:13, 1952
19. Classen JN: Neurotrophic arthroplasty with ulceration. Ann Surg 891, 1964
20. Mott V: A case of circular callus ulcer in the bottom of the foot. Med Surg Rev (New York) 1:129, 1818
21. Brand PW: Insensitive Feet, A Practical Handbook on Foot Problems in Leprosy. p. 17. The Leprosy Mission, London, 1967
22. Block P: The diabetic foot ulcer, a complex problem with a simple treatment approach. Mil Med 146:644, 1981
23. Coleman W: Shoegear for the insensitive foot. Clin Podiatr Med Surg 4:459, 1987
24. Habershaw G, Donovan JC: Biomechanical consideration in the diabetic foot. In Kozak, GP (ed): Management of Diabetic Foot Problems. WB Saunders, Philadelphia, 1984
25. Harkless LB, Kennick D: The Role of the Podiatrist from The Diabetic Foot. 4th Ed. In Levin M, O'Neal L, CV Mosby, St. Louis, 1988
26. Bowker JH. Amputation. Diabetes Forecast, 42:56, 1989
27. ADA Principles of Nutrition and Dietary Recommendations for Individuals with Diabetes Mellitus. Diabetes 28:1027, 1979
28. Simpson RW, Mann JI, Eaton J et al: Improved glucose control in maturity-onset diabetes treated with high carbohydrate-modified fat diet. Br Med J 1:1753, 1979
29. Curran JE: Nutrition and Management of the Diabetic Foot. Ch. 14. Williams & Wilkins, Baltimore, 1987
30. Pollack SV: Wound Healing: A Review. Ch. 3, Nutritional factors affecting wound healing. J Dermatol Surg Oncol 5:615, 1979
31. Wolback SB, Howe PR: Intercellular substances in experimental scorbutus. Arch Pathol 1:1, 1926
32. Levenson S, Seifter E, Van Winkle, Jr, et al: p. 310. In Hunt TK, Dunphy JE (eds): Fundamentals of Wound Management. Appleton-Century-Crofts, New York, 1979
33. Axelrod AE: Modern nutrition in health and disease. p. 493. In Goodhart RS, Shils ME (eds): Nutrition in Relation to Acquired Immunity. Lea Febiger, Philadelphia, 1973
34. Walterlow JC, Golden M, Picou D: The measurement of rates of protein turnover, synthesis and breakdown in man and effects of nutritional status and surgical injury. Am J Clin Nutr 30:1333, 1977
35. Marks J: A Guide to Vitamins: Their Role in Health and Disease. Technical, Lancaster, England, 1975
36. Logerfo FW, Coffman JD: Vascular and microvascular diseases of the foot in diabetes. N Engl J Med 311:1615, 1984
37. Delbridge L, Appleberg M, Reeve TS: Factors associated with development of foot lesions in the diabetic. Surgery 93:78, 1943
38. Levin ME: The Diabetic Foot: Pathophysiology, Evaluation and Treatment. p. 8. In: The Diabetic Foot. 4th Ed. CV Mosby, St. Louis, 1988
39. Allison RD, Roth GM: Central and peripheral vascular effects during cigarette smoking. Arch Environ Health 19:189, 1969
40. Eisen ME, Tyson MC, Michael S, Bauman F: Adhesiveness of blood platelets in arteriosclerosis obliterans, thromboangiitis obliterans, acute thrombophlebitis, chronic venous insufficiency and arthersclerotic heart disease. Circulation 3:271, 1951
41. Coffman JD: The attenuation by reserpine and guanethidine of the cutaneous vasconstriction caused by tobacco smoking. Am Heart J 74:229, 1967
42. Astrup P, Kjeldsen K. Carbon monoxide, smoking and atherosclerosis. Med Clin North Am 58:323, 1974
43. Beach KW, Strandness DE, Jr: Arteriosclerosis obliterans and associated risk factors in insulin dependent and non-insulin dependent diabetics. 29:822, 1980
44. Frykberg RG: Podiatric problems in diabetes. In Kozak GP: Management of Diabetic Foot Problems. WB Saunders, Philadelphia, 1984
45. Lang-Stevenson AI, Sharrard WJW, Betts RP et al: Neuropathic Ulcers of the Foot. J Bone Joint Surg (Br) 67:438, 1985
46. Brand PW: Management of the insensitive limb. Phys Ther 59:8, 1979
47. Hetherington VJ: The insensitive foot. In McGlamry ED (ed): Fundamentals of Foot Surgery. Williams & Wilkins, Baltimore, 1987
48. Beach RB, Thompson DE: Selected soft tissue research. Phys Ther 59:30, 1979
49. Bergtholdt HT: Temperature assessment of the insensitive foot. Phys Ther 59:18, 1979
50. Bergtholdt HT: Measurement in tissue response in rat footpad from repetitive mechanical stress. In Brand PW, Mooney V (eds): The Effects of Pressure

on Human Tissues. Report III. Rehabilitation Service Administration, Washington, DC, 1977
51. Eliashiv A et al: Depression of cell-mediated immunity in diabetes. Arch Surg 113:1180, 1978
52. Robertson HD: Polk HC: The mechanism of infection in patients with diabetes mellitus: a review of leukocyte function. Surgery 75:123, 1974
53. Repine JE, Clauson CC, Goetz FC: Bactericidal function of neutrophils from patients with acute bacterial infection and from diabetics. J Infect Dis 142:869, 1980
54. Nolan CM, Beaty HN, Bagdade JD: Further characterization of the impaired bactericidal function of granulocytes in patients with poorly controlled diabetes. Diabetes 27:889, 1978
55. Bagdade JD, Steward M, Walters E: Impaired granulocyte adherence: a reversible defect in host defense in patients with poorly controlled diabetes. Diabetes 27:677, 1978
56. Bagdade JD, Root RK, Bulger RJ: Impaired leukocyte function in patients with poorly controlled diabetes. Diabetes 23:9, 1974
57. Rayfield EF, Ault MJ, Keuson GT et al: Infection and diabetes: the case for glucose control. Am J Med 72:439, 1982
58. Goodson WH, Hunt TK: Wound healing and the diabetic patient. Surg Gynecol Obstet 149:600, 1979
59. Hunt TK, Van Winkle W, Jr: Normal repair. p. 4. In: Fundamentals of Wound Management. Appleton-Century-Crofts, Norwalk, CT, 1979
60. Hunt TK: Burns. p. 582. In: Fundamentals of Wound Management. Appleton-Century-Crofts, Norwalk, CT, 1979
61. Levin M, Sprutt I: To soak or not to soak: that is the question. Clinical Diabetes Mar/Apr, 1986
62. Bergtholdt WT: Temperature assessment of the insensitive foot. Phys Ther 59:18, 1979
63. Ryan J: Thermography. Australas Radiol 13:23, 1969
64. O'Neal LW: Surgical pathology of the foot and clinicopathological correlations. p. 203. In Levin M (ed): The Diabetic Foot. 4th Ed. CV Mosby, St. Louis, 1988
65. Frost LA: Root resection for incurvated nail: J Am Podiatry Assoc 40:19, 1950
66. Winograd AM: A Modification in the Technic of Operation for Ingrown Toenail. JAMA 91:229, 1929
67. Zadik FR: Obliteration of the nail bed of the great toe without shortening of the terminal phalanx. J Bone Joint Surg 32B:66, 1950
68. Ellenberg M: Diabetic neuropathic ulcer. J Mt Sinai Hosp 35:585, 1968
69. Stokes IAF, Faris IB, Hutton WC: The neuropathic ulcer and loads on the foot in diabetic patients. Acta Orthop Scand 46:839, 1975
70. Stokes IAF, Hutton WC: The effect of the diabetic ulcer on the load-bearing function of the foot. p. 245. In Kenedi RM, Cowden JM (eds): Bedsore Biomechanics. University Park Press, Baltimore, 1976
71. Holewski J, Moss KM, Stess RM et al: Prevalence of foot pathology and lower extremity complications in a diabetic outpatient clinic. J Rehabil Res Dev 26:35, 1989
72. Jimenez AL, McGlamry ED, Green DR: Lesser ray deformities. Ch. 3. In McGlamry ED (ed): Comprehensive Textbook of Foot Surgery Vol. 1. Williams & Wilkins, Baltimore, 1987
73. Kelikian H: Hallux Valgus Allied Deformities of the Forefoot and Metatarsalgia, WB Saunders, Philadelphia, 1965
74. Gooding GAW, Stess RA, Graft PM et al: Sonography of the sole of the foot: evidence of loss of foot pad thickness in diabetes and its relationship to ulceration of the foot. Invest Radiol 21:45, 1986
75. Ctercteko GC, Dhanendran M, Hutton WC et al: Vertical forces acting on the feet of diabetic patients with neuropathic ulceration. Br J Surg 68:608, 1981

27

Medicolegal Implications of Diabetic Foot Disease

Isidore Steiner, D.P.M., J.D., D.A.B.P.S., F.A.C.F.S.

Diabetes mellitus is a disease process that affects the feet of a large percentage of patients. The foot specialist should be aware of the legal ramifications involved in the treatment of diabetic patients and the peripheral issues that affect them. Diabetes affects the neurologic and vascular status of the digits and feet in a manner that causes patients much hardship and discomfort. Many times patients seek out physicians for diagnosis and treatment of foot conditions, not realizing that a systemic condition is the underlying cause of their problems. A foot specialist, therefore, may act as the primary care physician in diagnosing diabetes and may subsequently be responsible for referring an individual to a qualified primary care family physician, internist, or endocrinologist. Legal issues abound on this very situation, such as when a physician fails to diagnose a condition and subsequently treats a patient improperly, or when the condition is diagnosed correctly, but the patient is referred to a physician whose treatment causes the patient damage. Issues of malpractice are of particular importance to diabetic patients, and a large percentage of successful malpractice cases are caused by negligent and improper treatment of the diabetic foot. There are numerous duties that the referring physician owes to the patient and to third parties related to that patient.

There are multiple elements involved in a diabetic malpractice lawsuit and varied theories of malpractice that need to be understood by the physician prior to undertaking the treatment of the diabetic patient. New emerging issues such as discrimination against the diabetic patient in employment, drug problems caused by the prescription or injection of a drug, social security, disability claims of diabetic individuals, and worker's compensation related to diabetes also need to be addressed.

No single description can adequately cover the numerous potential liabilities that a physician faces when treating a diabetic patient. The timing and severity of the condition, its duration, and resulting complications can easily affect the outcome of treatment and the decision whether to treat and how to treat. However, whether the doctor manages a condition properly really depends upon knowledge of medicine and law. Whether to treat or not to treat, whether to prescribe medication or inject a particular substance into a diabetic patient's body, whether to operate or not, and whether to refer or not are issues of critical importance that can create major legal consequences. In this chapter we will examine those consequences and attempt to provide some solutions to problems and recommendations to particular situations.

BASIC AREAS OF LAW THAT AFFECT THE MALPRACTICE ARENA

Before discussing specifically how medical malpractice relates to diabetes, several basic areas of law must be addressed. Two distinct areas that directly affect the medical malpractice arena are contracts and torts. Contracts deal with the formative relationship between the physician and the diabetic patient. Torts deal with issues of assault and battery and how an invalid consent can lead to both criminal and civil sanctions.

Contracts

A contract is a transaction that involves a binding legal relationship between at least two parties. In general, contractors form an agreement, which can be either written or oral, that will be enforceable by the courts if the parties fail to do what they have agreed to do. A contract is formed at a particular time during a relationship. Once a contract begins, it imposes specific obligations upon the parties to act in good faith and abide by the terms of the contract. There are certain essential elements that prove the existence of a contract.

A contract includes an offer and an acceptance. The offer is a communication by one party to another that demonstrates a specific intent to perform. Usually the offer must be specific enough for the parties to understand what their obligations will be if they agree to accept the offer. An acceptance is a communication by which the recipient of an offer expresses his or her intention to be bound by the offer as it was presented. Acceptance must be established in a manner that is requested by the offerer.

Certain contracts are unenforceable by the courts. These are contracts that violate public policy. Any contract that violates the law is considered a violation of public policy and is therefore unenforceable. Also, contracts are not enforceable against parties who are either minors or mentally deficient. For example, if you are treating a juvenile diabetic patient for foot conditions and the parent leaves the patient unaccompanied at your office, you run the risk of treating that patient illegally. Should you decide to perform a minor surgical procedure on that patient and do not have the specific consent of the parent, you have violated a contract law and performed a battery on this particular patient.

When one of the parties violates an agreement, breach of contract has occurred. Courts look upon breaches in two different ways. A material breach is one that is so serious that it will excuse the nonbreaching party from its obligation under the contract. A nonmaterial breach can still maintain the contractural relationship, if the breach can be rectified.

When a contract is broken there are different types of remedies that are available. The obvious remedy is monetary damage. If you make a contract with a patient to provide surgical care for a particular deformity, you are obligated to perform that care within the standard appropriate for your community. If your performance is inferior to that standard and the patient is damaged, then you have breached the contract. The patient can subsequently sue you for monetary damages.

Equitable relief is another type of remedy that has three very familiar legal solutions: specific performance, injunctions, and restitution.

Specific performance is when the court orders a party to actually perform the contractural obligations. An injunction is awarded for the purpose of requiring a party to refrain from a particular activity. Restitution is based on the principle that if one party has been unjustly enriched at the expense of another person, the enriched person is required to make restitution to the other party.

Torts

Torts are invoked for injuries to persons or things. They are considered to be private or civil wrongs that are independent of any contract violation that might have transpired between parties. The individual performing a tort must bring about some harm to another party; however, malicious intent need not necessarily be present. Also, in many cases, the person does not even have to commit a particular harmful action in order to be held responsible for committing a tort; simply having intended to perform the act knowing that there was a substantial likelihood that injury might occur can cause the intending party to be held responsible.

The most common type of tort physicians deal with is battery. Battery is the intentional infliction of harmful or offensive contact on another person. Harmful contact usually means damage to one's body in the form of pain, bruises, tissue contact, or surgical incisions. However, battery may also occur if the offensive contact caused injury not to the person per se, but to the individual's clothing, walking stick, etc.

An assault differs from a battery in that no contact is necessary. An assault is an intentional causing of an apprehension of harmful or offensive contact. The injured party must have believed he or she would be injured or offended by the potential contact of the assailant. It must be proved that the person responsible intended to cause that particular fear in the harmed party.

Other torts that are applicable in the diabetic setting include false imprisonment, intentional affliction of emotional distress, negligence, intentional misrepresentation, and disclosure of private facts.

False imprisonment is the intentional confining of a person against his or her will. Infliction of an emotional distress is the intentional harming of a patient by using extreme and outrageous conduct to affect the patient's mental condition. A physician must have reasonably known that his or her behavior would cause a patient mental anguish to be liable under this tort.

Negligence is a tort that differs from the ones discussed above in that it is not intentional. Negligence is the *failure to appreciate the risks of one's behavior*. A physician has a duty to act as would any reasonable physician under like or similar circumstances. Duty also includes taking actions with caution to avoid unreasonable risk to one's patients. Physicians are held to a certain minimum standard of care regarding their actions, and that standard relates to what exists in similar communities. To have a successful claim of negligence, actual damages must be present. These include economic losses, lost wages, medical bills, pain and suffering, disability, and disfigurement.

Intentional misrepresentation, also known as fraud, is another tort of which physicians must be aware. Fraud is a misrepresentation of a past or present fact that would have influenced a reasonable person in making a decision. The physician must know that he or she is misrepresenting a fact to the patient. The physician must have intended to convince the patient to rely on this false information, and the patient must prove that he or she relied on this information and, due to this reliance, was injured.

If a podiatric physician schedules a diabetic patient for bunion surgery, that physician has a duty to determine medically if the patient is a good surgical risk. If, after performing blood studies, a physician is aware that the patient's blood sugar is at an extremely high level and does not cancel the surgery or advise the patient of this result, the physician runs the risk of being sued for this tort. The physician has fraudulently convinced the patient that he or she is healthy enough to undergo surgery. Should the patient develop a postoperative infection or sustain worse injuries, the surgeon is liable for intentional misrepresentation.

DUTIES EXPECTED OF THE FOOT SPECIALIST

Duty of Expert

Foot specialists consider themselves experts in foot care. This is particularly true for someone who portrays himself or herself as a specialized practitioner who can handle diabetic foot conditions better than the average general practitioner. When a general practitioner or orthopaedist refers a diabetic patient to a foot specialist, the patient is under the impression that the specialist's expertise is superior to that of the average practitioner. Accordingly, the duty of this physician is measured by a higher standard of skill than the average general practitioner. The duty is compared to those who possess a similar degree of learning and skill in the same specialized field and in the same locality.[1]

Duty to Educate

There are two aspects of the duty-to-educate doctrine that concern the treatment of diabetic patients. A physician has a duty to educate patients regarding their illness and the risks inherent in their condition. To do this effectively, the physician must also engage in self-education.

Diabetes presents a life-long condition to a patient, the patient's family, and the practitioners who treat the disease. It is imperative for practitioners to continually update their knowledge and skills. New discoveries are being made daily in the field of diabetes, and the duty rests upon the physician to seek out information about new avenues of therapy through continuing education. Although most physicians and podiatrists are required to be able to diagnose and treat diabetes, no formalized standard has been set by medical organizations as to what constitutes appropriate educational requirements.[2]

Once a practitioner is knowledgeable about a disease, that physician has a duty to educate his or her patients. Patient education begins with the diagnosis of a condition or the acceptance of a patient with a certain condition or disease. Patients need to know the characteristics of the condition, how serious the disability will be, how treatment will proceed, and how the disease and the treatment will affect their ability to maintain a normal life-style. A physician must integrate information obtained during the history and physical examination to assess the condition and to determine the amount of education necessary. When a diabetic patient is encountered, the physician must provide special forms regarding proper foot care and teach the patient proper care and treatment of nails and calluses. It is also helpful to explain to the patient how diabetes can result in infections and ulcerations, and to instruct the patient in ways to avoid these problems.

Physician-Patient Relationships

In order for a physician to be liable for malpractice a relationship must exist between the doctor and the patient. This relationship is based on contract, express or implied, that the doctor will treat the patient with the best possible available skill and care, and that the patient will pay for these services. The physician-patient relationship must be based on some legal principle, and usually the courts find that the contractural aspect of the law fits this criterion.

When the professional services of a physician are accepted for the purpose of treatment, the relationship becomes contractural, and courts have found that a physician-patient relationship exists.[3] There are many ways in which this relationship can be invoked. The contractural arrangement whereby a patient seeks a physician, engages the physician to render services, and the physician accepts the patient is the most common situation.[4]

There are situations where no contractural agreement exists, and the physician is absolved of liability in a malpractice case. A physician is not bound to render services to anyone who asks and, by advising the patient, can limit the extent or scope of his treatment.[5] A physician may even refuse to treat a patient, and that refusal cannot be held against him.[6]

Other situations have occurred in which a defendant physician was called into a hospital room as a consultant to evaluate a patient. The courts found that a physician-patient relationship was established with the consultant and the duties and liabilities of a physician were invoked.

MEDICAL MALPRACTICE ISSUES

A claim of malpractice can call into question any number of legal issues at any point in the physician-patient relationship—from initial contact, through diagnosis and treatment, to ultimate discharge of the patient by a treating physician. The rules regarding treatment of diabetic individuals are consistent with all general rules of medical malpractice. In addition, there are special rules prescribed for dealing with the diabetic patient. The following sections will discuss in general the kinds of situations that can lead to malpractice claims, with specific emphasis on special rules for diabetes. Points of law will be illustrated with actual case citations.

Improper Diabetes Treatment

Failure to Diagnose

Very often, a diabetic patient is improperly treated, and due to that negligence, the patient ultimately suffers either an amputation or severe infection. It is imperative to be aware that improper treatment can lead to a malpractice action. Once a physician accepts a diabetic patient, it is the physician's duty to treat that patient with utmost care at the level of standard of other physicians in the same geographic area.

Failure to diagnose a case of diabetes can lead to liability. Podiatrists who consider themselves general diagnosticians competent to discover systemic conditions are held to the same degree of skill and care as are medical doctors in this diagnostic procedure. Therefore, if a patient presents with symptoms indicating a potential for diabetes, the podiatrist is under a duty to test blood sugar to determine whether diabetes exists.[7] This is all the more necessary if this physician determines that some type of surgical treatment is indicated. Failure to determine whether that patient suffers from an infection, diabetes, or any other systemic condition prior to performing surgery is negligence.

Improper treatment of a diabetic patient that ultimately results in leg amputation can create damages predicated not only on negligence but also on pain and suffering caused by improper treatment. Loss of consortium can also be sustained if a physician improperly diagnoses a diabetic condition or improperly treats a diabetic individual, and that person sustains iatrogenic injury.

Failure to Refer

One of the major areas to which practitioners fall prey with regard to medical malpractice is their failure to refer a diabetic patient to an endocrinologist or peripheral vascular specialist in a timely manner. Physicians have a duty to advise patients to consult specialists when they are unqualified to give the necessary treatment. This is even more relevant when the physician knows that the patient would receive better treatment from another physician.[8]

The standard to which a physician is held with regard to a failure-to-refer malpractice case is whether a reasonably careful and skillful physician under like and similar circumstance would have referred that particular patient to a specialist.[1] A physician has a duty to understand at what point treatment becomes ineffectual and whether referral to another more qualified specialist is in order. This duty arises when the physician knows or should have known that he or she does not posses the necessary skill, common knowledge, or equipment to properly treat a patient's condition.[9] Similarly, when a physician realizes that the treatment regimen is not providing effective relief or cure, then the physician must refer that patient to someone whose knowledge is superior.[10]

It is my recommendation that whenever one sees a diabetic person for treatment of a vascular-related condition, that patient should immediately be sent to a vascular specialist for a complete examination and consultation. Following the examination, when the patient returns to the practice, treatment for any diabetes-related condition should be continued on a regular and persistent basis. An open line of communication with the consultant should be established. Discussion of the problem should occur regularly, and if any change in the patient's condition occurs, immediate action can be taken. It has been my experience that in most cases the peripheral vascular specialist determines that the patient's condition is severe and provides adequate documentation that, should an amputation be necessary, makes the first treating physician's liability negligible. It is also possible that the vascular specialist may elect to perform one of many surgical procedures to improve circulation for the diabetic patient. Subsequent to these surgeries, patients may return to the office for successful treatment of their pedal conditions. Not to refer for a vascular consultation can ultimately result in a successful claim of negligence against the primary care physician.

Failure to Obtain Informed Consent

It is essential that every physician have a patient's consent before rendering any type of treatment or care. Performing any procedure on a patient without consent results in a battery.

In a medical situation, any patient must approve any treatment or operation. Any unauthorized surgical procedure or unauthorized extension of a procedure can be considered a violation of the doctor-patient relationship and recognized as negligence. Several states still allow a patient to sue a physician for unauthorized treatment, using the theory of assault or battery. Most states use negligence theory of consent.

The negligence theory of consent involves failure to meet the standard of disclosure to a patient, which causes the patient to undergo a procedure to which they have not agreed and because of an inadequate explanation of what will be happening, the patient is injured. This strategy requires patients to prove that, had they been given all relevant and important information, they would not have agreed to the procedure that caused them injury. Contrary to popular belief, under the negligent theory of consent, it is not easy for plaintiffs to establish adequate evidence for a successful case. The difficulty arises because plaintiffs have to prove causality and establish that they would have refused the procedure had disclosure been totally rendered.

In order to have a valid consent between patient and physician, the patient must be capable of giving consent. The patient must be given sufficient information to reach a reasonable decision regarding treatment. Patients who have been coerced into accepting a procedure or who have been unduly influenced are considered incapable of giving consent.

Certain patients, such as those under the legal age or guardianship or conservatorship, do not have the legal capacity to give consent for medical treatment. It is essential in those cases to obtain the consent of the guardian or conservator, because only they have the power to act for their wards. Many jurisdictions have different age requirements regarding a minor's capacity for consent. Some states use the term *mature minor*.[11] Other states have a concept of *emancipated minor*. Physicians should be aware of what their state considers to be the appropriate age of consent.

Mental illness is another situation in which an individual is considered unable to give consent. Use of drugs and alcohol may also create a similar situation wherein someone does not have the capacity to give consent. Similarly, certain patients have periods of disorientation or confusion, either due to their mental conditions or some physical disability, that would preclude them from giving consent. Some psychotic individuals have lucid and irrational cycles of behavior. During lucid cycles they have the capacity for consent, whereas during irrational cycles they may not. This type of capacity is very difficult to prove, because if the physician realizes he or she is dealing with a psychotic, then the physician treats this patient only in emergency-type situations.

Consent is a dialogue between the patient and physician that leads to an exchange of information. A patient needs to be apprised of all the details of a procedure and must thoroughly understand them in order to give consent. The doctor requires adequate information about the patient before the total picture can be presented. Thus, consent is a process whereby an agreement is reached between patient and doctor, and that agreement need not necessarily be in writing. It takes place any time a doctor examines a patient. Most of the treatment physicians render to their patients is through an oral understanding.

Written consent can take many forms. The two most common are the long and short written consent forms. The long written consent form is a highly detailed document that contains the risks, benefits, and alternatives of the treatment. A short consent form lacks details and contains only succinct statements that the patient understands and freely accepts the procedure. Even though a physician has either of the two consent forms documented in a patient's chart, it is still necessary to make a medical record of the consent in the chart as a progress note.

The question arises as to what constitutes adequate disclosure for consent. A patient must be informed of the probable benefits, risks, and natures of the proposed diagnostic, medical, or surgical intervention. A doctor is not held responsible for withholding information that was unknown or could not have reasonably been known at the time consent was given. Reasonable alternatives to the recommended procedure must be disclosed, but remote risks need not be told to the patient.

The language of the consent form must be in layperson's terms. Explanations must be in a language that patients understand. The doctor must also gear discussion to the level of the patient's intelligence. Language barriers must be overcome by using interpreters or foreign language consent forms. It is not a valid excuse for a physician in a negligent consent lawsuit to claim a valid consent if that consent is in a language that the patient does not understand.

Failure to Inform of Risks

Any physician contemplating surgery on a diabetic patient has an obligation to inform that patient of the risks of the surgery and any potential problems that may occur subsequent to surgery. When treating a diabetic individual, the physician must also inform the patient of the known risks or dangers inherent in that disease process that may affect the proposed potential treatment. The patient will then be able to make an intelligent decision about whether he or she wishes to submit to this treatment or seek care elsewhere.

This is particularly important when dealing with patients with peripheral vascular compromise and diabetes. Patients should be given specialized consent forms so they are aware that additional complications may arise due to their medical condition. These consents should be written and there should also exist an oral understanding between patient and physician. It is helpful under some circumstances to have the patient write in their own words within the body of the physician's chart that they understand the specialized risks that a diabetic patient confronts, that they are fully aware that potential complications may arise, and that no guarantees have been made.

Courts have found that there are occasions when this duty to inform is limited. Physicians may not have to reveal the complete nature and risks of a treatment; however, the patient must be given sufficient information such that the consent to treatment or surgery is an informed consent.

Failure to Advise Patient of the Outcome of an Examination

Once a physician has made an unfavorable diagnosis regarding a patient's case, whether this be through diagnostic testing or clinical examination, a duty exists to inform the patient of this result. This is based on the common principle that every person is in control of his or her body and is entitled to sufficient information regarding the hazards of proposed courses of treatment. A physician who intentionally withholds diagnostic information from a patient can be judged negligent. The failure to inform is considered an intentional concealment and has also been actionable as a misrepresentation in addition to negligence. If a physician determines for some reason that he or she does not wish to convey the results of a test to a patient, it is the physician's duty to place in the patient's chart a brief written record of the factual basis of this decision. If a physician cannot inform a patient in person, he or she must take whatever steps are reasonable to do so otherwise.[12] Reasonable steps include sending registered letters and telephoning the patient. It is in the physician's best interest to always write a note in the patient's chart if he or she is unsuccessful in contacting a patient to inform of a diagnosis or test result. It is also beneficial to make a small notation in the chart that a patient was advised of any result.

There are several examinations we can perform on known diabetic patients who present with significant pathology. The arterial Doppler, venous Doppler, and plethysmography are useful tools in determining the presence of circulatory compromise in some patients.

Another important situation is the initial diagnosis of diabetes. Very frequently patients are unaware that they have this potentially debilitating condition. It is the primary care physician who, on clinical examination and family history, determines that a fasting blood glucose or even a finger blood sugar test is indicated. Prior to any surgery it is the duty of the surgeon to check for the presence of increased blood sugar. If this test is performed subsequent to treatment but the patient is not informed of the results and a severe problem results, that physician is liable for any damages the patient sustains.

Lack of Diligence

Lack of diligence includes all cases in which a physician or surgeon failed to exercise proper diligence in attending to a patient. Lack of diligence can be involved when the physician fails to give proper attention to a case, makes an omission in the course or treatment, or temporarily withdraws from the case. Situations of permanent withdrawal will be discussed under the section on abandonment.

A practitioner has a duty to give a patient the necessary care as long as a particular case warrants that care. Any lack of diligence in attending to the patient after the physician has accepted the case and begins treatment opens the door for malpractice.

One important element involved in establishing a cause of action in a lack of diligence claim is the presence of a physician-patient relationship, which results in a duty being established between the parties. The injured patient must show that lack of diligence was the proximate cause of the injury for which compensation is sought. There has to be negligence on the part of the physician, but the negligence must have led directly to the injury and the patient must have sustained compensable injuries. Also, in most cases an opinion by an expert medical witness is necessary to establish what constitutes due care under the circumstances in question, and whether the treatment given or not given was the proximate cause of the injury involved.

A surgeon has a special duty regarding postoperative care. Following an operation, the relationship between the physician and the patient continues until *both* parties mutually consent to the cessation of this relationship, the physician withdraws after giving the patient reasonable notice, or the patient dismisses the surgeon. The surgeon must not only use reasonable, ordinary care and skill in performance of an operation; that same care in the postoperative relationship and subsequent treatment must be exercised.[13]

The most common omission by a physician that gives rise to a lack of diligence complaint is failure to make a timely response to the call of a patient, or to visit the patient with necessary frequency after the doctor-patient relationship has been established. Inadequate visitation can occur when the physician fails to attend to the patient at the patient's home or hospital bed.

A physician has a duty to give a patient postoperative instructions, and any failure to do so can raise the claim of lack of diligence.

With a diabetic patient, the importance of postoperative instructions is compounded, because of the potential failure to heal in these patients. Therefore, it is incumbent upon a physician to give instructions that are clear, and that enable the patient or the patient's family to act intelligently in postoperative care and be able to contact the appropriate parties should an emergency arise.

Another situation that can lead to the claim of lack of diligence is when the physician prematurely discharges a patient from the hospital or permits the patient to leave on his or her own free will. It should be noted that if the patient decides to leave the hospital against the better judgment of a physician, the patient must sign a release that he or she has been told that the physician disagrees with the decision and recommends follow-up by the physician at the office. Should the doctor-patient relationship be disrupted after such an incident, the physician still has a duty to refer the patient to another physician of like kind. Once this referral is made, it is preferable that the physician send a certified, return receipt requested letter to the patient describing the situation and confirming the name of the referred physician.

Abandonment of a Patient by a Physician

Abandonment usually means that a physician unilaterally severs professional relationship with a patient without giving the patient reasonable notice. Usually the situation is such that continuing treatment is necessary.

Abandonment can only occur if the relationship is terminated by a unilateral act of the physician. Should the relationship be terminated by mutual consent or by physician dismissal by the patient, then the claim of abandonment usually fails.[14]

The law regarding abandonment is very well stated in a Utah case[15]:

> Upon undertaking an operation on another, a physician or surgeon is under the duty, in the absence of an agreement limiting his service, to continue his attention after the first operation or first treatment, so long as the case requires attention. The obligation of continuing attention can be terminated only by cessation of the necessity which gave rise to the relationship, by the discharge of the physician by the patient, or by withdrawal of the physician from the case after giving the patient reasonable notice, to enable the patient to secure other medical attention. A physician has the right to withdraw from a case, but if the case still requires further medical or surgical attention, he must, before withdrawing, give the patient sufficient notice, so the patient can procure other medical attention if he desires.

There is a proper way for a physician to withdraw from a case and give sufficient notice. When a physician determines that his or her services are no longer helpful to a patient, the physician must give that patient a reasonable time to procure other services.[16] The physician must continue to treat the patient until that time. Sending of a certified return receipt letter to the patient explaining the reasons for withdrawal as well as recommending several alternative physicians is prudent.

Abandonment — The Proximal Cause Issue

In order for a patient to successfully recover on a claim of abandonment, it must be shown that the abandonment was the proximate cause of the patient's injury. Usually, merely showing negligence on the part of the physician is not sufficient for this action to be successful. Occasionally, a physician treating a diabetic patient for a severe paronychia negligently treats that paronychia and the patient subsequently loses a digit through amputation; a question then arises as to whether the doctor is negligent. If the complaint served on the physician specifies only that the patient died several months later due to an overdose of self-administered insulin, and that the death was aggravated by the negligence of the treating physician, such a claim usually fails. The appropriate response by the plaintiff's attorney would be to include a special paragraph regarding the specific negligence in the treatment of this infection as separate from the ultimate demise of the patient.

There are several situations that have been identified as acts that constitute abandonment. The clearest form of abandonment is when the physician openly expresses to the patient that the physician wishes to cease attending that patient's care. Another form of abandonment is when a physician refuses to attend to a patient's needs, even though no oral declaration is made to the patient regarding withdrawal from the case.

Another type of abandonment occurs when the physician leaves the patient during or immediately after a treatment never to appear again. If a physician promises a patient that he or she will return and subsequently fails to do so, the area of abandonment is triggered. Courts have held that if a physician promises to return, then a duty to do so exists unless the physician is notified by the patient that the physician's services are not required. An omission of this kind establishes a lack of reasonable care and diligence on the physician's part.[17]

Res Ipsa Loquitur

The doctrine of *res ipsa loquitur* means that the thing speaks for itself. It is usually a reasonable conclusion drawn from the circumstances of an unusual event that an injury was a result of the physician's fault or negligence. This kind of injury ordinarily does not occur in the absence of someone's negligence, but is caused by an agency or instrument within the exclusive control of the physician and not due to a voluntary action or contribution on the part of the injured patient.

The doctrine can be raised when a physician gives a patient an injection into an ankle, and the patient subsequently develops an osteomyelitis of the bone directly below the injection site. It can be inferred that the injection by the doctor caused the osteomyelitis. In another diabetic scenario, let us say a physician treats a diabetic patient for digital ulcerations over a long period of time, and the patient subsequently develops a severe cellulitis followed by amputation. It can be inferred that the doctor was the cause of the ulcer not healing, and the doctrine of *res ipsa loquitur* can be applied.

Loss of Chance

One of the most interesting forms of negligence is the claim of loss of chance. The essence of this claim is that the injured patient believes the doctor failed to properly diagnose or treat a condition and thus deprived the patient of a possible cure. There are several elements involved in this type of claim. First, there must be a pre-existing condition. The patient must have had a health problem that is treatable by a medical specialty. Second, the patient's opportunity of recovery from the condition must be diminished by the attending physician's improper care. Finally, the lost chance must be forever lost. The doctrine can easily be applied when dealing with a diabetic patient, because if a patient ultimately loses a limb because of the direct action of a physician, the ability to cure that limb is forever lost.

Defenses to Malpractice

Defense to Abandonment

Although a malpractice complaint can cite many different potential areas of liability, the reply submitted by a defense attorney must attack and provide specified defenses for each arena. A defense is an argument that absolves the physician from liability. The simplest type of defense is an assertion that no causal connection can be established between the claim and the result.

If a physician becomes ill during a doctor-patient relationship, courts have excused that physician only if the patient is notified of the physician's inability to continue giving treatment. This will enable the patient to have a reasonable opportunity to obtain the services of another competent physician. This defense will be successful if the patient's condition was not detrimentally affected by the first treating physician.[18]

If a patient fails to cooperate with a physician, this may justify the physician's right to terminate a relationship. This occurs very frequently with diabetic patients in that many are given specific treatment regimens and regularly fail to follow instructions. It is the duty of the physician either to cease that relationship or have the patient sign a release indicating that the physician has recommended a particular mode of therapy and the patient has refused to follow those instructions.[19]

A defense that usually fails regarding the refusal of a physician to treat a patient is lack of patient payment. Should a doctor be in the middle of a treatment regimen for diabetic ulceration and aware that if treatment ceases that patient would be unlikely to continue treatment elsewhere, the physician has a duty to continue treatment without compensation. This is due to the general rule that failure of the patient to pay for services does not justify terminating the patient-physician relationship if the patient still needs medical treatment. The physician has a right to refuse to respond to the call of a patient who cannot pay for services; however, once that physician begins treatment, the patient is owed the same degree of care and skill that is required for any paying patient.[20]

It has also been noted that physicians can limit themselves to the type of care they wish to render to their patients. "A physician or surgeon may agree to perform an operation without undertaking or rendering himself responsible for the subsequent treatment of the case."[21] Some physicians limit themselves only to office treatment; others may limit themselves to performing surgery but not subsequent treatment.

There are certain situations where a physician is called upon to render services on a one-time basis only. This type of situation rarely leaves the physician open for a malpractice lawsuit should the patient worsen after the initial visit. Of course, if the physician fails to adequately act within the scope of service he or she has been called upon to provide, then the physician can be guilty of negligence. This falls within the general rule that a doctor may not, after accepting a patient, abandon that patient without giving sufficient opportunity to find another physician. The patient should understand that the physician is only rendering services for that one particular time. A failure by the physician to explain that to the patient can lead to a charge of negligence. The most common situation in a diabetic scenario is when the treating physician recommends a podiatric consultation, and the podiatrist is called upon to render a one-time visit. The podiatrist examines the patient and usually makes recommendations on a consultation sheet. It is a duty of the treating physician to read the sheet and either follow the recommendations of the podiatrist or not. The podiatrist, however, must make perfectly clear to the patient that he or she will not be continuing treatment, or that the podiatrist was only called upon to render an opinion.

Contributory Negligence

Recovery for an injured patient can be denied or lessened if that patient has contributed to the injury. The burden of proof with such a defense rests with the patient. The patient must prove the absence of his or her own negligence once the physician has claimed as a defense that the patient's actions ultimately affected the result. If a patient is found guilty of negligence that was an active and contributing cause of the injury in question, that patient is not entitled to recovery. Contributory negligence, simultaneous and cooperating with the fault of the physician, and entering into creation of the cause of action and forming an element in the transaction that constitutes the cause of action, will bar recovery.[22] In some jurisdictions the jury award may be reduced, depending upon what percentage of the negligence the patient contributed.

There are several acts by a patient that can be considered as contributing to an injury. The most obvious type of situation arises when a patient negligently administers, or prescribes for self-administration, medication without the authorization of a physician.[23]

If a defendant physician had instructed a patient on how to ambulate following surgery, and that patient does not comply with the instructions and subsequently fractures a hip, it is possible that the jury would find the physician not guilty because of contributory negligence of the patient. This category is labeled disobedience of physician's instructions and is a very common occurrence with noncompliant patients. The patient has a duty to follow the instructions of a physician and to submit to the treatment as prescribed. If the patient fails to follow instructions, patient negligence is considered to directly contribute to the ultimate injury. The patient therefore cannot maintain an action for malpractice against a physician in these circumstances.[24] If a patient has departed from the instructions in any material aspect or has submitted to treatment by other physicians without the consent and knowledge of the original treating physician, it is also possible that the courts will find that patient to have contributed to his or her injury.[25]

Another category of potential patient contribution is when the patient refuses the suggested treatment by the physician. This frequently is seen when it is suggested to a diabetic patient that he or she cease employment until the ulceration or infection is resolved. Unfortunately, because of economic circumstances, the patient cannot cease employment, continues to work wearing the same work shoe that originally caused the problem, and ultimately the infection spreads, resulting in extended ulceration or amputation. Also, if a patient has a severe infection and the physician recommends a surgical debridement, which is refused, the patient can be held to be contributorily negligent. In one Missouri case, the jury was left with the question whether the patient refused to submit to the operation recommended by the physician. If the patient's condition deteriorated because of this refusal, then the physician would be absolved from liability. The jury had to determine whether the physician did in fact recommend an operation and whether the condition did in fact deteriorate following that recommendation.[26]

The fact that a patient fails to return to a physician or seeks care elsewhere does not necessarily constitute contributory negligence on the patient's part. It is accepted that if a patient engages a physician to treat a condition and the physician provides skillful and careful treatment but the patient fails to return to the office for further recommended treatment prior to discharge, then that patient may be held contributorily negligent should an injury be suffered. In this condition, the patient would not be entitled to recover against the physician for injury. It is also understood that if the patient dismisses a physician who had rendered proper treatment until the point of discharge, the physician's liability ends at that time. However, a patient has the right to leave a physician at any time and may hold that physician liable for any injuries suffered, if it can be proven that the physician rendered improper treatment. This is so regardless of whether or not the patient's continued treatment with the physician would have allowed the doctor to recognize any deficiencies and change or correct the treatment pattern.[27]

Negligence on the part of a patient that occurs following the physician's act of malpractice but that causes additional injury is not a guaranteed defense for a physician. It does, however, serve to mitigate the damages, limiting the recovery to the patient of the injury sustained due to the negligence of the physician only.

Defending a Lack of Diligence Claim

A physician can avoid a claim of lack of diligence by contacting a patient by telephone to receive reports of the patient's state of health. Also, a physician-surgeon can instruct patients and their families as to necessary and proper care, even though the physician does not personally attend to those particular patients.

In cases where a physician temporarily leaves a practice, the claim of lack of diligence can be avoided if the physician makes the following necessary arrangements. The physician should make provisions for the attendance of a second, competent physician during the absence, and inform the patients of his or her unavailability and how to contact the substitute provided. Alternatively, patients could find their own substitute. This situation occurs regularly with diabetic patients as they need continuous and consistent care. A diabetic ulceration usually requires weekly care and observation; by leaving a patient unattended, serious damage can occur. Furthermore, when operating on a diabetic patient, it is essential that postoperative contact be made with the patient on a regular basis and visits be scheduled without fail, so that the patient does not have the opportunity to miss required treatment. Should a physician decide to take a vacation or attend a seminar, it is the physician's duty either to refer the patient to another colleague during that time or make arrangements for someone to cover the office. The physician should also notify staff that a certain patient must be followed, make a distinct effort to confirm the patient's appointments, and emphasize to the patient the importance of regular visits. Should the patient fail to keep scheduled appointments, the office staff must chart when they made the confirmatory call and on which dates the patient failed to keep the appointment.

Assumption of Risk

An area of the law that is very similar to contributory negligence is assumption of risk. A patient who is advised by a physician that there are different modalities of treatment and that one that may have a better result also has a larger risk can accept the extra risk and absolve the physician from liability. In one case a defendant physician asserted that he had advised the plaintiff that due to his diabetic condition there was risk of bone infection following an operation on his leg. The court found that the assumption of risk doctrine was applicable. The court noted that if a patient has full knowledge of an open and visible condition, appreciates the dangers involved, and voluntarily acts, that patient assumes the risks of those dangers. The court found in this case that the plaintiff assumed a risk of the consequences growing out of his diabetic condition.[28]

Statute of Limitations

Statute of limitations is a time period within which injured patients can file their lawsuits. Filing after the statute has run out will not be successful, because the courts will not accept such a case. The time period for the statute varies in different jurisdictions. For example, in Michigan, medical malpractice claims must be filed either 2 years from the date of injury or 6 months from the date the cause of action was discovered. In most jurisdictions, the statute starts to run from the time the negligent treatment was given. Many states allow parties to file within a specified period of time from the date that the injury is recognized or when a reasonably diligent person would have recognized the negligence. Certain situations can never be barred by the statute of limitations. Fraudulent concealment by the treating physician usually extends the time of the statute until a period following the discovery of that concealment. Foreign objects that were negligently left in a patient's body do not fall under the statute's limiting action; instead they toll the statute until discovery.

There are special situations regarding the statute of limitations. Children usually have until their eighteenth birthday or age of majority to bring a malpractice lawsuit against a physician. Insane individuals are also given a grace period for which they may bring a lawsuit after the statute of limitations has expired. If an injured patient is unable to bring a lawsuit because of a war, then the statute of limitations is also tolled.

Defensive Medicine When Treating Diabetic Patients

Medical History

A diabetic patient must be treated in a special manner. The treatment phase begins as soon as a patient schedules an appointment with a receptionist. The receptionist is under an obligation to obtain the initial medical history and insurance information. Subsequent to the initial care of a patient, my office mails out a brochure that describes our practice and how our office is run on a daily basis. It advises the patient of the hours a doctor is available and emergency phone numbers where the doctor can be reached. Included in this brochure is an initial history form the patient must complete and present at the first visit.

A thorough medical history should include the names of any physicians who have treated the patient prior to this date, including other podiatrists, general practitioners, endocrinologists, general surgeons, physical therapists, chiropractors, and any other medical care provider that has attended to the patient. The purpose in obtaining this information is to enable the treating physician to have easy access to the names and addresses of physicians in order to obtain oral consultations or records of other health care providers as necessary. One should also determine what conditions were treated by each previous physician, the type and duration of treatment rendered by each physician, and the success or failure of the treatment.

A discussion of the patient's diabetes should always be included in history-taking. Questions that should be asked include the following: Is the patient currently taking any medication, and for what period of time? Are other medications for different medical conditions also being used? Have different diabetic medications been taken in the past? What effects have these diabetic medications had, in conjunction with other prescriptions, on the patient's well-being, physical condition, and mental attitude? What dosages and frequencies have been prescribed, and has the patient fully complied with the medication regimen? Have there been periods of time during which the patient has failed to take the medications prescribed by other physicians, and what damage resulted due to this noncompliance? The approximate date of onset of the diabetes, and the individuals who care for the patient and who are responsible for administering or observing the affects of ingested medications should also be known.

Physical Examination

The physical examination of diabetic patients is critical in determining the medical condition that caused them to seek professional care. The diabetic physical examination must be extremely comprehensive and must be re-evaluated on each subsequent visit. The four important aspects of this examination include dermatologic, orthopaedic, neurologic, and vascular findings. Each of these should be recorded on a history and physical sheet and also in the body of the chart as a progress note.

The amount of time a physician invests in performing all the required tests is indicative of the time that will not have to be invested at a later date should the patient suffer a potential negligent act that will cause a lawsuit to be brought against either the treating or another physician. The attorney for the plaintiff will find this type of documentation a hindrance toward the success of the case. The physician's defense attorney will appreciate this type of documentation and will be aware that the physician is an individual who is totally concerned with treatment of patients and is intelligent enough to take protective steps to avoid potential liability.

Laboratory Testing

Under the category of laboratory tests are included various vascular examinations, as well as any type of examination that produces a report or form. This can include a radiographic examination performed by the physician, provided a full report is subsequently dictated and attached to the chart. On the first visit, it is essential for the physician to assess the patient's present blood sugar. This can be done either through the finger-stick method or phlebotomy. On each subsequent visit the physician should perform the most noninvasive blood sugar test to determine if the glucose level has significantly changed. Any open wound or skin infection should be cultured and a bacterial sensitivity should be performed. Complete blood analysis as well as other tests that the physician deems necessary should be obtained from the previous treating physician.

Specialized Testing

There are several other tests and examinations that one may be called upon to perform on a diabetic patient. A common finding in diabetic malpractice lawsuits is failure to perform either a vascular or bone study examination.

It may also be essential for the patient to have a special consultation with a vascular surgeon. The purpose of this examination is to give ample documentation that the patient's medical condition is deteriorating, the vascular status is poor, and the vascular surgeon has assessed and made the necessary recommendations to the patient. Thus, if the worst scenario should occur and the patient should lose a limb and ultimately sue the treating physician, then at least he can proclaim in his defense that he did everything possible, including consulting with a vascular specialist.

Patient Education

The diabetic patient needs to be educated. The patient's family should be instructed how to care for the diabetic patient. It cannot be assumed that the diabetic patient is knowledgeable on general foot care even though the patient has had diabetes for many years. The physician has a duty to explain to the patient the results of all the tests performed and to interpret those tests in conjunction with the changes present in the diabetic foot. The metabolic changes associated with diabetes should be explained to both patient and family, especially those changes that can affect circulation. The worst possible scenario regarding skin breaks or infections should be described to the patient so that he or she will be fully aware of the need to engage in a strict regimen of diabetic foot care. The poor prognosis of diabetic foot ulcerations and infections should be emphasized, as should the potential for digital, pedal, and even leg amputation if the condition proceeds unabated. The different types of treatments available for various diabetic conditions should be discussed with the patient, including the use of debridements, oral and intravenous antibiotics, specialized digital protectors, diabetic shoes, and the conservative and surgical treatments available.

The neurologic changes that take place in diabetes should be explained to both family and patient. In particular, emphasis should be placed upon neuropathy, whereby the digits lose all sensation and the patient becomes unaware of infections and potentially damaging digital conditions. Patients must be instructed to examine their feet on a daily basis without fail, because the warning system of pain may be not available to them, and any slight irritation to the digits can become a major problem.

Diabetic retinopathy should be discussed with the family and referral to or evaluation by an ophthalmologist should be considered. Our office presents the diabetic patient with a written instruction sheet that details the care required for proper foot maintenance. Our office staff discusses these instructions with both patient and family. If we believe a patient is not complying with the instructions, that patient is required to sign a written statement that he or she was presented with instructions and has been negligent in following the details, thus causing the condition to deteriorate. It is the task of the entire practice to make sure that all patients with diabetes or vascular compromise be completely educated in the care and treatment of their feet. Staff should telephone family members to discuss this care. In addition to being a special gesture, it protects the physician from the claim of failure to educate.

Record Documentation

The physician needs to maintain accurate and complete records. These should include references to a patient's past conditions, present treatment and evaluation, as well as prognosis of the particular condition. It is impossible for physicians to recall what occurred on a visit several weeks earlier. Record keeping is imperative for several reasons. The physician needs the prior evaluation to determine the present treatment plan and projections. Records become an issue should inquiries be made about what transpired during a specific visit or prior to a particular time. The records can be reviewed by medical insurance auditors to determine whether proper and necessary treatments were rendered or whether fraud or abuse occurred. During depositions and trials, health care professionals must refer to their handwritten or typed progress notes to enable them to answer specific questions.

There are certain notations that should not be recorded. It is essential to exclude any reference to monetary charges or collections in the body of the patient's chart. Medical-related notations, as well as suggestions from associates or staff regarding treatment, should not be found in the progress notes, borders, margins, or headings of the progress page. Thought processes of the physician should be left in the mind and not recorded, as well as errors in judgment that may have been committed. The record should reflect the physician's findings upon examination, the treatment, and the prognosis.

The office staff should also have the right to make specific recordings in the medical chart. Telephone conversations between the staff and patients should be documented, especially if a patient is not following the physician's recommendations or failing to keep scheduled appointments. Each phone call should be documented as to date and time, and the physician's response should be written directly below the staff's notations. When instructions are given to the patient, or when a consultation is performed, the date and time of those meetings, as well as the content reviewed and discussed, should be documented. Phone calls the physician makes to the patient or family, either because of lack of compliance or for postoperative checks, should also be documented. Any referrals made by the doctor should be written in the chart, noting the name, location, date, and time of appointment. All laboratory testing performed in the office should be charted, either in the body of the progress page or in a separate laboratory section. Should a physician believe that a patient's condition is deteriorating because of the contributory negligence of that individual, then a certified, return receipt letter should be sent to the patient describing the physician's concern for the patient's noncompliance in treatment and failure to keep scheduled appointments. Any correspondence, sent either to the patient, a referring doctor, a referred-to-doctor, insurance companies, attorneys, state agencies, or anyone else, should become part of the permanent chart.

Medical Records

There are three parties to each lawsuit: the plaintiff, the defendant, and the medical record. I consider the medical record to be just as important as the physician or the injured patient. This record will ultimately testify for or against the physician in every malpractice lawsuit; therefore, it is essential that clear, legible, and comprehensive medical records be kept.

Furthermore, the standard of care in many communities requires a specific type of medical record. Most of us have been trained in the S.O.A.P. method, in which the patient's complaints are described in the subjective section, followed by the physician's objective findings, assessment of the condition, and a list of the problematic elements of that visit. The projection includes the treatment phase and any recommendations or further indicated treatments. The S.O.A.P. record-keeping system allows for the most complete and thorough records.

Records are a permanent part of a patient's chart and should never be tampered with or changed. Laws in various states make tampering either a misdemeanor or felony. In some jurisdictions, licensure can be revoked if tampering of charts is proven. Thus, it is essential to write complete records at the appropriate time. Should a physician forget to include in a record some valuable and important information, that information may be added to the record at a later date, but only if the physician dates and initials the addition. This will prove to anyone reviewing the chart that no intent to defraud was involved.

Records should be written as close in spatial time to the visit as possible, because it is difficult to recant the exact words of a patient's subjective complaints if the record is written several days following the visit. Also, physicians who see many patients cannot remember every detail of every visit and may tend to forget or misrepresent treatment or findings if the records are not written as soon as possible. Records should be very complete. Any type of information that the patient relays should be recorded. This is particularly important when dealing with diabetic patients who may be noncompliant in their treatment. If a patient's dressing appears wet or dirty, this needs to be charted. If the patient is not applying medication as regularly as prescribed, this should also be recorded. The patient may be missing appointments. It is the duty of the physician's staff to contact that patient and emphasize the importance of keeping regular and consistent appointments. It should be charted in the record that the staff contacted the patient, advised the patient of the missed appointment, and stressed that the patient's condition warrants regular appointments. Also, the staff can record that they advised a patient that the physician cannot be responsible for the outcome of the condition if the patient fails to keep appointments.

Records may serve as *prima facie* evidence of negligence. In one case, failure of hospital records to contain nurses' observations about the condition of a patient's toes led a jury to draw the inference that no such observations were made and to conclude that the loss of the patient's leg was the proximate result.[29] Thus, if a physician treating a diabetic patient fails to record the vascular status of a patient's digits and the patient subsequently goes on to lose those digits, that physician may be held liable for negligence based on the record.

The most common method of using records by plaintiffs' attorneys is as supportive evidence. Hospital records frequently play an important part in a patient's case regarding substandard surgical care or postoperative care. Records may indicate that a necessary consultation was not ordered, that a physician failed to visit a patient in the hospital, or failed to arrestively treat a postoperative hospital complication. Thus, the entire picture of treatment, post-treatment, and identification of substandard treatment in the record is used when bringing a malpractice action against a physician. As diabetic persons tend to suffer numerous circulatory problems, it is essential that the records of diabetic patients be as thorough and complete as possible.

CONCLUSION

There is no known cure for diabetes mellitus. Thus, physicians should expect a portion of their practices to be made up of diabetic individuals. Understanding the legal ramifications of diabetes treatment can only aid in preventing improper medical treatment of these patients. The different theories of malpractice explain what type of treatment is expected of the practitioner. It was attempted to cover only a small portion of the legal issues affecting diabetic patients. It behooves each of us to think of these issues when treating our patients.

REFERENCES

1. *Valentine v. Kaiser Foundation Hospital*, 194 Cal App 2d 282, 15 Cal Rptr 26 (1961)
2. Third Annual Report of the National Diabetes Advisory Board, October 9-12, 1979. Appendix A. United States Department of Health and Human Services, Washington, D.C., April 1980
3. *Osborne v. Frazor*, 58 Tenn App 15, 425 SW 2d 768 (1968)
4. *Buttersworth v. Swint*, 53 Ga App 602, 186 SE 770 (1936)
5. *Childers v. Frye*, 201 NC 42, 158 SE 744 (1931)
6. *Hiser v. Randolph*, 126 Ariz 608, 617 P 2d 774 (1980)
7. *Dowell v. Mossberg*, 226 Or 173, 355 P 2d 624 (1960)
8. *King v. Flann*, 442 SW 2d 679 (Tex 1969); *Jansen v. Mulder* 232 Mich 183, 205 NW 159 (1925); *Morgan v. Engles*, 372 Mich 514, 127 NW 2d 382 (1964)
9. *Mallen v. Boynton*, 132 Mass 463 (1882)
10. 61 Am Jur 2d, Physicians, Surgeons, and Other Healers, Sec. 138
11. *Ark. Stat. Ann.*, Sec. 82-363 (1973)
12. *Ray v. Wagner*, 286 Minn 354, 176 NW 2d 101 (1970)
13. *Reed v. Laughlin*, 332 Mo 424, 58 SW 2d 440 (1933)
14. *MuGulpin v. Bessmer*, 241 Iowa 119, 43 NW 2d 121 (1950); *Brown v. Dark* 196 Ark 724, 119 SW 2d 529 (1938)
15. *Ricks v. Budge*, 91 Utah 307, 64 P 2d 208 (1937)
16. *Fortner v. Koch*, 272 Mich 273, 261 NW 762 (1935)
17. *Ritchey v. West*, 23 Ill 385 (1960)
18. *Warwick v. Bliss*, 46 SD 622, 195 NW 501 (1923)
19. *Dashiell v. Griffith*, 84 Md 363, 35 A 1094 (1896)
20. *Becker v. Janinski*, 27 App NYC 45, 15 NYS 675 (1891)
21. *Nash v. Roister*, 189 NC 408, 127 SE 356 (1925)
22. *Wesley v. Allen*, 235 Ill App 322 (1925)
23. *Los Alamos Medical Center v. Coe* 58 NM 686, 275 P 2d 175 (1954)
24. *Merrill v. Odiorne*, 113 Me 424, 94 A 753 (1915)
25. *McIlwain v. Gaebe*, 128 Ill App 209 (1906)
26. *Richeson v. Roebber*, 349 Mo 132, 159 SW 2d 658 (1941)
27. *Williams v. Wurdemann*, 71 Wash 390, 128 P 639 (1912)
28. *Mainfort v. Giannestras*, 49, Ohio Ops 440, Ill NE 2d 692 (1951)
29. *Collins v. Westlake Community Hospital*, 57 Ill 2d 388, 312 NE 2d 614 (1974)

Index

Page numbers followed by f indicate figures; those followed by t indicate tables.